MEDICAL RADIOLOGY
Radiation Oncology

Editors:
L. W. Brady, Philadelphia
H.-P. Heilmann, Hamburg
M. Molls, Munich
C. Nieder, Bodø

M. Molls · P. Vaupel · C. Nieder
M. S. Anscher (Eds.)

The Impact of Tumor Biology on Cancer Treatment and Multidisciplinary Strategies

With Contributions by

M. S. Anscher · S. T. Astner · M. J. Atkinson · M. Baumann · C. Belka · N. Cordes
J. Dahm-Daphi · P. Dent · E. Dikomey · J. Drevs · I. Eke · S. Grant · P. R. Graves
A.-L. Grosu · S. Hehlgans · M. Hiraoka · G. Iliakis · S. Itasaka · I. L. Jackson
A. M. Kaindl · C. A. Klein · T. Klonisch · M. Krause · M. Los · M. P. Mehta · M. Gužvić
M. Molls · G. Multhoff · U. Nestle · C. Nieder · J. Norum · K. Oexle · S. Panigrahi
A. Pawinski · I. Rashedi · H. C. Rischke · V. Schneider · K. Schulze-Osthoff · S. Song
S. Tapio · K. Valerie · P. Vaupel · Z. Vujaskovic · W. A. Weber · D. Zips

Foreword by
L. W. Brady, H.-P. Heilmann, M. Molls, and C. Nieder

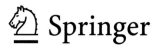 Springer

MICHAEL MOLLS, MD
Professor, Direktor, Klinik und Poliklinik für
Strahlentherapie und Radiologische Onkologie
Klinikum rechts der Isar der Technischen
Universität München
Ismaninger Straße 22
81675 München
Germany

PETER VAUPEL, Dr. med., MA/Univ. Harvard
Professor of Physiology and Pathophysiology
Institute of Physiology and Pathophysiology
University Medical Center
Duesbergweg 6
55099 Mainz
Germany

CARSTEN NIEDER, MD
Professor
Department of Internal Medicine – Oncology
Nordlandssykehuset HF Hospital
8092 Bodø
Norway

MITCHELL S. ANSCHER, MD, FACR, FACRO
Florence and Hyman Meyers Professor and Chair
Department of Radiation Oncology
Virginia Commonwealth University School
of Medicine
401 College Street
P. O. Box 980058
Richmond, VA 23298-0058
USA

MEDICAL RADIOLOGY · Diagnostic Imaging and Radiation Oncology
Series Editors:
A.L. Baert · L.W. Brady · H.-P. Heilmann · M. Knauth · M. Molls · C. Nieder

Continuation of Handbuch der medizinischen Radiologie
        Encyclopedia of Medical Radiology

ISBN   978- 3-540-74385-9   e-ISBN 978-3-540-74386-6

DOI 10.1007/978-3-540-74386-6

Library of Congress Control Number: 2008928298

Cover design: Verlagsservice Teichmann, Mauer, Germany
Production, reproduction and typesetting: le-tex publishing services oHG, Leipzig, Germany

Printed on acid-free paper

9 8 7 6 5 4 3 2 1

springer.com

Foreword

The rapidly changing concepts in radiation oncology with the development of more precise instrumentation for delivery of radiation therapy and a greater emphasis on hypofractionation technologies require a very intimate knowledge of tumor biology and the influence of various biologic factors on dose distribution within the tumor in terms of homogeneity as well as prevention of any late effects on normal tissue surrounding the tumor itself. Not only are these major factors in clinical practice but also the known factors of inhomogeneity of cancer cells, the impact of microenvironment in terms of radiation effect, and host factors make it mandatory to design therapeutic strategies to improve the outcome and to diminish any potential short-term or long-term risks from the radiation therapy.

The authors have developed an outstanding text that deals with these strategies and how they would impact on established and emerging new technologies and treatment. The context of the presentations within a multidisciplinary combined modality therapy program is incredibly important.

In this volume, various topics are reviewed including tumor genesis, cell proliferation, angiogenesis, the physiologic characteristics of malignant tissues, invasion and adhesion, the route and role pursued in the development of metastasis, and the role of the human immune system in cancer prevention and development.

Important chapters focus on cancer diagnosis and treatment along the basic principles of chemotherapy, radiotherapy, and molecularly targeted therapy. The presented rational adaptations allow for the design of translational studies and become increasingly more important as a better understanding is gained of gene expression profiling, gene transfer and silencing, proteomics and molecular imaging and their impact on the development of treatment programs.

The authors' aim is to educate and inspire those who devote most of their work to research in cancer and its clinical treatment. It represents an outstanding presentation in these regards.

Philadelphia	LUTHER W. BRADY
Hamburg	HANS-PETER HEILMANN
Munich	MICHAEL MOLLS
Bodø	CARSTEN NIEDER

Preface

Numerous developments in molecular biology and information technology over the past decade have led to an explosive growth in cancer biology research. Much of the research has focused on the underlying mechanisms of carcinogenesis, tumor progression and metastasis. Knowledge gained from this research has led to the development of new classes of drugs that target specific pathways known to be involved in one or more of the processes that may be altered as part of the malignant phenotype.

Radiation oncology as a specialty has benefited from this technological revolution, and it is now possible to target therapies much more precisely and safely than in the past. It is critically important, however, that the radiation oncologist becomes knowledgeable not only about new developments in radiation biology, but also about cancer biology in general. In fact, radiation biology has embraced molecular biology to such a degree that there are now few classically trained radiobiologists remaining on the faculties of many radiation oncology departments.

The purpose of this book is to provide the practicing radiation oncologist, as well as those in training, with a concise overview of the most important and up-to-date information pertaining to tumor biology as it impacts on cancer treatment. This information is not limited to that directly related to the interaction of radiation with cells and tissues, for it is important that the radiation oncologist have a broader understanding of tumor biology.

It is the intent of the editors to provide chapters from experts in not only the basic sciences, but also in the translational application of key basic biological concepts. Thus, the book contains chapters on the fundamental basic principles of cancer biology, such as tumorigenesis, cell growth and proliferation, angiogenesis, tumor physiology, the biology of metastasis and the role of the immune system. More clinically related topics, such as molecular and biological imaging and molecular targeted therapies for both cancer treatment and normal tissue injury, are also included. In order to be able to read and understand the latest literature, it is important to have an understanding of the principles behind some of the latest tools employed by scientists to conduct their research. To that end, chapters describing techniques such as gene expression profiling, gene transfer and gene silencing are also included.

We hope that the reader will find this book a useful guide to the molecular era of cancer biology and to the implications of increasing biology knowledge of personalized cancer therapy, particularly as it applies to the field of radiation oncology.

Munich	MICHAEL MOLLS
Mainz	PETER VAUPEL
Bodø	CARSTEN NIEDER
Richmond	MITCHELL S. ANSCHER

Contents

Tumorigenesis

Michael J. Atkinson and Soile Tapio

CONTENTS

M. J. Atkinson, PhD
Professor, Institute of Radiobiology, Helmholtz Centre
Munich, German Research Centre for Environmental Health,
Ingolstädter Landstraße 1, 85764 Neuherberg, Germany

S. Tapio, PhD
Institute of Radiobiology, Helmholtz Centre Munich, German Research Centre for Environmental Health, Ingolstädter
Landstraße 1, 85764 Neuherberg, Germany

KEY POINTS

- Analysis of the DNA of tumor cells reveals that a finite number of gene mutations are responsible for the transmission of the phenotypic changes characteristic of the tumor. These mutations may have arisen sporadically through misrepair of endogenous DNA damage from oxidative stress and DNA replication errors, or through mistakes in somatic recombination events. Alternatively, they may be induced exogenously through the DNA-damaging action of environmental agents such as ionising radiation and UV light.

- Failure of the damage control processes to correct the damage before it is incorporated permanently into the genome during replication is critical.

- In addition to the intragenic mutations, there is a range of additional mechanisms whereby the genome may become perturbed during tumor development. Alterations in the copy number of cellular genes are common in human tumors. Both allelic gains and losses are encountered. Amplification of genetic regions may take the form of intrachromosomal duplications, leading to the in situ amplification of a gene with oncogenic properties at its normal chromosomal location. Transcription of the amplified gene complex subsequently leads to overexpression of the gene product. Alternatively, the amplification may occur extrachromosomally, leading to the formation of multiple copies of chromosomal fragments (double minutes).

- The spectrum of mutational events in tumor cells can also include chromosomal translocation and inversion events leading to the structural rearrangement of parts of the genome. This may result in a fusion of two unrelated gene fragments, creating a chimeric gene instructing production of a protein with abnormal function. Alternatively, the rearrangement may transpose an endogenously active promoter with coding sequences from a gene that is normally either tightly regulated or transcriptionally silent in the tissue. This form of mutation leads to the inappropriate expression of the protein.

- Two non-mutational events are also implicated in the changes in gene expression during oncogenesis. In the first situation, transcriptional silencing of an essential tumor suppressor gene is associated with non-mutational changes to the structure of the gene promoter region. Changes in the methylation status of individual nucleotides of the DNA as well as to the methylation and acetylation status of the DNA-binding histone core proteins are involved in regulating local gene expression. A second non-mutational event is gene silencing through endogenous RNA-binding microRNA molecules.

- Oncogenes are genes that, through the action of the proteins they encode, cause cancer when transcribed. Oncogenes arise through the mutation of normal cellular genes with regulatory activities called proto-oncogenes.

- Tumor suppressor genes encode proteins that are responsible for control processes essential to limiting cell proliferation. They act upon pathways involved in growth control, cell cycle regulation and the maintenance of cell integrity (DNA repair and apoptosis).

- Carcinogens include a number of different substances that are directly involved in the initiation or promotion of cancer in humans. The nature of carcinogens varies from radiation to chemical substances, bacteria and viruses.

- Evolving concepts of tumor stem cells, the regulation of coordinated expression programmes by non-translated microRNAs and the role of the tumor microenvironment are just three areas where new knowledge is opening up possibilities for the diagnosis and treatment of malignant disease.

Abstract

Tumor cells possess a range of inherited phenotypic features that distinguish them from normal cells. They acquire the ability to undergo almost continual unregulated growth, resist cytotoxic chemicals and are able to metastasise from their initial locations to proliferate in inappropriate tissue compartments. This chapter describes the early stages of tumorigenesis, starting with genetic mutations and alterations in gene expression and biological signalling, and finally discusses inherited or environmental factors accelerating the initiative process to malignancy.

1.1 Introduction

The scientific search for the cause of cancer can be traced back to Hippocrates. His suggestion that an imbalance in the bodily fluids was the cause of cancer predated both the cellular theory of Johannes Müller and Rudolf Virchow and the oncogenetics of Vogelstein and colleagues. The Hippocratic view remained the conventional wisdom for generations, but was rapidly discarded in favour of more evidence-based models (Fig. 1.1). Maybe, given the importance now ascribed to the local tissue microenvironment in cancer, we should give more credit to Hippocrates.

After cancer was recognized as a cell-based disease, scientific effort focussed on understanding the processes involved in the genesis and behaviour of the abnormal cells. Whilst the origins of the cellular building blocks of tumors can be traced back to an apparently normal parental tissue, cancer cells clearly evolve unique phenotypic characteristics. Insight into potential mechanisms behind this process came from the early epidemiological studies by Percival Pott, Bernardino Ramazzini and others, who demonstrated exogenous causes for some cancer through infection, wounding or noxious chemicals (McDermott et al. 2007; Aronson 2007; Breasted 1922). The seminal study of Theodor Boveri, suggesting that tumors arise through abnormal distribution of chromosomes, focussed attention upon the genome (Manchester 1995; Harris 2008). Although Peyton Rous almost simultaneously established that the malignant phenotype could be transferred to normal cells in tumor cell extracts (Vogt 1996), the discovery of the central role of genetic material in the process had to await the explosion of interest in molecular biology that followed the clarification of the structure of DNA. This new era saw the identification of tumor-inducing genes within the genome of oncogenic viruses, the discovery that these viral genes were in fact mutated derivatives of cellular genes and that endogenous mutation of these very same cellular genes could give rise to cancers.

Although it was comforting to assume that a simple gene mutation underlies the development of cancer,

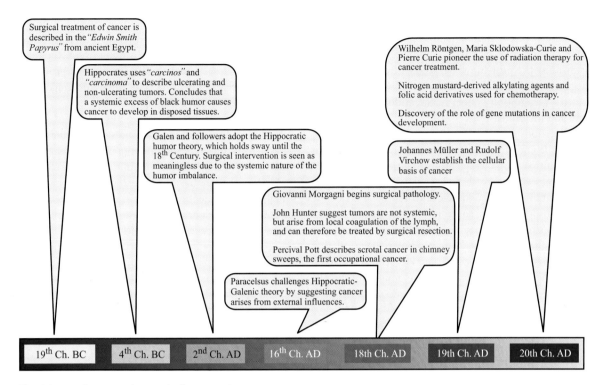

Fig. 1.1. Development of cancer biology over the centuries

more recent developments suggest that the reality is much more complex. Thus, the last decade has seen the realization that a host of other factors, such as epigenetic regulation, inherited susceptibility and changes in the local microenvironment, can all play a role in the development of a cancer. This expansion of our understanding of the carcinogenic process has many implications for the application and development of therapeutic strategies.

1.2
Early Mutational Events in Carcinogenesis

1.2.1
Alterations of the Genetic Code

Analysis of the DNA of tumor cells reveals that a finite number of gene mutations are responsible for the transmission of the phenotypic changes characteristic of the tumor from one cell to the other during cell division. These mutations may have arisen sporadically in a somatic cell through misrepair of endogenous DNA damage arising from oxidative stress and DNA replication errors, or through mistakes in somatic recombination

events. Alternatively, they may be induced exogenously through the DNA-damaging action of environmental agents, such as ionising radiation, UV, and mutagenic alkylating or intercalating agents. Failure of the damage control processes to correct the damage before it is incorporated permanently into the genome during replication is critical.

Infrequently, the critical alteration in gene function may be transmitted to an individual from a parent through the germ line, in which case the mutation can result in a familial (heritable) cancer syndrome, such as retinoblastoma or one of the multiple endocrine neoplasias.

Mutations involving damage to only small regions of the genome that result in phenotypic change are usually intragenic and are limited to only a single gene. The smallest mutations involve a single base, either resulting in a nucleotide exchange or insertion/deletion of one base (frame-shift mutation). The consequences for the gene sequence of such mutations are determined by the context of the altered base. If it is present within a codon, the genome-encoded amino acid may be substituted, which may sometimes result in catastrophic changes to the protein sequence through substitution of an inappropriate amino acid into the protein chain. Some substitutions may have only a modest effect upon phenotype or may even leave the encoded amino acid unchanged (silent mutations). Occasionally, the single base change may generate a premature stop codon, truncating the protein, which frequently leads to rapid degradation of the abnormal protein by the misfolded protein recognition system in the endoplasmic reticulum and the proteasome.

Insertions and deletions of a single base alter the reading frame of the gene. As most genes have evolved with multiple stop codons protecting the two non-coding frames, the frame-shifted sequence will most probably contain a stop codon close to the position of the insertion/deletion. In some infrequent instances, the mutated single base may lie in a critical structural element of the gene, such as the promoter site regulating gene activity, or in a recognition site critical for RNA processing, for example splice site mutations resulting in exon skipping deletions in the E-cadherin gene (BECKER et al. 1993).

In addition to the intragenic mutations described above, there is a range of additional mechanisms whereby the genome may become perturbed during tumor development. Alterations in the copy number of cellular genes are commonly described in human tumors. Both allelic gains and losses are encountered, and their biological consequences are described elsewhere in this review. Amplification of genetic regions may take the form of intrachromosomal duplications, leading to the in situ amplification of a gene with oncogenic potential. Transcription of the amplified gene complex subsequently leads to overexpression of the gene product. Alternatively, the amplification may occur extrachromosomally, leading to the formation of multiple copies of chromosomal fragments (double minutes) containing one or more transcriptionally active genes with an oncogenic capacity.

The spectrum of mutational events in tumor cells can also include chromosomal translocation and inversion events leading to the structural rearrangement of parts of the genome. This may result in a fusion of two unrelated gene fragments, creating a chimeric gene instructing production of a protein with abnormal function. Alternatively, the rearrangement may transpose an endogenously active promoter to coding sequences from a gene that is normally either tightly regulated or transcriptionally silent in the tissue. This form of mutation leads to the inappropriate expression of the protein, for example, in parathyroid tissue where the CCND1 (cyclin D1) gene is placed under the control of the highly active parathyroid hormone gene promoter (ARNOLD et al. 2002). This is also seen in thyroid tissue where the transcriptionally inactive glial-derived neurotrophic factor receptor (RET) tyrosine kinase gene is placed under the control of one of a number of different promoters active in thyroid tissue (SANTORO et al. 2004). As a result of this translocation event, the neuroendocrine tissue-restricted RET protein is produced in thyroid cells and delivers cell proliferation signals in a ligand-independent manner (see below).

Functional translocations are also frequent in the lymphoid and myeloid lineages, presumably due to the propensity of these cells to undergo chromosomal rearrangements during immunoglobulin and T cell receptor maturation. Failure to restrict the high level of chromosomal rearrangement activity to the correct locus may explain the abundance of such alterations in immature stages of the lineages. In solid tumors translocations are seen primarily in the endocrine tissues mentioned above and in the paediatric tumors rhabdomyosarcoma and Ewing's sarcoma, both of which involve activation of genes regulating developmental pathways. Translocations are reported less frequently in other solid tumors, and here their biological relevance remains uncertain. Significantly, in none of the solid tumor types showing translocations is there any evidence for endogenous chromosomal rearrangement processes that could explain the phenomena.

Two non-mutational events are also implicated in the changes in gene expression during oncogenesis. In the first situation, transcriptional silencing of an essential tumor suppressor gene is associated with non-mutational changes to the structure of the gene promoter region. Changes in the methylation status of individual nucleotides of the DNA, as well as to the methylation and acetylation status of the DNA-binding histone core proteins, are involved in regulating local gene expression. A second non-mutational event is discussed below, where gene silencing through endogenous RNA-binding microRNA molecules has been suggested to be an additional step in transcriptional control, leading to silencing in a post-transcriptional manner.

An altogether different mutational mechanism is seen almost exclusively in animal model systems, where insertion of retroviral sequences or retroviral-like elements into the genome results in the disruption of cellular genes. In humans, the role of insertional mutagenesis is less clear. Retroviral insertion leading to proto-oncogene overexpression has been implicated in the development of retroviral gene therapy-associated lymphoproliferative malignancies in a small number of cases. Nevertheless, the general applicability of this mutational mechanism for human cancer is unclear, and it is certainly uncommon. In addition to retroviral insertion, viruses have evolved a range of strategies for productive infection of mammalian cells that subvert defence and regulatory pathways. As a consequence of these actions, the viral proteins elicit an oncogenic action through growth stimulation, suppression of apoptosis or inactivation of endogenous tumor suppressor gene function.

1.2.2
Events Accompanying Progression

Mathematical and molecular studies on tumor tissues have each established that tumors can arise and develop through a series of intermediate stages. The clonal expansion paradigm suggests that discrete stages arise through evolutionary selection of appropriate phenotypes that are themselves defined by mutational events. Histopathological studies deliver a partially convergent concept, where morphologically distinct stages of tumor formation and development are discernable in almost all tumor entities. The combination of the morphological models of tumor development and analysis of molecular events suggests that tumor development indeed follows a series of steps from pre-cancerous lesions (hyperplasia, atypical hyperplasia) that lead either directly or indirectly to full neoplasia (infiltrative and metastatic growth). During this progression, the normally differentiated phenotype may become either partially or completely lost (WALCH et al. 2000).

Estimates of the number of mutations and steps that are required to create a full malignant phenotype vary wildly. In vitro studies suggest that mutation of as few as three key genes is sufficient, whilst massive DNA resequencing studies of tumor cell genomes have revealed hitherto undiscovered complexity in the magnitude and diversity of DNA alterations; however, it remains unclear which of these, if any, are required for the acquisition of a malignant phenotype (SJOBLOM et al. 2006). Three conceptual models can help in partly reconciling these differences. Kinzler and Vogelstein suggested, at least for the model of colon carcinogenesis, that there is a linear evolution of the cells within the developing tumor, which follows a well-circumscribed and sequential series of events (VOGELSTEIN et al. 1988; VOGELSTEIN and KINZLER 2004). Each step in their model is represented by the mutation of a single key gene. However, the analysis of the gene alterations present in different areas of some tumors shows that some clones lack the full compliment of gene mutations. This may indicate that a simple linear monoclonal evolution is not always followed (KUUKASJARVI et al. 1997). An alternate view to the Vogelstein model is that mutations are acquired in a cumulative manner, with some clones in the tumor acquiring mutations that lead to them branching off to an evolutionary dead end and others only being re-

quired at specific points in the tumor development. HANAHAN and WEINBERG (2000) have suggested that key cellular pathways related to functional changes in tumor cell biology are individually targeted by mutational events, explaining how the development of malignancy can result from a finite number of mutations. Finally, systems theory and pathway analysis suggest that each functional activity of the cell described by Hanahan and Weinberg requires multiple hits to remove back-up and alternative pathways. It is, however, worthy of note that tumor cells cannot tolerate wholesale genomic alterations; consequently, there cannot be an unlimited number of mutations as some functional pathways are essential for continued cell survival.

A discrepancy of orders of magnitude between the sporadic rate of mutational activity observed in cells and the level of mutations found in tumors has prompted LOEB (2001) to suggest that a key process in tumor cell development must be the acquisition of a mutational activity (mutator phenotype, loss of caretaker function). Although tumor suppressor and apoptosis genes could be considered candidate mutator genes, no convincing evidence for a specific increase in mutation rate due to loss of these genes has been presented. Genes involved in maintaining genomic integrity, such as the DNA mismatch repair genes, whilst implicated in cancer susceptibility, provide no clear evidence of mutator-gene driven genome changes.

1.2.3
Proliferation Modifying Genes

A major category of the genes influencing cell proliferation contains members of signalling pathways involved in the regulation of cellular growth. At the cell surface this can be seen by the uncontrolled production of stimulatory growth factors, the abnormal expression of growth factor receptors or the production of a mutated form of the receptor that has acquired the capacity to autonomously engage and activate the downstream intracellular signalling cascade. A related functional set of tumor genes is that involved in the transmission of the growth-regulating signal to the transcriptional apparatus, which includes signal-transducing kinases and transcription factors.

An additional group of proliferation genes plays a role in steering the transit of cells into, through and out of the cell cycle. Inappropriate functioning of these genes leads to uncontrolled cell cycle activity and the failure of proliferating cells to differentiate. In the case of cell cycle checkpoint control genes, this can allow cells with non-repaired DNA damage or chromosomal aberrations to continue through the cycle, yielding genetically aberrant daughter cells. Failure to eliminate damaged cells is an additional feature of the mutations influencing a further set of cancer genes, those involving the cellular pathways regulating programmed cell death (apoptosis and anoikis, a form of apoptosis that is induced in anchorage-dependent cells detaching from the surrounding cells and/or matrix). The failure of tumor cells to initiate a normal apoptotic death response after stress and/or mutation of DNA, or to initiate apoptosis after loss of cell–cell and cell–matrix contact, can involve inactivation of the intrinsic (mitochondrial) pathway and extrinsic (ligand-receptor) apoptosis-inducing pathways. This can be brought about by inappropriate overexpression of anti-apoptotic proteins or by inactivation of pro-apoptotic proteins. More recently, the protective sequestration of cells bearing oncogenic gene mutations into a pathway of oncogene-induced senescence (OIS) has been described. The regulation of this pathway is poorly understood, but escape from growth restrictions imposed by the activation of the senescence programme appears to be a critical step in oncogenesis and may involve overcoming cell cycle arrest by removing expression of the p16 cyclin-dependent kinase inhibitor. It remains to be seen which other protein activities regulate entry and exit from OIS and how mutations of these genes influence tumorigenesis.

1.2.4
Acquisition of the Invasive/Metastatic Phenotype

Although changes in proliferative regulation pathways are critically important, the acquisition of an invasive/metastatic phenotype is a major step in solid tumor formation. The necessary changes in gene expression may occur through mutation or through changes in more global programmes of cell regulation, such as the epithelial to mesenchymal phenotypic transition (EMT). Tumor invasion into surrounding tissues requires distinct phenotypic alterations. Loss of cell-specific adhesion allows tumor cells to detach from neighbouring cells and the underlying extracellular matrix. This may be accompanied by upregulation of an alternative programme of adhesion, allowing the tumor cell to adhere to anomalous cells or matrixes (e.g. a switch from epithelial-specific E-cadherin to the mesenchymal-cell specific cadherins in breast cancer) (Sarrio et al. 2008). At the same time as acquiring an abnormal adhesive profile, the tumor cells may also develop a programme allowing for the degradation of the surrounding matrix proteins.

Here, overexpression of specific proteases may facilitate local destruction of matrix that allows the non-adherent tumor cell to exit the parental tissue and migrate (Wagner et al. 1995). Recent evidence suggests that the mobilisation of tumor cells may be driven by local gradients of cell- and tissue-specific chemokine molecules. Changes in the expression pattern of surface chemokine receptors of tumor cells may permit them to respond to a different chemokine milieu and has been suggested to be partly responsible for homing of tumor cells to specific distant sites such as bone marrow (Kulbe et al. 2004). Separation of the tumor cell from surrounding parental tissue would normally be expected to initiate the anoikis programme of apoptosis, but as described above, this pathway is inactivated as part of the loss of proliferative regulation. The final stage in malignant growth, the acquisition of the capacity to generate new blood vessels that infiltrate the tumor and oxygenate the expanding cell mass, angiogenesis, is discussed in other chapters of this book.

1.3
Inherited Susceptibility

Within a population there is a proportion of individuals who are predisposed to develop cancer, either as an apparently sporadic disease or in response to an environmental challenge, such as exposure to tobacco smoke or ionising radiation. The abnormally high frequency of some tumor types within related members of large families provided evidence that cancer is, in some circumstances, a heritable disease. Genetic linkage studies of these families has revealed that a number of these cancer syndromes occur as simple Mendelian traits, usually with a highly penetrant dominant pattern of inheritance.

Many hereditary cancer susceptibility genes, such as breast cancer 1 and 2 (BRCA1/2) and the group of DNA mismatch repair genes, have a known function in the DNA repair. Incomplete functioning of DNA repair appears to render somatic cells highly susceptible to carcinogenetic noxae and spontaneous DNA mutations, leading to an accumulation of genetic damage and ultimately transformation. Other susceptibility genes involving impaired DNA repair lead to cancer-prone syndromes such as xeroderma pigmentosa, Bloom's disease and hereditary nonpolyposis colorectal cancer (HNPCC), also known as Lynch syndrome. Yet, there are inherited susceptibility genes having no direct function in DNA repair, but still showing an autosomal dominant familial pattern. Von-Hippel-Lindau syndrome is a dominantly inherited hereditary cancer syndrome predisposing to a variety of malignant and benign tumors of the eye, brain, spinal cord, kidney, pancreas and adrenal glands. Other inherited cancer syndromes include ataxia telangiectasia, Li-Fraumeni syndrome, retinoblastoma, Wilms' tumor, familial adenomatous polyposis, multiple endocrine neoplasia 1 and 2, just to mention a few.

The hereditary mutations associated with cancer syndromes only have a big impact on the risk of a population if they are common. Thus, whilst mutations in the breast cancer susceptibility genes BRCA1 and BRCA2 are found in almost 10% of women with breast cancer, the PTCH1 gene mutation responsible for the Gorlin/basal nevus syndrome occurs in less than 1 per 50,000 of the population. However, it must be appreciated that the gene mutation frequencies vary considerably between populations, especially if the populations are isolated for geographical, religious or other reasons. Good examples in this context are BRCA2 mutations in Iceland and BRCA1/2 mutations among the Ashkenazi Jewish population. Inaccuracies in population estimates may bias clinical judgement and allocation of diagnostic resources (HEMMINKI et al. 2008).

Susceptibility to many diseases has been shown to be polygenic, with a multitude of low-penetrance common polymorphisms contributing to the risk of developing disease. These complex trait genes may contribute significantly to risk estimations of certain cancers. Therefore, it is useful to quantify the relative importance of known genes in the burden of disease by using the population attributable fraction (PAF) that states the contribution of the studied gene to disease aetiology, independent of the environmental or other genetic factors that may interact with the gene in question (HEMMINKI and BERMEJO 2007). New approaches, such as genome-wide association studies (GWAS) using single nucleotide polymorphism (SNP) arrays, have provided tools to map and potentially identify some of the low-penetrance hereditary cancer-susceptibility genes. Future developments here will require large-scale multinational collaborations, similar to those conducted on breast cancer (EASTON et al. 2007).

1.4
Oncogenes

Oncogenes are genes that, through the action of the proteins they encode, cause cancer when transcribed (Table 1.1). Oncogenes arise through the mutation of normal cellular genes with regulatory activities called proto-oncogenes. Recent data indicate that small RNA molecules called microRNAs (miRNAs) may control the expression of proto-oncogenes and that mutations in these may lead to oncogene activation (see Sect. MicroRNAs in human cancer) (WIEMER 2007; NEGRINI et al. 2007).

The first evidence for the existence of oncogenes was provided by the study of viral oncogenesis. In 1910, Peyton Rous prepared cell-free filtrates from sarcomas arising in chickens. Injection of the filtrate into other chickens resulted in the development of the same tumors in the recipient birds (VOGT 1996). The aetiological agent was identified as an avian RNA virus and subsequently named Rous sarcoma virus (RSV). Comparisons between the genomes of oncogenic and non-oncogenic RNA viruses quickly established that the oncogenic genomes uniquely harboured specific cancer-inducing genes. This led to the discovery of the first oncogene, the *src* gene in RSV (*v-src*). Its cellular homologue, *c-src*, was identified soon after, leading to the realisation that the viral oncogene was in fact a derivative of the cellular oncogene that had in an unknown manner, presumably during viral retrotransposition or during viral genome replication, been integrated into the viral genome and subsequently underwent rapid molecular evolution to acquire transforming potential. The final confirmation of the tumor-inducing role of oncogenes came from cell transfection studies, where genomic DNA from tumor cells containing active oncogenes was shown to be capable of transferring the malignant phenotype into recipient cells.

Studies with animal viruses have been essential in elucidating how the activation of oncogenes takes place and leads to cellular carcinogenesis. Even if our knowledge of human viruses causing cancer is based on in vitro studies and epidemiological data, it is reasonable to assume that transformation mechanisms in humans are closely related to those in animals. Some human pathogenic viruses causing cancer are listed in Table 1.2.

A typical example of a proto-oncogene translocation is the membrane tyrosine kinase receptor RET [see review (SANTORO et al. 2004)]. The outer membrane part consists of four cadherin-like domains; the inner membrane domain has the tyrosine kinase activity. The gene was discovered in 1985 and was found to be activated by a DNA rearrangement, a mechanism giving the gene its name (Rearranged during Transfection). RET protein has several tyrosine residues that are auto-phosphorylated. The phosphorylation of the tyrosine 905 is suggested to act as a key in switching on the kinase activity. Other tyrosines serve as docking sites for signalling factors in their phosphorylated form. RET-mediated signalling pathways are shown in Fig. 1.2.

The RET gene, located in the long arm of chromosome 10 (10q11.2), is normally silent in thyrocytes. Due to a chromosomal inversion or translocation event taking place in a subpopulation of human papillary thyroid carcinomas (PTC), the tyrosine kinase-encoding part of the RET gene falls under the control of active promoter regions of several heterologous genes. The chromosomal rearrangements lead to a formation of chimeric RET/PTC oncoproteins that express constitutive tyrosine kinase activity. Different RET/PTC variants have been isolated that differ in the RET fusion partner. RET/PTC3, the fusion between RET and the RFG/Ncoa4 gene, is the most prevalent variant in radiation-associated paediatric PTCs. Data are accruing suggesting that the formation of RET/PTC oncogenes is causative in thyroid tumorigenesis. Thyroid follicular cells are transformed in vitro by RET/PTC. Furthermore, RET/PTC transgenic mice develop malignancy of the thyroid.

Table 1.1. Some oncogenes, their function and the pathways affected

Oncogene	Function	Pathway
Aurora A	Self-sufficiency growth signals	DNA repair
HPV-E6	Evading apoptosis	
MDM2	Evading apoptosis	
Abl	Self-sufficiency growth signals	Cell cycle control
CDK2	Self-sufficiency growth signals	
CDK4	Self-sufficiency growth signals	
Cyclin D	Self-sufficiency growth signals	
Cyclin E	Self-sufficiency growth signals	
HPV-E7	Self-sufficiency growth signals	
Gli	Evading apoptosis; self-sufficiency growth signals	Hedgehog signalling
Hedgehog	Evading apoptosis; self-sufficiency growth signals	
Smo	Evading apoptosis; self-sufficiency growth signals	
Akt	Evading apoptosis	Akt signalling
Bax	Evading apoptosis	
FKHR/FOXO	Evading apoptosis	
JAK	Evading apoptosis; self-sufficiency growth signals	
PI3K	Evading apoptosis	
B-Raf	Self-sufficiency growth signals	Ras signalling
Fos/Jun	Evading apoptosis; self-sufficiency growth signals	
ILK	Self-sufficiency growth signals; tissue invasion and metastasis	
Ras	Self-sufficiency growth signals	
RTKs	Evading apoptosis; self-sufficiency growth signals Tissue invasion and metastasis; sustained angiogenesis	
β-catenin	Self-sufficiency growth signals	Wnt signalling
RAR	Self-sufficiency growth signals	
SOX	Self-sufficiency growth signals	
Wnt1	Self-sufficiency growth signals	
Myc	Self-sufficiency growth signals	TGFβ signalling
Fas	Evading apoptosis	Death receptor
Notch	Evading apoptosis	Notch signalling
Gα	Self-sufficiency growth signals	GPCR signalling
GPCR	Self-sufficiency growth signals	

Table 1.2. Human viruses involved in cancer development

Virus	Non-tumor diseases	Tumor caused by infection
Human immunodeficiency virus	Acquired immune deficiency syndrome	Kaposi's sarcoma Non-Hodgkin's lymphoma Cervical cancer
Human papillomavirus	Warts	Cervical carcinoma Head and neck cancer
Hepatitis B	Hepatitis, liver cirrhosis	Liver cancer
Hepatitis C virus	Hepatitis, liver cirrhosis	Liver cancer
Epstein-Barr virus	Infectious mononucleosis	Burkitt's lymphoma Non-Hodgkin's lymphoma Hodgkin's disease Nasopharyngeal carcinoma
Human herpes virus 8	Castleman's disease	Kaposi's sarcoma Body cavity lymphoma
Human thymus-derived-cell leukaemia/lymphoma virus-1	Tropical spastic paraparesis	Adult T cell leukaemia

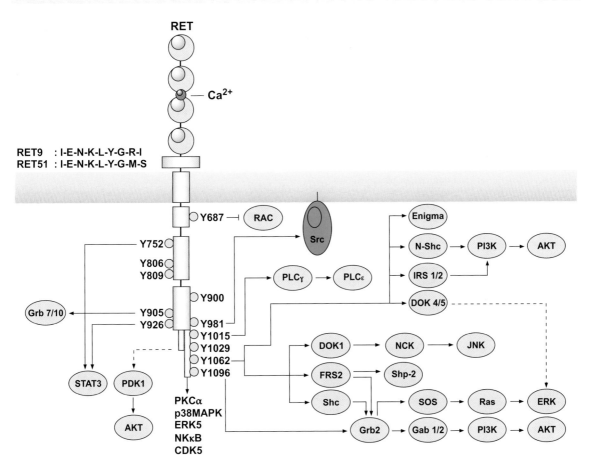

Fig. 1.2. The network of RET-mediated signalling events. RET auto-phosphorylation sites are shown with their direct targets. *Dotted lines* indicate pathways not yet fully elucidated. The amino acid sequences of RET9 and RET51 at the point in which they start to diverge at glycine 1063 are shown. With the courtesy of Dr. Massimo Santoro

Tumor Suppressor Genes

Our knowledge of tumor suppressor genes comes from seminal studies on the familial tumor syndrome retinoblastoma. Analysis of the frequency and age of onset of the disease in affected children revealed that bilateral disease had a much earlier onset than unilateral disease. The bilateral form of the disease is inherited by a germ-line mutation and is therefore present in all tissues, including both retinas, whereas the unilateral disease is due to a locally restricted somatic mutation affecting one eye only. To explain the earlier age of onset of the bilateral disease, it was proposed by KNUDSON (1996) that there must be a second event (subsequently proven to be loss of the remaining wild-type allele) that occurs earlier in the inherited form and later in the sporadic form. This two-hit model of inactivation of a tumor suppressor gene has remained a mainstay of our understanding of tumor suppressor gene inactivation. Inherited or sporadic mutation of one copy of the suppressor gene is postulated to confer a selection advantage to the cell clone, which through an undefined mechanism inactivates the remaining tumor suppressor allele. Many varieties of processes have been shown to

Table 1.3. Some tumor suppressors, their function and the pathways affected

Tumor suppressor	Function	Pathway
ARF	Self-sufficiency growth signals	DNA repair
ATM/ATR	Insensitivity to anti-growth signals	
BRCA1	Self-sufficiency growth signals; insensitivity to anti-growth signals	
Chk1	Insensitivity to anti-growth signals	
Chk2	Insensitivity to anti-growth signals	
DNA-PK	Insensitivity to anti-growth signals	
FANCD2	Insensitivity to anti-growth signals	
HIPK2	Evading apoptosis; self-sufficiency growth signals	
NBS1	Insensitivity to anti-growth signals	
P53	Evading apoptosis; insensitivity to anti-growth signals	
P15	Self-sufficiency growth signals	Cell cycle control
P16	Self-sufficiency growth signals	
Rb	Self-sufficiency growth signals	
Ptch	Evading apoptosis; self-sufficiency growth signals	Hedgehog signalling
Su(Fu)	Evading apoptosis; self-sufficiency growth signals	
Bcl-2	Evading apoptosis	Akt signalling
LKB1	Self-sufficiency growth signals	
PTEN	Evading apoptosis	
TSC1/TSC2	Self-sufficiency growth signals	
Integrin	Tissue invasion and metastasis	Ras signalling
NF1	Self-sufficiency growth signals	
VHL	Sustained angiogenesis	
APC	Self-sufficiency growth signals	Wnt signalling
Axin	Self-sufficiency growth signals	
α-catenin	Tissue invasion and metastasis	
E-cadherin	Self-sufficiency growth signals; insensitivity to anti-growth signals	
	Insensitivity to anti-growth signals	
Wnt5A	Self-sufficiency growth signals	
BMPR	Insensitivity to anti-growth signals	TGFβ signalling
Smad2/3	Insensitivity to anti-growth signals	
Smad4	Insensitivity to anti-growth signals	
TGFβ R	Insensitivity to anti-growth signals	

be responsible for loss of the second allele (second hit), including copying the inactive mutant allele into the locus of the wild-type allele, interstitial deletion of the wild type allele, deletion of a chromosomal fragment or the entire chromosomal arm containing the allele. Inconveniently, a number of suppressor gene loci do not show loss of both alleles, leading to a number of models of how these non-classical suppressor genes are involved in cancer. Ideas range from inactivation of the second allele through epigenetic mechanisms, the presence of hypomorphic alleles at the remaining wild-type locus, gene dosage effects, etc. In all probability, each model may have its validity in explaining the tumor suppressor inactivation of a specific gene in a specific tumor type.

Tumor suppressor genes encode proteins that are responsible for control processes essential to limiting cell proliferation. They act upon pathways involved in growth control, cell cycle regulation and the maintenance of cell integrity (DNA repair and apoptosis).

Since the pioneering work by Knudson in the early 1970s, a correlation between mutated tumor suppressor genes and different cancers has been found in several cases, such as BRCA1 (cancers of breast, ovary, colon and prostate), BRCA2 (cancers of breast, ovary, pancreas and prostate), CDK4 (melanoma) and PMS1 and PMS2 (colorectal cancer), just to mention a few. Representative tumor suppressor genes, their functions and the pathways affected are listed in Table 1.3.

In addition to an increased risk of cancer, individuals with germ-line mutations in tumor suppressor genes frequently show an increased susceptibility to radiation, with Li-Fraumeni (TP53), Gorlin (PTCH1) and retinoblastoma (RB1) syndromes being frequently encountered (Evans et al. 2006). The majority of reported cases with radiation-induced cancers carry mutations in RB1, with almost 40% of affected individuals developing radiotherapy-associated tumors compared to a sporadic rate of 20% in non-radiotherapy cases (Aerts et al. 2004; Kleinerman et al. 2005).

The retinoblastoma protein, Rb1, is a tumor suppressor found to be dysfunctional in several human cancers (Murphree and Benedict 1984). The gene RB1 encodes a factor that controls the progression of the cell cycle through the G1 phase and into S phase. The function of Rb1 depends on its phosphorylation state; Rb can actively inhibit cell cycle progression in its dephosphorylated form by binding and thereby inhibiting transcription factors of the E2F family (Korenjak and Brehm 2005). Rb-E2F complex stalls the cell cycle progression and allows repair of DNA damage before the cell enters the S-phase. Rb is initially phosphorylated by cyclin D1/CDK4/6 (Fig. 1.3), followed by additional phosphorylation by cyclin E/CDK2, allowing the cell to enter the S-phase. Rb1 remains phosphorylated throughout S, G2 and M phases and is again dephosphorylated near the end of G1 phase, allowing it to bind E2F (Vietri et al. 2006).

1.6
MicroRNAs in Human Cancer

MicroRNAs (miRNAs) are evolutionary conserved small non-coding RNAs, ranging in length from 16 and 29 nucleotides. The miRNAs are postulated to form an endogenous system to regulate and coordinate the expression of genes on a post-transcriptional level (Wiemer 2007; Negrini et al. 2007). They are able to bind complementary sequences in target messenger RNAs (mRNAs) and thus prevent their translation. Each miRNA may potentially target several hundreds different mRNA molecules, suggesting they may exert a one-step control over cellular processes (Lewis et al. 2005).

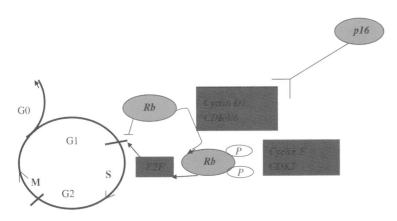

Fig. 1.3. The regulation of the cell cycle by the phosphorylated and non-phosphorylated forms of Rb1 protein. *Green ovals* represent proteins with tumor suppressor funktion, *red squares* proteins acting as oncogenes

The exact mechanism of the translational "silencing" is not known, but recently the target mRNAs were found to be sequestered in the so-called processing bodies (P bodies) distant from the translating ribosomes (COLLER and PARKER 2005; LIU et al. 2005; SEN and BLAU 2005).

At the moment, more than 4,000 different miRNAs are identified or predicted in the genomes of viruses, plants and animals, of which some 700 may occur in man (GRIFFITHS-JONES et al. 2006). Some mammalian miRNAs are located within gene introns and appear to be transcribed within the primary transcript, only to be released during RNA processing (SHIVDASANI 2006).

In recent years, miRNAs have been shown to influence a variety of cellular processes of key importance, including cellular differentiation and maintenance of a differentiation state, developmental timing, proliferation and apoptosis (ALVAREZ-GARCIA and MISKA 2005; ZHANG et al. 2007). Since deregulated cell death and proliferation are hallmarks of many types of carcinomas, it is not surprising that, on the one hand, alterations in miRNA may lead to carcinogenesis, and, on the other hand, many miRNAs are found to be abnormally expressed in clinical cancer samples.

The first study showing involvement of miRNA in human cancer was done by CALIN et al. (2002). In search of a tumor suppressor gene in chronic lymphocytic leukaemia (CLL) cases, they found that the smallest common lesion of a 30-kb region located at chromosome 13q14 coded for two miRNAs, miR15 and miR16. Furthermore, both genes were found to be deleted or downregulated in a majority (approximately 68%) of CLL cases. The discovery of a germ-line point mutation in two CLL patients that resulted in downregulation of both miRNAs and the induction of apoptosis by miR15 and miR16 by negatively regulating anti-apoptotic oncogene BCL2 in the leukaemic cell line MEG-01 supported the putative tumor suppressor role of these miRNAs (CALIN et al. 2005; CIMMINO et al. 2005).

MiRNAs may also act in an oncogene-like manner. The amplification of the miRNA gene cluster miR-17-92 on chromosome 13 in human B-cell lymphomas leads to upregulation of several miRNAs that together with MYC oncogene accelerate tumor development (HE et al. 2005). Transcription of this cluster is induced by MYC itself. Similarly, overexpression of miR-155 in B-lymphocytes of transgenic mice leads to pre-leukaemic pre-B cell polyclonal expansion followed by B-cell malignancy (COSTINEAN et al. 2006).

Considering how rapidly data have been accruing in the last years, it is reasonable to believe that the next decade will bring new insights about the role of miRNAs in carcinogenesis and their therapeutic tools.

1.7
Lifestyle, Environmental and Occupational Factors Causing Cancer

Known carcinogens include a number of different substances, mixtures and exposure circumstances that are directly involved in the initiation or promotion of cancer in humans. The nature of carcinogens varies from radiation to chemical substances, bacteria and viruses. Based on epidemiological data and biological data from both human and animal material, the International Agency for Research on Cancer (IARC) has classified agents, mixtures and exposures into five categories (IARC): Category 1: carcinogenic to humans; category 2A: probably carcinogenic to humans; category 2B: possibly carcinogenic to humans; category 3: not classifiable as to carcinogenicity in humans; category 4: probably not carcinogenic to humans.

Some examples of different types of category 1 carcinogens include gamma radiation (lung, liver, skeletal and other solid cancers) and underground mining with exposure to radon (lung cancer); arsenic compounds (cancers of skin, lung, bladder and liver); aflatoxin B1 produced by the fungus *Aspergillus flavus* growing on grains and nuts (liver cancer); various viruses such as hepatitis B and C (liver cancer), Epstein-Barr virus (Burkitt's lymphoma, non-Hodgkin's lymphoma, Hodgkin's disease) and human papilloma virus (cervical cancer); and bacteria, such as *Helicobacter pylori* (gastric cancer), just to mention a few.

To what extent populations come into contact with different carcinogens depends largely on cultural and socioeconomic factors such as diet, and tobacco and alcohol consumption. Populations of less-developed countries are to a much greater extent exposed to indoor pollution caused by cooking fumes and solid heating fuels than those in developed countries (LISSOWSKA et al. 2005). On the other hand, the broiling and barbecuing meat at high temperatures typical for western civilisations lead to the formation of polycyclic aromatic hydrocarbons (PAH) and tars that are potent carcinogens (FELTON et al. 1997; SUGIMURA et al. 2004). However, apart from consumption of alcohol or aflatoxin-contaminated food (IARC 1993), no single dietary factor can be pinpointed as a definite cause of cancer. More importantly, lifestyle factors leading to obesity and increased tobacco and alcohol consumption are probably causing more cancer cases, either directly or as co-factors, than any single factor alone (DOLL et al. 2005; PETO 2001).

The carcinogenic effect of cigarette smoking is by far the most important discovery of modern epidemiology

(IARC 1986). The steep rise in the cigarette consumption among the Western European male population after the First World War and among the North American male population after the Second World War was tracked by increase in carcinomas of the lung (Peto 2001).

There are about a dozen occupational exposure situations known to increase the risk of cancer, mostly carcinomas of the lung. In many cases the carcinogens are in airborne complex mixtures with other carcinogens and co-factors. Especially in underground mining, the workers may be heavily exposed to several carcinogens, such as coal, dust, asbestos, radon and arsenic (Taylor et al. 1989; Tapio and Grosche 2006; Grosche et al. 2006; Wichmann et al. 2005; Liu et al. 2002).

Asbestos is a naturally occurring fibrous silicate that has been widely used for insulation. Epidemiological data show a strong correlation between asbestos and pleural and peritoneal mesotheliomas as well as lung cancer (Boffetta 2007; Becklake et al. 2007). Due to the long latency of about 30 years and more, incidence rates are still rising, and it is estimated that occupational exposure prior to 1980 will eventually cause 250,000 cases of mesothelioma and the same amount of lung cancer cases in Western Europe (Peto et al. 1999). According to the WHO, 5% of the European population are environmentally exposed to asbestos, leading annually to approximately 1,500 additional cases of mesothelioma and lung cancer (WHO 1987; Boffetta and Nyberg 2003).

Arsenic is a widely distributed semi-metallic compound that causes several types of cancer due to both environmental and occupational exposure situations (Tapio and Grosche 2006). The primary route of environmental exposure is drinking water contaminated with inorganic arsenic. Contrarily to the organic arsenic compounds frequently present in seafood, inorganic arsenic, especially in its trivalent forms, is a group 1 carcinogen (IARC 2004). Inhalation of arsenic-contaminated dust is a common problem in tin, gold and uranium mines (Chen and Chen 2002; Taylor et al. 1989; Kusiak et al. 1991; Grosche et al. 2006). Whilst inhalation of airborne arsenic in glass and copper smelters or arsenic-contaminated dust in mines causes mostly lung cancer, arsenic in drinking water increases additionally the risk of bladder, liver, skin and kidney cancers. Both inhalation and ingestion of inorganic arsenic compounds are correlated with the increased occurrence of squamous cell carcinomas of the lung and skin in comparison to other types of lung and skin carcinomas (Tapio and Grosche 2006).

In China, Bangladesh and India, millions of people have been exposed to arsenic-contaminated drinking water since the 1980s (Table 1.4). Formerly, shallow well water or surface water was used in households, causing other health problems. The effort to improve the quality of drinking water by drilling deeper wells led to the unanticipated opposite effect by increasing the amount of arsenic in the water leaking from the surrounding soil.

Table 1.4. Countries with arsenic-contaminated drinking water (from Tapio and Grosche 2006)

Country	Number of people affected	Arsenic concentration (µg/l)
Bangladesh	50–75 Million	<10->1,000
West Bengale (India)	>6 Million	3–3,700
China	>2 Million	50–2,000
Taiwan	120,000 (1982)	200–2,500
Thailand	n.d.	1–5,114
Vietnam	11 Million	1–3,050
Mexico	400,000	8–624
Chile	250,000	470–770
Argentina	2 Million	>100
United States	350,000	1–1,160
Finland	10,000	17–980
Hungary	n.d.	1–174

In large areas of endemic arsenic poisoning, the rate of malignancies is expected to explode within the next decades.

1.8
Cancer Stem Cell Hypothesis and Microenvironment

Stem cells are pluripotent undifferentiated cells capable of undergoing a self-renewing cell division in contrast to embryonic stem cells that are omnipotent. The asymmetric division of a stem cell, by definition, yields one daughter cell that can differentiate along multiple lineages and a daughter stem cell with all the properties of the parental stem cell. A spectrum of cells with varying degrees of stemness is recognised by phenotypic markers. These cells are presumed to represent the second or third generation of stem cells that have undergone some preliminary commitment to one or more of the tissue lineages. Thus, a mesenchymal stem cell may differentiate to produce adipocytes, fibroblasts, osteoblasts and a host of other mesenchymal cells, but it is committed to the mesenchymal lineage.

In 1926, Bailey and Cushing proposed that cancer was initiated and maintained by a subpopulation of transformed precursor cells. However, it was not until recently that Dick (2005) and co-workers showed that only a few (0.1–1%) of the tumor cells present within an acute myeloid leukaemia (AML) sample had the capacity to initiate AML growth after transplantation into NOD/SCID mice. Since then, small populations of cells with self-renewing capacity have been isolated from most leukaemias, solid cancers such as medulloblastoma and glioblastoma, as well as carcinomas of different organs. These putative cancer stem cells are defined as cancer cells with stem-like properties, such as the ability to remain quiescent for long periods of time and the capacity for asymmetric cell division giving rise to one cancer stem cell and one differentiated progeny. However, they differ from normal stem cells by demonstrating unregulated proliferation, probably due to acquired gene mutations that render them less responsive to negative growth signals or to the loss of contact inhibition and gap junction intercellular communication. They display the same cell surface markers as their normal tissue counterparts, allowing their isolation and enrichment.

The definition of cancer stem cells directly implies that a cancer treatment can only be successful if all cancer stem cells are killed. A subset of cancer stem cells

expresses multidrug resistance transporters ABCB1 and ABCG2 (Mimeault and Batra 2007); others express constitutively vascular endothelial growth factor receptors (VEGFR2) and seem to be the source of intrinsic vasculature building for the tumor (Shen et al. 2008). Studies with glioblastoma and breast cancer stem cells indicate an increased radioresistance due to a more efficient DNA damage repair compared to non-stem cancer cells (Baumann et al. 2008). The development of approaches to radiosensitise tumor stem cells remains an important future challenge.

Although many fruitful studies on cancer biology have been performed in monotypic cell culture, the basic structural unit of living tissues remains a highly complex three-dimensional mixture of cell types. In 1959, Letterer defined the morphology of this complex mixture as a histion; more recently, the term microenvironment has been used. It is important to note that the microenvironment includes not only different cell types, such as fibroblasts, endothelial cells, tissue macrophages, leucocytes, nerve cells, etc., but also extracellular matrix, serum and lymph proteins, and a whole host of locally- and systematically-acting secreted molecules. Within the microenvironment, tumors develop and interact with the different components. It seems unwise to assume that tumor stem cells are immune from the influence of this microenvironment (Kenny et al. 2007).

1.9
Radiation-Induced Cancers

Ionising radiation is an effective carcinogen, causing malignant transformation of many different tissues. The shape of the dose-response relationship for cancer induction is currently assumed to be best represented by a linear no-threshold relationship. This also describes the dose response observed for the accumulation of damage to cellular macromolecules, in particular DNA. Although not universally accepted, it is considered that a failure to repair DNA damage leads to the permanent accumulation of gene mutations in irradiated tissues that then lead to alterations in the regulatory pathways described above. Alternative views give more weight to non-targeted effects of radiation damage, including local inflammatory and stress responses, which are postulated to lead to more global changes in mutational activity characterised by genomic instability.

Evidence for a direct, targeted, mutational event in radiation-induced cancers is lacking, even for alpha-radiation, which would be expected to induce characteristic large deletions in critical genes, which should then be present in all progeny cells.

A number of studies have reported either specific gene alterations (e.g. RET/PTC3 translocations in radiation-induced thyroid cancer, AML-ETO alterations in radiation-associated myeloid leukaemia) or a specific profile of gene expression changes (e.g. in radiation-induced osteosarcoma and papillary thyroid cancer). However, the specificity of these changes may reflect the histopathological uniqueness of the radiation-induced tumors, which suggests that they may be derived from different progenitor cells than those giving rise to sporadic cancers in these tissues. An additional complication is that many radiation-induced cancers arise in genetically predisposed individuals who have inherited a germ-line mutation (e.g. in the RB1 gene). The mechanisms behind the development of therapy-associated cancers in such an individual may well be quite different from those in sporadic cancers.

1.10
Conclusions

The underlying molecular mechanism responsible for the development of a tumor cell may vary (e.g. inactivation of a tumor suppressor gene by a virally encoded protein, inheritance of a germ-line mutation or sporadic point mutation of an oncogene). Nevertheless, all of the mutational events target a common set of regulatory nodes within the cell, such as the cell cycle checkpoints, growth factor independence and prevention of apoptosis. The wide spectrum of genetic alterations, even within one tumor type, reflects the multiple points at which key processes may be subverted and camouflages a much more simple biological process involving only a set of critical processes.

Evolving concepts of tumor stem cells, the regulation of coordinated expression programmes by non-translated microRNAs and the role of the tumor microenvironment are just three areas where new knowledge is opening up possibilities for the diagnosis and treatment of malignant disease. In all three situations, the role of ionising radiation is, at best, poorly understood, and harnessing them for therapeutic purposes requires that considerable effort be expended to define their interaction with radiation.

References

Aerts I, Pacquement H, Doz F, Mosseri V, Desjardins L, Sastre X, Michon J, Rodriguez J, Schlienger P, Zucker JM, Quintana E (2004) Outcome of second malignancies after retinoblastoma: a retrospective analysis of 25 patients treated at the Institut Curie. Eur J Cancer 40: 1522–1529

Alvarez-Garcia I, Miska EA (2005) MicroRNA functions in animal development and human disease. Development 132: 4653–4662

Arnold A, Shattuck TM, Mallya SM, Krebs LJ, Costa J, Gallagher J, Wild Y, Saucier K (2002) Molecular pathogenesis of primary hyperparathyroidism. J Bone Miner Res 17 (Suppl 2): N30–36

Aronson SM (2007) Galen and the causes of disease. Med Health R I 90: 375

Bailey P, Cushing H (1926) A classification of the tumors of the glioma group on a histogenetic basis with a correlated study of prognosis. JB Lippincott, Philadelphia

Baumann M, Krause M, Hill R (2008) Exploring the role of cancer stem cells in radioresistance. Nat Rev Cancer 8: 545–554

Becker KF, Atkinson MJ, Reich U, Huang HH, Nekarda H, Siewert JR, Hofler H (1993) Exon skipping in the E-cadherin gene transcript in metastatic human gastric carcinomas. Hum Mol Genet 2: 803–804

Becklake MR, Bagatin E, Neder JA (2007) Asbestos-related diseases of the lungs and pleura: uses, trends and management over the last century. Int J Tuberc Lung Dis 11: 356–369

Boffetta P (2007) Epidemiology of peritoneal mesothelioma: a review. Ann Oncol 18: 985–990

Boffetta P, Nyberg F (2003) Contribution of environmental factors to cancer risk. Br Med Bull 68: 71–94

Breasted JH (1922) The Edwin Smith Papyrus

Calin GA, Dumitru CD, Shimizu M, Bichi R, Zupo S, Noch E, Aldler H, Rattan S, Keating M, Rai K, Rassenti L, Kipps T, Negrini M, Bullrich F, Croce CM (2002) Frequent deletions and down-regulation of micro-RNA genes miR15 and miR16 at 13q14 in chronic lymphocytic leukemia. Proc Natl Acad Sci U S A. 99: 15524–15529

Calin GA, Ferracin M, Cimmino A, Di Leva G, Shimizu M, Wojcik SE, Iorio MV, Visone R, Sever NI, Fabbri M, Iuliano R, Palumbo T, Pichiorri F, Roldo C, Garzon R, Sevignani C, Rassenti L, Alder H, Volinia S, Liu CG, Kipps TJ, Negrini M, Croce CM (2005) A MicroRNA signature associated with prognosis and progression in chronic lymphocytic leukemia. N Engl J Med 353: 1793–1801

Chen W, Chen J (2002) Nested case-control study of lung cancer in four Chinese tin mines. Occup Environ Med 59: 113–118

Cimmino A, Calin GA, Fabbri M, Iorio MV, Ferracin M, Shimizu M, Wojcik SE, Aqeilan RI, Zupo S, Dono M, Rassenti L, Alder H, Volinia S, Liu CG, Kipps TJ, Negrini M, Croce CM (2005) miR-15 and miR-16 induce apoptosis by targeting BCL2. Proc Natl Acad Sci U S A 102: 13944–13949

Coller J, Parker R (2005) General translational repression by activators of mRNA decapping. Cell 122: 875–886

Costinean S, Zanesi N, Pekarsky Y, Tili E, Volinia S, Heerema N, Croce CM (2006) Pre-B cell proliferation and lymphoblastic leukemia/high-grade lymphoma in E(mu)-miR155 transgenic mice. Proc Natl Acad Sci U S A 103: 7024–7029

Dick JE (2005) Acute myeloid leukemia stem cells. Ann N Y Acad Sci 1044: 1–5

Doll R, Peto R, Boreham J, Sutherland I (2005) Mortality in relation to alcohol consumption: a prospective study among male British doctors. Int J Epidemiol 34: 199–204

Easton DF, Pooley KA, Dunning AM, Pharoah PD, Thompson D, Ballinger DG, Struewing JP, Morrison J, Field H, Luben R, Wareham N, Ahmed S, Healey CS, Bowman R, Meyer KB, Haiman CA, Kolonel LK, Henderson BE, Le Marchand L, Brennan P, Sangrajrang S, Gaborieau V, Odefrey F, Shen CY, Wu PE, Wang HC, Eccles D, Evans DG, Peto J, Fletcher O, Johnson N, Seal S, Stratton MR, Rahman N, Chenevix-Trench G, Bojesen SE, Nordestgaard BG, Axelsson CK, Garcia-Closas M, Brinton L, Chanock S, Lissowska J, Peplonska B, Nevanlinna H, Fagerholm R, Eerola H, Kang D, Yoo KY, Noh DY, Ahn SH, Hunter DJ, Hankinson SE, Cox DG, Hall P, Wedren S, Liu J, Low YL, Bogdanova N, Schurmann P, Dork T, Tollenaar RA, Jacobi CE, Devilee P, Klijn JG, Sigurdson AJ, Doody MM, Alexander BH, Zhang J, Cox A, Brock IW, MacPherson G, Reed MW, Couch FJ, Goode EL, Olson JE, Meijers-Heijboer H, van den Ouweland A, Uitterlinden A, Rivadeneira F, Milne RL, Ribas G, Gonzalez-Neira A, Benitez J, Hopper JL, McCredie M, Southey M, Giles GG, Schroen C, Justenhoven C, Brauch H, Hamann U, Ko YD, Spurdle AB, Beesley J, Chen X, Mannermaa A, Kosma VM, Kataja V, Hartikainen J, Day NE, Cox DR, Ponder BA (2007) Genome-wide association study identifies novel breast cancer susceptibility loci. Nature 447:1087–1093

Evans DG, Birch JM, Ramsden RT, Sharif S, Baser ME (2006) Malignant transformation and new primary tumors after therapeutic radiation for benign disease: substantial risks in certain tumor prone syndromes. J Med Genet 43: 289–294

Felton JS, Malfatti MA, Knize MG, Salmon CP, Hopmans EC, Wu RW (1997) Health risks of heterocyclic amines. Mutat Res 376: 37–41

Griffiths-Jones S, Grocock RJ, van Dongen S, Bateman A, Enright AJ (2006) miRBase: microRNA sequences, targets and gene nomenclature. Nucleic Acids Res 34(Database issue): D140–144

Grosche B, Kreuzer M, Kreisheimer M, Schnelzer M, Tschense A (2006) Lung cancer risk among German male uranium miners: a cohort study, 1946–1998. Br J Cancer 95: 1280–1287

Hanahan D, Weinberg RA (2000) The hallmarks of cancer. Cell 100: 57–70

Harris H (2008) Concerning the origin of malignant tumors by Theodor Boveri. Translated and annotated by Henry Harris. J Cell Sci 121 (Suppl 1): 1–84

He H, Jazdzewski K, Li W, Liyanarachchi S, Nagy R, Volinia S, Calin GA, Liu CG, Franssila K, Suster S, Kloos RT, Croce CM, de la Chapelle A (2005) The role of microRNA genes in papillary thyroid carcinoma. Proc Natl Acad Sci U S A 102: 19075–19080

Hemminki K, Bermejo JL (2007) Constraints for genetic association studies imposed by attributable fraction and familial risk. Carcinogenesis 28: 648–656

Hemminki K, Forsti A, Lorenzo Bermejo J (2008) Etiologic impact of known cancer susceptibility genes. Mutat Res 658: 42–54

IARC. http://monographs.iarc.fr/ENG/Classification/index

IARC (1986) Tobacco smoking. IARC, Lyon

IARC (1993) Some naturally occurring substances: Food items and constituents, heterocyclic aromatic amines and myotoxins. IARC, Lyon

IARC (2004) Some drinking-water disinfectants and contaminants, including arsenic. IARC, Lyon

Kenny PA, Lee GY, Bissell MJ (2007) Targeting the tumor microenvironment. Front Biosci 12: 3468–7344

Kleinerman RA, Tucker MA, Tarone RE, Abramson DH, Seddon JM, Stovall M, Li FP, Fraumeni JF Jr (2005) Risk of new cancers after radiotherapy in long-term survivors of retinoblastoma: an extended follow-up. J Clin Oncol 23: 2272–2279

Knudson AG (1996) Hereditary cancer: two hits revisited. J Cancer Res Clin Oncol 122: 135–140

Korenjak M, Brehm A (2005) E2F-Rb complexes regulating transcription of genes important for differentiation and development. Curr Opin Genet Dev 15: 520–527

Kulbe H, Levinson NR, Balkwill F, Wilson JL (2004) The chemokine network in cancer—much more than directing cell movement. Int J Dev Biol 48: 489–496

Kusiak RA, Springer J, Ritchie AC, Muller J (1991) Carcinoma of the lung in Ontario gold miners: possible aetiological factors. Br J Ind Med 48: 808–817

Kuukasjarvi T, Karhu R, Tanner M, Kahkonen M, Schaffer A, Nupponen N, Pennanen S, Kallioniemi A, Kallioniemi OP, Isola J (1997) Genetic heterogeneity and clonal evolution underlying development of asynchronous metastasis in human breast cancer. Cancer Res 57: 1597–1604

Letterer E (1959) Allgemeine Pathologie. Thieme, Stuttgart

Lewis BP, Burge CB, Bartel DP (2005) Conserved seed pairing, often flanked by adenosines, indicates that thousands of human genes are microRNA targets. Cell 120: 15–20

Lissowska J, Bardin-Mikolajczak A, Fletcher T, Zaridze D, Szeszenia-Dabrowska N, Rudnai P, Fabianova E, Cassidy A, Mates D, Holcatova I, Vitova V, Janout V, Mannetje A, Brennan P, Boffetta P (2005) Lung cancer and indoor pollution from heating and cooking with solid fuels: the IARC international multicentre case-control study in Eastern/Central Europe and the United Kingdom. Am J Epidemiol 162: 326–333

Liu J, Valencia-Sanchez MA, Hannon GJ, Parker R (2005) MicroRNA-dependent localization of targeted mRNAs to mammalian P-bodies. Nat Cell Biol 7: 719–723

Liu J, Zheng B, Aposhian HV, Zhou Y, Chen ML, Zhang A, Waalkes MP (2002) Chronic arsenic poisoning from burning high-arsenic-containing coal in Guizhou, China. Environ Health Perspect 110: 119–122

Loeb LA (2001) A mutator phenotype in cancer. Cancer Res 61: 3230–3239

Manchester KL (1995) Theodor Boveri and the origin of malignant tumors. Trends Cell Biol 5: 384–387

McDermott C, O'Sullivan R, McMahon G (2007) An unusual cause of headache: Pott's puffy tumor. Eur J Emerg Med 14: 170–173

Mimeault M, Batra SK (2007) Interplay of distinct growth factors during epithelial mesenchymal transition of cancer progenitor cells and molecular targeting as novel cancer therapies. Ann Oncol 18: 1605–1619

Murphree AL, Benedict WF (1984) Retinoblastoma: clues to human oncogenesis. Science 223: 1028–1033

Negrini M, Ferracin M, Sabbioni S, Croce CM (2007) MicroRNAs in human cancer: from research to therapy. J Cell Sci 120(Pt 11): 1833–1840

Peto J (2001) Cancer epidemiology in the last century and the next decade. Nature 411: 390–395

Peto J, Decarli A, La Vecchia C, Levi F, Negri E (1999) The European mesothelioma epidemic. Br J Cancer 79: 666–672

Santoro M, Carlomagno F, Melillo RM, Fusco A (2004) Dysfunction of the RET receptor in human cancer. Cell Mol Life Sci 61: 2954–2964

Sarrio D, Rodriguez-Pinilla SM, Hardisson D, Cano A, Moreno-Bueno G, Palacios J (2008) Epithelial-mesenchymal transition in breast cancer relates to the basal-like phenotype. Cancer Res 68: 989–997

Sen GL, Blau HM (2005) Argonaute 2/RISC resides in sites of mammalian mRNA decay known as cytoplasmic bodies. Nat Cell Biol 7: 633–636

Shen R, Ye Y, Chen L, Yan Q, Barsky SH, Gao JX (2008) Precancerous stem cells can serve as tumor vasculogenic progenitors. PLoS ONE 3: e1652

Shivdasani RA (2006) MicroRNAs: regulators of gene expression and cell differentiation. Blood 108(12): 3646–3653

Sjoblom T, Jones S, Wood LD, Parsons DW, Lin J, Barber TD, Mandelker D, Leary RJ, Ptak J, Silliman N, Szabo S, Buckhaults P, Farrell C, Meeh P, Markowitz SD, Willis J, Dawson D, Willson JK, Gazdar AF, Hartigan J, Wu L, Liu C, Parmigiani G, Park BH, Bachman KE, Papadopoulos N, Vogelstein B, Kinzler KW, Velculescu VE (2006) The consensus coding sequences of human breast and colorectal cancers. Science 314: 268–274

Sugimura T, Wakabayashi K, Nakagama H, Nagao M (2004) Heterocyclic amines: Mutagens/carcinogens produced during cooking of meat and fish. Cancer Sci 95: 290–299

Tapio S, Grosche B (2006) Arsenic in the aetiology of cancer. Mutat Res 612:215–246

Taylor PR, Qiao YL, Schatzkin A, Yao SX, Lubin J, Mao BL, Rao JY, McAdams M, Xuan XZ, Li JY (1989) Relation of arsenic exposure to lung cancer among tin miners in Yunnan Province, China. Br J Ind Med 46: 881–886

Vietri M, Bianchi M, Ludlow JW, Mittnacht S, Villa-Moruzzi E (2006) Direct interaction between the catalytic subunit of protein phosphatase 1 and pRb. Cancer Cell Int 6: 3

Vogelstein B, Fearon ER, Hamilton SR, Kern SE, Preisinger AC, Leppert M, Nakamura Y, White R, Smits AM, Bos JL (1988) Genetic alterations during colorectal-tumor development. N Engl J Med 319: 525–532

Vogelstein B, Kinzler KW (2004) Cancer genes and the pathways they control. Nat Med 10: 789–799

Vogt PK (1996) Peyton Rous: homage and appraisal. Faseb J 10: 1559–1562

Wagner SN, Atkinson MJ, Thanner S, Wagner C, Schmitt M, Wilhelm O, Rotter M, Hofler H (1995) Modulation of urokinase and urokinase receptor gene expression in human renal cell carcinoma. Am J Pathol 147: 183–192

Walch AK, Zitzelsberger HF, Bruch J, Keller G, Angermeier D, Aubele MM, Mueller J, Stein H, Braselmann H, Siewert JR, Hofler H, Werner M (2000) Chromosomal imbalances in Barrett's adenocarcinoma and the metaplasia-dysplasia-carcinoma sequence. Am J Pathol 156: 555–566

WHO (1987) Air quality guidelines for Europe. Copenhagen, World Health Organization Regional Office for Europe

Wichmann HE, Rosario AS, Heid IM, Kreuzer M, Heinrich J, Kreienbrock L (2005) Increased lung cancer risk due to residential radon in a pooled and extended analysis of studies in Germany. Health Phys 88: 71–79

Wiemer EA (2007) The role of microRNAs in cancer: no small matter. Eur J Cancer 43: 1529–1544

Zhang B, Wang Q, Pan X (2007) MicroRNAs and their regulatory roles in animals and plants. J Cell Physiol 210: 279–289

Tumor Growth and Cell Proliferation

Marek Los, Iran Rashedi, Soumya Panigrahi, Thomas Klonisch, and Klaus Schulze-Osthoff

CONTENTS

M. Los, MD, PhD
BioApplications Enterprises, 34 Vanier Drive, Winnipeg, MB R2V2N6, Canada

KEY POINTS

- Several checkpoint mechanisms within the cell cycle are responsible for the monitoring of individual steps during cell division and mitosis. While cell proliferation normally is tightly controlled, cancer might be viewed as a manifestation of uncontrolled, "selfish" cell divisions.
- A family of proteins called cyclin-dependent serine/threonine protein kinases (CDKs) constitutes pivotal regulator proteins governing the transition from one cell cycle phase to the next. CDKs are activated at specific cell cycle points. Positive regulation of CDK activity occurs through association with proteins called cyclins. Cyclins are produced at each of the cell cycle phases and form protein complexes with their CDK partners. Mutations within genes encoding for CDKs and/or associated cyclins have been often found in tumors.

I. Rashedi, MD
Manitoba Institute of Cell Biology, CancerCare Manitoba and, Department of Biochemistry and Medical Genetics, University Manitoba, ON 6009-675 McDermot Ave., Winnipeg, MB, R3E0V9, Canada

S. Panigrahi, MD
Manitoba Institute of Cell Biology, CancerCare Manitoba, and Department of Physiology, University of Manitoba, ON6009-675 McDermot Avenue, Winnipeg, MB R3E0V9, Canada

T. Klonisch, MD, PhD
Department of Human Anatomy and Cell Science, University of Manitoba, Winnipeg, MB, Canada

K. Schulze-Osthoff, PhD
Institute of Molecular Medicine, University of Düsseldorf, Building 23.12 Universitätsstraße 1, 40225 Düsseldorf, Germany

- Malfunction of critical organelles or structures (e.g., faulty mitotic spindle) and/or DNA damage prompts checkpoints to activate cell cycle arrest and trigger apoptotic cell death cascades if the damage is not repaired.
- Cell cycle entry (G0/G1–S phase transition) is controlled by two major pathways: (1) Rb (Rb, cyclin D1, and p16^{INK4A}) cell cycle pathway, and (2) p53/p21^{Waf1} G1–S checkpoint arrest pathway.
- The p53 molecule appears to be the most important guardian of genome stability, and its multiple functions unite the regulation of cell cycle progression, DNA damage detection, and apoptosis induction. p53 has tumor suppressor activity, and about 50% of tumors display inactivation of this gene. If p53 detects DNA damage, it will stop cell cycle progression and allow time for DNA repair. If the repair mechanisms fail, then it will activate the expression of several genes involved in apoptosis in an attempt to counteract uncontrolled cell division, leading to tumorigenesis.
- Stem cells attracted significant attention in recent years, due to their enormous potential in regenerative medicine. Their capacity for endless self-renewal and plasticity makes them ideal tools for the treatment of a number of diseases. Unfortunately, the same qualities make them precursors for the development of cancer cells if their cell cycle control fails and/or their differentiation programs go astray. Thus, cancer could be perceived as a disease of stem cells.
- The phosphoinositol-3-kinase (PI3-K)/Akt signaling pathway is a major prosurvival pathway within the cell. Activated by a number of cellular stimuli and external signals, this pathway regulates key cellular functions such as proliferation, growth, transcription, translation, cell cycle, and apoptosis. Notably, PI3-K/Akt signaling is frequently disrupted in human cancers and plays a major role not only in tumor growth, but also in the response to cancer treatment.
- Epidermal growth factor (EGF) promotes survival and stimulates growth and differentiation of epithelial cells. Enhanced tumor malignancy and shorter survival periods are positively correlated with the expression of EGF-like ligands and ErbB and are poor prognostic markers for a number of malignancies of epithelial origin.
- Therapeutic approaches based on targeting growth and survival signaling pathways, including but not limited to PI3-K/Akt and EGF, have been established. Novel targeted cancer therapies aim at the correction (mostly inhibition) of signaling pathways, which are dysregulated in cancer, e.g., by interfering with tyrosine kinases.

Abstract

The regulation of cell proliferation, cell death, and cell survival must be tightly controlled in multicellular organisms where different tissues fulfill specialized functions. Uncontrolled overgrowth of a single tissue or even organ within the organism would be fatal for the existence of the whole organism. Thus, in multicellular organisms, decisions about cell divisions can no longer rest within a single cell, but rather must be undertaken collectively so that they serve the organism as a whole. Failure of these mechanisms will lead to developmental abnormalities and/or cancer. Thus, cancer could be viewed as diseases of cell proliferation and cell death. In this chapter, we discuss various aspects and interconnections between cell survival, proliferation, and death. We also introduce the basic information about (cancer) stem cells and their physiology, since mutations within stem cells that affect the regulation of their proliferation, survival, and differentiation can potentially lead to cancer development. While the focus of the chapter is on the interconnection between cell proliferation and cell death, a significant part of the chapter is dedicated to major survival/proliferation pathways frequently mutated in cancer, like ErbB2/Her2/Neu, ABL, and PI3-K/AKT, used here as examples. In the last part of the chapter, we emphasize the potential of regulators of cell survival and proliferation as pharmacologic targets for the development of targeted anticancer therapies.

2.1
Introduction: Tumor Development and Growth Characteristics

Tumor development can be viewed in several aspects. In this chapter we discuss tumorigenesis in the context of: (1) a disease of tissue-committed stem cells caused by disturbances in their homeostasis and differentiation (cancer stem cell concept) (HOMBACH-KLONISCH et al. 2008), and (2) a dysequilibrium of homeostasis between cell proliferation and cell death (the removal of supernumerary or damaged cells) (MADDIKA et al. 2007a). Both scenarios may reflect a manifestation of disturbed cell cycle control, are not mutually exclusive, and can co-exist within cells.

The eukaryotic cell cycle is divided into four non-overlapping phases: G1 (gap 1), S (DNA synthesis), G2 (gap 2), and M (mitosis, cell division) phases, respectively. Once committed to enter the S phase, a healthy cell will complete the entire cell cycle. If the cell encounters unmanageable obstacles during cell cycle progression, then this cell will undergo programmed cell death (apoptosis). Several checkpoint mechanisms within the cell cycle are responsible for the monitoring of individual steps during cell division and mitosis. We focus on three important control mechanisms involving cyclin-dependent kinases, retinoblastoma (Rb), and p53.

2.2
Brief Overview of the Cell Cycle

Unlike in a single-cell organism where the decision to divide rests largely on the availability of sufficient energy supply, the decision for individual cells to divide in multicellular organisms is the result of intricate intercellular networking in a collective attempt to preserve tissue integrity and function and sustain the existence of the organism as a whole. Cancer is a manifestation of uncontrolled, "selfish" cell divisions.

The G1 phase is the first phase of the cell cycle and serves to prepare cells for DNA synthesis. Diploid cells contain $2n$ chromosomes (COLLINS and GARRETT 2005; SCHAFER 1998) and in the subsequent S phase, this DNA is duplicated to reach $4n$. Before undergoing mitosis, cells prepare for cell division in G2 phase. During mitosis, the genome composed of $4n$ chromosomes is equally divided into two daughter cells, each receiving two copies of the genome ($2n$). Non-cycling/quiescent cells remain in G0 phase (COLLINS and GARRETT 2005). Cell proliferation is tightly controlled. A family of proteins called cyclin-dependent serine/threonine protein kinases (CDKs) constitute pivotal regulator proteins governing the transition from one cell cycle phase to the next. CDKs are activated at specific cell cycle points (COLLINS and GARRETT 2005; VERMEU-

LEN et al. 2003). Positive regulation of CDK activity occurs through association with proteins called cyclins. Cyclins are produced at each of the cell cycle phases and form protein complexes with their CDK partners. The levels of activating cyclins fluctuate at different stages of the cell cycle, whereas the CDK protein levels remain fairly stable (VERMEULEN et al. 2003). Cyclins D1, D2, D3, and C regulate G0/G1- to S-phase transition. Cyclins D1, D2, and D3 interact with CDK4 and CDK6, whereas cyclin C interacts with CDK8. On receiving a growth signal and being prompted to enter the cell cycle, cyclins D1, D2, and D3 are the first to be expressed in cells exiting G0 state. The progression through G1 is governed by cyclin D isoforms and CDKs -2, -4, and -6 (SCHWARTZ and SHAH 2005; VERMEULEN et al. 2003). Cyclin E is associated with G1- to S-phase transition and activates CDK2. Cyclin A is expressed during the S-phase transition and it interacts with CDK1 and -2. B-type cyclins are expressed in the end of G2 and mitosis, and they interact with CDK1 (COQUERET 2003). G- and T-type cyclins activate CDK5 and CDK9, respectively (JOHNSON and WALKER 1999).

The activity of CDKs is tightly regulated by inhibitory phosphorylation and by inhibitory molecules. The inhibitory phosphorylation is mediated by the Wee1 and MYT1 kinases (PARK and LEE 2003). In addition, two classes of protein-based inhibitors the INK4 group such as $p16^{Ink4a}$ or $p15^{Ink4b}$ and the CIP/KIP class such as $p21^{waf1}$ or $p27^{kip1}$ may negatively regulate the activity of CDKs (PARK and LEE 2003; SCHWARTZ and SHAH 2005).

Each phase of the cell cycle contains checkpoints that will arrest cell cycle progression and allow activation of repair mechanisms (PARK and LEE 2003). Malfunction of critical organelles or structures (e.g., faulty mitotic spindle) and/or DNA damage prompts these checkpoints to activate cell cycle arrest and trigger apoptotic cell death cascades if the damage is not repaired (ROWINSKY 2005; SIEGEL 2006). The apoptotic machinery is an important part of cell cycle checkpoints, protects the integrity of multicellular organisms, and allows for selective removal of unwanted or damaged cells (KHOSRAVI-FAR and ESPOSTI 2004; LOS and GIBSON 2005; LOS et al. 1999). The induction of apoptosis leads to cell blebbing, exposure of phosphatidylserine at the cell surface, shrinkage in cell size, DNA condensation, and the formation of apoptotic bodies (DARZYNKIEWICZ et al. 1997; KHOSRAVI-FAR and ESPOSTI 2004).

2.3
Reciprocal Control
of Cell Proliferation and Cell Death

Tumor suppressor genes like *p53*, *Rb*, and *E2F* appeared during evolution, probably to protect the integrity of the organism from uncontrolled cell proliferation within multicellular specialized tissues. This concept is supported by the observation that the respective proteins or pathways are mutated or inactivated in most human cancers. Cell cycle entry (G0–G1- to S-phase transition) is controlled by two major pathways: (1) the Rb (Rb, cyclin D1, and p16^{Ink4a}) cell cycle pathway and (2) the p53/p21^{Waf1} G1–S checkpoint arrest pathway. Although both pathways act largely independently, they are interconnected (Burke et al. 2005; Hsieh et al. 2002).

2.3.1
Rb Tumor Suppressor

Rb was the first tumor suppressor gene to be identified (Lee et al. 1987) and has a major role in controlling cell cycle entry. Besides the control of G1–S transition, Rb is critical for tissue regeneration, stem cell maintenance, differentiation, and developmental programs. Rb is a 928–amino acid nuclear phosphoprotein that may weakly bind DNA. Rb interacts with a number of proteins, which mostly play a role in transcription control. Among these proteins, E2Fs and its partner DP are key regulators of cell cycle-related gene expression. These heterodimers directly modulate the expression of genes involved in DNA replication, DNA repair, and G2–M progression (Knudsen and Knudsen 2006).

Rb and its homologues RBL1/p107 and RBL2/p130 mediate cell cycle arrest by antagonizing transcription factor E2F/DP. This event is regulated by the phosphorylation status of Rb family proteins. Only hypophosphorylated Rb protein family members can interact with E2Fs and function as cell cycle inhibitors (Hsieh et al. 2002; Jackson and Pereira-Smith 2006). Rbs are phosphorylated by the CDK/cyclin complexes. Mitogenic signals (e.g., growth factors) lead to the activation of CDK/cyclin complexes, while antimitogenic conditions (e.g., cell confluence or nutrient depletion) inhibit activation of the G1 CDK/cyclins. Phosphorylation of Rb turns off its transcription repressor function, thus releasing the E2F/DP transcription factor complex and allowing expression of *E2F* target genes essential for entry into S phase. Rb is held in a hyperphosphorylated/inactive state throughout the rest of the cell cycle (S, G2, and M phases) (Knudsen and Knudsen 2006).

Rb family members may also regulate gene expression by affecting chromatin structure. These chromatin changes are invoked by the recruitment of histone deacetylases (HDACs), histone methyltransferases, SWI/SNF complex members, and, less well-characterized DNA methyltransferases and polycomb proteins (Jackson and Pereira-Smith 2006). The integrity of the Rb pathway can influence the activity of p53 and vice versa (Hsieh et al. 2002).

In tumors, downregulation or complete inhibition of Rb function is achieved by a variety of mechanisms: (1) high expression of CDK4 or cyclin D, which maintains Rb in an inactive/phosphorylated state; (2) loss or mutation of p16^{Ink4a} CDK-inhibitor; (3) sequestration of Rb by oncoproteins, e.g., the human papilloma virus E7 protein; and (4) mutations of the *Rb* gene (Knudsen and Knudsen 2006).

E2F/DP complexes are key downstream mediators of the p16^{Ink4a}/RB pathway. Six E2F-like proteins (E2F1 to 6) have so far been identified and can be classified into two subgroups: (1) activating E2Fs (E2F1, E2F2, and E2F3 are strong transcriptional activators), and (2) repressive E2Fs (E2F4, E2F5, and E2F6) that repress gene transcription. E2F/DP activity is essential for cell proliferation, and its malfunction immediately provokes a senescence-like cell cycle arrest (Maehara et al. 2005). Overexpression of E2F1 induces apoptosis that is independent of p53 (Holmberg et al. 1998).

2.3.2
p53 and p53-Dependent Cell Cycle Checkpoints

The p53 molecule appears to be the most important guardian of genome stability, and its multiple functions unite the regulation of cell cycle progression, DNA damage detection, and apoptosis induction. p53 has tumor-suppressor activity, and about 50% of tumors display inactivation of this gene. If p53 detects DNA damage, then it will stop cell cycle progression and allow time for DNA repair. If the repair mechanisms fail, then it will activate the expression of several genes involved in apoptosis in an attempt to counteract uncontrolled cell division, leading to tumorigenesis (Kim et al. 2006; Rowinsky 2005). Induction of p53-dependent apoptosis proceeds through the activation of mitochondrial apoptotic pathways with the release of cytochrome *c* from mitochondria, an event that triggers the apoptotic proteolytic cascade.

How does the p53-dependent pathway become activated? In response to stress stimuli, p53, which normally resides in the cell at a low level, accumulates as a result of increased protein stability (Finlan and Hupp 2005; Hsieh et al. 2002). The accumulation of p53 can be triggered by various signals, including DNA damage, hypoxia, and increased expression/activity of (proto-) oncogenes. This initiates various cellular responses that lead to cell cycle arrest, senescence, differentiation, DNA repair, apoptosis, and/or inhibition of angiogenesis (Finlan and Hupp 2005; Giono and Manfredi 2006). Most of these p53-mediated responses are carried out via its activity as a transcription factor. p53 (1) induces cell growth arrest via the expression of p21, 14-3-3s, Cdc25C, and GADD45; (2) activates DNA repair by inducing the expression of p21, GADD45, and the p48 xeroderma pigmentosum protein; and (3) triggers apoptosis by upregulating the transcription of Bax, PUMA, Noxa, p53-AIP, PIG3, Fas/APO1/CD95, and KILLER/DR5. These responses are regulated through different pathways and are highly dependent on the type and abundance of the specific trigger. For example, low levels of stress or DNA damage will secure levels of p53 that induce growth arrest genes, but under aggravated cellular stress higher p53 levels will activate apoptotic pathways. Furthermore, posttranslational modifications of p53 are important for the final outcome of p53-mediated responses.

In tumor cells, p53 may cooperate with E2F1 to induce apoptosis. This capacity is independent of the transactivational function of E2F1, and may occur on interaction of E2F1 with p53 via its cyclin A domain. Cyclin A competes for this binding and, thus, the level of cellular cyclin A will affect the interaction between E2F1 and p53. In normal cells and in the presence of Rb, which downregulates E2F1, p53 stabilization induced by DNA damage is unable to trigger apoptosis by proteins like E2F. In addition, mitogen-induced E2F will transcriptionally activate genes like cyclin A, and increased cyclin A protein content prevents E2F binding to p53. This explains why in normal cells a predominantly p53-dependent G1 arrest occurs but not apoptosis (Hsieh et al. 2002).

In cells with damaged DNA, p53 prevents the initiation of DNA replication at the G1–S checkpoint by activating the expression of the CDK-inhibitor $p21^{Waf1}$, which inhibits Rb phosphorylation (Finlan and Hupp 2005; Giono and Manfredi 2006). In addition, expression of $p21^{Waf1}$ induces growth arrest at G1 and G2 phases (Giono and Manfredi 2006). DNA damage-induced G1 arrest consists of two phases with the first phase being independent of p53. The second

p53-dependent phase involves the p53-activating kinases ATM, ATR, and Chk2. Thus, it is proposed that p53 is more important for the maintenance rather than for the induction of G1 arrest. p53-dependent arrest in G1 extends the Cdc25A-mediated delay in cell cycle progression and provides the cell with sufficient time to repair damaged DNA. During the S phase, an isoform of p53 (Δp53) causes cell cycle arrest by binding to $p21^{Waf1}$ and *14-3-3s* growth arrest genes, but not the apoptotic *PIG3* gene (Giono and Manfredi 2006). p53 also prevents aneuploidy by blocking endoreduplication of tetraploid cells that result from mitotic failure (Giono and Manfredi 2006). p53 can directly interact with proteins involved in DNA repair and a variety of DNA structures, acting as a sensor of damage or mismatch. Furthermore, p53 binds to double-stranded and single-stranded DNA in a nonspecific way, to ends of double-strand breaks, to Holliday junctions, and to DNA bulges caused by DNA mismatches (Giono and Manfredi 2006).

2.3.3
Role of Cyclin-Dependent Kinases in the Regulation of Cell Cycle and Apoptosis

CDKs form a group of heterodimeric serine/threonine kinases that regulate cell cycle progression. CDKs form complexes with cyclins, which act as activating partners. CDKs, cyclins, and CDK inhibitors act in a coordinated manner to achieve cellular homeostasis. Mutations within genes encoding for CDKs and/or associated cyclins have been often found in tumors and neurodegenerative disorders, since CDKs have also cell cycle-unrelated functions in neurons.

CDK1 is the only nonredundant CDK family member. It is involved in the G2–M transition and has a function in mitosis. Inhibitors of CDK1 arrest the cell cycle at the G2–M transition (Gray et al. 1999). CDK1 exerts its effects on the cell cycle by phosphorylating a number of protein substrates involved in cell cycle regulation.

CDK2 form complexes with E-type and A-type cyclins. CDK2/cyclin E plays a redundant role in the G1–S transition. Unlike CDK1$^{-/-}$ mice, CDK2 knockout mice are viable, though females and males remain infertile, which indicates that CDK2 plays a nonredundant role in gametogenesis and meiosis, whereas its role in cell proliferation appears redundant (Berthet et al. 2003; Ortega et al. 2003). Hence, it has been described recently that CDK1/cyclin E complexes can compensate for the absence of CDK2 activity (Aleem et al. 2005; Kaldis and Aleem 2005).

Beside their role in cell cycle, some CDKs are also involved in cell death. CDK1 activity has been observed in cells triggered to die with granzyme B (Shi et al. 1996), perforin, fragmentin-2, and camptothecin (Borgne and Golsteyn 2003; Shimizu et al. 1995). Exposure of tumor cells to CDK1 inhibitors for longer than 24 h induces apoptosis (Vassilev et al. 2006). In noncycling G1, CD4⁺CD8⁺ thymocytes triggered to die by various stimuli such as dexamethasone, heat shock, γ-irradiation, or Fas/CD95 cross-linking, CDK2 activity was increased indicating its role in thymocyte selection (Hakem et al. 1999). CDK2 also plays a key role in tumor cell-selective induction of apoptosis triggered by the viral protein apoptin, which is also phosphorylated and activated by CDK2 (Maddika et al., unpublished).

2.4
Stem Cell Proliferative Potential and Plasticity, and Their Contribution to Tumor Development

Stem cells have attracted significant attention in recent years due to their enormous potential in regenerative medicine. Their capacity for endless self-renewal and plasticity makes them ideal tools for the treatment of a number of diseases. Unfortunately, the same qualities make them precursors for the development of cancer cells if their cell cycle control fails and/or their differentiation programs go astray. Thus, cancer could be perceived as a disease of stem cells (Hombach-Klonisch et al. 2008). So far, stem cells are still largely defined by their capacity to (re-)colonize a given tissue niche, or initiate tumor growth (cancer stem cells), as only few molecular markers of "stemness" exist. Among them, the transcription factors Oct3/4 (POU5F1/Oct 4) is perceived as one of the best indicators of stemness (de Jong and Looijenga 2006). Apart from its presence in the embryo and germ cells, Oct3/4 expression in non-malignant cells is restricted to tissue-committed pluripotent cells. Oct3/4, together with Nanog and Sox2, are reliable markers in germ cell tumor diagnostics. These markers are widely expressed in lesions that may initiate gonadoblastoma and carcinoma in situ, as well as in invasive embryonal carcinoma and seminomas. Other markers worth considering, especially with respect to hematopoietic stem cells are the members of SLAM family, CD150 and CD48.

Pluripotency and plasticity are prominent properties of embryonic stem cells. Adult stem cells are thought to be restricted in their differentiation potential to the progeny of the tissue in which they reside. When parts of an organ are transplanted to a new site, the transplanted tissue preserves its original character. Similarly, cells dissociated from an organ or tissue, tend to maintain elements of their previous phenotype in culture. Despite losing some of their properties, these cells tend to preserve characteristics of the original differentiated cell lineage. However, plasticity in the differentiation potential of stem cells derived from adult tissues has recently been reported (Wagers and Weissman 2004). Moreover, murine bone marrow-derived cells may give rise to skeletal muscle cells when transplanted into damaged mouse muscle (Ferrari et al. 1998). Thus, transplanted bone marrow cells can generate a wide spectrum of different cell types, including endothelial, myocardial (Lin et al. 2000; Orlic et al. 2001), hepatic (Petersen et al. 1999), neuronal, and glial cells (Brazelton et al. 2000; Mezey et al. 2000; Priller et al. 2001). Furthermore, hematopoietic stem cells may produce cardiac myocytes and endothelial cells (Jackson et al. 2001), epithelial cells of the liver, gut, lung, and skin (Krause et al. 2001), and even functional hepatocytes (Lagasse et al. 2000). Mesenchymal stromal cells of the bone marrow are able to generate brain astrocytes (Kopen et al. 1999), and enriched stem cells from murine adult skeletal muscle can produce blood cells (Gussoni et al. 1999; Jackson et al. 1999; Pang 2000).

In the majority of these plasticity studies performed in the murine system, genetically marked cells from one organ apparently gave rise to cell type characteristics of other organs, after transplantation. This suggests that even cell types once perceived as terminally differentiated exhibit considerable plasticity in their developmental potential. Pluripotent primitive stem cells present in a very low number in most tissues may explain the acquisition of an unexpected phenotype. Recently, non-hematopoietic cell populations from bone marrow and umbilical cord blood were enriched by in vitro culture and had the potential to differentiate into derivatives of all three germline layers with meso-, endo-, and ecto-dermal characteristics (D'Ippolito et al. 2004; Kogler et al. 2004; Yoon et al. 2005). Known as multipotent adult progenitor cells, these cells contributed to most if not all somatic cell lineages, including brain cells, when injected into a murine blastocyst (Jiang et al. 2002; Reyes et al. 2001). They express Oct4, a transcription factor required for undifferentiated embryonic stem cells maintenance (Nichols et al. 1998), at levels approaching those of embryonic stem cells. Multipotent adult progenitor cells do not express the two transcription factors Nanog and Sox2, which play a major role in embryonic stem cell pluripotency (Boyer et al. 2005; Chambers et al. 2003). This expression profile may help to explain the fact that the use of embryonic stem cells, but not multipotent adult progenitor cells, carries the risk of tumor development post-transplantation.

2.5
Cell Survival and Proliferation Signaling Pathways Active in Cancer and Their Role in Tumor Growth

Several pathways, when deregulated may induce uncontrolled proliferation. Due to the space constrains, we use Abl, PI3-K/Akt, and EGFR pathways as examples to illustrate common phenomena related to uncontrolled proliferation and malignancy development.

2.5.1
Abl Pathway

The Abl kinase is encoded on the long arm of chromosome 9, a locus frequently involved in a translocation with chromosome 22. This Philadelphia translocation (Ph1) t(9; 22) (q34, q11) leads to the development of chronic myeloid leukemia (CML) (Bartram et al. 1983; Heisterkamp et al. 1988). Abl is a 145-kD protein with two isoforms derived by alternative splicing of the first exon. It is highly homologous to the kinase encoded by the Abelson murine leukemia virus (Abelson and Rabstein 1970). Human Abl is ubiquitously expressed, localizes to different cellular compartments (Baltimore et al. 1995; Laneuville 1995), and as a multidomain protein, is engaged in different functions (Fig. 2.1). At its NH$_2$ terminus, Abl protein contains three SRC homology domains (SH1–SH3). The SH1 domain of Abl

has tyrosine kinase activity, whereas the SH2 and SH3 domains serve as protein–protein interaction motifs. The proline-rich sequences in the central part of the Abl molecule can interact with SH3 domains and have inhibitory roles (Alexandropoulos et al. 1995; Feller et al. 1994). Nuclear localization signals and the DNA-binding and actin-binding motifs are found close to the C-terminal part of the Abl molecule (McWhirter and Wang 1993; Van Etten et al. 1989).

The Abl protein is involved in numerous processes, including cell cycle regulation, the response to genotoxic stress, and integrin signaling relaying information on cell density and other cellular environment-related signals (Kipreos and Wang 1990; Van Etten 1999). Numerous domains within the Abl molecule allow formation of multiprotein complexes. For example, the Cables protein links Abl to CDK5 and to *N*-cadherin-dependent signaling pathways (Rhee et al. 2007; Zukerberg et al. 2000). Thus, within cells Abl protein acts as an integrating element for complex extra- and intracellular environmental scenarios, thus, significantly influencing the cellular decision making with respect to cell cycle progression and apoptosis.

Abl is a highly regulated kinase. In its inactive form, the SH3 domain interacts with its internal proline rich region ("internal substrate" binding) (Goga et al. 1993). Concurrently, structural alterations occur as a consequence of the formation of Bcr-Abl chimeric protein rendering this chimeric kinase constitutively active.

Several proteins have been identified that bind to the SH3 domain of Abl (Cicchetti et al. 1992; Shi et al. 1995). Two proteins, Abi-1 and Abi-2 (Abl interacting proteins 1 and 2) were shown to have inhibitory functions on Abl by interacting with the SH3 domain of Abl protein. Activated Abl normally counteracts their inhibitory action by promoting proteasome-mediated

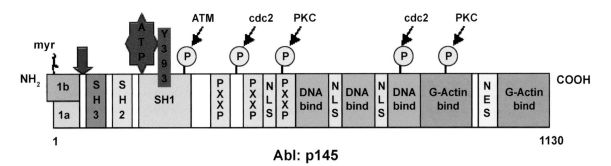

Abl: p145

Fig. 2.1. ABL protein—structural features. Both isoforms of p145-ABL are indicated. Type 1b ABL has a myristoylation (*myr*) consensus site. The three SRC-homology (*SH*) domains situated near the NH$_2$ terminus. In ABL, the Tyr-393 (*Y393*) is a major site for autophosphorylation within the kinase domain. The proline-rich regions (*PxxP*) are capable of binding to SH3 domains of other proteins. The position of the breakpoint in the BCR-ABL fusion protein is indicated by a *blue arrow*. (See main text for detailed description)

degradation of Abi-1 and Abi-2 (Dai et al. 1998). It has also been reported that the degradation of Abi-1 and Abi-2 occurs in Philadelphia chromosome positive acute leukemia but not in the Philadelphia-negative disease phenotype. Abl may also be inhibited by Pag/Msp23 that becomes oxidized and dissociates from Abl on exposure of cells to oxidative stress and/or ionizing radiation (Wen and van Etten 1997).

2.5.1.1
BCR-ABL Chimeric Oncoprotein and Its Oncogenic Effects

BCR-ABL is the causative oncogenic factor in Philadelphia chromosome–positive chronic myelocytic leukemias. In this fusion protein, the N terminus of BCR (*breakpoint cluster region*) is joined head-to-tail with the N-terminal portion of ABL, creating the P210BCR-ABL phosphoprotein with tyrosine kinase activity. The breakpoints within the *Abl* gene at 9q43 may occur anywhere within a region spanning about 300 kb at the 5' end of *Abl* either downstream or upstream of the first alternative exon Ib (Melo 1996). Regardless of the precise location of the breakpoint, the primary hybrid transcript yields an mRNA in which *Bcr* sequences are fused to *Abl* exon a2 (Melo 1996). In a sharp contrast to *Abl* splicing, the breakpoints within *Bcr* localize to three breakpoint cluster regions (BCR). These breaks may occur in an area spanning 5.8 kb in the *Bcr* exons 12–16 (exons b1–b5) and is called the major breakpoint cluster region (*M-Bcr*). Because of this alternative splicing, fusion transcripts with either b2a2 or b3a2 junctions can be formed (Fig. 2.2). This chimeric mRNA is translated into a 210-kDa chimeric protein (p210BCR-ABL) in patients with

Ph⁺ CML and about one third of the patients with Ph⁺ acute lymphatic leukemia (ALL) (van Rhee et al. 1996). In the remaining Ph⁺ ALL patients (and a small number of patients with CML), the breakpoints are in the alternative *Bcr* exons e2′ and e2 (minor breakpoint cluster region, or *m-BCR*), and the *e1a2* fusion mRNA is translated into a 190-kDa protein kinase (p190BCR-ABL) responsible for the characteristic disease phenotype (Ravandi et al. 1999; van Rhee et al. 1996).

The fusion of BCR protein fragment to the ABL SH3 domain interferes with the physiological negative regulatory signals of ABL (Afar et al. 1994). The BCR-ABL fusion protein is a potent tyrosine kinase that may also undergo autophosphorylation resulting in higher affinity for the SH2 domains of interaction partners. A number of substrates are phosphorylated by BCR-ABL largely in a tissue-dependent manner. For example, CRKL is the major tyrosine-phosphorylated protein in neutrophils of CML patients, whereas phosphorylated p62-DOK is predominantly found in early hematopoietic progenitor cells (Clarkson et al. 1997; Oda et al. 1994). Other examples of BCR-ABL substrates are listed in Table 2.1.

ABL, and to a lesser extend BCR-ABL, are regulated by tyrosine phosphatases like PTP1B, Syp83, and Shp1. The PTP1B levels increase in a kinase-dependent manner, and in fibroblasts, the transforming effect of BCR-ABL is impaired by the overexpression of PTP1B. PTP1B recognizes p210BCR-ABL as a substrate, disrupts the formation of a p210BCR-ABL/Grb2 complex, and inhibits downstream signaling events (LaMontagne et al. 1998). Shp1, which interacts with ABL/BCR-ABL via SH2 domain, is a major inhibitory mediator of BCR-ABL. Shp1 levels are markedly decreased in blast crisis or advanced phase of CML due to posttranscriptional modifications (Amin et al. 2007).

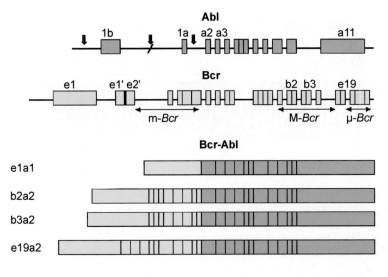

Fig. 2.2. BCR-ABL fusion proteins. Positions of the fusions between *Bcr* and *Abl*, and schematic depiction of the generated chimeric mRNA

Table 2.1. BCR-ABL substrates and their key functions

Substrate	Phosphorylated site	Description	Literature
Bap-1	–	14-3-3 protein	REUTHER ET AL. 1994
Cbl	–	Unknown	ANDONIOU ET AL. 1994
Caspase 9	Tyr-153	Apoptosis	RAINA ET AL. 2005
CD19	Tyr-508	BCR co-receptor	ZIPFEL ET AL. 2000
CrkL	–	Adapter protein	ODA ET AL. 1994
Crk	Tyr-221	Adapter protein	FELLER ET AL. 1994
DNA-PK	Not mapped	Protein kinase	KHARBANDA ET AL. 1997
Dok1	Tyr-361	Docking protein	WOODRING ET AL. 2004
Fak	–	Cytoskeleton/cell membrane	GOTOH ET AL. 1995
Fes	–	Myeloid differentiation	ERNST ET AL. 1994
Fe65	Tyr-547	Adapter protein	PERKINTON ET AL. 2004
GAP-associated proteins	–	Ras activation	DRUKER ET AL. 1992
Hdm2, Mdm2	Tyr-394	Cell cycle regulation	GOLDBERG ET AL. 2002
HPK1/p62DOK	Not mapped	Hematopoietic progenitor kinase	ITO ET AL. 2001
MEKK1, MAP3K1	Not mapped	Serine/threonine kinase	KHARBANDA ET AL. 2000B
Paxillin	–	Cytoskeleton/cell membrane	SALGIA ET AL. 1995B
PLCγ	Tyr-69/Tyr-74	Phospholipase	GOTOH ET AL. 1994A
PI3-K p85	–	Serine kinase	SKORSKI ET AL. 1995
PKD	Tyr-463	Protein kinase	STORZ ET AL. 2003
p73	–	Transcription activation	AGAMI ET AL. 1999
Rad9	Tyr-28	DNA damage repair	YOSHIDA ET AL. 2002
Rad51	Tyr-54	DNA damage repair	YUAN ET AL. 1998
Ras-GAP	–	Ras-GTPase	GOTOH ET AL. 1994B
RNA-Pol II	C terminus	RNA polymerase	BASKARAN ET AL. 1993
RAFT1, FRAP1	Not mapped	Rapamycin associated protein	KUMAR ET AL. 2000
Shc	–	Adapter	MATSUGUCHI ET AL. 1994
Syp		Cytoplasmic phosphatase	TAUCHI ET AL. 1994
Talin	–	Cytoskeleton/cell membrane	SALGIA ET AL. 1995A
hTERT	Not mapped	Telomerase reverse transcriptase	KHARBANDA ET AL. 2000A
p95-Vav	–	Hematopoietic differentiation	MATSUGUCHI ET AL. 1995

BCR-ABL plays the key role in CML pathogenesis, wherein the ABL kinase activity is deregulated (see above) and the fusion protein BCR-ABL is hyperautophosphorylated and active (Skorski et al. 1998). Thus, the activity of a number of downstream signal transduction pathways is altered, leading to a series of changes in the cell behavior, which include altered adhesion properties, degradation of inhibitory proteins, activation of mitogenic signaling, and inhibition of apoptosis (Bedi et al. 1994; Gordon et al. 1987). CML progenitor cells adhere only loosely to bone marrow stromal cells and extracellular matrix, thus, are less sensitive to stromal negative proliferative signals (Gordon et al. 1987). Depending on the specific extracellular environment, integrins initiate defined signaling events in cells (Lewis et al. 1996). In CML, an adhesion-inhibitory variant of β-integrin is expressed that is not found in normal progenitor cells (Verfaillie et al. 1997). Therefore, in CML cells, the expression of this abnormal integrin variant prevents inhibitory signaling and facilitates tumor cell proliferation. Adding to this vicious cycle, in the presence of active BCR-ABL the inhibitory endogenous proteins Abi-1 and Abi-2 are more rapidly degraded via proteasome-dependent pathway (Dai et al. 1998).

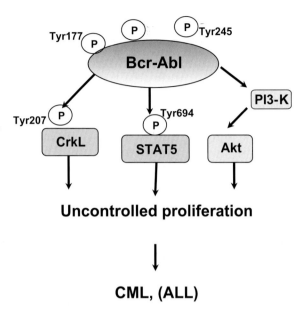

Fig. 2.3. Major signaling pathways activated by BCR-ABL. Multiple signaling pathways become activated by the constitutively active chimeric fusion oncoprotein. (See main text for further details)

2.5.1.2
Major Signal Transduction Pathways Activated by ABL/BCR-ABL

BCR-ABL undergoes uncontrolled autophosphorylation and activates downstream cell growth, proliferation, and anti-apoptotic pathways (Fig. 2.3; Table 2.1). CRK and CRKL are among the most prominent tyrosine-phosphorylated proteins in *BcrAbl*-transformed cells (ten Hoeve et al. 1994). The stromal cell-derived factor-1α (SDF-1α) is a potent chemoattractant for hematopoietic progenitor cells. Modulation of VLA-4-mediated CD34+ bone marrow cell adhesion by SDF-1α plays a key role in the migration of hematopoietic progenitor cells within and to the bone marrow. BCR-ABL markedly inhibits SDF-1α-mediated chemotactic response by a downregulation of the seven transmembrane-spanning SDF-1α receptor CXCR4 (Geay et al. 2005; Hidalgo et al. 2001). Activation of the Sapk/Jnk pathway by BCR-ABL is also required for malignant transformation (Kang et al. 2000). Constitutive phosphorylation of the STATs, particularly STAT5 activation, contributes to the clonal malignant transformation (Danial and Rothman 2000). Also, PI3-K is phosphorylated by BCR-ABL, leading to transactivation of the serine/threonine kinase AKT (Fig. 2.3) (Arslan et al. 2006; Burchert et al. 2005).

2.5.2
PI3-K/Akt Pathway

The phosphoinositol-3-kinase (PI3-K)/Akt signaling pathway is a major prosurvival pathway within the cell. Activated by a number of cellular stimuli and external signals, this pathway regulates key cellular functions such as proliferation, growth, transcription, translation, cell cycle, and apoptosis (Cantley 2002; Maddika et al. 2007a). Notably, PI3-K/Akt signaling is frequently disrupted in human cancers and plays a major role not only in tumor growth, but also in the response to cancer treatment (Vivanco and Sawyers 2002). PI3-K is a heterodimer composed of a catalytic subunit (p110) and a regulatory subunit (p85). The p85 subunit and the p85/p110 dimer can both repress or activate kinase activity of the complex, depending on its conformation. PI3-K may be activated by several mechanisms. The most common ones involve signals generated by receptor tyrosine kinase dimerization; alternatively, activation is achieved by intracellular nonreceptor tyrosine kinases. PI3-K converts the lipid phosphatidylinositol(4,5) P2 to phosphatidylinositol(3,4,5) (PIP3) P3. The serine/threonine kinases PDK1 (3'-phosphoinositide-dependent kinase 1) and AKT (PKB) are than recruited to PIP3 via their PH domains. Subsequently, AKT is activated by PDK1 through phosphorylation at Ser-473 and Thr-308 (CUEVAS et al. 2001; FRUMAN et al. 1998). PTEN (phosphatase and tensin homolog, also known as MMAC1, for *mutated in multiple advanced cancers*) negatively regulates the PI3-K/AKT pathway by dephosphorylating PIP3 to PIP2 (STAMBOLIC et al. 1998). PTEN is very frequently mutated in cancer (ALI et al. 1999). Activated AKT regulates numerous pathways and likely interacts with up to about 900 potential substrates in a cell, both in the cytoplasm and the nucleus. Here we discuss only selected AKT substrates that are involved in survival, cell cycle, and apoptosis.

2.5.2.1
Anti-Apoptotic Actions of AKT

AKT regulates cell survival by phosphorylating different substrates that directly or indirectly regulate the apoptotic program. The targets for AKT in this context involve the phosphorylation of BAD (a pro-apoptotic Bcl2 family member), caspase-9, IKK, FKHRL1 (a fork-head transcription factor), MDM2 (negative regulator of p53), and cyclic AMP response element-binding protein. When phosphorylated at Ser-136, BAD no longer efficiently interacts with anti-apoptotic Bcl2 family members such as Bcl-xL (DATTA et al. 1997). Phosphorylation of caspase-9 at Ser-196 causes the inhibition of its proteolytic activity (CARDONE et al. 1998). Phosphorylated fork-head transcription factor FKHRL1 can no longer support the transcription of its pro-apoptotic targets FasL, Bim, IGFBP1, and Puma (BRUNET et al. 1999; GUO et al. 1999; KOPS et al. 1999; YOU et al. 2006). On the other hand, AKT promotes cell survival by phosphorylating IKKα, leading to the activation of NF-κB, which in turn phosphorylates and triggers the degradation of IκB, an NF-κB inhibitor (KANE et al. 1999; ROMASHKOVA and MAKAROV 1999). This leads to further elevation in transcription of NF-κB-dependent survival genes (*Bcl-xL, Bcl2, c-FLIP, c-IAPs*) (CATZ and JOHNSON 2001; LEE et al. 1999). Furthermore, AKT-mediated phosphorylation of cyclic AMP-response-element-binding protein (CREB) enhances survival by increasing transcription of prosurvival genes like *Mcl-1, Bcl2*, and *Akt* itself (PUGAZHENTHI et al. 2000; REUSCH and KLEMM 2002). In addition, Akt phosphorylation of p53 enhances its degradation, promotes p53 nuclear localization and its binding to its inhibitor MDM2 (MAYO and DONNER 2001).

2.5.2.2
Role of PI3-K/Akt
Pathway in Cell Cycle Progression

The activity of PI3-K pathway occurs at two phases of the cell cycle, during the early G1 phase and in the late S phase (JONES et al. 1999; MADDIKA et al. 2007a). During G1–S phase transition, the PI3-K/Akt pathway phosphorylates multiple substrates including cyclin D, c-Myc, p27[Kip1], and p21[Waf1]. GSK3β, a kinase downstream in PI3-K/Akt pathway, phosphorylates cyclin D1 at Thr-286 (DIEHL et al. 1998) and c-Myc at Thr-58 (GREGORY et al. 2003), which direct them for degradation via the ubiquitin-dependent pathway. By phosphorylating and inactivating GSK3β, AKT prevents the degradation and cytoplasmic relocation of cyclin D1 and c-Myc, thus, facilitating G1–S transition. Another way for AKT to regulate G1–S transition is by affecting at the transcriptional and the posttranslational levels the presence of the cell cycle inhibitors p27[Kip1] and p21[Waf1]. AKT enhances degradation of p27 in a proteasome-dependent manner by upregulating *Skp2* mRNA levels, a key component of the SCF/SKP2 ubiquitin ligase that mediates p27 degradation in a cyclin E/CDK2-dependent phosphorylation (HARA et al. 2001; PAGANO et al. 1995). AKT-mediated phosphorylation of p27 at Thr-157 also causes the relocation of p27 to the cytoplasm. This relieves nuclear substrates like CDK1 from p27-mediated inhibition and enhances cell cycle progression (SHIN et al. 2002). Degradation of p27 is also regulated and dependent on AKT-mediated phosphorylation of its Thr-157 residue (MADDIKA and LOS, unpublished). AKT phosphorylates FKHRL1 and inhibits its transcriptional activity, which results in the downregulation of p27 transcription (MEDEMA et al. 2000). AKT also phosphorylates another cell cycle inhibitor, p21, at neighboring residues Thr-145 and Ser-146, promoting cell cycle progression. Phosphorylation of Thr-145 residue in p21 by AKT results in the cytoplasmic localization of p21 (ZHOU et al. 2001). Phosphorylation of p21 at Ser-146 enhances the stability of the protein and increases the assembly of cyclin D/CDK4 complexes, thus, supporting G1–S transition (LI et al. 2002b). Regulation of p21 at the transcription level by AKT also involves FKHRL1 (MADDIKA and LOS, unpublished). In addition, AKT plays the role in S/G2 transition by phosphorylation of CDK2 at Thr-39. This AKT-mediated phosphorylation event enhances cyclin A binding but is dispensable for CDK2 basal binding and kinase activity (MADDIKA et al. 2008b). Although the PI3-K/Akt pathway is mostly reported to be required for G1–S progression, there have been few studies suggesting a role for this pathway in G2–M progression (SHTIVELMAN et al. 2002). It was shown that AKT activation could overcome a G2–M cell cycle checkpoint induced by DNA damage (KANDEL et al. 2002). Though PI3-K/AKT activity might be important for G2–M progression, it must be transiently inactivated later for proper mitotic exit. The constitutive activation of this pathway leads to G2–M cell cycle arrest in an FKHRL1/cyclin B/PLK dependent manner (ALVAREZ et al. 2001).

2.5.2.3
Role of PI3-K/Akt
Pathway in Cell Death

Although the PI3-K/Akt pathway is a promoter of cell proliferation and cell survival, under defined conditions, the PI3-K/Akt pathway is also involved in promoting cell death. The activation of PI3-K/Akt has been observed in some experimental systems on induction of apoptosis by selected stimuli like CD95, cisplatin, arsenite, TNF, serum withdrawal, hypoxia (AKI et al. 2001, 2003; BAR et al. 2005; LEE et al. 2005; LU et al. 2006; NIMBALKAR et al. 2003; ONO et al. 2004; SHACK et al. 2003). Recent data also indicate that apoptin, a viral protein that selectively kills cancer cells, requires for its toxicity both PI3-K/Akt activation and the phosphorylation by CDK2 (MADDIKA et al. 2008a).

2.5.3
ErbB Pathway

Epidermal growth factor (EGF) promotes survival and stimulates growth and differentiation of epithelial cells. EGF receptor signaling is also involved in cardiac and neural development, glial cell development, and later stages of mammary gland development during pregnancy (YARDEN 2001). The EGF-like growth factor family includes heparin-binding EGF (HB-EGF), transforming growth factor-alpha (TGF-α), heregulin/neuregulins 1–4, betacellulin, cripto, epiregulin, epigen, and amphiregulin (BELL et al. 1986). EGF family ligands preferably bind to specific EGF receptors, named ErbB1 to -4, and induce homo- and heterodimerization and autophosphorylation. The tissue-specific expression pattern of the EGF-like ligands and ErbB1 to -4 determine the effects on cell growth and differentiation (MASSAGUE and PANDIELLA 1993). Enhanced tumor malignancy and shorter survival periods are positively correlated with the expression of EGF-like ligands and ErbB and are poor prognostic markers for a number of malignancies of epithelial origin (NORMANNO et al. 2006).

The ErbB family includes four closely related transmembrane tyrosine kinases: ErbB1/EGFR, ErbB2/HER2/neu, ErbB3/HER3, and ErbB4/HER4. On interaction with their ligands, ErbB receptors form either homo- or heterodimers that activate the receptor tyrosine kinases. EGF-like ligands interact with ErbB1, heregulin/neuregulin-like ligands interact with ErbB3 and ErbB4, and EGF, and neuregulin-like ligands interact with ErbB1 and ErbB4. ErbB2 has only been detected in heterodimer combinations, and ErbB3 possesses no endogenous autophosphorylation activity, thus, requires one of the other ErbB receptors for phosphorylation (MASSAGUE and PANDIELLA 1993).

Mice lacking EGF receptors developed defects in the epithelium of various organs. ErbB1 deficiency leads to embryonic or perinatal lethality with ErbB1$^{-/-}$ mice showing abnormalities in multiple organs. ErbB2 knockout mice die during midgestation, due to malformation of the heart. Similarly, ErbB3 knockout mice die due to defective valve formation in the heart as well as neural crest defects and lack of Schwann cell precursors (OLAYIOYE et al. 2000).

EGF receptors show homology with the v-*erbB* oncogene. Amplification or overexpression of ErbB2 is observed in breast and ovarian cancer, and correlates with poor clinical outcome. Abnormal ErbB2 activation is associated with drug resistance through the impairment of both the extrinsic and intrinsic apoptotic signaling pathways, and may promote micrometastatic bone marrow disease. Activating mutations within the ErbB tyrosine kinase domain also have transforming potential. Found in certain breast and ovarian cancers, a point mutation within the transmembrane region of the *ERBB2* gene facilitates dimerization in the absence of ligand (MENDELSOHN and BASELGA 2000). This induces ligand-independent autophosphorylation with constitutive receptor activation and autonomous prosurvival and proliferation-enhancing signal transduction.

2.6
Tumor Biology and Future Therapies

Therapeutic approaches based on targeting growth and survival signaling pathways have been established. Novel targeted cancer therapies aim at the correction (mostly inhibition) of signaling pathways, which are dysregulated in cancer. Tyrosine kinases are frequently deregulated in cancer cells, making them attractive therapeutic targets. Table 2.2 provides examples of anticancer agents aimed at targeted therapeutic intervention in cancer. The kinase inhibitor Gleevec® (Imatinib mesy-

Table 2.2. Anticancer drugs that target growth factor-mediated cell survival pathways

Target	Drug name	Drug type
ABL, BCR-ABL, KIT, PDGFR	Gleevec® (Imatinib)	Small-molecule tyrosine kinase inhibitor
CDK1, CDK2	Roscovitine (CYC202)	Small-molecule serine/threonine kinase inhibitor
ErbB2 (HER2/neu)	Trastuzumab (Herceptin®)	Monoclonal antibody
ErbB1 (EGFR; HER1)	Cetuximab (IMC-C225)	Monoclonal antibody
ErbB1 (EGFR; HER1)	ABX-EGF	Small-molecule tyrosine kinase inhibitor
ErbB1 (EGFR; HER1)	Iressa® (ZD1839)	Small-molecule tyrosine kinase inhibitor
ErbB1 (EGFR; HER1)	Tarceva® (CP358)	Small-molecule tyrosine kinase inhibitor
All ErbB receptors (pan-HER inhibitor)	CI-1033	Small-molecule tyrosine kinase inhibitor
HDAC	SAHA or Depsipeptide	Modified peptide
PDGFR	SU-101	Small-molecule tyrosine kinase inhibitor
PKC	UNC-01	Small-molecule kinase inhibitor
PKC-α	ISIS-321	Antisense oligonucleotide
VEGF, PDGFR	PTK787 or SU11248	Small-molecule kinase inhibitor

late, STI571) is an example of selective targeting of the constitutively active fusion oncoprotein BCR-ABL for the treatment of CML. The Gleevec® molecule occupies the active site of the ABL protein, thus, preventing ATP from binding. Without ATP as a phosphate donor, ABL is unable to phosphorylate its substrates (KANTARJIAN and TALPAZ 2001). Gleevec may also be used in cancers with hyper-activated platelet-derived growth factor receptor (PDGFR). Angiogenesis is essential for tumor growth and disrupting angiogenesis is an effective approach to reduce tumor mass, although complete cure is impossible with anti-angiogenic therapy alone. In a squamous cell carcinoma model, endostatin a natural anti-angiogenic protein that inhibits vascular endothelial growth factor (VEGF) was much more effective in combination with other chemotherapeutic drugs than was each of these components alone (LI et al. 2002a). PTK787 (vatalanib, VEGF inhibitor) is at the stage of clinical trials, while SU11248 (sunitinib malate, VEGF, and PDGF inhibitor) has been approved for treatment of metastatic kidney cancer. These drugs have anti-angiogenic effects because in many types of tumors VEGF and PDGF promote the development of new blood vessels. Since ErbB signaling is also involved in regulation of VEGF and angiogenesis, ErbB inhibitors such as Herceptin®, a monoclonal blocking antibody against ErbB2,

have anti-angiogenic and anti-proliferative properties (IZUMI et al. 2002). Competitive tyrosine kinase inhibitors for EGF receptors have been designed as experimental anticancer drugs. Quinazoline compounds competitively inhibit ATP-binding sites and are orally active, potent, and selective tyrosine kinase inhibitors. Breast cancer patients with ErbB2 overexpression have a poor prognosis and, therefore, tyrosine kinase inhibitors have been tested for the treatment of breast cancer. Kinase inhibitors ZD1839 and OSI-774 (EGFR specific) and the pan-Her inhibitor CI-1033, which inhibits all four ErbB receptors, have intensively been studied. Blockage of EGFR by ZD1839 (Gefitinib, Iressa®) prevents transactivation of ErbB2 and improves response rates to Herceptin® in the treatment of Herceptin®-resistant tumors. Phase I/II clinical studies showed partial responses for colon and renal cancer and stable disease in prostate, cervical, and head and neck cancers (NAHTA et al. 2003a). ZD1839 also has been shown to block the action of the EGF receptors in non-small cell lung cancer, where it has been tested in phase III studies. When used in combination with radiotherapy on human colorectal cancer xenograft models, ZD1839 showed significant tumor growth inhibition (WILLIAMS et al. 2002). Other tyrosine kinase inhibitors have been tested for inhibition of ErbB receptor kinases. CI-1033 irreversibly inhibits a catalytic site present in all ErbB1 to -4 receptors. Both CI-1033 and PD168393 are effective against the ErbB1 and ErbB2 receptors. Clinical trials with CI-1033 are being conducted on metastatic breast cancer patients resistant to Herceptin® therapy. PD153035, CP-358,774, and AG1478 also inhibit receptor tyrosine kinase activity and proliferation of tumor cells that highly express EGF receptors (MENDELSOHN 2001). SU-101 inhibits the kinase activity of the PDGF receptor and is in phase II of clinical trial, e.g., for the treatment of glioblastomas (GIBBS 2000).

Since PTEN phosphatase is among the most frequently inactivated proteins in cancer, the PI3-K/Akt pathway inhibitors have been investigated for cancer treatment. Most likely due to the versatility of the pathway, targeting of the PI3-K/Akt pathway has only been of very limited success. Wortmannin, a fungal metabolite, is a potent inhibitor of PI3-K. When administered to SCID mice harboring xenografts of human or murine mammary carcinoma cells or pancreatic carcinoma cells, wortmannin was able to reduce tumor sizes (WEST et al. 2002). However, wortmannin is unstable in aqueous solutions and more stable derivates need to be developed. STI571, an AKT inhibitor, caused transcriptional downregulation of the prosurvival proteins Bcl-2, and c-IAP when tested in vitro (WEST et al. 2002).

Attempts have been made to target CDKs in the course of cancer therapy. Compounds such as roscovitine/CYC202, flavopiridol, olomoucine, and SU9516 represent a group of very specific CDKs inhibitors, which are able to stop the cell cycle by inhibiting CDK1 and -2. Roscovitine, flavopiridol, and SU9516 all induce apoptosis. SU9516-mediated CDK2-inhibition leads to a decrease in Rb protein phosphorylation (GOLSTEYN 2005).

These targeted anticancer therapeutics serve as examples of approaches targeting signaling pathways in cancer for the development of novel therapeutics. A more comprehensive compilation of selected therapies portrayed both from an experimental and clinical point of view can be found in other chapters of this book.

References

Abelson HT, Rabstein LS (1970) Lymphosarcoma: virus-induced thymic-independent disease in mice. Cancer Res 30:2213–2222

Afar DE et al (1994) Genetic approaches to defining signaling by the CML-associated tyrosine kinase BCR-ABL. Cold Spring Harb Symp Quant Biol 59:589–594

Agami R et al (1999) Interaction of c-Abl and p73alpha and their collaboration to induce apoptosis. Nature 399:809–813

Aki T et al (2001) Phosphoinositide 3-kinase accelerates necrotic cell death during hypoxia. Biochem J 358:481–487

Aki T et al (2003) Phosphoinositide 3-kinase accelerates autophagic cell death during glucose deprivation in the rat cardiomyocyte-derived cell line H9c2. Oncogene 22:8529–8535

Aleem E et al (2005) Cdc2-cyclin E complexes regulate the G1/S phase transition. Nat Cell Biol 7:831–836

Alexandropoulos K et al (1995) Proline-rich sequences that bind to Src homology 3 domains with individual specificities. Proc Natl Acad Sci USA 92:3110–3114

Ali IU et al (1999) Mutational spectra of PTEN/MMAC1 gene: a tumor suppressor with lipid phosphatase activity. J Natl Cancer Inst 91:1922–1932

Alvarez B et al (2001) Forkhead transcription factors contribute to execution of the mitotic programme in mammals. Nature 413:744–747

Amin HM et al (2007) Decreased expression level of SH2 domain-containing protein tyrosine phosphatase-1 (Shp1) is associated with progression of chronic myeloid leukemia. J Pathol 212:402–410

Andoniou CE et al (1994) Tumour induction by activated *abl* involves tyrosine phosphorylation of the product of the *cbl* oncogene. EMBO J 13:4515–4523

Arslan MA et al (2006) Protein kinases as drug targets in cancer. Curr Cancer Drug Targets 6:623–634

Baltimore D et al (1995) A nuclear tyrosine kinase becomes a cytoplasmic oncogene. Ann N Y Acad Sci 758:339–344

Bar J et al (2005) The PI3K inhibitor LY294002 prevents p53 induction by DNA damage and attenuates chemotherapy-induced apoptosis. Cell Death Differ 12:1578–1587

Bartram CR et al (1983) Translocation of c-abl oncogene correlates with the presence of a Philadelphia chromosome in chronic myelocytic leukaemia. Nature 306:277–280

Baskaran R et al (1993) Tyrosine phosphorylation of mammalian RNA polymerase II carboxyl-terminal domain. Proc Natl Acad Sci USA 90:11167–11171

Bedi A et al (1994) Inhibition of apoptosis by BCR-ABL in chronic myeloid leukemia. Blood 83:2038–2044

Bell GI et al (1986) Human epidermal growth factor precursor: cDNA sequence, expression in vitro and gene organization. Nucleic Acids Res 14:8427–8446

Berthet C et al (2003) Cdk2 knockout mice are viable. Curr Biol 13:1775–1785

Borgne A and Golsteyn RM (2003) The role of cyclin-dependent kinases in apoptosis. Prog Cell Cycle Res 5:453–459

Boyer LA et al (2005) Core transcriptional regulatory circuitry in human embryonic stem cells. Cell 122:947–956

Brazelton TR et al (2000) From marrow to brain: expression of neuronal phenotypes in adult mice. Science 290:1775–1779

Brunet A et al (1999) Akt promotes cell survival by phosphorylating and inhibiting a forkhead transcription factor. Cell 96:857–868

Burchert A et al (2005) Compensatory PI3-kinase/Akt/mTor activation regulates imatinib resistance development. Leukemia 19:1774–1782

Burke L et al (2005) Prognostic implications of molecular and immunohistochemical profiles of the Rb and p53 cell cycle regulatory pathways in primary non-small cell lung carcinoma. Clin Cancer Res 11:232–241

Cantley LC (2002) The phosphoinositide 3-kinase pathway. Science 296:1655–1657

Cardone MH et al (1998) Regulation of cell death protease caspase-9 by phosphorylation. Science 282:1318–1321

Catz SD, Johnson JL (2001) Transcriptional regulation of bcl-2 by nuclear factor kappa B and its significance in prostate cancer. Oncogene 20:7342–7351

Chambers I et al (2003) Functional expression cloning of Nanog, a pluripotency sustaining factor in embryonic stem cells. Cell 113:643–655

Cicchetti P et al (1992) Identification of a protein that binds to the SH3 region of Abl and is similar to Bcr and GAP-rho. Science 257:803–806

Clarkson BD et al (1997) New understanding of the pathogenesis of CML: a prototype of early neoplasia. Leukemia 11:1404–1428

Collins I, Garrett MD (2005) Targeting the cell division cycle in cancer: CDK and cell cycle checkpoint kinase inhibitors. Curr Opin Pharmacol 5:366–373

Coqueret O (2003) New targets for viral cyclins. Cell Cycle 2:293–295

Cuevas BD et al (2001) Tyrosine phosphorylation of p85 relieves its inhibitory activity on phosphatidylinositol 3-kinase. J Biol Chem 276:27455–27461

D'Ippolito G et al (2004) Marrow-isolated adult multilineage inducible (MIAMI) cells, a unique population of postnatal young and old human cells with extensive expansion and differentiation potential. J Cell Sci 117:2971–2981

Dai Z et al (1998) Oncogenic Abl and Src tyrosine kinases elicit the ubiquitin-dependent degradation of target proteins through a Ras-independent pathway. Genes Dev 12:1415–1424

Danial NN, Rothman P (2000) JAK-STAT signaling activated by Abl oncogenes. Oncogene 19:2523–2531

Darzynkiewicz Z et al (1997) Cytometry in cell necrobiology: analysis of apoptosis and accidental cell death (necrosis). Cytometry 27:1–20

Datta SR et al (1997) Akt phosphorylation of BAD couples survival signals to the cell-intrinsic death machinery. Cell 91:231–241

Diehl JA et al (1998) Glycogen synthase kinase-3beta regulates cyclin D1 proteolysis and subcellular localization. Genes Dev 12:3499–3511

Druker B et al (1992) Tyrosine phosphorylation of rasGAP and associated proteins in chronic myelogenous leukemia cell lines. Blood 79:2215–2220

Ernst TJ et al (1994) p210Bcr/Abl and p160v-Abl induce an increase in the tyrosine phosphorylation of p93c-Fes. J Biol Chem 269:5764–5769

Feller SM et al (1994) SH2 and SH3 domains as molecular adhesives: the interactions of Crk and Abl. Trends Biochem Sci 19:453–458

Ferrari G et al (1998) Muscle regeneration by bone marrow-derived myogenic progenitors. Science 279:1528–1530

Finlan LE and Hupp TR (2005) The life cycle of p53: a key target in drug development. In: Los M, Gibson SB (eds) Apoptotic pathways as target for novel therapies in cancer and other diseases. Springer, Berlin Heidelberg New York

Fruman DA et al (1998) Phosphoinositide kinases. Annu Rev Biochem 67:481–507

Geay JF et al (2005) p210BCR-ABL inhibits SDF-1 chemotactic response via alteration of CXCR4 signaling and down-regulation of CXCR4 expression. Cancer Res 65:2676–2683

Gibbs JB (2000) Anticancer drug targets: growth factors and growth factor signaling. J Clin Invest 105:9–13

Giono LE, Manfredi JJ (2006) The p53 tumor suppressor participates in multiple cell cycle checkpoints. J Cell Physiol 209:13–20

Goga A et al (1993) Oncogenic activation of c-ABL by mutation within its last exon. Mol Cell Biol 13:4967–4975

Goldberg Z et al (2002) Tyrosine phosphorylation of Mdm2 by c-Abl: implications for p53 regulation. EMBO J 21:3715–3727

Golsteyn RM (2005) Cdk1 and Cdk2 complexes (cyclin dependent kinases) in apoptosis: a role beyond the cell cycle. Cancer Lett 217:129–138

Gordon MY et al (1987) Altered adhesive interactions with marrow stroma of haematopoietic progenitor cells in chronic myeloid leukemia. Nature 328:342–344

Gotoh A et al (1994a) Potential molecules implicated in downstream signaling pathways of p185BCR-ABL in Ph+ ALL involve GTPase-activating protein, phospholipase C-gamma 1, and phosphatidylinositol 3⊠-kinase. Leukemia 8:115–120

Gotoh N et al (1994b) Epidermal growth factor-receptor mutant lacking the autophosphorylation sites induces phosphorylation of Shc protein and Shc-Grb2/ASH association and retains mitogenic activity. Proc Natl Acad Sci USA 91:167–171

Gotoh A et al (1995) Tyrosine phosphorylation and activation of focal adhesion kinase (p125FAK) by BCR-ABL oncoprotein. Exp Hematol 23:1153–1159

Gray N et al (1999) ATP-site directed inhibitors of cyclin-dependent kinases. Curr Med Chem 6:859–875

Gregory MA et al (2003) Phosphorylation by glycogen synthase kinase-3 controls c-myc proteolysis and subnuclear localization. J Biol Chem 278:51606–51612

Guo S et al (1999) Phosphorylation of serine 256 by protein kinase B disrupts transactivation by FKHR and mediates effects of insulin on insulin-like growth factor-binding protein-1 promoter activity through a conserved insulin response sequence. J Biol Chem 274:17184–17192

Gussoni E et al (1999) Dystrophin expression in the mdx mouse restored by stem cell transplantation. Nature 401:390–394

Hakem A et al (1999) The cyclin-dependent kinase Cdk2 regulates thymocyte apoptosis. J Exp Med 189:957–968

Hara T et al (2001) Degradation of p27(Kip1) at the G_0–G_1 transition mediated by a Skp2-independent ubiquitination pathway. J Biol Chem 276:48937–48943

Heisterkamp N et al (1988) The first *BCR* gene intron contains breakpoints in Philadelphia chromosome positive leukemia. Nucleic Acids Res 16:10069–10081

Hidalgo A et al (2001) Chemokine stromal cell-derived factor-1alpha modulates VLA-4 integrin-dependent adhesion to fibronectin and VCAM-1 on bone marrow hematopoietic progenitor cells. Exp Hematol 29:345–355

Hoeve J ten et al (1994) Cellular interactions of CRKL, and SH2-SH3 adaptor protein. Cancer Res 54:2563–2567

Holmberg C et al (1998) E2F-1-induced p53-independent apoptosis in transgenic mice. Oncogene 17:143–155

Hombach-Klonisch S et al (2008) Cancer stem cells as targets for cancer therapy: selected cancers as examples. Arch Immunol Ther Exp 56:165–180

Hsieh JK et al (2002) Novel function of the cyclin A binding site of E2F in regulating p53-induced apoptosis in response to DNA damage. Mol Cell Biol 22:78–93

Ito Y et al (2001) Interaction of hematopoietic progenitor kinase 1 and c-Abl tyrosine kinase in response to genotoxic stress. J Biol Chem 276:18130–18138

Izumi Y et al (2002) Tumour biology: herceptin acts as an anti-angiogenic cocktail. Nature 416:279–280

Jackson JG, Pereira-Smith OM (2006) Primary and compensatory roles for RB family members at cell cycle gene promoters that are deacetylated and downregulated in doxorubicin-induced senescence of breast cancer cells. Mol Cell Biol 26:2501–2510

Jackson KA et al (2001) Regeneration of ischemic cardiac muscle and vascular endothelium by adult stem cells. J Clin Invest 107:1395–1402

Jackson KA et al (1999) Hematopoietic potential of stem cells isolated from murine skeletal muscle. Proc Natl Acad Sci USA 96:14482–14486

Jiang Y et al (2002) Pluripotency of mesenchymal stem cells derived from adult marrow. Nature 418:41–49

Johnson DG, Walker CL (1999) Cyclins and cell cycle checkpoints. Annu Rev Pharmacol Toxicol 39:295–312

Jong J de, Looijenga LH (2006) Stem cell marker OCT3/4 in tumor biology and germ cell tumor diagnostics: history and future. Crit Rev Oncog 12:171–203

Jones SM et al (1999) PDGF induces an early and a late wave of PI 3-kinase activity, and only the late wave is required for progression through G1. Curr Biol 9:512–521

Kaldis P, Aleem E (2005) Cell cycle sibling rivalry: Cdc2 vs. Cdk2. Cell Cycle 4:1491–1494

Kandel ES et al (2002) Activation of Akt/protein kinase B overcomes a G_2/M cell cycle checkpoint induced by DNA damage. Mol Cell Biol 22:7831–7841

Kane LP et al (1999) Induction of NF-κB by the Akt/PKB kinase. Curr Biol 9:601–604

Kang CD et al (2000) The inhibition of ERK/MAPK not the activation of JNK/SAPK is primarily required to induce apoptosis in chronic myelogenous leukemic K562 cells. Leuk Res 24:527–534

Kantarjian HM, Talpaz M (2001) Imatinib mesylate: clinical results in Philadelphia chromosome-positive leukemias. Semin Oncol 28:9–18

Kharbanda S et al (1997) Functional interaction between DNA-PK and c-Abl in response to DNA damage. Nature 386:732–735

Kharbanda S et al (2000a) Regulation of the hTERT telomerase catalytic subunit by the c-Abl tyrosine kinase. Curr Biol 10:568–575

Kharbanda S et al (2000b) Activation of MEK kinase 1 by the c-Abl protein tyrosine kinase in response to DNA damage. Mol Cell Biol 20:4979–4989

Khosravi-Far R, Esposti MD (2004) Death receptor signals to mitochondria. Cancer Biol Ther 3:1051–1057

Kim R et al (2006) Role of mitochondria as the gardens of cell death. Cancer Chemother Pharmacol 57:545–553

Kipreos ET, Wang JY (1990) Differential phosphorylation of c-Abl in cell cycle determined by cdc2 kinase and phosphatase activity. Science 248:217–220

Knudsen ES, Knudsen KE (2006) Retinoblastoma tumor suppressor: where cancer meets the cell cycle. Exp Biol Med (Maywood) 231:1271–1281

Kogler G et al (2004) A new human somatic stem cell from placental cord blood with intrinsic pluripotent differentiation potential. J Exp Med 200:123–135

Kopen GC et al (1999) Marrow stromal cells migrate throughout forebrain and cerebellum, and they differentiate into astrocytes after injection into neonatal mouse brains. Proc Natl Acad Sci USA 96:10711–10716

Kops GJ et al (1999) Direct control of the Forkhead transcription factor AFX by protein kinase B. Nature 398:630–634

Krause DS et al (2001) Multi-organ, multi-lineage engraftment by a single bone marrow-derived stem cell. Cell 105:369–377

Kumar V et al (2000) Functional interaction between RAFT1/FRAP/mTOR and protein kinase Cδ in the regulation of cap-dependent initiation of translation. EMBO J 19:1087–1097

Lagasse E et al (2000) Purified hematopoietic stem cells can differentiate into hepatocytes in vivo. Nat Med 6:1229–1234

LaMontagne KR Jr et al (1998) Protein tyrosine phosphatase 1B antagonizes signalling by oncoprotein tyrosine kinase p210 bcr-abl in vivo. Mol Cell Biol 18:2965–2975

Laneuville P (1995) Abl tyrosine protein kinase. Semin Immunol 7:255–266

Lee HH et al (1999) NF-κB-mediated up-regulation of Bcl-x and Bfl-1/A1 is required for CD40 survival signaling in B lymphocytes. Proc Natl Acad Sci USA 96:9136–9141

Lee SB et al (2005) Serum withdrawal kills U937 cells by inducing a positive mutual interaction between reactive oxygen species and phosphoinositide 3-kinase. Cell Signal 17:197–204

Lee WH et al (1987) Human retinoblastoma susceptibility gene: cloning, identification, and sequence. Science 235:1394–1399

Lewis JM et al (1996) Integrin regulation of c-Abl tyrosine kinase activity and cytoplasmic-nuclear transport. Proc Natl Acad Sci USA 93:15174–15179

Li M et al (2002a) Enhanced antiangiogenic therapy of squamous cell carcinoma by combined endostatin and epidermal growth factor receptor-antisense therapy. Clin Cancer Res 8:3570–3578

Li Y et al (2002b) AKT/PKB phosphorylation of p21Cip/WAF1 enhances protein stability of p21Cip/WAF1 and promotes cell survival. J Biol Chem 277:11352–11361

Lin Y et al (2000) Origins of circulating endothelial cells and endothelial outgrowth from blood. J Clin Invest 105:71–77

Los M, Gibson S (2005) Apoptotic pathways as target for novel therapies of cancer and other diseases. Springer, Berlin Heidelberg New York

Los M et al (1999) The role of caspases in development, immunity, and apoptotic signal transduction: lessons from knockout mice. Immunity 10:629–639

Lu B et al (2006) Phosphatidylinositol 3-kinase/Akt positively regulates Fas (CD95)-mediated apoptosis in epidermal Cl41 cells. J Immunol 176:6785–6793

Maddika S et al (2007a) Cell survival, cell death and cell cycle pathways are interconnected: implications for cancer therapy. Drug Resist Updat 10:13–29

Maddika S et al (2007b) Akt is transferred to the nucleus of cells treated with apoptin, and it participates in apoptin-induced cell death. Cell Prolif 40:835–848

Maddika S et al (2008a) Interaction with PI3-kinase contributes to the cytotoxic activity of apoptin. Oncogene 27:3060–3065

Maddika S et al (2008b) Akt-mediated phosphorylation of CDK2 regulates its dual role in cell cycle progression and apoptosis. J Cell Sci 121:979–988

Maehara K et al (2005) Reduction of total E2F/DP activity induces senescence-like cell cycle arrest in cancer cells lacking functional pRB and p53. J Cell Biol 168:553–560

Massague J, Pandiella A (1993) Membrane-anchored growth factors. Annu Rev Biochem 62:515–541

Mathew P et al (2004) Combination docetaxel and platelet-derived growth factor receptor inhibition with imatinib mesylate in prostate cancer. Semin Oncol 31:24–29

Matsuguchi T et al (1994) Shc phosphorylation in myeloid cells is regulated by granulocyte macrophage colony-stimulating factor, interleukin-3, and steel factor and is constitutively increased by p210BCR/ABL. J Biol Chem 269:5016–5021

Matsuguchi T et al (1995) Tyrosine phosphorylation of p95Vav in myeloid cells is regulated by GM-CSF, IL-3 and steel factor and is constitutively increased by p210BCR/ABL. EMBO J 14:257–265

Mayo LD, Donner DB (2001) A phosphatidylinositol 3-kinase/Akt pathway promotes translocation of Mdm2 from the cytoplasm to the nucleus. Proc Natl Acad Sci USA 98:11598–11603

McWhirter JR, Wang JY (1993) An actin-binding function contributes to transformation by the Bcr-Abl oncoprotein of Philadelphia chromosome-positive human leukemias. EMBO J 12:1533–1546

Medema RH et al (2000) AFX-like Forkhead transcription factors mediate cell-cycle regulation by Ras and PKB through p27kip1. Nature 404:782–787

Melo JV (1996) The diversity of BCR-ABL fusion proteins and their relationship to leukemia phenotype. Blood 88:2375–2384

Mendelsohn J (2001) The epidermal growth factor receptor as a target for cancer therapy. Endocr Relat Cancer 8:3–9

Mendelsohn J, Baselga J (2000) The EGF receptor family as targets for cancer therapy. Oncogene 19:6550–6565

Mezey E et al (2000) Turning blood into brain: cells bearing neuronal antigens generated in vivo from bone marrow. Science 290:1779–1782

Nahta R et al (2003a) Growth factor receptors in breast cancer: potential for therapeutic intervention. Oncologist 8:5–17

Nahta R et al (2003b) Signal transduction inhibitors in the treatment of breast cancer. Curr Med Chem Anticancer Agents 3:201–216

Nichols J et al (1998) Formation of pluripotent stem cells in the mammalian embryo depends on the POU transcription factor Oct4. Cell 95:379–391

Nimbalkar D et al (2003) Cytokine activation of phosphoinositide 3-kinase sensitizes hematopoietic cells to cisplatin-induced death. Cancer Res 63:1034–1039

Normanno N et al (2006) Epidermal growth factor receptor (EGFR) signaling in cancer. Gene 366:2–16

Oda T et al (1994) Crkl is the major tyrosine-phosphorylated protein in neutrophils from patients with chronic myelogenous leukemia. J Biol Chem 269:22925–22928

Olayioye MA et al (2000) The ErbB signaling network: receptor heterodimerization in development and cancer. EMBO J 19:3159–3167

Ono K et al (2004) Contribution of caveolin-1α- and Akt to TNF-α-induced cell death. Am J Physiol 287:L201–L209

Orlic D et al (2001) Mobilized bone marrow cells repair the infarcted heart, improving function and survival. Proc Natl Acad Sci USA 98:10344–10349

Ortega S et al (2003) Cyclin-dependent kinase 2 is essential for meiosis but not for mitotic cell division in mice. Nat Genet 35:25–31

Pagano M et al (1995) Role of the ubiquitin-proteasome pathway in regulating abundance of the cyclin-dependent kinase inhibitor p27. Science 269:682–685

Pang W (2000) Role of muscle-derived cells in hematopoietic reconstitution of irradiated mice. Blood 95:1106–1108

Park MT, Lee SJ (2003) Cell cycle and cancer. J Biochem Mol Biol 23:60–65

Perkinton MS et al (2004) The c-Abl tyrosine kinase phosphorylates the Fe65 adaptor protein to stimulate Fe65/amyloid precursor protein nuclear signaling. J Biol Chem 279:22084–22091

Petersen BE et al (1999) Bone marrow as a potential source of hepatic oval cells. Science 284:1168–1170

Priller J et al (2001) Neogenesis of cerebellar Purkinje neurons from gene-marked bone marrow cells in vivo. J Cell Biol 155:733–738

Pugazhenthi S et al (2000) Akt/protein kinase B up-regulates Bcl-2 expression through cAMP-response element-binding protein. J Biol Chem 275:10761–10766

Raina D et al (2005) c-Abl tyrosine kinase regulates caspase-9 autocleavage in the apoptotic response to DNA damage. J Biol Chem 280:11147–11151

Ravandi F et al (1999) Chronic myelogenous leukaemia with p185(BCR/ABL) expression: characteristics and clinical significance. Br J Haematol 107:581–586

Reusch JE, Klemm DJ (2002) Inhibition of cAMP-response element-binding protein activity decreases protein kinase B/Akt expression in 3T3-L1 adipocytes and induces apoptosis. J Biol Chem 277:1426–1432

Reuther GW et al (1994) Association of the protein kinases c-Bcr and Bcr-Abl with proteins of the 14-3-3 family. Science 266:129–133

Reyes M et al (2001) Purification and ex vivo expansion of postnatal human marrow mesodermal progenitor cells. Blood 98:2615–2625

Rhee J et al (2007) Cables links Robo-bound Abl kinase to N-cadherin-bound β-catenin to mediate Slit-induced modulation of adhesion and transcription. Nat Cell Biol 9:883–892

Rhee F van et al (1996) p190 BCR-ABL mRNA is expressed at low levels in p210-positive chronic myeloid and acute lymphoblastic leukemias. Blood 87:5213–5217

Romashkova JA, Makarov SS (1999) NF-κB is a target of AKT in anti-apoptotic PDGF signalling. Nature 401:86–90

Rowinsky EK (2005) Targeted induction of apoptosis in cancer management: the emerging role of tumor necrosis factor-related apoptosis-inducing ligand receptor activating agents. J Clin Oncol 23:9394–9405

Salgia R et al (1995a) Increased tyrosine phosphorylation of focal adhesion proteins in myeloid cell lines expressing p210BCR/ABL. Oncogene 11:1149–1155

Salgia R et al (1995b) Molecular cloning of human paxillin, a focal adhesion protein phosphorylated by P210BCR/ABL. J Biol Chem 270:5039–5047

Schafer KA (1998) The cell cycle: a review. Vet Pathol 35:461–478

Schwartz GK, Shah MA (2005) Targeting the cell cycle: a new approach to cancer therapy. J Clin Oncol 23:9408–9421

Shack S et al (2003) Caveolin-induced activation of the phosphatidylinositol 3-kinase/Akt pathway increases arsenite cytotoxicity. Mol Cell Biol 23:2407–2414

Shi Y et al (1995) Abl-interactor-1, a novel SH3 protein binding to the carboxy-terminal portion of the Abl protein, suppresses v-abl transforming activity. Genes Dev 9:2583–2597

Shi L et al (1996) Granzyme B induces apoptosis and cyclin A-associated cyclin-dependent kinase activity in all stages of the cell cycle. J Immunol 157:2381–2385

Shimizu T et al (1995) Unscheduled activation of cyclin B1/Cdc2 kinase in human promyelocytic leukemia cell line HL60 cells undergoing apoptosis induced by DNA damage. Cancer Res 55:228–231

Shin I et al (2002) PKB/Akt mediates cell-cycle progression by phosphorylation of p27(Kip1) at threonine 157 and modulation of its cellular localization. Nat Med 8:1145–1152

Shtivelman E et al (2002) A role for PI 3-kinase and PKB activity in the G2/M phase of the cell cycle. Curr Biol 12:919–924

Siegel RM (2006) Caspases at the crossroads of immune-cell life and death. Nat Rev Immunol 6:308–317

Skorski T et al (1995) Phosphatidylinositol-3 kinase activity is regulated by BCR/ABL and is required for the growth of Philadelphia chromosome-positive cells. Blood 86:726–736

Skorski T et al (1998) The SH3 domain contributes to BCR/ABL-dependent leukemogenesis in vivo: role in adhesion, invasion, and homing. Blood 91:406–418

Stambolic V et al (1998) Negative regulation of PKB/Akt-dependent cell survival by the tumor suppressor PTEN. Cell 95:29–39

Storz P et al (2003) Tyrosine phosphorylation of protein kinase D in the pleckstrin homology domain leads to activation. J Biol Chem 278:17969–17976

Tauchi T et al (1994) SH2-containing phosphotyrosine phosphatase Syp is a target of p210bcr-abl tyrosine kinase. J Biol Chem 269:15381–15387

Van Etten RA (1999) Cycling, stressed-out and nervous: cellular functions of c-Abl. Trends Cell Biol 9:179–186

Van Etten RA et al (1989) The mouse type IV c-abl gene product is a nuclear protein, and activation of transforming ability is associated with cytoplasmic localization. Cell 58:669–678

Vassilev LT et al (2006) Selective small-molecule inhibitor reveals critical mitotic functions of human CDK1. Proc Natl Acad Sci USA 103:10660–10665

Verfaillie CM et al (1997) Integrin-mediated regulation of hematopoiesis: do BCR/ABL-induced defects in integrin function underlie the abnormal circulation and proliferation of CML progenitors? Acta Haematol 97:40–52

Vermeulen K et al (2003) The cell cycle: a review of regulation, deregulation and therapeutic targets in cancer. Cell Prolif 36:131–149

Vivanco I, Sawyers CL (2002) The phosphatidylinositol 3-Kinase AKT pathway in human cancer. Nat Rev Cancer 2:489–501

Wagers AJ, Weissman IL (2004) Plasticity of adult stem cells. Cell 116:639–648

Wen ST, van Etten RA (1997) The *PAG* gene product, a stress-induced protein with antioxidant properties, is an Abl SH3-binding protein and a physiological inhibitor of c-Abl tyrosine kinase activity. Genes Dev 11:2456–2467

West KA et al (2002) Activation of the PI3K/Akt pathway and chemotherapeutic resistance. Drug Resist Updat 5:234–248

Williams KJ et al (2002) ZD1839 ("Iressa"), a specific oral epidermal growth factor receptor-tyrosine kinase inhibitor, potentiates radiotherapy in a human colorectal cancer xenograft model. Br J Cancer 86:1157–1161

Woodring PJ et al (2004) c-Abl phosphorylates Dok1 to promote filopodia during cell spreading. J Cell Biol 165:493–503

Yarden Y (2001) The EGFR family and its ligands in human cancer: signalling mechanisms and therapeutic opportunities. Eur J Cancer 37:S3–S8

Yoon YS et al (2005) Clonally expanded novel multipotent stem cells from human bone marrow regenerate myocardium after myocardial infarction. J Clin Invest 115:326–338

Yoshida K et al (2002) c-Abl tyrosine kinase regulates the human Rad9 checkpoint protein in response to DNA damage. Mol Cell Biol 22:3292–3300

You H et al (2006) FOXO3a-dependent regulation of Puma in response to cytokine/growth factor withdrawal. J Exp Medicine 203:1657–1663

Yuan ZM et al (1998) Regulation of Rad51 function by c-Abl in response to DNA damage. J Biol Chem 273:3799–3802

Zhou BP et al (2001) Cytoplasmic localization of p21Cip1/WAF1 by Akt-induced phosphorylation in HER-2/neu-overexpressing cells. Nat Cell Biol 3:245–252

Zipfel PA et al (2000) The c-Abl tyrosine kinase is regulated downstream of the B cell antigen receptor and interacts with CD19. J Immunol 165:6872–6879

Zukerberg LR et al (2000) Cables links Cdk5 and c-Abl and facilitates Cdk5 tyrosine phosphorylation, kinase upregulation, and neurite outgrowth. Neuron 26:633–646

Tumor Angiogenesis

Vesile Schneider, Hans Christian Rischke, and Joachim Drevs

CONTENTS

V. Schneider, MD
Tumorklinik SanaFontis, Alpine GmbH, An den Heilquellen 2, 79111, Freiburg, Germany

H. C. Rischke, MD
Diagnostische Radiologie und PET/CT-Zentrum, Tumorklinik SanaFontis, Alpine GmbH, An den Heilquellen 2, 79111 Freiburg, Germany

J. Drevs, MD
Chefarzt und Ärztliche Direktion, Tumorklinik SanaFontis, Alpine GmbH, An den Heilquellen 2, 79111 Freiburg, Germany

KEY POINTS

- To grow over a certain size of a few millimeters in diameter, solid tumors need a blood supply from surrounding vessels.
- Small tumors can stay dormant for a very long time period until the so-called angiogenic switch occurs.
- Tumor-induced angiogenesis is mainly sustained by the production and secretion of angiogenic factors originating from tumor and stroma cells.
- The VEGF family of growth factors and the receptor tyrosine kinases play a key role in tumor angiogenesis and targeted therapy strategies.
- High VEGF expression promotes vascular permeability, leading to high interstitial and intratumoral pressure.
- The chaotic layout of tumor vasculature leads to inconsistent oxygen delivery within the tumor and creates regions of hypoxia.
- It is assumed that antiangiogenic drugs 'normalize' the tumor vasculature.
- Inhibiting tumor angiogenesis is a rational and potentially valuable therapeutic strategy.
- The available preclinical and clinical data strongly support the introduction of antiangiogenic drugs into combined modality treatment regimens that include radiation therapy.

Abstract

Since the first description of angiogenesis and the discovery of its crucial role in tumor growth, extensive efforts have been made to develop antiangiogenic drugs. Some targeted therapies have been established as the first-line therapy in certain tumor types. However, the pathophysiological principles are not fully understood, and little is known about the interaction of antiangiogenic drugs in combination with other classical antitumoral therapies like chemotherapy or radiation. A combination of all three strategies represents a very powerful tool to treat cancer aggressively, but also increases the risk of side effects. To understand the rationale of these combinational therapies, it is critically important to understand the angionesis and pathophysiology of antiangiogenic drugs on the one hand and the effects of radiation and chemotherapy on the other.

A correlation between malignant tumors and surrounding blood vessels was first described at the annual meeting of Internal Medicine in 1908 by Elia Metschnikoff, a Russian clinician and noble prize winner. In 1971, the hypothesis that tumor growth was angiogenesis-dependent was raised by JUDAH FOLKMAN (1971): To grow over a certain size of a few millimeters in diameter, solid tumors need a blood supply from surrounding vessels.

Solid tumors of up to 2–3 mm³ can grow without a blood vessel supply. Nutrition and oxygen are provided via diffusion from the surrounding tissue. Above this size, diffusion becomes insufficient due to the negative surface/volume ratio. Based on a good balance between angiogenic and anti-angiogenic growth factors, a tumor of this size can stay dormant for a very long time period

until the so-called angiogenic switch occurs. Based on several possible stimuli, a misbalance between angiogenic and anti-angiogenic factors in favor of pro-angiogenic factors leads to the proliferation of new blood vessels that originate from the existing vascular system. These blood vessels grow into the tumor and thus provide the necessary nutrients and growth factors for tumor progression. At the same time, the newly formed blood vessels allow tumor cells to disseminate and form metastases in distant organs (Fig. 3.1). Normally, vascular homeostasis is regulated by a balance of angiogenic and antiangiogenic mechanisms. Tumor-induced angiogenesis is mainly sustained by the production and secretion of angiogenic factors originating from tumor and stroma cells.

3.2
VEGF and Tumor Growth

The VEGF family of growth factors and the receptor tyrosine kinases play a key role in tumor angiogenesis and targeted therapy strategies. The VEGF family includes VEGF-A, VEGF-B, VEGF-C, VEGF-D, and placental growth factor (PlGF), and they bind with different affinity and signaling response to VEGF receptors 1 (VEGFR-1), VEGF receptor 2 (VEGFR-2), and VEGF-receptor 3 (VEGFR-3) (Fig. 3.2).

VEGF promotes the growth of tumor vasculature to allow oxygen and nutrients to reach the rapidly dividing cancer cells. However, this tumor vasculature is abnor-

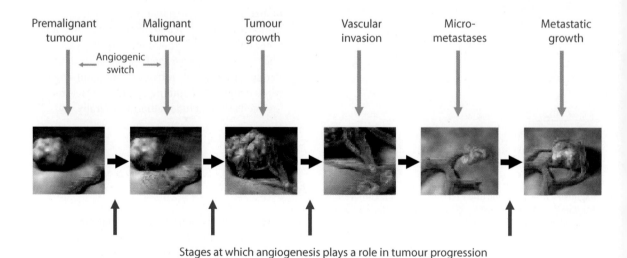

Fig. 3.1. Principles of tumor angiogenesis

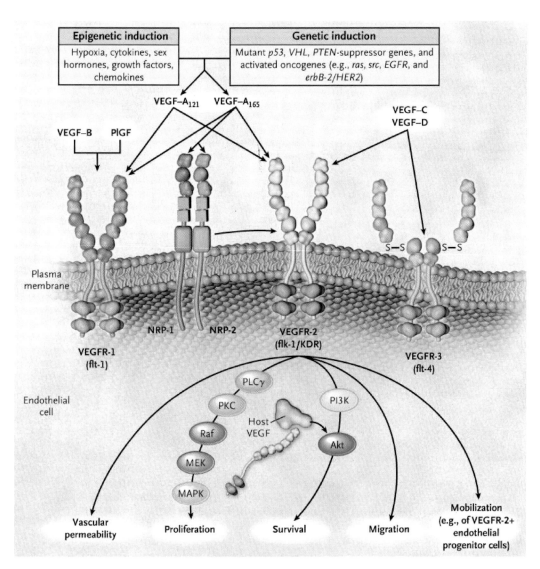

Fig. 3.2. The VEGF-receptor family. Binding and activation of VEGF-receptors and induction of intracellular signaling pathways. *VEGF121* and *VEGF165*: isoforms of VEGF; *VEGFR-2* VEGF receptor 2; *KDR* kinase-insert domain–containing receptor; *Flk-1* fetal liver kinase 1; *PLC* phospholipase C; *PKC* protein kinase; *MAPK* mitogen-activated protein kinase; *PI3K* phosphatidylinositol 3'–kinase; *EGFR* epidermal growth factor receptor; *flt-1* fms-like tyrosine kinase 1; *PlGF* placental growth factor; *PTEN* phosphatase and tensin homologue; *S–S* disulfide bond; *VHL* von Hippel–Lindau. Adapted from: Kerbel 2008 (N Engl J Med 2008;358:2039–49)

mal both in structure and function, with the vessels being immature, leaky, and tortuous, with a reduction or absence of supporting cells. The effect of VEGF on endothelial cells is important in the development of these abnormal vessels. High VEGF expression also promotes vascular permeability, leading to high interstitial and intratumoral pressure, which may allow tumor cells to enter the bloodstream and metastasizes, and which impairs the delivery of chemotherapy to the tumor (Jain 2001, 2003). The chaotic layout of tumor vasculature leads to inconsistent oxygen delivery within the tumor; this creates regions of hypoxia, which are resistant to radiotherapy (Brown 2002). Tumor blood vessels also have a reduction or absence of supporting pericyte and smooth muscle cells, which are essential to the functioning of the vasculature by stabilizing vessel walls and helping to regulate microcirculatory blood flow, as well as influencing endothelial permeability, proliferation, survival, migration, and maturation. An absence of pericytes sensitizes tumor vessels to VEGF inhibi-

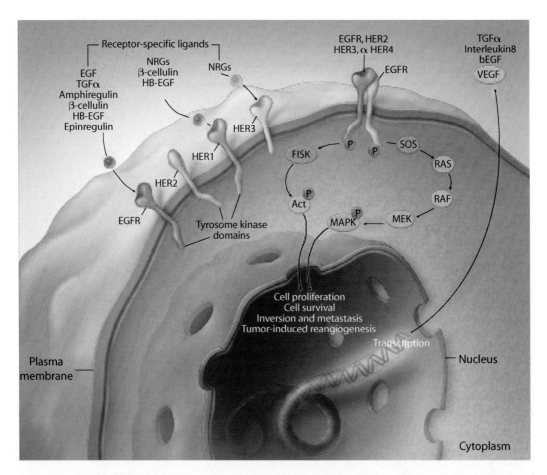

Fig. 3.3. The EGFR signal transduction pathway. After binding of a receptor-specific ligand to the extracellular portion of the EGFR or of one of the EGFR-related receptors (HER2, HER3, or HER4), the receptors build functionally active homodimers or heterodimers and cause the ATP-dependent phosphorylation of specific tyrosine residues in the EGFR intracellular domain. The two major intracellular pathways activated by EGFR are the RAS–RAF–MEK–MAPK pathway, which controls gene transcription, cell-cycle progression from the G1 phase to the S phase, and cell proliferation, and the PI3K–Akt pathway, which activates a cascade of anti-apoptotic and prosurvival signals. *bFGF* basic fibroblast growth factor, *HB-EGF* heparin-binding EGF, *MAPK* mitogen-activated protein kinase, *P phosphate* PI3K phosphatidylinositol 3,4,5-kinase, *TGF* transforming growth factor, *VEGF* vascular endothelial growth factor. Adapted from (Ciardiello and Tortora 2008)

tors, as shown in a number of mouse xenograft models (Abramsson et al. 2002; Morikawa et al. 2002; Baluk et al. 2005).

Further, endothelial cells and circulating bone-marrow-derived endothelial progenitor cells mainly express VEGFR-2 and, activated by VEGF-A, play a key role in tumor angiogenesis. In contrast, the role of VEGFR-1 remains uncertain in respect to VEGF-induced angiogenesis. In breast cancer cells, an intracellular intracrine mechanism of receptor and ligand interaction was postulated, giving VEGF and VEGFR-1 an autocrine function. VEGFR-1 is also associated with vascular development, and it may have a function in quiescent endothelium of mature vessels not related to cell growth. Some tumor cells produce VEGF, but due to a lack of VEGF receptors on their own surface, they do not respond to VEGF directly. Recent findings also suggest that the amount of VEGF produced by platelets and muscle cells are sufficient to induce tumor angiogenesis.

EGFR and Intracellular Signaling

Epidermal growth factor receptor (EGFR) is a member of the ErbB family of receptors, a subfamily of four closely related receptor tyrosine kinases: EGFR (ErbB-1), HER2/c-neu (ErbB-2), Her 3 (ErbB-3), and Her 4 (ErbB-4). In tumor cells overexpression of EGFR is associated with more aggressive disease, increased resistance to radiation therapy and chemotherapy, and finally with more aggressive spread of metastases and overall with a poor prognosis. After binding of receptor-specific ligands like epidermal growth factor (EGF), transforming growth factor α (TGFα), or further ligands, a functionally active dimer of EGFR with EGFR, HER2 HER4, or HER 3 occurs, and intracellular signaling cascades are initiated. EGFR mainly induces two pathways: the RAS–RAF–MAP–MAPK-pathway, which controls gene transcription and cell proliferation, and the PI3K-Akt-pathway, which activates a cascade of antiapoptotic and prosurvival signals (Fig. 3.3).

In patients with metastatic colorectal cancer, the success of anti-EGFR therapy with cetuximab depends on the nonmutated KRAS status. In patients with mutant KRAS, the intracellular signaling continues despite EGFR therapy. Mutated KRAS genes have been detected in about 40% of metastatic colorectal cancer patients. A retrospective analysis of tumor types revealed that patients with wild-type KRAS respond to cetuximab in combination with leucovorin, fluoruracil, and irinotecan (FOLFIRI) with an increase in progression-free survival from 25% without cetuximab to 43% (Van Cutsem et al. 2008). These results also describe a further step to individualized and customized treatment of cancer with targeted therapies.

Inhibiting tumor angiogenesis by targeting VEGF and also EGFR signaling is therefore a rational and potentially valuable therapeutic strategy. Approaches include the development of anti-VEGF-antibodies, anti-VEGF-receptor antibodies, antibodies to EGFR, small molecule inhibitors of receptor tryrosine kinases, and soluble VEGF-receptors.

Pathophysiology of Angiogenesis and Radiation

Blood vessels play a crucial role in the reaction to radiation exposure. Endothelial cells that line capillary blood vessels are situated very close to normal tissue cells, for example, such as epithelial cells in the gut mucosa. This close apposition enables endothelial cells and epithelial cells to communicate with each other by release of growth factors and hormones. Epithelial cells are also able to derive oxygen and nutrients from blood vessels. In contrast, tumor cells form multiple layers around a capillary blood vessel such that the most remote tumor cells are oxygen-deprived (hypoxic or anoxic) (Folkman and Camphausen 2001). The acute vascular reaction is mediated in a dose-dependent manner by the release of inflammatory substances, which in the literature are described as functional radiation effects. Already after the first or a few fractions of a conventional fractionated radiotherapy scheme, inflammatory cytokines such as interleukin-1 and TNF-alpha are expressed. Further the synthesis of prostaglandins and the activity of the nitric oxide (NO)-synthase are found to be increased in endothelial cells (Dörr and Trott 2000).

Sonveaux and colleagues (2003) specifically examined the effects of irradiation on endothelial cells to identify signaling cascades induced by ionizing radiation that could lead to alterations in endothelial cell phenotype and changes in angiogenesis. Earlier studies of several investigators had confirmed that treatment with growth factor antibodies or tyrosine kinase inhibitors can indeed increase the antitumoral effect of ionizing radiation and that such a combination could have super-additive effects, allowing a gain in efficacy by acting on two different targets, namely, tumor cells and endothelial cells (Gorski et al. 1999; Lee et al. 2000; Geng et al. 2001; Hess et al. 2001; Kozin et al. 2001; Camphausen and Menard 2002; Griffin et al. 2002; Huang et al. 2002).

Addressing the impact of irradiation on endothelial cells and the tumor vasculature, they demonstrated that the potentiation of the nitric oxide (NO) signaling pathway after irradiation induces profound alterations in the endothelial phenotype leading to tumor angiogenesis and that the inhibition of NO production suppresses these provascular effects of irradiation.

It has also been shown that NO modulates VEGF-induced angiogenesis and vascular permeability in vivo (Fukumura et al. 2001). There are three differently distributed and regulated isoforms of NO synthase (NOS): neuronal NOS (nNOS, also referred to as type I NOS), inducible NOS (iNOS, type II NOS), and endothelial NOS (eNOS, type III NOS). Endothelial NOS predominantly mediates this process, and iNOS appears to have a small, but additive effect. Thus, selective modulation of eNOS activity by targeting the VEGF pathway alters angiogenesis and vascular permeability in vivo. Other physiologic vascular changes mediated by NO are blood flow and vessel diameter, respectively, vasorelaxation (FUKUMURA et al. 2001).

Endothelial cells react differently to radiation, depending on the inflammation. In inflammation endothelial cells are in a special physiologic condition, rapidly proliferating, actively synthesizing many pro-inflammatory and other peptides and proteins and responding differently to radiation than resting endothelial cells. The functional consequences of radiation exposure of these activated endothelial cells might be different from those induced in endothelial cells in healthy normal tissues studied (TROTT and KAMPRAD 1999).

NO is also known as an important mediator in the status of inflammation in addition to its wide range of physiological and pathophysiological activities, including the regulation of vessel tone and angiogenesis in wound healing, inflammation, ischemic cardiovascular diseases, and malignant diseases. Depending on the dose and fractionation schedule, in the status of inflammation low-dose radiation attenuates the acitivity of iNOS and therefore mediates the acute inflammation in vivo. This appears to be one of the possible pathways explaining the well-known anti-inflammatory effect of low-dose radiotherapy (Review by RISCHKE et al. 2007).

Other effects of irradiation on endothelial cells are cytotoxic effects that participate in the antitumor treatment. As a chronic effect of radiation exposure to blood vessels, histopathologic investigation reveals a capillary rarefication, which means a markedly reduced density of capillaries in irradiated tissues, which can occur, depending on the tissue type, even after many years. The depletion of capillaries and mircrovessels is supposed to be the consequence of an impaired cellular function leading to destruction of capillaries. The exact mechanisms are still not known (TROTT 2002).

An interesting approach postulates that angiogenic growth factors such as platelet-derived growth factor, insulin-like growth factor-1, and vascular endothelial growth factor lead to reduced long-term toxicity in the spinal cord in pre-clinical studies in a spinal-cord irradiation rat model (ANDRATSCHKE et al. 2005).

3.5
Antiangiogenic Substances

Anti-VEGF-therapies can lead to regression of already existing tumor vascularization. VEGF is essential for tumor vessel cells to survive; it protects them from apoptosis and promotes tumor growth. Without a continuing supply of VEGF, endothelial cell apoptosis occurs, and newly developed tumor microvessels decay. VEGF inhibition also can lead to both structural and functional changes on surviving vessels, a phenomenon described as vessel normalization (JAIN 2005).

3.5.1
Bevacizumab (Avastin™)

Bevacizumab (Avastin™) is a recombinant humanized monoclonal antibody directed against VEGF. Bevacizumab binds to VEGF and inhibits VEGF receptor binding. A precursor antibody to Bevacizumab was A4.6.1, a murine antibody cloned by Ferrara (LEUNG et al. 1989) and bound with high affinity to different isoforms of VEGF. It inhibited cell growth in immortalized tumor cell lines by a significant reduction of vascular density. As a murine protein, it provoked anaphylactic reactions and needed to be humanized.

In preclinical studies, the combination of Bevacizumab with chemotherapy led to synergistic activity. In xenotransplants, the combination of Bevacizumab with capecitabine inhibited tumor growth more effectively and longer than any other tested substance (SACHSENMAIER 2001). It also showed synergistic effects in combination with paclitaxel and Trastuzumab (Herceptin™), a humanized monoclonal antibody that acts on the HER2/neu (erbB2) receptor. In further invivo studies, the application of Bevacizumab to animals previously treated with capecitabine, topotecan, or cisplatin showed more successful tumor suppression. Also, repeated application of Bevacizumab proved to be safe and well tolerated.

3.5.2
Cetuximab (Erbitux ™)

Cetuximab (Erbitux ™), a monoclonal antibody, binds to the extracellular domain of EGFR, competing with its specific ligands and inhibiting intracellular signaling. Further, as an IgG1 immunoglobulin, it could elicit host antitumor immune responses such as cell-mediated antibody-dependent cytotoxicity and also EGFR internalization, down-regulation, and finally receptor degradation.

Among the EGFR targeting substances, Cetuximab has been approved for combination with radiotherapy for the treatment of locally advanced squamous-cell carcinoma of the head and neck (SCCHN) or as a single agent in patients who have had prior platinum-based therapy. Side effects of Cetuximab treatments include acne-like skin affections, fever, and chills, asthenia, and nausea.

3.5.3
Small Molecule Tyrosine Kinase Inhibitors

Small molecule tyrosine kinase inhibitors (TKI), such as sorafenib (Nexavar™) and sunitinib (Sutent™), also represent antiangiogenic agents. Sorafenib is a potent orally available protein kinase inhibitor. Originally identified as a Raf kinase inhibitor, Sorafenib also inhibits VEGFR-1 and 2, platelet-derived-growth factor receptor (PDGFR-β), and c-Kit-Protein. Sorafenib has a dual antitumoral target affecting the tumor cell and its blood vessels. In human endothelial cells and in smooth muscle cells, VEGFR-2 signaling and activation of extracellular signal-regulated kinase (ERK) are induced.

Sunitinib (Sutent™) is also an orally available multi-targeted TKI. Especially in renal cell carcinoma and in gastrointestinal stroma tumors (GIST), sunitinib proved to be superior to earlier therapy strategies and is now established as first-line treatment.

Sorafenib and sunitinib are both approved for the treatment of renal cell carcinoma. A clinical phase III trial studying sunitinib compared to sorafenib or placebo in treating patients with kidney cancer that has been removed by surgery (ClinTrails.gov NCT00326898) is currently recruiting patients.

3.5.4
Cediranib (Recentin™)

Cediranib (Recentin™), known as AZD2171, is an oral, highly potent, inhibitor of VEGF signaling that selectively inhibits all known VEGFR tyrosine kinase activity (VEGFR-1, -2 and -3; Fig. 3.4). Encouraging results obtained to date with Cediranib in a range of clinical studies show its potential as a new antiangiogenic drug in combination with radiotherapy.

The ability of Cediranib to inhibit growth factor-stimulated receptor phosphorylation was determined in a range of cell lines (WEDGE et al. 2005). Furthermore, this effect was also associated with inhibition of MAP kinase phosphorylation, a downstream marker of VEGF signaling. These data suggest that Cediranib can selectively inhibit VEGFR-dependent proliferation, but appreciable functional selectivity is evident versus other targets, including EGFR, FGFR, and PDGFR-α.

The in vivo activity of Cediranib was also investigated in a model of vascular sprouting. In nude mice implanted with a VEGF-containing Matrigel plug, Cediraninb completely abolished VEGF-induced vessel formation (WEDGE et al. 2005). Furthermore, Cediranib

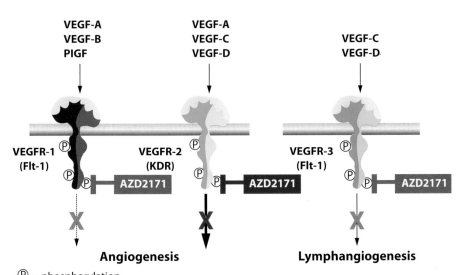

P = phosphorylation

PGF: placental growth factor; VEGF: vascular endotherial growth factor; VEGFR: VEGF receptor

Fig. 3.4. Intracellular signaling inhibition by Cediranib

has demonstrated antitumor efficacy in a number of in vivo preclinical studies, including xenograft, orthotopic, metastatic, and spontaneous models of human cancer (WEDGE et al. 2005).

Administration of Cediranib produced dose-dependent inhibition of tumor growth in a range of histologically distinct human tumor xenografts (lung, colon, breast, prostate, and ovarian) and also decreased primary tumor growth, metastasis, and microvessel density in an orthotopic model of murine renal cell carcinoma (DREVS et al. 2004).

Taken together, Cediranib has shown anti-tumor activity in a range of preclinical in vivo models consistent with inhibition of VEGF signaling and an antiangiogenic mode of action rather than a direct antiproliferative effect on tumor cells. In an extensive phase I program, Cediranib was tested as monotherapy in prostate cancer, with carboplatin and paclitaxel in non-small cell lung cancer (NSCLC), with selected chemotherapy regimens in advanced cancer, and with gefitinib in advanced cancer.

Cediranib is one of the most potent inhibitors of VEGFR-2 tyrosine kinase activity in development. Preclinical studies have demonstrated that Cediranib inhibits VEGF-dependent signaling, angiogenesis, and neovascular survival. Cediranib is also a potent inhibitor of VEGFR-1 and -3 tyrosine kinases, and shows selectivity for VEGFRs versus a range of other kinases. Consistent with an antiangiogenic effect, once-daily treatment with Cediranib produced dose-dependent inhibition of tumor growth in a broad range of established human tumor xenografts.

A series of phase I studies have been conducted to investigate Cediranib in patients with cancer, both as monotherapy and in combination with certain other anticancer strategies. These investigations have shown Cediranib to be generally well tolerated, with a side effect profile that is tolerable and manageable. Currently available pharmacokinetic data are supportive of a once-daily oral dosing schedule for Cediranib. Furthermore, preliminary efficacy data demonstrate that Cediranib has potential antitumor activity in multiple tumor types. Recruitment to a number of clinical trials has been initiated to further determine the activity of Cediranib in a wide range of tumors. Currently ongoing trials address the effect of Cediranib on metastatic colorectal cancer in combination with different chemotherapies. Encouraging preliminary results were reported for Cediranib in patients with glioblastoma suggesting an increase in overall survival (BATCHELOR 2008).

3.6
Chemotherapy and Antiangiogenic Therapy

Bevacizumab in combination with certain chemotherapy regimens has demonstrated clinically relevant improvements in survival or in progression-free survival in patients with colorectal, lung, and breast cancer.

Bevacizumab in combination with IFL (Irinotecan, 5-FU, and leukovorin) was studied as first-line therapy for patients with metastatic colorectal cancer. Eight hundred thirteen patients were randomly assigned, and 402 patients received IFL with bevacizumab. The addition of bevacizumab to fluorouracil-based combination chemotherapy results in statistically significant and clinically meaningful improvement in survival (HURWITZ et al. 2004).

Bevacizumab was also evaluated in patients with non-squamous NSCLC also chemotherapy naive. Four hundred thirty-four patients received bevacizumab in combination with carboplatin and paclitaxel versus 444 patients with carboplatin and paclitaxel alone. Overall survival was also significantly improved by addition of bevacizumab (COHEN et al. 2007).

A trial focusing on patients with HER2-negative and chemotherapy naive metastatic breast cancer comparing treatment with bevacizumab in combination with paclitaxel versus paclitaxel alone showed significant improvement of progression-free survival (median of 11.8 versus 5.9 months). In contrast, overall survival was not improved. As the reason for this discrepancy, the authors discuss possible rebound effects on subsequent treatments after ending the therapy or a correlation between bevacizumab resistance and resistance to other therapeutic attempts. Interestingly, progression-free survival and high response rates were seen early in metastatic disease, suggesting that development of metastases as a VEGF-dependent event is more vulnerable to bevacizumab treatment, and the question of bevacizumab effects in an adjuvant setting needs to be answered (MILLER et al. 2007). Based on this trial the FDA granted an accelerated approval for bevacizumab in combination with paclitaxel.

However, the observation that antiangiogenic drugs combined with chemotherapeutic agents improve antitumoral effects is surprising, because one would expect the intratumoral delivery of drugs to be suppressed. Different models have been discussed to explain the chemosensitizing activity of antiangiogenic drugs. It is assumed that antiangiogenic drugs 'normalize' the tumor vasculature, enhancing the efficacy of chemotherapeutic drugs. Tumor vessels in general are structurally abnormal, showing absence of hierarchically structured patterns such as reduced basement membranes and dilated vessels, making them leaky and resulting in altered perfusion or blood flow. Even highly vascularized tumors can be hypoxic, which again is known as being an angiogenesis-inducing factor. Antiangiogenic therapy can reverse these alterations, a phenomenon known as vessel normalization, and thus enhance antitumor effects of chemotherapeutic agents. After vessel normalization, a synergistic effect of bevacizumab with chemotherapy is assumed regarding the tumor cell recovery and repopulation. The rate of tumor cell repopulation after MTD of conventional chemotherapy or radiation does not necessarily decline in proportion to the number of treatment cycles. In fact, the observed trend suggests the opposite effect. Consequently, exposing the tumor to an antiangiogenic drug during the break periods between courses of chemotherapy is sought to reduce oxygenization and delivery of nutrients to repopulating cells. Taking those hypotheses into consideration, the timing of combinational therapies needs to be optimized. This also supports the suggestion to apply bevacizumab between chemotherapy cycles when tumor cell repopulation after cytotoxic chemotherapy is increased and repopulating cells demand for oxygen is high.

Further, for cytotoxic chemotherapy itself, antiangiogenic effects enhancing antitumoral activity have been described. It has been hypothesized that these drugs could damage endothelial cells that proliferate during the formation of new blood vessels, and also destruction of circulating bone marrow cells leads to impaired tumor angiogenesis. These endothelial cells include circulating endothelial progenitor cells (EPCs) that can incorporate into the lumen of nascent vessels and differentiate into mature endothelial cells (Asahara et al. 1997; Shaked et al. 2005). Given the well-established myelosuppressive effects of cytotoxic chemotherapy, one might predict that at least some of these proangiogenic bone marrow cell types would be sensitive to chemotherapy. Many of these cell populations can be mobilized into the peripheral blood by growth factors such as VEGF; thus, the combination of a VEGF-targeting agent with chemotherapy would be expected to have an additive, if not synergistic, suppressive effect on these cells.

Because of its low toxicity, metronomic chemotherapy, continuously administered low doses of chemotherapeutic drugs below toxicity levels, may be well suited for long-term combination with antiangiogenic drugs; such combinations have had marked antitumor effects in preclinical models (Klement et al. 2000; Kerbel and Kamen 2004; Pietras and Hanahan

2005). Both antibody-based and small-molecule antiangiogenic drugs enhance the effects of metronomic chemotherapy in preclinical models. Phase II trials of metronomic chemotherapy (Colleoni et al. 2002; Kieran et al. 2005), sometimes used in combination with antiangiogenic drugs, have yielded encouraging results in patients with advanced cancer (Canady 2005), but larger randomized trials are needed to validate the concept. There is also a need for surrogate markers to help determine the optimal biologic dose of this therapy. Circulating EPCs have been used successfully as a marker in preclinical studies (Shaked et al. 2005), but are not yet validated clinically.

3.7
Radiation and Antiangiogenic Therapy

Because of the encouraging results of antiangiogenic therapy combined with chemotherapy, consequently combinational therapies including antiangiogenesis and radiation with or without chemotherapy are becoming the focus of clinical interest. Besides developing new therapeutic strategies to improve curative cancer treatment, also the safety of combinational therapies needs to be addressed since tumor patients receiving antiangiogenic drugs might also receive radiation therapy for palliation.

The rationale for combining radiation with antiangiogenic drugs is based on several pathophysiological considerations. Tumor response to radiation therapy is caused by DNA damage to tumor cells and also depends on intracellular pathways controlling apoptosis, autophagy, and cell death induced by radiation. Oxygene is a potent radiosensitizer, and its interaction with radicals formed by radiation induces DNA damage. Hypoxia leads to radiation resistance. Radiation induces the secretion of cytokines that inhibit apoptosis in endothelial cells. Hypoxia inducible factor (HIF)-1α is activated when cells are hypoxic, it dimerizes with HIF-1β, and this leads to an increase in VEGF transcription. This is associated with a lower radiation response and tumor progression, mainly experienced in head and neck tumors, uterine cervix tumors, and sarcomas. Radiation itself also induces hypoxia and thus increases VEGF production and VEGFR expression. Hypoxia can be measured directly by determination of oxygen pressure or more recently by PET using misonidazol or 2nitroimidazole as tracers (Koch and Evans 2003; Rischin et al. 2006; Thorwarth et al. 2007). Again, vessel normalization enhances oxygenation and thus radiosensitivity in tumor cells. In preclinical studies antiangiogenic therapy has been shown to enhance radiation-induced cell death (LEE et al. 2000; HESS et al. 2001).

Factors known to control angiogenesis, such as fibroblast growth factor 2 (FGF2), EGF, VEGF, the alpha-vβ3 and alpha-vβ5 integrins, and some GTPase proteins, have been clearly demonstrated to be involved in controlling intrinsic radiation resistance.

The induction of this radiation resistance is also mediated by a small G protein, RhoB, known to be activated by various stresses, such as UV, but also ionizing radiation or hypoxia as well as by growth factors, such as EGF or FGF2 (MOYAL 2008). Normalization of tumor vasculature by anti-VEGFR-2 antibody has also led to enhanced radiation-induced tumor response (WINKLER et al. 2004). This study demonstrated the necessity to optimize timing of radiation and chemotherapy and supports the advantage of this therapy during the normalization phase.

There are also several trials ongoing, studying antiangiogenic drugs in combination with radiotherapy in patients with rectal cancer, pancreatic cancer, head and neck tumors, and brain tumors, e.g., with bevacizumab, imatinib (Gleevec™), and sunitinib.

The use of cetuximab in combination with radiotherapy is approved by the FDA for squamous cell carcinoma of the head and neck (SCCHN). Four hundred twenty-four patients with untreated SCCHN entered a phase III trial (BONNER et al. 2006) and were randomly assigned to radiotherapy alone or in combination with cetuximab. Overall survival and progression-free survival were significantly increased in the experimental arm (24.4 vs. 14.9 months). Interestingly, this trial also showed that radiation side effects were not increased. It has been noted critically that this trial did not compare chemoradiation as standard therapy with radiotherapy and cetuximab. Cetuximab has been studied in combination with chemotherapy, including 5-FU, paclitaxel, and cisplatin (BURTNESS et al. 2005; BOURHIS et al. 2006) in patients with SCCHN. In a small number of patients, cetuximab has reverted cisplatin resistance, and it was suggested that cetuximab is the only second-line treatment with significant response rates available.

The widespread use of bevacizumab in multimodal attempts to treat different tumor entities logically demands an extension to address the advantages of bevacizumab in combination with radiation with or without chemotherapy. To date, no phase III studies have been completed, so that the extent of the benefit that bevacizumab seems to have remains to be determined. In patients with rectal carcinoma, WILLET and colleagues (2007) demonstrated in a continuation of a dose-escalation phase I trial in addition to the dose limiting toxicity

of bevacizumab that the combination of bevacizumab with chemoradiation may have high response rates. In this study, two consecutive cohorts of three patients with locally advanced rectal carcinoma were treated with bevacizumab (10 mg/kg), and concurrent administration of bevacizumab with 5-FU chemotherapy and pelvic radiation therapy. Surgery was scheduled 7 to 9 weeks after completion of therapy. Functional, cellular, and molecular studies were performed before and after initial bevacizumab monotherapy. Following the National Cancer Institute trial guidelines, they terminated the dose-escalation component of their study when two consecutive patients developed dose-limiting toxicities (DLT) of diarrhea and colitis during the combined treatment. Following recovery from toxicity, these patients were able to resume and complete radiation therapy and 5-FU. Because of these DLT, only five patients were enrolled at the 10 mg/kg dose. All the patients underwent surgery. Of considerable interest in respect of combining antiangiogenic substances with radiation or chemoradiation has been the fact that the patients receiving 10 mg/kg bevacizumab showed two complete pathologic responses, as compared to no complete pathologic response in the 5 mg/kg bevacizumab group (WILLETT et al. 2004, 2007). These tumor responses were also detected on computed tomography (CT) and positron emission tomography (PET) scans after completion of chemoradiation therapy, stressing that PET/CT-scans may be a valuable tool acting as an appropriate surrogate marker, while it is a non-invasive, sensitive, semi-quantitative, and reproducible method.

The few phase I publications studying toxicity of antiangiogenics in association with radiotherapy mainly investigated the acute effects. One study combined radiotherapy and 15 mg/kg bevacizumab with oxaliplatin and capecitabine in escalating doses in patients with rectal adenocarcinoma and showed that the antiangiogenics increased the toxicity of the combination of capecitabine, oxaliplatin, and radiotherapy, the DLT being grade 4 diarrhea (CZITO et al. 2007). The combination of bevacizumab with radiotherapy and capecitabine in patients with pancreatic carcinoma showed grade 3 ulcerations with bleeding or perforation in four patients. These events occurred up to 20 weeks after the end of the combination of radiation with chemotherapy, particularly in patients whose tumor invaded the duodenum (CRANE et al. 2006).

The available recent preclinical and clinical data strongly support the introduction of antiangiogenics into combined modality treatment schemes that include radiotherapy. The ultimate benefit of these therapeutic combinations needs to be determined with longer follow-up of the effect of these antiangiogenic agents and by studying surrogate markers by metabolic and functional imaging (perfusion MRI, PET/CT–FDG, PET/CT-misonidazole) in early clinical studies, notably concerning the effect on tumor oxygenation and vascularization, in order to choose the optimal sequence and administration time of these drugs compared to radiotherapy. Elucidating the mechanisms by which radiosensitization is obtained and the molecular interplay between radiation toxicity to normal organs and antiangiogenics is also important to facilitate the design and testing of clinical strategies aimed at minimizing toxicity.

References

Abramsson A, Berlin O et al. (2002) Analysis of mural cell recruitment to tumor vessels. Circulation 105(1): 112–117

Andratschke NH, Nieder C et al. (2005) Potential role of growth factors in diminishing radiation therapy neural tissue injury. Semin Oncol 32(2 Suppl 3): S67–70

Asahara T, Murohara T et al. (1997) Isolation of putative progenitor endothelial cells for angiogenesis. Science 275(5302): 964–967

Baluk P, Hashizume H et al. (2005) Cellular abnormalities of blood vessels as targets in cancer. Curr Opin Genet Dev 15(1): 102–111

Batchelor T, Sorensen A et al. (2008) A multidisciplinary phase II study of AZD2171 (cediranib), an oral Pan-VEGF receptor tyrosine kinase inhibitor, in patients with recurrent glioblastoma. Proc Am Assoc Cancer Res (AACR) 2008 Annual Meeting. Abstract LB-247

Batchelor TT, Sorensen AG et al. (2007) AZD2171, a pan-VEGF receptor tyrosine kinase inhibitor, normalizes tumor vasculature and alleviates edema in glioblastoma patients. Cancer Cell 11(1): 83–95

Bonner J A, Harari PM, et al. (2006) Radiotherapy plus cetuximab for squamous-cell carcinoma of the head and neck. N Engl J Med 354(6): 567–578

Bourhis J, Rivera F et al. (2006) Phase I/II study of cetuximab in combination with cisplatin or carboplatin and fluorouracil in patients with recurrent or metastatic squamous cell carcinoma of the head and neck. J Clin Oncol 24(18): 2866–2672

Brown JM (2002) Tumor microenvironment and the response to anticancer therapy. Cancer Biol Ther 1(5): 453–458

Burtness B, Goldwasser MA et al. (2005) Phase III randomized trial of cisplatin plus placebo compared with cisplatin plus cetuximab in metastatic/recurrent head and neck cancer: an Eastern Cooperative Oncology Group study. J Clin Oncol 23(34): 8646–8654

Camphausen K, Menard C (2002) Angiogenesis inhibitors and radiotherapy of primary tumours. Expert Opin Biol Ther 2(5): 477–481

Canady C (2005) Metronomic chemo/Avastin may be effective in ovarian cancer. Oncol News Int 14:8–22

Ciardiello F, Tortora G (2008) EGFR antagonists in cancer treatment. N Engl J Med 358(11): 1160–1174

Cohen MH, Gootenberg J et al. (2007). FDA drug approval summary: bevacizumab (Avastin) plus Carboplatin and Paclitaxel as first-line treatment of advanced/metastatic recurrent nonsquamous non-small cell lung cancer. Oncologist 12(6): 713–718

Colleoni M, Rocca A et al. (2002) Low-dose oral methotrexate and cyclophosphamide in metastatic breast cancer: antitumor activity and correlation with vascular endothelial growth factor levels. Ann Oncol 13(1): 73–80

Crane CH, Ellis LM et al. (2006) Phase I trial evaluating the safety of bevacizumab with concurrent radiotherapy and capecitabine in locally advanced pancreatic cancer. J Clin Oncol 24(7): 1145–1151

Czito BG, Bendell JC et al. (2007) Bevacizumab, oxaliplatin, and capecitabine with radiation therapy in rectal cancer: Phase I trial results. Int J Radiat Oncol Biol Phys 68(2): 472–478

Dörr W, Trott KR (2000) Strahlenbiologie der Normalgewebe. München, Urban und Vogel

Drevs J, Konerding MA et al. (2004) The VEGF receptor tyrosine kinase inhibitor, ZD6474, inhibits angiogenesis and affects microvascular architecture within an orthotopically implanted renal cell carcinoma. Angiogenesis 7(4): 347–354

Van Cutsem E, D'haens G et al. (2008) KRAS status and efficacy in the first-line treatment of patients with metastatic colorectal cancer (mCRC) treated with FOLFIRI with or without cetuximab: The CRYSTAL experience. J Clin Oncol 26 suppl; abstract 2

Folkman J (1971) Tumor angiogenesis: therapeutic implications. N Engl J Med 285(21): 1182–1186

Folkman J, Camphausen K (2001) Cancer. What does radiotherapy do to endothelial cells? Science 293(5528): 227–228

Fukumura D, Gohongi T et al. (2001) Predominant role of endothelial nitric oxide synthase in vascular endothelial growth factor-induced angiogenesis and vascular permeability. Proc Natl Acad Sci USA 98(5): 2604–2609

Geng L, Donnelly E et al. (2001) Inhibition of vascular endothelial growth factor receptor signaling leads to reversal of tumor resistance to radiotherapy. Cancer Res 61(6): 2413–2439

Gorski DH, Beckett MA et al. (1999) Blockage of the vascular endothelial growth factor stress response increases the antitumor effects of ionizing radiation. Cancer Res 59(14): 3374–3378

Griffin RJ, Williams BW et al. (2002) Simultaneous inhibition of the receptor kinase activity of vascular endothelial, fibroblast, and platelet-derived growth factors suppresses tumor growth and enhances tumor radiation response. Cancer Res 62(6): 1702–1706

Hess C, Vuong V et al. (2001) Effect of VEGF receptor inhibitor PTK787/ZK222584 [correction of ZK222548] combined with ionizing radiation on endothelial cells and tumour growth. Br J Cancer 85(12): 2010–2016

Huang SM, Li J et al. (2002) Modulation of radiation response and tumor-induced angiogenesis after epidermal growth factor receptor inhibition by ZD1839 (Iressa). Cancer Res 62(15): 4300–4306

Hurwitz H, Fehrenbacher L et al. (2004) Bevacizumab plus irinotecan, fluorouracil, and leucovorin for metastatic colorectal cancer. N Engl J Med 350(23): 2335–2342

Jain RK (2001) Normalizing tumor vasculature with anti-angiogenic therapy: a new paradigm for combination therapy. Nat Med 7(9): 987–989

Jain RK (2003) Molecular regulation of vessel maturation. Nat Med 9(6): 685–963

Jain RK (2005) Normalization of tumor vasculature: an emerging concept in antiangiogenic therapy. Science 307(5706): 58–62

Kerbel RS, Kamen BA (2004) The anti-angiogenic basis of metronomic chemotherapy. Nat Rev Cancer 4(6): 423–436

Kerbel (2008) Tumor angiogenesis. N Engl J Med 358:2039–49

Kieran MW, Turner CD et al. (2005) A feasibility trial of antiangiogenic (metronomic) chemotherapy in pediatric patients with recurrent or progressive cancer. J Pediatr Hematol Oncol 27(11): 573–581

Klement G, Baruchel S et al. (2000) Continuous low-dose therapy with vinblastine and VEGF receptor-2 antibody induces sustained tumor regression without overt toxicity. J Clin Invest 105(8): R15–24

Koch CJ, Evans SM (2003) Non-invasive PET and SPECT imaging of tissue hypoxia using isotopically labeled 2-nitroimidazoles. Adv Exp Med Biol 510: 285–292

Kozin SV, Boucher Y et al. (2001) Vascular endothelial growth factor receptor-2-blocking antibody potentiates radiation-induced long-term control of human tumor xenografts. Cancer Res 61(1): 39–44

Lee CG, Heijn M et al. (2000) Anti-vascular endothelial growth factor treatment augments tumor radiation response under normoxic or hypoxic conditions. Cancer Res 60(19): 5565–5570

Leung DW, Cachianes G et al. (1989) Vascular endothelial growth factor is a secreted angiogenic mitogen. Science 246(4935): 1306–1309

Miller K, Wang M et al. (2007) Paclitaxel plus bevacizumab versus paclitaxel alone for metastatic breast cancer. N Engl J Med 357(26): 2666–2676

Morikawa S, Baluk P et al. (2002) Abnormalities in pericytes on blood vessels and endothelial sprouts in tumors. Am J Pathol 160(3): 985–1000

Moyal EC, Laprie A et al. (2007) Phase I trial of tipifarnib (R115777) concurrent with radiotherapy in patients with glioblastoma multiforme. Int J Radiat Oncol Biol Phys 68(5): 1396–1401

Moyal EC-J (2008) Optimizing antiangiogenic strategies: combining with radiotherapy. Targeted Oncol 3(1):51

Pietras K, Hanahan D (2005) A multitargeted, metronomic, and maximum-tolerated dose chemo-switch regimen is antiangiogenic, producing objective responses and survival benefit in a mouse model of cancer. J Clin Oncol 23(5): 939–952

Rischin D, Hicks RJ et al. (2006) Prognostic significance of [18F]-misonidazole positron emission tomography-detected tumor hypoxia in patients with advanced head and neck cancer randomly assigned to chemoradiation with or without tirapazamine: a substudy of Trans-Tasman Radiation Oncology Group Study 98.02. J Clin Oncol 24(13): 2098–2104

Rischke HC, Momm F et al. (2007) Does radiation prevent 5-fluorouracil-induced colitis in the early phase of radiochemotherapy? A case report and literature review. Strahlenther Onkol 183(8): 459–463

Sachsenmaier C (2001) Targeting protein kinases for tumor therapy. Onkologie 24(4): 346–355

Shaked Y, Bertolini F et al. (2005) Genetic heterogeneity of the vasculogenic phenotype parallels angiogenesis; Implications for cellular surrogate marker analysis of antiangiogenesis. Cancer Cell 7(1): 101–111

Shaked Y, Emmenegger U et al. (2005) Optimal biologic dose of metronomic chemotherapy regimens is associated with maximum antiangiogenic activity. Blood 106(9): 3058–3061

Sonveaux P, Brouet A et al. (2003). Irradiation-induced angiogenesis through the up-regulation of the nitric oxide pathway: implications for tumor radiotherapy. Cancer Res 63(5): 1012–1019

Thorwarth D, Eschmann SM et al. (2007). Hypoxia dose painting by numbers: a planning study. Int J Radiat Oncol Biol Phys 68(1): 291–300

Trott KR (2002) Strahlenwirkung auf Normalgewebe. München, Urban und Vogel

Trott KR, Kamprad F (1999) Radiobiological mechanisms of anti-inflammatory radiotherapy. Radiother Oncol 51(3): 197–203

Wedge SR, Kendrew J et al. (2005) AZD2171: a highly potent, orally bioavailable, vascular endothelial growth factor receptor-2 tyrosine kinase inhibitor for the treatment of cancer. Cancer Res 65(10): 4389–400

Willett CG, Boucher Y et al. (2004) Direct evidence that the VEGF-specific antibody bevacizumab has antivascular effects in human rectal cancer. Nat Med 10(2): 145–147

Willett CG, Duda DG et al. (2007) Complete pathological response to bevacizumab and chemoradiation in advanced rectal cancer. Nat Clin Pract Oncol 4(5): 316–321

Winkler F, Kozin SV et al. (2004) Kinetics of vascular normalization by VEGFR2 blockade governs brain tumor response to radiation: role of oxygenation, angiopoietin-1, and matrix metalloproteinases. Cancer Cell 6(6): 553–563

Pathophysiology of Solid Tumors

Peter Vaupel

CONTENTS

KEY POINTS

- The physiology of tumors is uniquely different to that of normal tissues and is characterized by adverse conditions that can be summarized as the "crucial Ps."
- The hostile pathophysiological microenvironment is largely determined by an abnormal tumor microcirculation.
- Blood flow can vary considerably despite similar histological classification and primary site.
- Blood flow is not regulated according to the metabolic demands as is the case in normal tissues.

P. Vaupel, Dr. med., M.A./Univ. Harvard
Professor of Physiology and Pathophysiology, Institute of Physiology and Pathophysiology, University of Mainz, Duesbergweg 6, 55099 Mainz, Germany

- Increased vascular permeability has been demonstrated, with extravasation of blood plasma expanding the interstitial fluid space and—because of the lack of functional lymphatics—drastically increasing the hydrostatic pressure in the tumor interstitium.

- Interstitial hypertension forms a "physiologic" barrier to the delivery of therapeutic macromolecules to the cancer cells.

- The tumor interstitial space is three to five times larger than in most normal tissues and contains a relatively large quantity of mobile (i.e., freely moving) fluid.

- A pH gradient exists across the cell membrane in tumors ($pH_i > pH_e$). Interestingly, this gradient is the reverse of that found in normal tissues.

- Lactate accumulation mirrors malignant potential in different types of human cancers.

- The presence of hypoxic tissue areas with oxygen tensions ≤ 2.5 mmHg is a characteristic pathophysiological property of locally advanced solid tumors.

- Pathogenesis of tumor hypoxia is multifactorial.

- Hypoxic and/or anoxic tissue areas are heterogeneously—both temporarily and spatially—distributed within the tumor mass.

- Hypoxia-induced changes in gene expression are mediated by a special set of transcription factors, mainly by the hypoxia-inducible factor-1 (HIF-1) and HIF-2.

- Downstream effects of HIF activation include modulation of glycolysis capacity ("Warburg effect"), cell survival, and increased angiogenesis.

- Tumor cell variants with adaptations favorable to survival under hypoxic conditions may have growth advantages over non-adapted cells in the hypoxic microenvironment and expand through clonal selection.

Abstract

It is generally accepted that tumor blood flow, microcirculation, oxygen and nutrient supply, tissue pH distribution, lactate levels, and the bioenergetic status—factors that are usually closely linked and that define the so-called pathophysiological microenvironment ("tumor pathophysiome")—can markedly influence the therapeutic response of malignant tumors to conventional irradiation, chemotherapy, other non-surgical treatment modalities, malignant progression, and the cell proliferation activity within tumors. Currently available information on the parameters defining the pathophysiological micromilieu in human tumors is presented in this chapter. According to these data, significant variations in these relevant factors are likely to occur between different locations within a tumor and between tumors of the same grading and clinical staging. Therefore, evaluation of the pathophysiological microenvironment in individual tumors before therapy and a corresponding "fine-tuning" of treatment protocols for individual patients may result in an improved tumor response to treatment.

4.1
Introduction

The physiology of tumors ("tumor pathophysiome") is uniquely different to that of normal tissues. It is characterized inter alia by O_2 depletion (hypoxia or anoxia), extracellular acidosis, high lactate levels, glucose deprivation, energy impoverishment, significant interstitial fluid flow, and interstitial hypertension, i.e., adverse conditions that can be summarized as the "crucial Ps" characterizing the metabolic tumor microenvironment (see Table 4.1) (SUTHERLAND 1988; VAUPEL et al. 1989, 1997; VAUPEL and JAIN 1991; VAUPEL 1992, 1994a,b; VAUPEL and KELLEHER 1999; BUSSINK 2000; MOLLS and VAUPEL 2000; VAUPEL and HÖCKEL 2000; GOODE and CHADWICK 2001). This hostile microenvironment is largely determined by an abnormal tumor microcirculation. When considering the continuous and indiscriminate formation of a vascular network in a growing tumor, five different pathogenetic mechanisms can be discussed: (1) angiogenesis by endothelial sprouting from preexisting venules, (2) co-option of existing vessels, (3) vasculogenesis (de novo vessel formation through incorporation of circulating endothelial precursor cells), (4) intussusception (splitting of the lumen of a vessel into two), and (5) formation of pseudo-vascular channels lined by tumor cells rather than endothelial cells ("vascular mimicry," for reviews see REINHOLD and VAN DEN BERG-BLOK 1983; REINHOLD 1987; RIBATTI et al. 2003; SIVRIDIS et al. 2003; VAUPEL 2004b; CAIRNS et al. 2006; FUKUMURA and JAIN 2007; TRÉDAN et al. 2007). The tumor vasculature is characterized by vigorous proliferation leading to immature, structurally defective and, in terms of perfusion, ineffective microvessels. "Tumor vessels lack the signals to mature"

Table 4.1. The dozen crucial **P**s characterizing the hostile pathophysiological tumor microenvironment ("tumor pathophysiome")

Perfusion inadequacies/vascular chaos	↑
Perfusion heterogeneities	↑
Permeability of tumor microvessels	↑
Pressure of interstitial fluid	↑
Production of lactate	↑
Production of adenosine	↑
Paucity of nutrients	↑
Partial pressure of CO_2 (pCO_2)	↑
Paucity of bicarbonate	↑
Partial pressure of O_2 (pO_2)	↓
Production of high-energy compounds	↓
pH of extracellular compartment	↓

↑ = increase, change for the worse, ↓ = decrease

and tumor vasculature is often described as an "aberrant monster" (SHCHORS and EVAN 2007). Consequently, tumor blood flow is chaotic and heterogeneous.

In this chapter, the consequences of the irregular structure and function of the tumor microcirculation and the self-perpetuating hostile pathophysiological microenvironment (via a vicious circle) will be described. This overview considers, inter alia, many metabolic, biophysical, and physico-biochemical parameters of the tumor microenvironment rather than focusing on the complex composition of the tumor stroma, the cells therein, and their factors secreted, the key components of the tumor stroma, and the interactions between tumor cells, the extracellular matrix, and stromal cells (for reviews see, e.g., MUELLER and FUSENIG 2004; WITZ and LEVY-NISSENBAUM 2006; WEINBERG 2008; ARIZTIA et al. 2006; CUNHA et al. 2003; PARK et al. 2000; LIOTTA and KOHN 2001; FIDLER 2002; UNGER and WEAVER 2003; DENKO et al. 2003).

4.2

Tumor Vascularity

As already mentioned, newly formed microvessels in most solid tumors do not conform to the normal morphology of the host tissue vasculature (Fig. 4.1). The

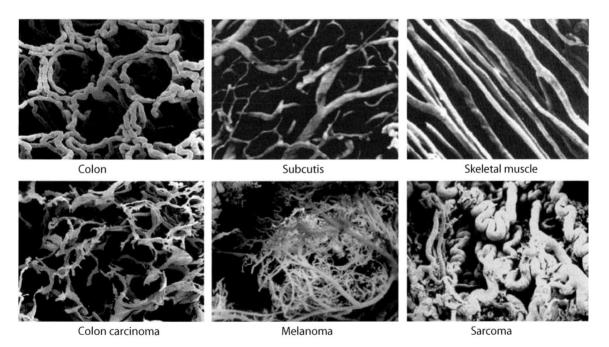

Colon	Subcutis	Skeletal muscle
Colon carcinoma	Melanoma	Sarcoma

Fig. 4.1. Differences in microvasculature between normal tissues (*upper panels*) and malignant tumors (*lower panels*; courtesy of Prof. Dr. M.A. Konerding, Department of Anatomy and Cell Biology, University of Mainz)

tumor vasculature can be described as a system that is maximally stimulated, yet only minimally fulfills the metabolic demands of the growing tumor that it supplies (HIRST and FLITNEY 1997).

Microvessels in solid tumors exhibit a large series of severe structural and functional abnormalities (see Table 4.2). They are often dilated, tortuous, elongated, and saccular. There is significant arterio-venous shunt perfusion (see Sect. 4.4) accompanied by a chaotic vascular organization that lacks any regulation matched to the metabolic demands or functional status of the tissue. Excessive branching is a common finding, often coinciding with blind vascular endings. Incomplete or even missing endothelial lining and interrupted basement membranes result in an increased vascular permeability with extravasation of blood plasma and of red blood cells expanding the interstitial fluid space and drastically increasing the hydrostatic pressure in the tumor interstitium (see Sect. 4.6). In solid tumors there is a rise in viscous resistance to flow caused mainly by hemoconcentration (increase in hematocrit of between 5 and 14%, BUTLER et al. 1975; VAUPEL and KALLINOWSKI 1987; SEVICK and JAIN 1989; Fig. 4.2, Table 4.2). Aberrant vascular morphology and a decrease in vessel density are responsible for an increase in geometric resistance to flow, which can lead to an inadequate perfusion. Substantial spatial heterogeneity in the distribution of tumor vessels and significant temporal heterogeneity in the microcirculation within a tumor (GILLIES et al. 1999) may result in a considerably anisotropic distribution of tumor tissue oxygenation and a number of other factors, which are usually closely linked and which define the so-called pathophysiological microenvironment. Variations in these relevant parameters between tumors are often more pronounced than differences occurring between different locations or microareas within a tumor (VAUPEL and HÖCKEL 2000; VAUPEL et al. 2001, 2003).

Tumor Blood Flow

A number of studies on blood flow through human tumors have been reported. Some of them are anecdotal reports rather than systematic investigations, and therefore definite conclusions cannot be drawn partly due to the use of non-validated techniques to measure flow in volume flow rate units. Considering the presently available data, the following conclusions can be drawn when flow data derived from different reports are pooled (for reviews see VAUPEL et al. 1989; VAUPEL and JAIN 1991; VAUPEL 1990, 1992, 1993, 1994a, 1998, 2004b, 2006):

1. Blood flow can vary considerably despite similar histological classification and primary site (0.01–2.9 ml/g/min; Fig. 4.3; VAUPEL 2006; LYNG et al. 2001; HAIDER et al. 2005).
2. Tumors can have flow rates that are similar to those measured in organs with a high metabolic rate such as liver, heart, or brain.
3. Some tumors exhibit flow rates that are even lower than those of tissues with a low metabolic rate such as skin, resting muscle, or adipose tissue.

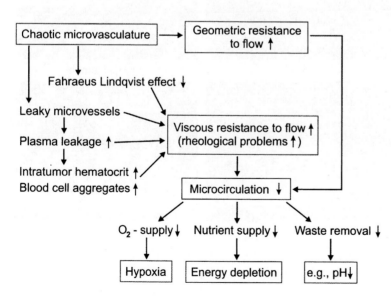

Fig. 4.2. Flow chart describing the mechanisms responsible for the increase in geometric and viscous resistance to flow caused by structural and functional abnormalities of the tumor microvasculature, which lead to a hostile tumor microenvironment

Table 4.2. Major structural and functional irregularities of tumor microvessels (updated from VAUPEL 2006)

1. Blood vessels	1. Blood vessels (*continued*)
Missing differentiation	Increased geometric resistance to flow
Loss of vessel hierarchy (disorganized vascular network)	Increase in hematocrit within tumor microvessels by 5–14%
Increased intervessel distances	Increased viscous resistance to flow
Existence of avascular areas	Unstable flow velocities (about 85% of all microvessels, REINHOLD and VAN DEN BERG-BLOK 1987, KIMURA et al. 1996)
Large diameter (sinusoidal) microvessels	
Elongated, tortuous (convoluted) vessels	Unstable direction of flow
Contour irregularities	Intermittent flow, regurgitation (about 5% of all microvessels, KIMURA et al. 1996)
Saccular microvessels, blind endings	
Aberrant branching (KONERDING et al. 2001)	Flow stasis (about 1% of all microvessels, KIMURA et al. 1996)
Haphazard pattern of vessel interconnection	
Incomplete endothelial lining, fenestrations	Plasma flow only (about 8% of all microvessels, KIMURA et al. 1996)
Interrupted or absent basement membranes	
Presence of lumen-less endothelial cell cords	Formation of platelet/leukocytes-clusters (BARONZIO et al. 2003)
Existence of vessel-like cavities not connected to the blood stream	Thrombus formations
Existence of tumor cell-lined vascular channels ("vascular mimicry")	Formation of RBC aggregates
Arterio-venous anastomoses (shunts)	Reduced Fahraeus-Lindqvist effect
Vessels originating from the venous side	Acidosis-induced rigidity of RBCs
Missing innervation	**2. Lymphatic vessels**
Lack of physiological/pharmacological receptors	Commonly infiltrated by tumor cells (periphery)
Lack of smooth muscle cells	Flattened vessels without lumen (center)
Poor or absent coverage by pericytes	VEGF-C- and VEGF-D-induced growth at tumor margin
Absence of vasomotion	
Absence of flow regulation	Inadequate lymphatic drainage in the tumor center
Increased vascular permeability, plasma leakage	Interstitial fluid flow
	Interstitial hypertension

It is not only the quantity of microvessels that counts, but also—or even more so—the quality of vascular function in terms of the tumor tissue supply or drainage!

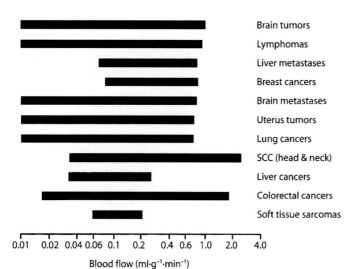

Fig. 4.3. Variability of blood flow rates in solid tumors (*SCC* = squamous cell carcinomas, modified from Vaupel and Höckel 2000)

4. Blood flow in human tumors can be higher or lower than that of the tissue of origin, depending on the functional state of the latter tissue (e.g., average blood flow in breast cancers is substantially higher than that of postmenopausal breast and significantly lower than flow data obtained in the lactating, parenchymal breast).

5. The average perfusion rate of carcinomas does not deviate substantially from that of soft tissue sarcomas.

6. Metastatic lesions exhibit a blood supply that is comparable to that of the primary tumor perhaps with the exception of those secondary lesions in the liver, which are preferentially supplied by the portal system (due to lower perfusion pressure).

7. In some tumor entities, blood flow in the periphery is distinctly higher than in the center, whereas in others, blood flow is significantly higher at the tumor center compared with the tumor edge.

8. Flow data from multiple sites of measurement show marked heterogeneity within individual tumors. In cervical cancer, the intratumor heterogeneity was similar to the intertumor heterogeneity (Lyng et al. 2001).

9. There is substantial temporal flow heterogeneity on a microscopic level within human tumors as shown by multichannel laser Doppler flowmetry (Hill et al. 1996; Pigott et al. 1996).

10. There is no association between tumor size and blood flow in many cancers (e.g., Wilson et al. 1992; Lyng et al. 2001).

11. Tumor blood flow is not regulated according to the metabolic demand as is the case in normal tissues.

4.4
Arterio-Venous Shunt Perfusion in Tumors

First rough estimations concerning the arterio-venous shunt flow in malignant tumors showed that at least 30% of the arterial blood can pass through experimental tumors without participating in the microcirculatory exchange processes (Vaupel et al. 1978; Weiss et al. 1979; Endrich et al. 1982). In patients receiving intraarterial chemotherapy for head and neck cancer, shunt flow is reported to be 8–43% of total tumor blood flow, the latter consistently exceeding normal tissue perfusion of the scalp (Wheeler et al. 1986). The mean fractional shunt perfusion of tumors was 23 ± 13% in studies utilizing ^{99m}Tc-labeled macroaggregated albumin (diameter of the particles, 15–90 μm). The significance of this shunt flow on local, intratumor pharmacokinetics, on the development of hypoxia, and on other relevant metabolic phenomena has not yet been systematically studied and remains speculative.

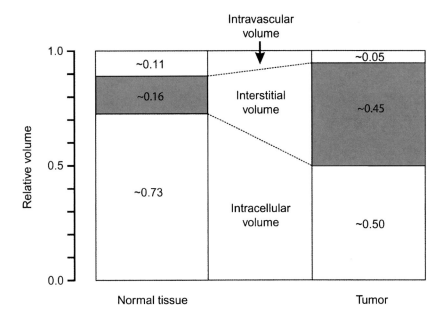

Fig. 4.4. Mean relative volumes of the intracellular fluid, the vascular compartment, and the interstitial fluid space in malignant tumors (*right panel*) and in normal tissue (*left panel*; adapted from Vaupel 1994a)

Volume and Characteristics of the Tumor Interstitial Space

The interstitial compartment of solid tumors is significantly different from that of most normal tissues (Vaupel and Mueller-Klieser 1983). In general, the tumor interstitial space is characterized by

1. an expansion of its volume, which is three to five times larger than in most normal tissues (Fig. 4.4),
2. high interstitial hydraulic conductivity and diffusivity,
3. a relatively large quantity of mobile, i.e., freely moving fluid in contrast to normal tissues where almost all of the fluid is in the gel phase, and
4. a quick spread of water-soluble agents (e.g., contrast agents) due to significant extravascular convection (Reinhold 1971).

Interstitial Fluid Pressure and Convective Currents into the Interstitial Space of Tumors

As already mentioned, the growing tumor produces new, often abnormally leaky (hyper-permeable) mi-

crovessels, but is unable to form its own functional lymphatics (Fukumura and Jain 2007). As a result, there is significant bulk flow of free fluid into the interstitial space. Whereas convective currents into the interstitial compartment are estimated to be about 0.5–1% of plasma flow in normal tissue, in human cancers water efflux into the interstitium can reach 15% of the respective plasma flow (Vaupel 1994a; see Fig. 4.5).

After seeping copiously out of the highly permeable tumor microvessels—an equilibrium is reached when the hydrostatic and oncotic pressures within the microvessels and the respective interstitial pressures become equal—fluid accumulates in the tumor extracellular matrix and a high interstitial fluid pressure (IFP) builds up in solid tumors (Young et al. 1950; Gutmann et al. 1992; Less et al. 1992; Milosevic et al. 2001, 2004).

Besides vessel hyper-permeability and lack of functional lymphatics, interstitial fibrosis and contraction of the interstitial space mediated by stromal fibroblasts may contribute to the development of interstitial hypertension (Heldin et al. 2004). Whereas in most normal tissues IFP is slightly subatmospheric ("negative") or just above atmospheric values (Guyton and Hall 2006), an interstitial hypertension with values up to 60–70 mmHg (Heldin et al. 2004; Lunt et al. 2008; Table 4.3) develops in cancers that forms a "physiologic" barrier to the delivery of therapeutic macromolecules to the cancer cells.

Table 4.3. Interstitial fluid pressure in normal tissues and in human tumors

Type of tissue	Mean interstitial fluid pressure (mmHg) [range]	Authors
A. Normal tissues		
Breast tissue	0	Jain (1994)
Skin	−2	Guyton and Hall (2006)
	−0.3	Nathanson and Nelson (1994)
	0.4	Jain (1994)
Subcutis	−3	Guyton and Hall (2006)
Fibrous tissue	−3	Gutmann et al. (1992)
Submucosa (paravaginal)	1	Milosevic et al. (1998)
Tightly encased tissues		
Brain	4 to 6	Guyton and Hall (2006)
Kidney	6	Guyton and Hall (2006)
B. Malignant tumors		
Renal cell carcinomas	38	Less et al. (1992)
Cervix cancers	16 [10–26]	Roh et al. (1991)
	19 [−6 to 76]	Milosevic et al. (1998)
	19 [3 to 48]	Milosevic et al. (2001)
	15 [6 to 40]	Haider et al. (2005)
	19 [−3 to 48]	Fyles et al. (2006)
Liver metastases (colorectal)	21 [4 to 45]	Less et al. (1992)
Head and neck carcinomas	15 [4 to 33]	Gutmann et al. (1992)
Breast carcinomas	17 [4 to 33]	Less et al. (1992)
Breast ca. (invasive, ductal)	29	Nathanson and Nelson (1994)
Melanomas	29 [0–110]	Curti et al. (1993)
Metastatic melanomas	14 [2–41]	Boucher et al. (1991)
	33 [20–50]	Less et al. (1992)
Non-Hodgkin's lymphomas	5 [1–12.5]	Curti et al. (1993)
Lung carcinomas	10	Jain (1994)

The tumor IFP is rather uniform throughout the center of the tumor, but drops steeply in the periphery. Fluid is squeezed out of the high- to the low-pressure regions at the tumor/normal tissue interface, carrying away antitumor drugs.

Despite increased overall leakiness, not all tumor microvessels are leaky. Vascular permeability varies from tumor to tumor and exhibits spatio-temporal heterogeneity within the same tumor as well as during tumor growth or regression. Furthermore, IFP in tumors fluctuates with changing microvascular pressures (Netti et al. 1995).

Transmural coupling between IFP and microvascular pressure due to the high permeability of tumor microvessels can abolish perfusion pressure differences between up- and down-stream tumor blood vessels and thus can lead to blood flow stasis in tumors without "physically" occluding (compressing) the vessels (Fukumura and Jain 2007). The equilibration of hydrostatic pressures between the interstitial and microvascular compartments is accompanied by a similar equilibration of oncotic pressures in both spaces (20.0 mmHg in plasma vs. 20.5 mmHg in solid tumors; Stohrer et al. 2000).

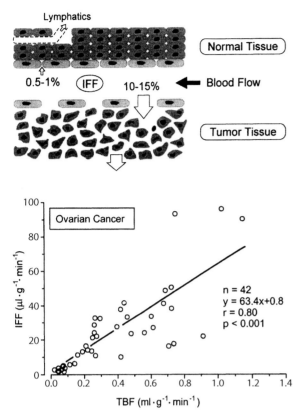

Fig. 4.5. Interstitial fluid flow (*IFF*) as a function of blood flow (*TBF*) in xenografted human ovarian cancers (*lower part*). Schematic representation of convective fluid currents in normal and tumor tissues (*upper part*; adapted from VAUPEL 2004b)

4.7
Tumor Hypoxia

In the following subsections (4.7.1–4.7.8), current knowledge concerning the oxygenation status of tumors and the occurrence of hypoxia in solid malignancies has been compiled, and the mechanisms causing tumor hypoxia are discussed. All data presented here are derived from clinical studies on the pretreatment oxygenation status of solid tumors using the computerized oxygen sensors (pO₂ histography system). This technique—based on a mechanically stable O₂ microsensor—is minimally invasive and allows the direct and reliable measurement of oxygen partial pressures (pO₂ values) in tissues. It provides quantitative measures and is (still) regarded as the "gold standard" for the assessment of the tissue oxygenation status (STONE et al. 1993).

4.7.1
Definition of Hypoxia

In pathophysiological terms, hypoxia is defined as a state of reduced O_2 availability or decreased O_2 partial pressures (O_2 tensions, pO_2 values) below critical thresholds, thus resulting in limitations of characteristic cellular or organ functions (HÖCKEL and VAUPEL 2001a). In contrast to normal tissues, malignant tumors obviously have no "physiological" functions. Thus, tumor hypoxia cannot be defined by functional deficits, although areas of necrosis—which are often found in tumors on microscopic examination—indicate the loss of vital cellular functions. In the following, the term hypoxia is used to describe critical O_2 levels below which clinical, biological, and/or molecular effects are progressively observed (e.g., acquired treatment resistance, ATP depletion, binding of hypoxic markers, slowing of proliferation rate, proteome and genome changes, metabolic hypoxic stress response, and development of an aggressive phenotype). In this discussion of hypoxic thresholds, it is important to note that, for any particular functional parameter, a sharp threshold between "hypoxia" (i.e., more hypoxic tumors) and "normoxia" (i.e., less hypoxic tumors) does not exist and should not be expected (HÖCKEL and VAUPEL 2001a). Generally, four descriptors of the tumor oxygenation status are used: the median tumor pO_2 value, the fraction of pO_2 values ≤ 2.5 mmHg (HF 2.5), the fraction of pO_2 values ≤ 5 mmHg (HF 5), and the fraction of pO_2 values ≤ 10 mmHg (HF 10).

Unfortunately, in an increasing number of reports on tumor oxygenation, the term hypoxia has been used in a somewhat unprecise manner, with clear definitions for the (experimental) conditions used and scientific questions being asked frequently not having been provided. As a result, discussions involving researchers and clinicians have often led to confusion since the single term hypoxia has been used by many groups to describe quite different conditions (HÖCKEL and VAUPEL 2001a). Anoxia describes the (patho-)physiological state where no O_2 is detectable (measurable) in the tissue ($pO_2 =$ 0 mmHg).

4.7.2
Pathogenesis of Tumor Hypoxia

Investigations carried out in the clinical setting over the last 2 decades demonstrated that the presence of hypoxic tissue areas with pO_2 values ≤ 2.5 mmHg is a characteristic pathophysiological property of locally advanced solid tumors, and such areas have been found in a wide range of human malignancies. Evidence has accumulated showing that at least 50–60% of locally advanced solid tumors may exhibit hypoxic and/or anoxic tissue areas that are heterogeneously distributed within the tumor mass. The hypoxic (or anoxic) areas arise as a result of an imbalance between the supply and consumption of oxygen. Whereas in normal tissues or organs the O₂ supply is matched to the metabolic re-

quirements, in solid tumors the O₂ consumption rate of neoplastic as well as stromal cells may outweigh an insufficient oxygen supply and result in the development of tissue areas with very low O₂ levels.

Tumor hypoxia predominantly results from an inadequate perfusion due to severe structural and functional abnormalities of the tumor microcirculation (see Fig. 4.6; for reviews see VAUPEL 1994a, 2004b, 2006, VAUPEL et al. 1989). Hypoxic (micro-) regions are heterogeneously

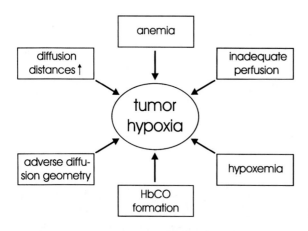

Fig. 4.6. Key factors in the pathogenesis of tumor hypoxia

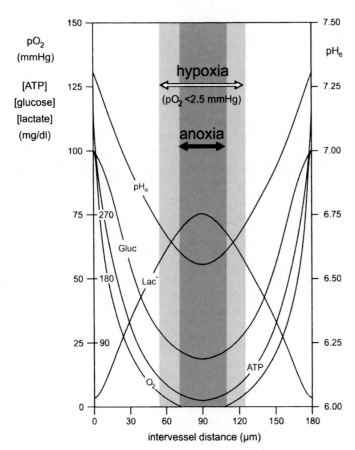

Fig. 4.7. Schematic representation of 2D profiles of relevant microenvironmental parameters within the intervessel space of tumors (adapted from VAUPEL 2004b)

distributed within the tumor mass and may be located adjacent to regions with O_2 tensions in the range of those found in the normal tissue neighboring the neoplastic lesion. Perfusion-limited O_2 delivery leads to ischemic hypoxia, which is often transient. For this reason, this type of hypoxia is also called "acute" hypoxia, a term that does not take into account the mechanisms underlying this condition (VAUPEL and MAYER 2005; VAUPEL et al. 2004). Alternatively, "acute" hypoxia often results as a consequence of transient flow with plasma only due to the very low O_2 content in plasma (GROEBE and VAUPEL 1988; VAUPEL et al. 1988).

Hypoxia in tumors can also be caused by an increase in diffusion distances, so that cells far away (>70 μm) from the nutritive blood vessel receive less oxygen than required (see Fig. 4.7). This condition is termed diffusion-limited hypoxia, also known as "chronic" hypoxia. In addition to enlarged diffusion distances, an adverse diffusion geometry (e.g., concurrent vs. countercurrent tumor microvessels) can also cause hypoxia (VAUPEL and HARRISON 2004).

Tumor-associated or therapy-induced anemia can lead to a reduced O_2 transport capacity of the blood, a major (systemic) factor contributing to the development of hypoxia (anemic hypoxia). This type of hypoxia is especially pronounced in tumors or tumor areas exhibiting low perfusion rates. A similar condition can be caused by carboxyhemoglobin (HbCO) formation in heavy smokers, which leads to a functional anemia, since hemoglobin blocked by carbon monoxide (CO) is no longer capable of transporting oxygen.

As already mentioned, tumor microvessels are frequently perfused (at least transiently) by plasma only. In this situation, hypoxemic hypoxia develops very rapidly around these vessels because only a few tumor cells at the arterial end can be supplied adequately. Similarly, hypoxia can rapidly develop in (primary or metastatic) liver tumors that are preferentially supplied by branches of the portal vein. There is abundant evidence for the existence of a substantial heterogeneity in the development and extent of tumor hypoxia due to pronounced intra-tumor (and inter-tumor) variabilities in vascularity and perfusion rates (for reviews see VAUPEL 1994a, 2004b; VAUPEL et al. 1989, 2007).

4.7.3
Oxygenation Status of Carcinomas of the Uterine Cervix

Current knowledge on the oxygenation status of primary cancers of the uterine cervix generally refers to pretherapeutic data obtained in pre- and postmenopausal, con-

scious women. Mean and median O_2 tensions obtained from >13,500 measurements in 150 primary carcinomas of the uterine cervix were, on average, distinctly lower than in normal tissues (see Fig. 4.8). Oxygen tensions measured in the normal cervix of nulliparous women revealed a median pO_2 of 42 mmHg, whereas in locally advanced cancers of the cervix (stages FIGO Ib-IVa), the median pO_2 was 10 mmHg (see Table 4.4). When tumors of different clinical sizes are compared, there is no evidence of a correlation between the maximum tumor diameter and the median pO_2, the fraction of pO_2 values ≤2.5 mmHg, or the fraction of pO_2 values ≤5 mmHg. In addition, there is no characteristic topological distribution of O_2 tensions within cervix cancers (i.e., as a function of the measurement site; e.g., tumor periphery vs. tumor center).

The oxygenation status and the extent of pretherapeutically measured hypoxic tissue areas are independent of the FIGO stage, histological type, and pathohistological grade. Similarly, there was no association between the oxygenation patterns and parity, menopausal status, smoking habits, or a series of other clinically relevant parameters. In cervical cancers, the median pO_2 values rose with increasing hemoglobin concentrations over the range from 10 to 13 g/dl. At Hb levels >14 g/dl, a worsening of the tumor oxygenation became apparent (VAUPEL and MAYER 2005; VAUPEL et al. 2002b, 2006a). These data suggest that an optimal cHb range exists with regard to the median pO_2. The rise in the median pO_2 is based on an increase in the O_2 transport capacity of the blood with increases in cHb values up to approximately 13 g/dl. At higher cHb values, this effect is counteracted by a substantial increase in the viscous resistance to flow (i.e., a deterioration of the blood's rheological properties) caused by a pronounced increase in blood viscosity within the chaotic microvasculature, which is further aggravated by a high vascular permeability (leaky blood vessel walls) that obligatorily leads to a severe intratumor hemoconcentration, finally leading to a net reduction in oxygen supply (VAUPEL and MAYER 2004; VAUPEL et al. 2006a). About 60% of locally advanced carcinomas of the uterine cervix (FIGO stages Ib-III) exhibited hypoxic (pO_2 ≤2.5 mmHg) and/or anoxic ($pO_2 = 0$ mmHg) tissue areas, which are heterogeneously distributed within the tumor mass.

From our systematic studies on the oxygenation status of locally advanced solid tumors, there was clear evidence that tumor-to-tumor variability in the oxygenation status was significantly greater than intra-tumor variability, both for squamous cell carcinomas and for adenocarcinomas of the uterine cervix (HÖCKEL and VAUPEL 2001a,b; HÖCKEL et al. 1999).

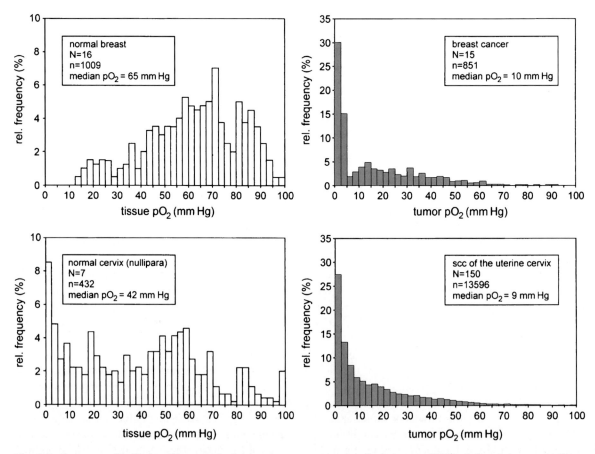

Fig. 4.8. Frequency distribution (*histograms*) of oxygen partial pressures (*pO₂*) measured in normal breast (*upper left panel*) and in locally advanced breast cancers (T1b-T4, *upper right panel*), in normal cervix of nullipara (*lower left panel*), and in squamous cell carcinomas (*SCC*) of the uterine cervix (*lower right panel*). N = number of patients; n = number of pO₂ values measured (reviewed in Vaupel et al. 2007)

In order to clarify whether the pathological tumor stage (pT) rather than the FIGO stage may have an impact on the oxygenation status, pathological tumor staging was performed based on histopathological investigation of the surgical specimens following radical hysterectomy or exenteration and lymph node dissection in a subgroup of 65 patients treated with primary surgery (with curative intent). This procedure identified a median maximum (histological) tumor diameter of 40 mm (Höckel and Vaupel 2001a, 2003). In tumors with a maximum extension <40 mm ($n = 37$), the median pO₂ was 11 mmHg, which was significantly higher than the respective pO₂ value in tumors with a maximum diameter >40 mm ($n = 28$, median pO₂ = 5 mmHg; $p < 0.05$). Median pO₂ values in stage pT1b tumors were significantly higher (18 mmHg) than in pT2b lesions (5 mmHg, $p < 0.05$). Hypoxic fractions were slightly lower in pT1b (bulky) tumors than in pT2b malignancies. From these data it can be concluded that only a detailed histopathological tumor staging using surgical specimens enables detection of stage- and size-related differences in the oxygenation status of primary cancers of the uterine cervix. Clinical tumor dimensions and FIGO staging are not sufficiently accurate to allow for the estimation and characterization of the tumor oxygenation (Höckel and Vaupel 2001a).

In an earlier study, Sundfør et al. (1998a) pointed out that adenocarcinomas (AC) of the uterine cervix were significantly better oxygenated than squamous cell carcinomas (SCC). In our studies, however, pO₂ values were comparable in tumors of both histologies: median pO₂ = 11 mmHg in SCC vs. 12 mmHg in AC, and mean pO₂ = 16 mmHg in SCC vs. 18 mmHg in AC. There were only slight differences in the fraction of pO₂ values ≤2.5 mmHg (25% in SCC vs. 16% in AC), in the fraction of pO₂ values ≤5 mmHg (38% in SCC vs. 32% in AC), and in the percentage of patients with tumor pO₂ values ≤2.5 mmHg (60% in SCC vs. 66% in AC). The better stage-for-stage prognosis for SCC than for AC of the uterine cervix thus cannot be explained by a substantially different oxygenation status between tumors with these histologies.

Measurements of intra-tumoral oxygenation in locally recurrent cervical carcinomas with a methodological approach similar to that developed for the primary disease showed a pronounced shift to more hypoxic oxygenation profiles in the recurrent tumors as compared to the primary lesions (Höckel et al. 1998). Median pO_2 values in 53 pelvic recurrences of SCC were significantly lower than the median pO_2 values of 117 primary tumors of comparable sizes (7 mmHg vs. 12 mmHg, $p < 0.001$).

In locally recurrent tumors, no significant differences in the oxygenation status between SCC and AC were observed. For both histologies the median pO_2 was lower, and the hypoxic fraction with pO_2 values ≤ 2.5 mmHg was higher in recurrent tumors than in the primaries. The percentage of patients with pO_2 values ≤ 2.5 mmHg in recurrent tumors was 77% for SCC ($n = 46$) and 87% for AC ($n = 14$), respectively.

An analysis of inter-group differences in tumor oxygenation indicated that the greater the extent of hypoxia in primary tumors, the higher the probability of local recurrence of cervix cancers.

When the available data on pretreatment tumor oxygenation of locally advanced cancers of the uterine cervix is summarized (Höckel and Vaupel 2001b; Vaupel and Höckel 2001; Höckel et al. 1991, 1998; Vaupel et al. 2007), there is evidence that

a) Oxygenation in tumors is heterogeneous and compromised as compared to normal tissues.

b) Tumor oxygenation is not regulated according to the metabolic demands as is the case in normal tissues.

c) Causative factors for the development of hypoxia are limitations in perfusion and diffusion as well as tumor-associated anemia.

d) On average, the median pO_2 values in primary cancers of the uterine cervix are lower than those in the normal cervix.

e) Many cervical cancers contain hypoxic tissue areas (at least 60% in SCC).

f) There is no characteristic topological distribution of O_2 tensions within cervix cancers.

g) Tumor-to-tumor variability in oxygenation is greater than intra-tumor variability.

h) Tumor oxygenation is independent of various patient demographics (e.g., age, menopausal status, parity).

i) Anemia (found in approximately 30% of patients at diagnosis) considerably contributes to the development of hypoxia, especially in low-flow tumor areas.

j) In cervix cancers of moderately/severely anemic patients, hypoxic areas are more frequently found than in non-anemic patients.

k) Tumor oxygenation and the extent of hypoxia are independent of clinical size, FIGO stage, histological type (SCC vs. AC), grade, and lymph node status.

l) Tumor oxygenation is weakly dependent on the pathological tumor stage (pT stage).

m) Local recurrences of cervix cancers have a higher hypoxic fraction than the primary tumors.

n) Hypoxia in cervical cancers has been found to be of prognostic significance in many investigations (see Table 4.4 and Fig. 4.9).

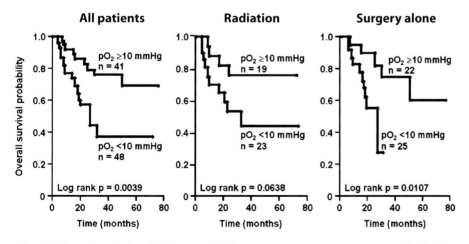

Fig. 4.9. Overall survival probabilities stratified by tumor oxygenation status, estimated by Kaplan-Meier methods for patients with advanced cancers of the uterine cervix (modified from Höckel et al. 1996b). n = number of patients

Table 4.4. Pretherapeutic oxygenation status of primary, locally advanced cancer of the uterine cervix and prognostic significance of tumor hypoxia (n = number of patients)

Center	n	Median pO$_2$ (mmHg) [range]	HF 2.5 (%)	HF 5 (%)	HF 10 (%)	Prognostic significance of tumor hypoxia — Endpoint	Oxygenation parameter	References
Mainz/ Leipzig	150	10 [2–34]	23	37	50	DFS, OS	pO$_2$ <10 mmHg	Höckel et al. (1993a,b, 1996a,b)
Toronto	135	5 [0–94]		50		DFS, PFS, DS[a]	pO$_2$ <5 mmHg	Doll et al. (2003), Fyles et al. (1998, 2002), Milosevic et al. (2001b), Pitson et al. (2001), Wong et al. (1997)
Halle	87	17 [0–81]	16	26				Dunst et al. (1999, 2003a), Hänsgen et al. (2001)
Leipzig	86	5 [1–57]						Leo et al. (2005)
Vienna	51	10 [0–60]	22	28	50	DFS, (LC)	pO$_2$ <10 mmHg	Knocke et al. (1999)
Oslo	49	4 [1–25]	47	64	76	DFS, OS, LC DS	HSV[b] pO$_2$ <5 mmHg pO$_2$ <10 mmHg	Lyng et al. (1997, 2000), Rofstad et al. (2000), Sundfør et al. (1997, 1998a,b, 2000)
Manchester	43	3 [0–42]	39	58	75			Airley et al. (2001), Cooper et al. (1999), Nordsmark et al. (2003), Cooper et al. (2000)
	30	6 [0–41]						
Paris	37	12	15	17	21			Lartigau et al. (1992a,b, 1999)
Aarhus	24	3 [0–19]	49	61	73			Nordsmark et al. (2003)
Vancouver	19	3 [0–34]	38	66	76			Acquino-Parsons et al. (2000), Nordsmark et al. (2003)
Vienna	10	17 [3–54]		42				Weitmann et al. (2003)
Durham	9	5		61				Brizel et al. (1995)
Overall	730	9	28	44	59			Vaupel et al. (2007)

[a] In node-negative patients

[b] Hypoxic subvolume calculated as the product of the total tumor volume and the relative frequency of hypoxic pO$_2$ readings <5 mmHg

There may be some overlaps in patients reported from the same institution. *Empty boxes* indicate lack of suitable information.

DFS = disease-free survival, *OS* = overall survival, *PFS* = progression-free survival, *DS* = distant spread, *LC* = local control

4.7.4
Oxygenation Status of Primary and Metastatic Cancers of the Head and Neck

The accessibility of primary and metastatic squamous cell carcinomas (SCC) of the head and neck for tumor oxygenation assessment has meant that these tumors have received considerable attention with a large number of studies already documented (see Table 4.5). Reliable O_2-sensitive polarographic electrodes for measurement of O_2 tensions in head and neck cancers were first used by GATENBY et al. (1985, 1988). These authors convincingly demonstrated that hypoxia in advanced tumors was associated with a poor prognosis.

Relevant oxygenation data derived from primary head and neck tumors (BECKER et al. 1998a,b, 2000; BRIZEL et al. 1997, 1999; FLECKENSTEIN et al. 1988; LARTIGAU et al. 1998; SAUMWEBER et al. 1995; STADLER et al. 1998, 1999) and from metastatic lesions of SCC of the head and neck (BECKER et al. 1998a,b, 2000; BRIZEL et al. 1997, 1999; EBLE et al. 1995; FÜLLER et al. 1994; LARTIGAU et al. 1993, 1994, 1998; MARTIN et al. 1993; NORDSMARK et al. 1996b; STADLER et al. 1999; STRNAD et al. 1997) were summarized in 1998 (see Fig. 4.10; VAUPEL et al. 1998) and in 2001 (see Fig. 4.9; VAUPEL 2001). The latter pO_2 measurements published between 1988 and 2000 confirm, in essence, the oxygenation pattern described for cancers of the uterine cervix.

For primary tumors the following descriptive parameters for the oxygenation status (pooled data) have been calculated: overall median $pO_2 = 13$ mmHg and overall HF 2.5 = 19%. A pronounced inter-institutional difference becomes obvious when the data from several centers are compared, with less hypoxic tumors being reported by the Stanford group (TERRIS 2000) and Durham (Duke) documenting more patients with more hypoxic tumors (BRIZEL et al. 1997, 1999).

For metastatic tumors, the following descriptive parameters for the oxygenation status have been assessed (pooled data collected between 1993 and 2000): overall median $pO_2 = 13.5$ mmHg and overall HF 2.5 = 17%. On comparing these latter data with pO_2 parameters of primary tumors, it becomes evident that no obvious difference between the oxygenation status of primary and metastatic tumors of the head and neck exists. Again, pronounced inter-institutional differences can be seen, with Stanford reporting relatively more patients with less hypoxic tumors and Durham more patients with more hypoxic tumors.

An updated summary of all major studies on the oxygenation status of head and neck cancers and on the relationship between pretreatment pO_2 measurements and survival in advanced tumors after primary radiotherapy has been published by NORDSMARK et al. (2005). In Table 4.5 tumor oxygenation data and survival in 397 primary head and neck cancers as summarized by NORDSMARK et al. (2005) and updated to include results communicated subsequently are shown (CLAVO et al. 2004; LE et al. 2003).

As was the case for cancers of the uterine cervix, pO_2 data clearly show that an optimal Hb level with regard to the median pO_2 values of head and neck cancers is seen at cHb values of between 12.5 and 14.5 g/dl (see Fig. 4.11; BECKER et al. 2000; NORDSMARK et al. 2005; VAUPEL and MAYER 2004; VAUPEL et al. 2005, 2006a). Furthermore, when comparing the parameters of the oxygenation status, there is a trend suggesting that can-

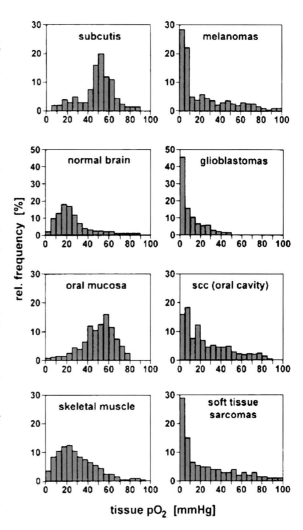

Fig. 4.10. Compilation of pO_2 histograms (i.e., frequency distributions of measured pO_2 values) for normal tissues (*left*) and for malignant tumors growing in the respective tissue site (*right*). *SCC* = squamous cell carcinomas (adapted from VAUPEL et al. 1998)

Table 4.5. Pretherapeutic oxygenation status of head and neck cancers[a] and prognostic significance of tumor hypoxia (n = number of patients)

Center	n	Median pO₂ (mmHg) [range]	HF 2.5 (%)	HF 5 (%)	Prognostic significance of tumor hypoxia — Endpoint	Oxygenation parameter	References
Halle/ Munich	125	9 [0–59]		33	OS	HSV[b]	Dunst et al. (2003)
Durham	86	5 [0–60]		51	DFS, OS, LC	pO₂ <10 mmHg	Brizel et al. (1997, 1999), Nordsmark et al. (2005)
Aarhus	67	13 [0–54]	22	32	LC	pO₂ <2.5 mmHg	Nordsmark and Overgaard (2000, 2004)
Stanford	65	12 [0–45]		25			Le et al. (2003)
Heidelberg	44	7 [0–60]	25	44	OS	pO₂ <2.5 mmHg	Rudat et al. (2000, 2001)
Paris	40	9 [0–55]	22	41			Lartigau et al. (1993), Martin et al. (1993), Nordsmark et al. (2005)
Stanford	37	19 [0–77]	16	21	LC	Median pO₂ (trend)	Adam et al. (1999)
Heidelberg	37	3	45	58	No evidence		Dietz et al. (2000, 2003)
Stanford	25	18 [0–51]	0	2	No evidence		Terris (2000)
Aachen	20	11 [0–22]	32	44			Di Martino et al. (2005)
Las Palmas	16	16	20	29			Clavo et al. (2004)
Leipzig/ Aachen	16	10					Scholbach et al. (2005)
Erlangen	14	16	19	35			Strnad et al. (1997)
Overall	592	10	21	32			Vaupel et al. (2007)

[a] Tumor oxygenation was measured in neck node metastases (predominantly) and in primary cancers

[b] Hypoxic subvolume calculated as the product of the total tumor volume and the relative frequency of hypoxic pO₂ readings <5 mmHg

There may be some overlaps in patients reported from the same institution. *Empty boxes* indicate lack of suitable information.

For further explanations, see Table 4.4.

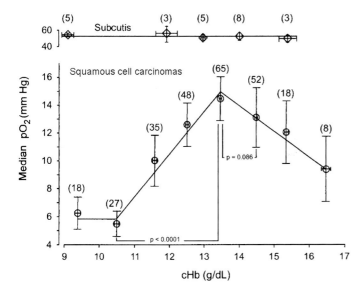

Fig. 4.11. Oxygenation status of squamous cell carcinomas of the head and neck and of the uterine cervix (*lower curve*) and of the normal subcutis (*upper curve*) as a function of hemoglobin levels (*cHb*). *n* = number of patients

cers of the head and neck may be slightly better oxygenated than cervical cancers (Tables 4.4 and 4.5), due primarily to the smaller hypoxic fractions found in head and neck tumors. Hypoxia in head and neck cancers is of prognostic significance in many investigations (see Table 4.5).

4.7.5
Oxygenation Status of Breast Cancers

Many breast cancers reveal hypoxic tissue areas that are heterogeneously distributed within the tumor mass. Mean and median O_2 tensions (pO_2) obtained from different pathological stages and histological grades are on average distinctly lower than in the normal breast or in fibrocystic disease (Fig. 4.8). Oxygen tensions measured in normal breast tissue revealed a mean (and median) pO_2 of 65 mmHg, whereas in breast cancers of stages T1b-T4, the median pO_2 was 28 mmHg (Vaupel et al. 1991). Nearly 60% of the primary breast cancers investigated exhibited pO_2 values ≤ 2.5 mmHg, i.e., tissue areas with less than half-maximum radiosensitivity. In contrast, in the normal breast, pO_2 values ≤ 12.5 mmHg were not found (Vaupel et al. 1991). In earlier studies on breast cancers, bimodal pO_2 distribution curves were obtained indicating a relevant contribution of pO_2 readings from the stromal compartment of breast cancers in these measurements, possibly due to partial inflammation. A contribution of pO_2 readings in the stromal

compartment is substantiated by the finding that pO_2 readings under ultrasound guidance are on average lower (Fig. 4.8). Thus, unintentional pO_2 measurements in the stromal compartment of breast cancer can cause a shift in the pO_2 histogram to higher values (Vaupel and Höckel 2004; Vaupel et al. 2002a).

When tumors of different clinical sizes are compared, there is no evidence of a correlation between the median pO_2 and the diameter of the tumor. This implies that the oxygenation in breast cancers and the occurrence of hypoxia and/or anoxia do not correlate with clinical stage (Vaupel and Höckel 1999, 2000, 2004; Vaupel et al. 1991). Similarly, there is no association between tumor size and blood flow (Grischke et al. 1994; Wilson et al. 1992). In addition, there is substantial evidence that the oxygenation patterns do not correlate with either histology (Falk et al. 1992; Vaupel et al. 1991) or a series of other clinically relevant parameters, e.g., hormone receptor status, parity, menopausal status, and smoking habits (Vaupel et al. 1991). In contrast, a significant correlation between the mean pO_2 values, fraction of hypoxic pO_2 readings, the degree of differentiation, and prognostic markers was found in a subsequent study (Hohenberger et al. 1998).

No significant differences were found between pre- and postmenopausal patients, between lobular and ductal carcinomas, and between tumors in the upper versus lower quadrants. No correlation between pathological staging or grading and the number of pO_2 readings at zero level, the pO_2 readings from 0 to 2.5 mmHg, the mean or median pO₂, and the 10th and 90th percentiles could be detected. Up to now, no correlations have been found between the oxygenation status of the tumors and the extent of necrosis or fibrosis (information based on qualitative evaluation). There is marked tumor-to-tumor variability, even when tumors of the same clinical size, stage (pT2), grade (G2), and histology (ductal carcinomas) are compared (VAUPEL et al. 1991). For this reason, tumor oxygenation is unpredictable in terms of clinical size, stage, grade, or histological type.

The pretreatment oxygenation status in breast cancers tended to be poorer and the occurrence of hypoxia and/or anoxia was more frequent in anemic patients than in nonanemic women (cHb > 12 g/dl; VAUPEL et al. 2002a, 2003a).

When comparing pO₂ data of breast cancers measured with the computerized pO₂ histography system by different institutions, significant inexplicable interinstitutional variation in the oxygenation status was observed (see Table 4.6).

As was the case with primary tumors, the oxygenation of metastatic lesions is generally heterogeneous and lower than that of normal tissues at the site of metastatic growth. Metastatic lesions of breast cancers tended to have a poorer oxygenation status than the primaries. Local recurrences of breast cancers also seem to have a higher hypoxic fraction than the primary tumors, although this information is based on only one communication (FÜLLER et al. 1994).

4.7.6
Oxygenation Status of Soft Tissue Sarcomas

As was the case with the tumor entities listed above, the oxygenation of soft tissue sarcomas (STS) was significantly lower than that of the skeletal muscle (VAUPEL et al. 1998; see Fig. 4.10; NORDSMARK et al. 1994) or of benign tumors (e.g., lipomas, schwannomas; BENTZEN et al. 2003). Tumor oxygenation was markedly het-

Table 4.6. Pretherapeutic oxygenation status of breast cancers (*n* = number of patients)[a]

Center	n	Median pO₂ (mmHg)	HF 2.5 (%)	HF 5 (%)	HF 10 (%)	References
Munich	41	2	68	87		RAAB et al. (2002)
Mainz/Leipzig	37	6	25	49		VAUPEL et al. (2003a)
Berlin[b]	32	44	7		17	HOHENBERGER et al. (1998)
Mainz	18	28	6	15	32	VAUPEL et al. (1991)
Mannheim	18	23	8	16	26	RUNKEL et al. (1994)
Durham	18	21		35		VUJASKOVIC et al. (2003)
Leipzig	15	10	30	45	50	VAUPEL et al. (2002a)
Durham	15	6				BRIZEL (1999)
Durham	13	14				JONES et al. (2004)
Oxford	5	24	5		13	FALK et al. (1992)
Overall	212	10[c]	30[c]	47[c]	50[c]	VAUPEL et al. (2007)

[a] No convincing data on the prognostic significance of tumor hypoxia in breast cancers available so far

[b] General anesthesia, inspiratory O₂ concentration = 30%

[c] Only pO₂ readings obtained under ultrasound guidance included

There may be some overlaps in patients reported from the same institution. *Empty boxes* indicate lack of suitable information.

erogeneous (NORDSMARK et al. 1996a, 1997) with the variation in oxygenation between tumors being significantly greater than that within tumors (BRIZEL et al. 1994; NORDSMARK et al. 1994, 1996a). No correlation was found between the oxygenation status and volume, histopathology, grade of malignancy, p53 status and other tumor features, or several patient characteristics (NORDSMARK et al. 1996a, 2001). In addition, no association with electrode position within tumors (i.e., between the depth from the tumor surface and measured pO_2 values) was seen (BRIZEL et al. 1994). In contrast to the tumor entities described above, no correlation with Hb levels was found (NORDSMARK et al. 1996a). Again, a pronounced inter-institutional variation becomes obvious when data from several centers are compared, with less hypoxic tumors reported by the Aarhus group (NORDSMARK et al. 1994, 1997) and the group

from Philadelphia (EVANS et al. 2001). In addition, pronounced intra-institutional differences are reported by the Duke (Durham) group when the median pO_2 is considered (6 mmHg vs. 21 mmHg; BRIZEL et al. 1994, 1996a,b). Factors that might be responsible for these differences have not yet been communicated. Hypoxia in STS is of prognostic significance in investigations involving large numbers of patients (see Table 4.7).

4.7.7
Oxygenation Status of Brain Tumors

Studies performed so far on primary brain tumors convincingly show the existence of areas of severe hypoxia in both high- and low-grade brain tumors (e.g., BEPPU et al. 2002; CRUICKSHANK et al. 1994; KAYAMA et al.

Table 4.7. Pretherapeutic oxygenation status of soft tissue sarcomas and prognostic significance of tumor hypoxia (n = number of patients)

Center	n	Median pO_2 (mmHg) [range]	HF 2.5 (%)	HF 5 (%)	HF 10 (%)	Prognostic significance of tumor hypoxia — Endpoint	Oxygenation parameter	References
Durham	45	10				DFS	pO_2 <10 mmHg	BRIZEL (1999)
Durham	34	6 [0–68]				DFS	Median pO_2	BRIZEL et al. (1996b)
Aarhus	31	19 [1–58]				DFS, OS	pO_2 <19 mmHg	NORDSMARK et al. (2001)
Durham	30	10				DFS	pO_2 <10 mmHg	BRIZEL et al. (1996a)
Durham	28	10						DEWHIRST et al. (2005)
Aarhus	25	22 [1–58]	5					NORDSMARK et al. (1997)
Aarhus	22	18		17				NORDSMARK et al. (1996a)
Aarhus	18	23		10				NORDSMARK et al. (1994)
Durham	15	18		31				BRIZEL et al. (1995)
Durham	9	21 [2–38]	19	29	44			BRIZEL et al. (1994)
Munich/ Essen	8			10				FÜLLER et al. (1994)
Munich/ Essen	7[a]		8					MOLLS et al. (1994)
Aarhus	6	10 [1–34]	18					BENTZEN et al. (2003)
Philadelphia	5		4	45	57	74		EVANS et al. (2001)
Overall	283		14	13	21			VAUPEL et al. (2007)

[a] Recurrent soft tissue sarcomas.

There may be some overlaps in patients reported from the same institution. *Empty boxes* indicate lack of suitable information.

1991; Moringlane 1994; Vaupel 1994b, 2002; see Table 4.8).

As was also seen in the other tumor entities characterized so far, pO₂ values varied widely among patients (Knisely and Rockwell 2002) and were distinctly lower than in the normal brain tissue (see. Fig. 4.10; Vaupel et al. 1998; Rampling et al. 1994; Vaupel 1994b). Hypoxia was not an artifact of general anesthesia (as it was also not in the before-mentioned tumor entities), since comparable hypoxic areas were also found in patients undergoing craniotomy under local anesthetics. An association between oxygenation status and clinical tumor size has so far not been found. There is evidence that hypoxia might be grade-dependent (Collingridge et al. 1999; Lally et al. 2004; Moringlane 1994) with high-grade gliomas exhibiting poorer oxygenation status than low-grade tumors.

Increasing hypoxia with increasing tumor aggressiveness and rapidity of growth was observed by Rampling et al. (1994). In contrast, Evans et al. (2004b)

failed to find correlations between oxygenation parameters (median pO₂, HF 2.5, HF 5, and HF 10) and histopathological grade. In a mixed group of metastatic brain tumors, marked hypoxia was also a common finding (Rampling et al. 1994). In five metastatic lesions within the brain (maximum tumor diameter: 38 mm), the median pO₂ was 10 mmHg (range: 3–24 mmHg), the hypoxic fraction of pO₂ values ≤2.5 mmHg being 26% (range: 1.5–46.5%). From these data it may be concluded that metastatic lesions in the brain do not substantially deviate from primary tumors in terms of oxygenation status.

4.7.8
Pretherapeutic Oxygenation Status of Miscellaneous Tumors

Quantitative data on the oxygenation status of several other tumor entities as assessed by pO₂ histography—

Table 4.8. Pretherapeutic oxygenation status of primary brain tumors and prognostic significance of tumor hypoxia (n = number of patients)

Center	n	Median pO₂ (mmHg) [range]	HF 2.5 (%)	HF 5 (%)	HF 10 (%)	References
Philadelphia	26	22	16	25	40	Evans et al. (2004b)
New Haven	25	5[e]				Lally et al. (2004)
	14[b]	3 [0–30]				
	11[c]	15 [0–40]				
New Haven[a]	23	11 [0–40]	40			Collingridge et al. (1999)
	13[b]	6	48			
	10[c]	17	31			
Glasgow	15	9 [0–42]	42			Rampling et al. (1994)
	10[d]	7	38	45	59	
Philadelphia	12[d]	22	6	16	37	Evans et al. (2004a)
Las Palmas	3[b]	13		28	49	Clavo et al. (2002)
Overall	104	13	26			Vaupel et al. (2007)

[a] Mean arterial O₂ tension: 200 mmHg

[b] High grade gliomas

[c] Low grade gliomas

[d] Glioblastomas

[e] No prognostic value of the median pO₂

There may be some overlaps in patients reported from the same institution. *Empty boxes* indicate lack of suitable information.

and not yet mentioned in this article—are compiled in Table 4.9. Again, there is clear evidence that the oxygenation of these tumors is distinctly poorer than that of the respective normal tissues (see Fig. 4.10; Vaupel et al. 1998; see Table 4.10). For prostate cancers, there are again pronounced inter-institutional and intra-institutional variations that cannot yet be explained. With the exception of prostate cancer, the number of patients is rather low so that further discussion of the data here is not appropriate at this time. Tumor oxygenation measurements in 28 tumors summarized by Aquino-Parsons et al. (1999) are not included here since 12 different histologies were listed, making a systematic evaluation impossible. The overall median pO_2 value for all 28 tumors was 24 mmHg (range: 0–54 mmHg).

Considering all data of the oxygenation status of solid tumors, it can be concluded that all types of solid tumors contain tissue areas that are severely hypoxic with great inter- and intra-institutional variations. Tumor hypoxia mainly results from inadequate perfusion and diffusion within tumors and from a reduced O_2 transport capacity in anemic patients. Hypoxic areas are heterogeneously distributed within the tumors. The development, existence, and extent of hypoxia are usually independent of a series of patient and tumor characteristics. Tumor oxygenation is—as a rule—poorer than that of the respective normal tissue. The oxygenation status of cancers of the cervix and of the head and neck as well as oxygenation parameters of soft tissue sarcomas may be independent adverse prognostic factors and may help to select patients for individual and/or intensified treatment schedules. The significance of tumor oxygenation as an adverse prognostic factor is most probably based on acquired treatment resistance and on hypoxia-induced malignant progression (see Sects. 4.8 and 4.9).

Table 4.9. Pretherapeutic oxygenation status of miscellaneous human tumors (n = number of patients)

Center	n	Median pO_2 (mmHg) [range]	HF 2.5 (%)	HF 5 (%)	HF 10 (%)	References
Prostate cancer						
Philadelphia	57	2 [0–68]				Movsas et al. (2002)
	55	10				Movsas et al. (2000)
Toronto	55	5 [0–57]		60		Parker et al. (2004)
Philadelphia	13	21 [0–45]				Cvetkovic et al. (2001)
	10	11 [2–38]	45	49		Movsas et al. (1999)
Vulvar cancer						
Mainz/Leipzig	29	11	25	40		Vaupel et al. (2002b)
	15[a]	13	25	37		Vaupel et al. (2006b)
	19[b]	11	25	45		
Vancouver	20	10	29			Stone et al. (2005)

[a]Primaries

[b]Recurrencies

There may be some overlaps in patients reported from the same institution. *Empty boxes* indicate lack of suitable information. For a review see Vaupel et al. (2007)

Table 4.9. (*continued*) Pretherapeutic oxygenation status of miscellaneous human tumors (*n* = number of patients)

Center	n	Median pO$_2$ (mmHg) [range]	HF 2.5 (%)	HF 5 (%)	HF 10 (%)	References
Non Hodgkin's lymphoma						
London	8	18	36		43	Powell et al. (1999)
Malignant melanoma (metastatic)						
Paris	18	12	5	17	40	Lartigau et al. (1997)
Lung cancer						
Cambridge	6	14	13	24	36	Falk et al. (1992)
Stanford	20	17				Le et al. (2006)
Pancreatic adenocarcinoma						
Stanford	7[c]	2	59			Koong et al. (2000)
Lund	1	2				Graffman et al. (2001)
Renal cell carcinoma						
Heidelberg (Australia)	3	10				Lawrentschuk et al. (2005)
Rectal carcinomas						
Heidelberg (Germany)	14	32		10		Kallinowski and Buhr (1995a,b) Mattern et al. (1996)
	15	19				
Liver tumors (metastatic)						
Heidelberg (Germany)	4	6			75	Kallinowski and Buhr (1995a,b)

[c] All patients were anemic

There may be some overlaps in patients reported from the same institution. *Empty boxes* indicate lack of suitable information. For a review see Vaupel et al. (2007)

Table 4.10. Oxygenation status of normal tissues

Tissue	Median pO$_2$ (mmHg)	HF 2.5 (%)	HF 5 (%)	HF 10 (%)	References
Pancreas	57	2			Koong et al. (2000)
Breast	52	0	0	0	Vaupel et al. (2003a)
Rectal mucosa	52				Kallinowski and Buhr (1995a)
Subcutis	51	0	0	4	Vaupel et al. (2003a)
Cervix	42	8	13	20	Höckel et al. (1991)
Kidney	31	3		8	Lawrentschuk et al. (2005)
Skeletal muscle	30				Movsas et al. (2002)
	25		4	12	Vaupel et al. (2003b)
Liver	30		5	13	Kallinowski and Buhr (1995b)
Brain	24		3	13	Vaupel (2002)
	27		8	13	Clavo et al. (2002)

Empty boxes indicate lack of suitable information. For a review see Vaupel et al. (2007)

4.8
Hypoxia and Aggressive Tumor Phenotype

4.8.1
The Janus Face of Tumor Hypoxia

Cells exposed to hypoxia respond by reducing their overall protein synthesis, which in turn leads to restrained proliferation and subsequent cell death (see Fig. 4.12). Chronically hypoxic cells usually have a lifetime within the range of 1 to 10 days (Durand and Sham 1998; Ljungkvist et al. 2005). Hypoxia can hinder or even completely inhibit tumor cell proliferation in vitro. Sustained hypoxia can also change the cell cycle distribution and the relative number of quiescent cells leading to alterations in the response to radiation and many drugs. The degree of inhibition depends on the severity and duration of hypoxia. Under anoxia, most cells undergo immediate arrest in whichever cell cycle phase they are presently in. Additionally, hypoxia can induce programmed cell death (apoptosis) both in normal and in neoplastic cells. p53 accumulates under hypoxic conditions through a HIF-1α-dependent mechanism and induces apoptosis. However, hypoxia also initiates p53-independent apoptosis pathways including those involving genes of the BCL-2 family. Below a critical energy state, hypoxia may result in necrotic cell death. Hypoxia-induced proteome changes leading to cell cycle arrest, differentiation, apoptosis, and necrosis may explain delayed recurrences, dormant micrometastases, and growth retardation, which can occur in large tumors. In contrast, hypoxia has been recognized as an important driving force in malignant progression (Höckel and Vaupel 2001a; see Fig. 4.12).

Experimental findings have revealed that hypoxia—as an inherent consequence of unregulated growth—promotes local invasion, intravasation of cancer cells, and finally metastatic spread to distant sites and that this occurs in a cooperative manner:

a) On the proteome/metabolome level through adaptive gene expression, posttranscriptional and posttranslational modifications,

b) on the genome/epigenome level by increasing genomic and epigenomic instability, and

c) on the level of cell populations by clonal selection and clonal expansion according to phenotype fitness (Harris 2002).

'Janus Face' of tumor hypoxia

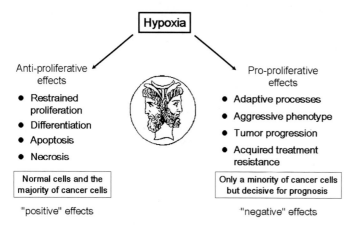

Fig. 4.12. The Janus face of tumor hypoxia. Tumor cells exposed to O_2 depletion can either respond with restrained proliferation and cell death (*left*) or with changes in the proteome and/or genome (*right*), favoring tumor progression and acquired treatment resistance, both of which result in poor clinical outcome and prognosis

4.8.2
Hypoxia-Induced Changes in Gene Expression

4.8.2.1
The HIF System

Hypoxia-induced changes in gene expression at tumor O_2 concentrations <1% (pO_2 <7 mmHg) are coordinated mainly by the hypoxia-inducible factor-1 (HIF-1) and HIF-2 (GIACCIA 1996; SEMENZA 2000, 2002a,b, 2003; LEO et al. 2004; CHAN and GIACCIA 2007; BRAHIMI-HORN and POUYSSEGUR 2006; VAUPEL 2004a; VAUPEL and HARRISON 2004; VAUPEL et al. 2004). Downstream effects of HIF activation, which contribute to increased malignancy, include modulation of glucose metabolism through increased cellular glucose uptake via glucose transporter-1 (GLUT-1) and enhanced glycolysis by up-regulation of key glycolytic enzymes, increased proton-extrusion capacity by overexpression of carbonic anhydrase IX (CA IX), increased angiogenesis by up-regulation of vascular endothelial growth factor, and the activation of the c-MET/HGF system characterized by cell proliferation, cell-cell dissociation, migration, and apoptosis protection (see Fig. 4.13a).

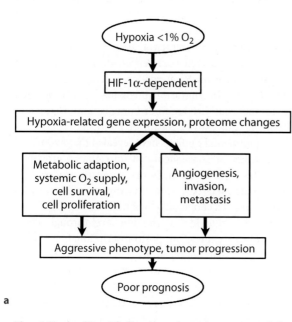

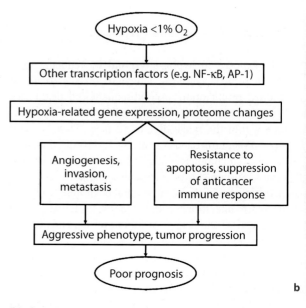

Fig. 4.13a,b. (Simplified) schematic representation of the pivotal role of hypoxia in malignant progression of solid tumors through HIF-1α-dependent (**a**) and HIF-1α-independent (**b**) alterations in gene expression with subsequent changes of the proteome, indicating redundancy in biological mechanisms in malignant tumors

A role of HIF-1α, GLUT-1, or CA IX as endogenous markers of tumor hypoxia is currently not supported by the available experimental data (VORDERMARK and BROWN 2003; MAYER et al. 2006). The same is true for a variety of other endogenous markers (e.g., VEGF).

4.8.2.2
HIF-Independent Hypoxia-Induced Proteins

Many other proteins have been implicated in the genetic response to hypoxia, among them nuclear factor κB (NF-κB), activator protein-1 (AP-1; see Fig. 4.13b), and members of the unfolded protein response (e.g., GRP78). Their exact role in hypoxia-induced tumor progression is less clear. For example, "hypoxic" induction of NF-κB is likely to be the consequence of reoxygenation-induced reactive oxygen species. Overexpression of osteopontin (OPN) has been demonstrated to be involved in metastasis formation. OPN is overexpressed during hypoxia, and the transcriptional control seems to be independent of HIF-1α.

4.9
Hypoxia-Induced Changes in the Genome and Clonal Selection

Tumor cell survival and proliferation or, alternatively, growth impairment, stasis, and cell death are not solely dependent on proteomic changes. Mutations in oncogenes and/or tumor suppressor genes are generally thought to be of crucial importance for the development of tumor aggressiveness. Hypoxia at O_2 concentrations ≤0.1% (pO$_2$ ≤0.7 mmHg) promotes genomic instability, thereby increasing the number of mutations (genetic variants). Hypoxia concomitantly exerts a strong selection pressure (REYNOLDS et al. 1996; YUAN et al. 2000; GRAEBER et al. 1996; KIM et al. 1997; KONDO et al. 2001; VAUPEL 2004a; VAUPEL et al. 2004; BRISTOW and HILL 2008). Tumor cell variants with adaptations favorable to survival under hypoxic conditions (e.g., lower capacity for cell-cycle arrest or apoptosis, greater angiogenic potential) may have growth advantages over nonadapted cells in the hypoxic microenvironment and expand through clonal selection (see Fig. 4.14). The expansion of cell clones with favorable proteomic and genomic adaptive changes can, in turn, exacerbate tumor hypoxia, thereby establishing a vicious circle of increasing hypoxia and subsequent malignant progression. At the clinical level, the consequences of this vicious circle are translated into more local recurrences, locoregional spread, distant tumor metastases, and greater resistance to radiation therapy and certain forms of chemotherapy (see Fig. 4.15).

In this context, it has to be mentioned that cycles of hypoxia and reoxygenation have been shown to be of importance for tumor progression, i.e., cyclic (intermittent, fluctuating, transient) hypoxia is the most powerful factor promoting an aggressive tumor phenotype (CAIRNS et al. 2001; CAIRNS and HILL 2004; WEINMANN et al. 2004; MAGAGNIN et al. 2007; ROFSTAD et al. 2007; TOFFOLI and MICHIELS 2008). Flat spatio-temporal oxygen gradients reflecting (although extreme) stable hypoxic microenvironments with low intra-tumoral variation may not be a prominent factor in terms of tumor progression (MAYER et al. 2008).

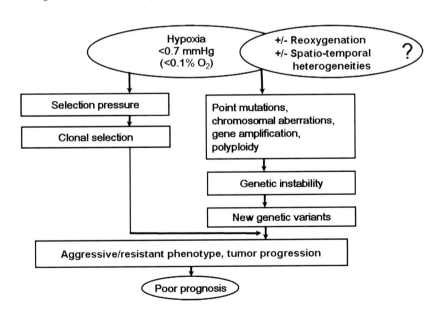

Fig. 4.14. (Simplified) schematic representation of the crucial role of hypoxia (± reoxygenation and/or spatio-temporal O$_2$ gradients) in malignant progression of solid tumors via changes in the genome and clonal selection

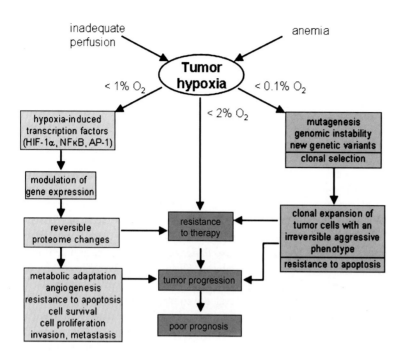

Fig. 4.15. Schematic representation of major pathogenetic factors causing tumor hypoxia and of the pivotal role of hypoxia in the development of therapeutic resistance via direct and indirect mechanisms

pH of Human Tumors

Warburg's classic work in the 1920s showed that cancer cells intensively convert glucose to lactic acid even in the presence of oxygen. Because of this excessive lactic acid production, it was assumed for many decades that tumors are acidic (WARBURG 1925, 1930; GULLINO et al. 1965; THISTLETHWAITE et al. 1985; VAN DEN BERG et al. 1982; WIKE-HOOLEY et al. 1984; VAUPEL et al. 1989; HELMLINGER et al. 1997; VAUPEL and JAIN 1991; ASHBY 1966). However, the unfolding story of tumor pH and its consequences has become clearer over the last 2 decades due to techniques that are able to preferentially measure intra- or extracellular pH in malignancies. Under many conditions, it has now been confirmed that the intracellular pH in tumor cells is neutral to alkaline as long as tumors are not oxygen- and energy-deprived (VAUPEL et al. 1994a,b; VAUPEL 1992). Tumor cells have efficient mechanisms for exporting protons into the extracellular space, which represents the acidic compartment in tumors (STUBBS et al. 2000; TANNOCK and ROTIN 1989; GOODE and CHADWICK 2001; NEWELL and TANNOCK 1991). For this reason, a pH gradient exists across the cell membrane in tumors ($pH_i > pH_e$). Interestingly, this gradient is the reverse of normal tissues where pH_i is lower than pH_e (Fig. 4.16) (for reviews

see VAUPEL et al. 1989; VAUPEL 1992; GRIFFITHS 1991; GERWECK 1998; SONG et al. 1993, 1999).

As already mentioned, cancer cells intensively split glucose to lactic acid (besides glucose oxidation). However, there are no longer any reasons to ascribe the aerobic glycolysis found as being specific to malignant growth, although the increased capacity for glycolysis still remains a key feature of tumors. Other relevant pathogenetic mechanisms yielding an intensified tissue acidosis are based on substantial ATP hydrolysis, glutaminolysis, ketogenesis, and CO_2/carbonic acid production (see Fig. 4.17).

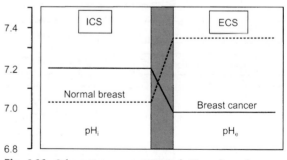

Fig. 4.16. Schematic representation of pH gradients between the intracellular space (*ICS*) and the extracellular space (*ECS*) of normal breast tissue and in breast cancer. pH_i = intracellular pH, pH_e = extracellular pH

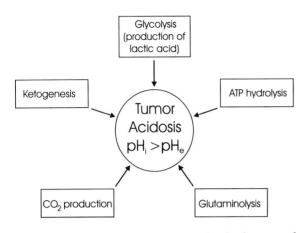

Fig. 4.17. Mechanisms contributing to the development of (extracellular) acidosis in solid tumors. pH_i = intracellular pH, pH_e = extracellular pH

Lactic acid production alone cannot explain the acidosis observed in the extracellular compartments. The other mechanisms may also play a relevant role. This is supported by experimental data of NEWELL et al. (1993) who suggested that production of lactic acid is not the only cause of tumor acidity. These results are based on experiments with glycolysis-deficient cells.

4.10.1
Tumor pH Values Measured with Electrodes

pH values measured with invasive electrodes (potentiometric pH measurements) preferentially reflect the acid-base status of the extracellular space (pH_e), which occupies ca. 45% of the total tissue volume in malignant tumors (see Sect. 4.5). This is in strong contrast to normal tissues where, on average, the extracellular compartment encompasses only approximately 16%. The pH_e values measured in malignancies are shifted to more acidic values with respect to normal tissues (0.2–0.5 units; Fig. 4.18). In some tumors, the pH_e may be as low as 5.6. A remarkable variability in measured values exists between tumors, which exceeds the heterogeneity observed within tumors. This intratumor heterogeneity, however, has not been studied in human tumors using pH electrodes in as much detail as it has been in animal tumors (for reviews see VAN DEN BERG 1991; VAUPEL et al. 1989; WIKE-HOOLEY et al. 1985). Since the lactic acid distribution on a microscale is rather heterogeneous in tumors (Fig. 4.19), distinct heterogeneities in the pH distribution within different microareas should occur. Intratumor pH heterogeneities are especially evi-

dent in partially necrotic tumors where tissue pH values even higher than the arterial blood pH can be observed in areas of longstanding necrosis. This latter pH shift is mostly due to proton-binding during protein denaturation, to accumulation of ammonia, which is generated through the catabolism of peptides and proteins, and to cessation of proton production from energy metabolism (KALLINOWSKI and VAUPEL 1988).

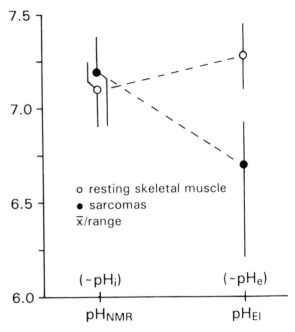

Fig. 4.18. Intracellular (pH_i measured with ^{31}P-NMR) and extracellular pH (pH_e assessed by pH sensitive electrodes) values in resting skeletal muscle (*open circles*) and in soft tissue sarcomas of patients (*filled circles*). Values shown are means ($\bar{x}$) and the range of pH data measured

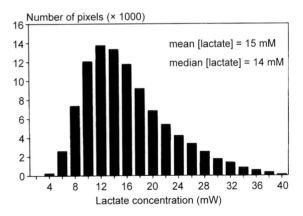

Fig. 4.19. Histogram of measured lactate concentrations in a cancer of the uterine cervix

4.10.2
Intracellular pH in Tumors

Tumors were thought for many years to have a more acidic intracellular pH (pH$_i$) than most normal tissues. However, the results of pH measurements using ^{31}P-nuclear magnetic resonance spectroscopy (^{31}P-NMR or ^{31}P-MRS) yielded quite a different picture. pH values derived from MRS (pH$_{NMR}$) appear to be very similar to those in normal tissues (Fig. 4.20). These values mainly

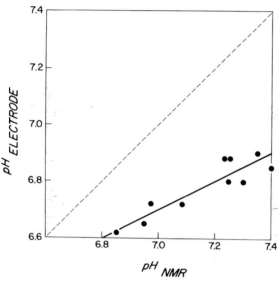

Fig. 4.20. Correlation between pH values assessed by ^{31}P-NMR spectroscopy (pH_{NMR}) and pH data obtained from microelectrode measurements ($pH_{Electrode}$) in C3H mouse mammary tumors of identical volumes (*broken line*: line of identity)

reflect intracellular pH (STUBBS et al. 1992) and suggest that the cell may keep its internal (cytosolic) pH at a relatively constant level, or at least above the extracellular level, over a considerable range of extracellular pH values, a feature already known from animal tumor studies. pH is neutral or slightly alkaline. This is most probably due to the fact that tumor cells—besides having intracellular buffer systems—also possess efficient mechanisms for exporting protons into the extracellular space (these include a rapid export of anionic lactate$^-$, which is accompanied by a movement of H$^+$) and for importing proton acceptors (e.g., HCO$_3^-$) into the cytosolic compartment. The subsequent inadequate removal of protons from the extracellular space in low-flow areas may result in an extracellular acidosis as often demonstrated by electrode measurements in many solid tumors. Acidic pH$_i$ values were found only in bulky, poorly oxygenated, energy- and nutrient-deprived tumors (e.g., in FsaII mouse tumors when tumor volumes exceeded 1.5% of the body weight). Another technique predominantly measuring pH$_i$ in solid tumors is positron emission tomography (PET) using ^{11}C-DMO (ARNOLD et al. 1985).

4.10.3
Extracellular-Intracellular pH Gradients in Tumors and in Normal Tissues

pH$_i$ in tumors and in normal tissues is relatively invariable ranging from 7.0 to 7.3, indicating that the pH$_i$ of human tumors and normal tissues is well-regulated. Extracellular pH values are on average 0.3–0.4 pH-units

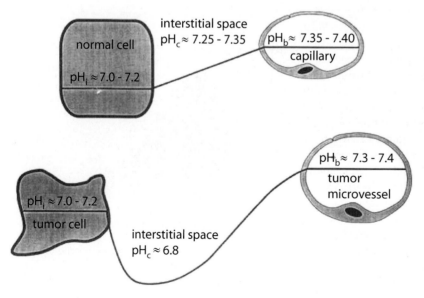

Fig. 4.21. Schematic representation of pH-profiles in the interstitial space of normal breast tissue (*upper panel*) and in breast cancer (*lower panel*). pH_i, intracellular pH measured with ^{31}P-NMR spectroscopy; pH_e, extracellular pH assessed by pH-sensitive microelectrodes; pH_b, blood pH (adapted from VAUPEL and HÖCKEL 2000)

lower. In soft tissue sarcomas, pH_e is roughly 0.45 pH-units lower than in the respective normal tissue. In breast cancer this difference is approximately 0.35 pH-units (see Fig. 4.21) and in primary brain tumors (glioblastomas) about 0.2 pH-units below normal brain tissue. As a rule, in solid human tumors pH_i values are on average 0.4 pH-units higher than pH_e, which is similar to differences obtained in experimental tumors (ΔpH = 0.2–0.6 pH-units). As already mentioned, the pH gradient is the reverse of normal tissues, where pH_i is somewhat lower than pH_e. This difference may provide an exploitable avenue for cancer treatment because weakly acidic drugs (e.g., 5-FU, melphalan, mitomycin C) may substantially accumulate within the tumor cells (STUBBS et al. 2000; GOODE and CHADWICK 2001; GERWECK 1998).

4.10.4
Bicarbonate Depletion in the Extracellular Compartment of Tumors

Exported H^+-ions from the intracellular space to the interstitial compartment promote extracellular acidification. The latter, together with a HIF-1α-induced upregulation of the membrane-bound ectoenzyme carbonic anhydrase (CA IX), finally leads to buffering of the exported protons by extracellular bicarbonate causing a bicarbonate depletion and an intensified CO_2 release, both characteric features of the tumor pathophysiome (Fig. 4.22) (GULLINO et al. 1965; GULLINO 1970, 1975; VAUPEL 2008).

4.10.5
Tumor Respiratory Quotients

Lactic acid production and metabolic acidosis not only lead to substantial proton accumulation, but also to elevated respiratory quotients (respiratory quotient RQ = CO_2 output/O_2 uptake) >1.3 in tumors caused by an intensified CO_2 release according to the equation:

$$H^+ + HCO_3^- \xrightarrow{CA} H_2O + CO_2 \qquad \text{(Eq. 4.1)}$$

Hypoxia-induced upregulation of the enzyme carbonic anhydrase (CA) is thus a meaningful physiological adaptation (VAUPEL et al. 2001). Carbonic anhydrase is a membrane-bound ectoenzyme that is activated at low pH (VAUPEL 2008). Experimental evidence for the occurrence of this reaction is provided by the very high CO_2 partial pressures (79 mmHg) and low bicarbonate concentrations (19 mmol/l) found in the interstitial fluid of solid tumors (GULLINO 1970, 1975). Because the total CO_2 output is greater than the metabolic formation of CO_2 (from substrate oxidation), the respiratory quotient can range from 1.29 to 1.95.

Strikingly high RQ values may thus be a further characteristic of the tumor pathophysiome (VAUPEL 2008) that quantitatively describes the pathophysiologic features of tumors. Finally, it has to be mentioned that "titration" of extracellular bicarbonate to CO_2 and H_2O is not the only cause of extremely high RQs, but also this condition may be caused by channeling of glycolytic end-products into lipogenesis (VAUPEL 2008).

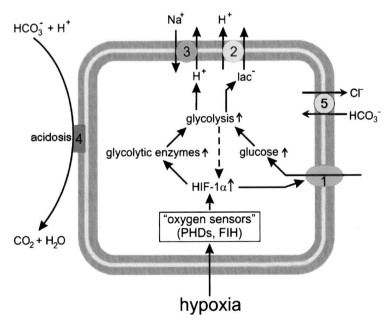

Fig. 4.22. Hypoxia-mediated metabolic adaptation for energy preservation. Activation of genes for glucose transporter-1 (GLUT-1 = 1) and glycolytic enzymes yields an increased glycolytic rate. H^+-ions produced are preferentially exported via a Na^+/H^+-antiporter (NHE-1 = 3) and a lactate$^-$/H^+-symporter (monocarboxylate transporter MCT-1 = 2) leading to a drop in extracellular pH (pH_e). Low extracellular pH activates the membrane-bound ectoenzyme carbonic anhydrase IX (CA IX = 4). Key mechanism regulating intracellular pH in tumor cells when protons are produced is also shown (Na^+-dependent HCO_3^-/Cl^--exchanger = 5). *HIF-1α* = hypoxia-inducible factor 1α, *PHDs* = prolyl hydroxylases, *FIH* = asparagyl hydroxylase, *lac$^-$* = lactic acid

Bioenergetic Status of Tumors

4.11.1
Human Tumor Bioenergetics Monitored by ³¹P-Nuclear Magnetic Resonance

³¹P-nuclear magnetic resonance (³¹P-NMR, ³¹P-MRS) is able to provide important biochemical information on living tissues. Since the MRS technique is noninvasive, nondestructive, and painless, it allows the patient to be repeatedly monitored throughout the course of tumor treatment (NEGENDANK 1992; VAUPEL 1994a; STUBBS 1999; STUBBS and GRIFFITHS 1999).

In vivo ³¹P-NMR spectroscopy has been employed in monitoring the energy metabolism of human tumors since 1983 (GRIFFITHS et al. 1983). From the studies available, information is provided that may be beneficial in the clinical treatment of cancer. Furthermore, there are indications that serial monitoring of tumor response can assist in optimizing the timing of treatments.

In Figs. 4.23 and 4.24, ³¹P-NMR spectra from normal tissues are compared with tumor spectra (spectra are redrawn from original recordings, VAUPEL 1994a). According to these exemplary spectra, in many human malignancies, other than brain tumors, very often high concentrations of phosphomonoesters (PME), phosphodiesters (PDE) and inorganic phosphate (P_i), and low phosphocreatine (PCr) levels are characteristically found. In contrast, studies on human brain tumors often fail to show any significant differences in the spectra of malignancies vs. normal brain tissue (VAUPEL 1994a).

The PME signal primarily includes phosphocholine and phosphoethanolamine, both of which are membrane phospholipid precursors. In addition, phosphorylated sugars (glucose-6-phosphate, fructose-6-phosphate, and fructose-1,6-diphosphate) might be present and fall in the PME region. The PDE peak in murine tumors was identified to be largely glycerophosphocholine and glycerophosphoethanolamine, both membrane phospholipid decomposition products (VAUPEL 1994a).

In order to describe the bioenergetic status of normal tissues and malignancies, relevant metabolite ratios

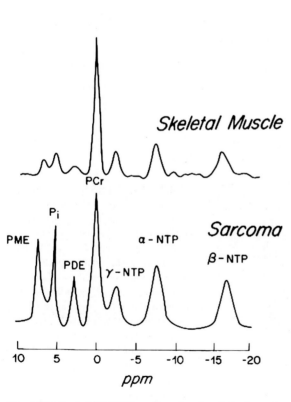

Fig. 4.23. Typical ³¹P-NMR spectra of resting skeletal muscle and a human sarcoma (spectra are redrawn from original recordings from VAUPEL 1994a)

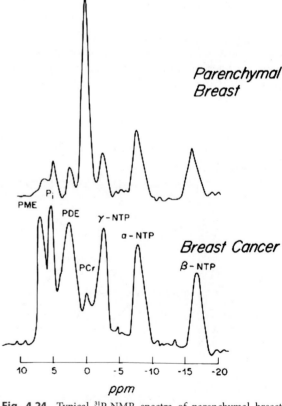

Fig. 4.24. Typical ³¹P-NMR spectra of parenchymal breast and a human breast cancer (spectra are redrawn from original recordings, from VAUPEL 1994a)

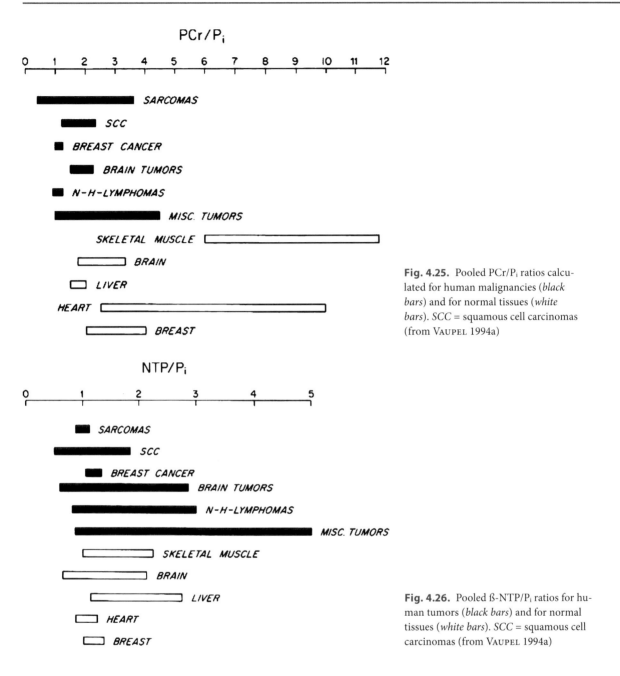

Fig. 4.25. Pooled PCr/P$_i$ ratios calculated for human malignancies (*black bars*) and for normal tissues (*white bars*). *SCC* = squamous cell carcinomas (from Vaupel 1994a)

Fig. 4.26. Pooled ß-NTP/P$_i$ ratios for human tumors (*black bars*) and for normal tissues (*white bars*). *SCC* = squamous cell carcinomas (from Vaupel 1994a)

are compiled in Figs. 4.25 and 4.26. PCr/P$_i$ ratios for various human malignancies and normal tissues are depicted in Fig. 4.25. The data show that PCr/P$_i$ in normal brain and in brain tumors is similar, whereas this ratio is significantly higher in skeletal muscle or myocardium relative to sarcomas, and in parenchymal breast vs. breast cancer.

ß-NPT/P$_i$ ratios for human tumors and normal tissues are presented in Fig. 4.26. Here again, no clear differences are seen between normal brain and brain tumors. The only significant differences evident were between sarcomas and skeletal muscle. From these data, the (cautious) conclusion can be drawn that, on average, the bioenergetic status may be similar in normal brain and brain tumors. The latter data confirm the results on ATP distribution obtained with quantitative bioluminescence (Vaupel 1994a).

4.11.2
Tumor Bioenergetics Assessed by High Performance Liquid Chromatography

Global ATP concentrations measured in experimental tumors with high performance (pressure) liquid chromatography (HPLC) are typically in the range of 0.4–2.0 mM (Vaupel 1994a; Vaupel et al. 1994b). As long as tumor masses did not exceed 1% of the body weight (i.e., biologically relevant tumor sizes), global ATP concentrations and adenylate energy charge only changed marginally (Vaupel 1994a; Vaupel et al. 1994a,b). This stable bioenergetic status coincides with a "physiological" tissue oxygenation (i.e., pO_2 distribution comparable with that of normal organs; median $pO_2 \geq 10$ mmHg), mean tissue glucose concentrations of approximately 2 mM, and mean lactate levels ≤ 10 mM (Vaupel 1994a).

Increased ATP hydrolysis with enlarging tumor mass is a typical finding observed during tumor growth. As a result of an increased ATP degradation, an accumulation of purine catabolites has to be expected together with a formation of protons and reactive oxygen species at several stages during degradation to the final product uric acid (Vaupel 1994a). The accumulation of the purine catabolites xanthine, hypoxanthine, and uric acid in experimental rat DS sarcomas is shown in Fig. 4.27.

4.11.3
Microregional ATP Distribution Assessed by Quantitative Bioluminescence

Owing to the heterogeneous microcirculation in tumors, the ATP concentration in vivo may be low in some distinct tumor regions containing viable cancer cells, and this has implications for metabolism, growth, and therapeutic response of the respective malignant cells. On the other hand, tumors are often characterized by necrotic areas where ATP is low due to its rapid hydrolysis upon cell death. Such regions will not contribute to the therapeutic behavior of tumors, e.g., to tumor regrowth after a certain treatment. Consequently, techniques are required that make it possible to image concentrations of metabolites, such as ATP, with a high spatial resolution in relation to the tissue architecture.

An ex vivo technique for imaging metabolites in tissues has been developed using quantitative bioluminescence, single photon imaging, and computerized image analysis. The method allows measurement of steady state concentrations of ATP, glucose, and lactate in absolute terms with a spatial resolution near the cellular level (Mueller-Klieser and Walenta 1993; Mueller-Klieser et al. 1988).

The microregional distribution of ATP has been assessed in cryobiopsies of cervix tumors taken from patients immediately after pO_2 measurements from

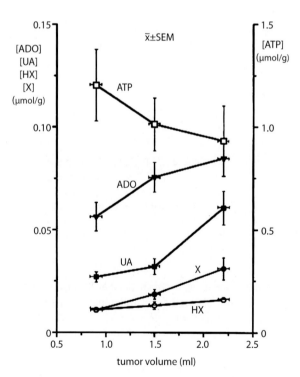

Fig. 4.27. Concentrations of ATP, adenosine (*ADO*), uric acid (*UA*), xanthine (*X*), and hypoxanthine (*HX*) in experimental rat DS sarcomas as a function of tumor volume. Values are means ± SEM (from Vaupel 1994a)

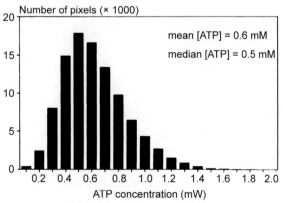

Fig. 4.28. Histogram of measured ATP concentrations in a cancer of the uterine cervix (from Vaupel 1994a)

sites adjacent to an O_2 electrode track (Fig. 4.28). Similar to the glucose (Fig. 4.29) and lactate distributions (Fig. 4.19), microregional concentrations of ATP were heterogeneous and comparable to findings in high-flow experimental tumors, and there was no clear-cut correlation between tumor oxygenation and regional ATP levels in the patient tumors investigated so far. Pronounced heterogeneity in ATP levels occurred, although extended necrosis was not visible in histological sections.

Distribution patterns of ATP, glucose, and lactate and the corresponding histological structure in a cervix cancer of a patient have been evaluated (VAUPEL 1994a, 2006). In some cervix tumors investigated, there was an obvious relationship between the distribution of metabolites and the histological architecture of the tissue. This is particularly evident in malignancies with circumscribed areas of densely packed, viable cancer cells surrounded by necrosis and stromal tissue with low packing density. A comparison of ATP and lactate distribution with the histological structure suggests that concentrations of these metabolites are relatively high in the viable tumor areas and lower in the vicinity of necrotic regions. As a consequence, one would expect that there is a positive correlation between both metabolites for each equivalent location within the tumor. Although such a correlation is not that obvious for the glucose distribution, one may suspect that this substrate is negatively correlated with the other two metabolites measured.

Quantitative pixel-to-pixel correlations for the different metabolites of interest have been performed. Data obtained show a positive linear correlation between ATP and lactate levels, and a negative linear correlation between ATP and glucose concentrations. Glu-

cose and lactate levels thus are negatively correlated in cancers of the uterine cervix (VAUPEL 1994a; WALENTA and MUELLER-KLIESER 2004). It is interesting to note that in cervix cancers measured mean glucose concentrations were never below 1 µmol/g (= 18 mg/dl), a level that has also been predicted for breast cancers (see Fig. 4.7).

Measurements of the regional ATP distribution with quantitative bioluminescence in experimental brain tumors have shown that ATP levels were similar to normal brain (2.6 vs. 2.5 µmol/g) with slightly lower glucose (2.4 vs. 2.8 µmol/g) and substantially higher lactate concentrations (6.4 vs. 1.2 µmol/g) in vital tumor tissue (VAUPEL 1994a; HOSSMANN et al. 1982, 1986; PASCHEN 1985; PASCHEN et al. 1987). In tumors, marked heterogeneity of these metabolites was present (HOSSMANN et al. 1982). By applying quantitative imaging bioluminescence, WALENTA et al. (1997, 2000, 2003; WALENTA and MUELLER-KLIESER 2004) have provided clinical evidence that lactate accumulation mirrors malignant potential in squamous cell carcinomas of the uterine cervix and of the head and neck, and in colorectal adenocarcinomas.

Acknowledgments

The valuable assistance of Dr. Debra K. Kelleher and Mrs. Anne Deutschmann-Fleck in preparing this manuscript is greatly appreciated. This work has continuously been supported by grants from the Deutsche Krebshilfe (M 40/91Va1 and 106758).

References

Adam MF, Gabalski EC, Bloch DA, Oehlert JW, Brown JM, Elsaid AA, Pinto HA, Terris DJ (1999) Tissue oxygen distribution in head and neck cancer patients. Head Neck 21:146–153

Airley R, Loncaster J, Davidson S, Bromley M, Roberts S, Patterson A, Hunter R, Stratford I, West C (2001) Glucose transporter Glut-1 expression correlates with tumor hypoxia and predicts metastasis-free survival in advanced carcinoma of the cervix. Clin Cancer Res 7:928–934

Aquino-Parsons C, Green A, Minchinton AI (2000) Oxygen tension in primary gynaecological tumours: The influence of carbon dioxide concentration. Radiother Oncol 57:45–51

Aquino-Parsons C, Luo C, Vikse CM, Olive PL (1999) Comparison between the comet assay and the oxygen microelectrode for measurement of tumor hypoxia. Radiother Oncol 51:179–185

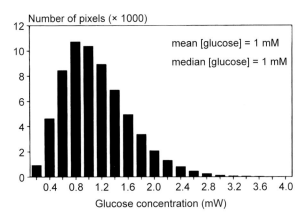

Fig. 4.29. Histogram of measured glucose concentrations in a cancer of the uterine cervix (from VAUPEL 1994a)

Ariztia EV, Lee CJ, Gogoi R, Fishman DA (2006) The tumor microenvironment. Crit Rev Clin Lab Sci 43:393–425

Arnold JB, Junck L, Rottenberg DA (1985) In vivo measurement of regional brain and tumor pH using [^{14}C]dimethyloxazolidinedione and quantitative autoradiography. J Cereb Blood Flow Metab 5:369–375

Ashby BS (1966) pH studies in human malignant tumours. Lancet 2:312–315

Baronzio G, Freitas I, Kwaan HC (2003) Tumor microenvironment and hemorheological abnormalities. Sem Thrombosis Hemostasis 29:489–497

Becker A, Hänsgen G, Bloching M, Weigel C, Lautenschläger C, Dunst J (1998a) Oxygenation of squamous cell carcinoma of the head and neck: Comparison of primary tumors, neck node metastases, and normal tissue. Int J Radiat Oncol Biol Phys 42: 35–41

Becker A, Hänsgen G, Richter C, Dunst J (1998b) Oxygenierungsstatus von Plattenepithelkarzinomen der Kopf-Hals-Region. Strahlenther Onkol 174:484–486

Becker A, Stadler P, Lavey RS, Hänsgen G, Kuhnt T, Lautenschläger C, Feldmann HJ, Molls M, Dunst J (2000) Severe anemia is associated with poor tumor oxygenation in head and neck squamous cell carcinomas. Int J Radiat Oncol Biol Phys 46:459–466

Bentzen L, Keiding S, Nordsmark M, Falborg L, Hansen SB, Keller J, Nielsen OS, Overgaard J (2003) Tumour oxygenation assessed by ^{18}F-fluoromisonidazole PET and polarographic needle electrodes in human soft tissue tumours. Radiother Oncol 67:339–344

Beppu T, Kamada K, Yoshida Y, Arai H, Ogasawara K, Ogawa A (2002) Change of oxygen pressure in glioblastoma tissue under various conditions. J Neuro-Oncol 58:47–52

Boucher Y, Kirkwood JM, Opacic D, Desantis M, Jain RK (1991) Interstitial hypertension in superficial metastatic melanomas in humans. Cancer Res 51:6691–6694

Brahimi-Horn C, Pouyssegur J (2006) The role of the hypoxia-inducible factor in tumor metabolism growth and invasion. Bull Cancer 93:E73–80

Bristow RG, Hill RP (2008) Hypoxia, DNA repair and genetic instability. Nat Rev Cancer 8:180–192

Brizel DM (1999) Human tumor oxygenation: The Duke University Medical Center Experience. In: Vaupel P, Kelleher DK (eds) Tumor hypoxia. Wissenschaftliche Verlagsgesellschaft, Stuttgart, pp 29–38

Brizel DM, Dodge RK, Clough RW, Dewhirst MW (1999) Oxygenation of head and neck cancer: Changes during radiotherapy and impact on treatment outcome. Radiother Oncol 53:113–117

Brizel DM, Rosner GL, Harrelson J, Prosnitz LR, Dewhirst MW (1994) Pretreatment oxygenation profiles of human soft tissue sarcomas. Int J Radiat Oncol Biol Phys 30:635–642

Brizel DM, Rosner GL, Prosnitz LR, Dewhirst MW (1995) Patterns and variability of tumor oxygenation in human soft tissue sarcomas, cervical carcinomas, and lymph node metastases. Int J Radiat Oncol Biol Phys 32:1121–1125

Brizel DM, Scully SP, Harrelson JM, Layfield LJ, Bean JM, Prosnitz LR, Dewhirst MW (1996a) Tumor oxygenation predicts for the likelihood of distant metastases in human soft tissue sarcoma. Cancer Res 56:941–943

Brizel DM, Scully SP, Harrelson JM, Layfield LJ, Dodge RK, Charles HC, Samulski TV, Prosnitz LR, Dewhirst MW (1996b) Radiation therapy and hyperthermia improve the oxygenation of human soft tissue sarcomas. Cancer Res 56:5347–5350

Brizel DM, Sibley GS, Prosnitz LR, Scher RL, Dewhirst MW (1997) Tumor hypoxia adversely affects the prognosis of carcinoma of the head and neck. Int J Radiat Oncol Biol Phys 38:285–289

Bussink J (2000) The tumor microenvironment and effects of hypoxia modification. Proefschrift, Katholieke Universiteit, Nijmegen

Butler TP, Grantham FH, Gullino PM (1975) Bulk transfer of fluid in the interstitial compartment of mammary tumors. Cancer Res 35:3084–3088

Cairns R, Papandreou I, Denko N (2006) Overcoming physiologic barriers to cancer treatment by molecularly targeting the tumor microenvironment. Mol Cancer Res 4:61–70

Cairns RA, Hill RP (2004) Acute hypoxia enhances spontaneous lymph node metastasis in an orthotopic murine model of human cervical carcinoma. Cancer Res 64:2054–2061

Cairns RA, Kalliomaki T, Hill RP (2001) Acute (cyclic) hypoxia enhances spontaneous metastasis of KHT murine tumors. Cancer Res 61:8903–8908

Chan DA, Giaccia AJ (2007) Hypoxia, gene expression, and metastasis. Cancer Metast Rev 26:333–339

Clavo B, Robaina F, Catalá L, Pérez JL, Camarés MA, Morera J, López L, Suárez G, Macías D, Rivero J, Hernández MA (2004) Effect of cervical spinal cord stimulation on regional blood flow and oxygenation in advanced head and neck tumours. Ann Oncol 15:802–807

Clavo B, Robaina F, Morera J, Ruiz-Egea E, Pérez JL, Macías D, Caramés MA, Catalá L, Hernández MA, Günderoth M (2002) Increase of brain tumor oxygenation during cervical spinal cord stimulation. J Neurosurg 96:94–100

Collingridge DR, Piepmeier JM, Rockwell S, Knisely JP (1999) Polarographic measurements of oxygen tension in human glioma and surrounding peritumoural brain tissue. Radiother Oncol 53:127–131

Cooper RA, Carrington BM, Loncaster JA, Todd SM, Davidson SE, Logue JP, Luthra AD, Jones AP, Stratford I, Hunter RD, West CML (2000) Tumour oxygenation levels correlate with dynamic contrast-enhanced magnetic resonance imaging parameters in carcinoma of the cervix. Radiother Oncol 57:53–59

Cooper RA, West CM, Logue JP, Davidson SE, Miller A, Roberts S, Statford IJ, Honess DJ, Hunter RD (1999) Changes in oxygenation during radiotherapy in carcinoma of the cervix. Int J Radiat Oncol Biol Phys 45:119–126

Cruickshank GS, Rampling RP, Cowans W (1994) Direct measurement of the pO_2 distribution in human malignant brain tumours. Adv Exp Med Biol 345:465–470

Cunha GR, Hayward SW, Wang YZ, Ricke WA (2003) Role of the stromal microenvironment in carcinogenesis of the prostate. Int J Cancer 107:1–10

Curti BD, Urba WJ, Alvord WG, Janik JE, Smith JW, Madara K, Longo DL (1993) Interstitital pressure of subcutaneous nodules in melanoma and lymphoma patients: Changes during treatment. Cancer Res 53:2204–2207

Cvetkovic D, Movsas B, Dicker AP, Hanlon AL, Greenberg RE, Chapman JD, Hanks GE, Tricoli JV (2001) Increased hypoxia correlates with increased expression of the angiogenesis marker vascular endothelial growth factor in human prostate cancer. Urology 57:821–825

Denko NC, Fontana LA, Hudson KM, Sutphin PD, Raychaudhuri S, Altman RB, Giaccia AJ (2001) Investigating hypoxic tumor physiology through gene expression patterns. Oncogene 22:5907–5914

Dewhirst MW, Poulson JM, Yu D, Sanders L, Lora-Michiels M, Vujaskovic Z, Jones EL, Samulski TV, Powers BE, Brizel DM, Prosnitz LR, Charles HC (2005) Relation between pO_2, ^{31}P magnetic resonance spectroscopy parameters and treatment outcome in patients with high-grade soft tissue sarcomas treated with thermoradiotherapy. Int J Radiat Oncol Biol Phys 61:480–491

Di Martino EFN, Gagel B, Schramm O (2005) Evaluation of tumor oxygenation by color duplex sonography: A new approach. Otolaryngol Head Neck Surg 132:765–769

Dietz A, Rudat V, Conradt C, Vanselow B, Wollensack P, Staar S, Eckel H, Volling P, Schröder M, Wannenmacher M, Müller RP, Weidenauer H (2000) Prognostischer Stellenwert des Hämoglobinwertes vor primärer Radiochemotherapie von Kopf-Hals-Karzinomen. HNO 48:655–664

Dietz A, Vanselow B, Rudat V, Conradt C, Weidauer H, Kallinowski F, Dollner R (2003) Prognostic impact of reoxygenation in advanced cancer of the head and neck during initial course of chemoradiation or radiotherapy alone. Head Neck 25:50–58

Doll CM, Milosevic M, Pintilie M, Hill RP, Fyles AW (2003) Estimating hypoxic status in human tumors: A simulation using Eppendorf oxygen probe data in cervical cancer patients. Int J Radiat Oncol Biol Phys 55:1239–1246

Dunst J, Hänsgen G, Lautenschläger C, Fuchsel G, Becker A (1999) Oxygenation of cervical cancers during radiotherapy and radiotherapy + cis-retinoic acid/interferon. Int J Radiat Oncol Biol Phys 43:367–373

Dunst J, Kuhnt T, Strauss HG, Krause U, Pelz T, Koelbl H, Hänsgen G (2003a) Anemia in cervical cancers: Impact on survival, patterns of relapse, and association with hypoxia and angiogenesis. Int J Radiat Oncol Biol Phys 56:778–787

Dunst J, Stadler P, Becker A, Lautenschläger C, Pelz T, Hänsgen G, Molls M, Kuhnt T (2003b) Tumor volume and tumor hypoxia in head and neck cancers. The amount of the hypoxic volume is important. Strahlenther Onkol 179:521–526

Durand RE, Sham E (1998) The lifetime of hypoxic human tumor cells. Int J Radiat Oncol Biol Phys 42:711–715

Eble MJ, Lohr F, Wannenmacher M (1995) Oxygen tension distribution in head and neck carcinomas after peroral oxygen therapy. Onkologie 18:136–140

Endrich B, Hammersen F, Goetz A, Messmer K (1982) Microcirculatory blood flow, capillary morphology, and local oxygen pressure of the hamster amelanotic melanoma A-Mel-3. J Natl Cancer Inst 68:475–485

Evans SM, Hahn SM, Magarelli DP, Zhang PJ, Jenkins WT, Fraker DL, Hsi RA, McKenna WG, Koch CJ (2001) Hypoxia in human intraperitoneal and extremity sarcomas. Int J Radiat Oncol Biol Phys 49:587–596

Evans SM, Judy KD, Dunphy I, Jenkins WT, Hwang W-T, Nelson PT, Lustig RA, Jenkins K, Magarelli DP, Hahn SM, Collins RA, Grady MS, Koch CJ (2004a) Hypoxia is important in the biology and aggression of human glial brain tumors. Clin Cancer Res 10:8177–8184

Evans SM, Judy KD, Dunphy I, Jenkins WT, Nelson PT, Collins R, Wileyto EP, Jenkins K, Hahn SM, Stevens CW, Judkins AR, Phillips P, Geoerger B, Koch CJ (2004b) Comparative measurements of hypoxia in human brain tumors using needle electrodes and EF5 binding. Cancer Res 64:1886–1892

Falk SJ, Ward R, Bleehan NM (1992) The influence of carbogen breathing on tumour tissue oxygenation in man evaluated by computerized pO_2 histography. Br J Cancer 66:919–924

Fidler IJ (2002) The organ microenvironment and cancer metastasis. Differentiation 70:498–505

Fleckenstein W, Jungblut JR, Suckfüll M, Hoppe W, Weiss C (1988) Sauerstoffdruckverteilungen in Zentrum und Peripherie maligner Kopf-Hals-Tumoren. Dtsch Z Mund Kiefer GesichtsChir 12:205–211

Fukumura D, and Jain RK (2007) Tumor microenvironment abnormalities: causes, consequences, and strategies to normalize. J Cell Biochem 101:937–949

Füller J, Feldmann HJ, Molls M, Sack H (1994) Untersuchungen zum Sauerstoffpartialdruck im Tumorgewebe unter Radio- und Thermoradiotherapie. Strahlenther Onkol 170:453–460

Fyles A, Milosevic M, Hedley D, Pintilie M, Levin W, Manchul L, Hill RP (2002) Tumor hypoxia has independent predictor impact only in patients with node-negative cervix cancer. J Clin Oncol 20:680–687

Fyles A, Milosevic M, Pintilie M, Syed A, Levin W, Manchul L, Hill RP (2006) Long-term performance of interstitial fluid pressure and hypoxia as prognostic factors in cervix cancer. Radiother Oncol 80:132–137

Fyles A, Milosevic M, Wong R, Kavanagh MC, Pintilie M, Sun A, Chapman W, Levin W, Manchul L, Keane T, Hill RP (1998) Oxygenation predicts radiation response and survival in patients with cervix cancer. Radiother Oncol 48:149–156

Gatenby RA, Coia LR, Richter MP, Katz H, Moldofsky PJ, Engstrom P, Brown DQ, Brookland R, Broder GJ (1985) Oxygen tension in human tumors: In vivo mapping using CT-guided probes. Radiology 156:211–214

Gatenby RA, Kessler HB, Rosenblum JS, Coia LR, Moldofsky PJ, Hartz WH, Broder GJ (1988) Oxygen distribution in squamous cell carcinoma metastases and its relationship to outcome of radiation therapy. Int J Radiat Oncol Biol Phys 14:831–838

Gerweck LE (1998) Tumor pH: Implications for treatment and novel drug design. Sem Radiat Oncol 8:176–182

Giaccia AJ (1996) Hypoxic stress proteins: survival of the fittest. Semin Radiat Oncol 6:46–58

Gillies RJ, Schornack PA, Secomb TW, Raghunand N (1999) Causes and effects of heterogeneous perfusion in tumors. Neoplasia 1:197–207

Goode JA, Chadwick DJ (eds) (2001) The tumour microenvironment: Causes and consequences of hypoxia and acidity. Novartis Foundation Symposium 240. John Wiley & Sons, Chichester, New York

Graeber TG, Osmanian C, Jacks T, Housman DE, Koch CJ, Lowe SW, Giaccia AJ (1996) Hypoxia-mediated selection of cells with diminished apoptotic potential in solid tumours. Nature 379:88–91

Graffman S, Björk P, Ederoth P, Ihse I (2001) Polarographic pO$_2$ measurements of intra-abdominal adenocarcinoma in connection with intraoperative radiotherapy before and after change of oxygen concentration of anaesthetic gases. Acta Oncol 40:105–107

Griffiths JR (1991) Are cancer cells acidic? Br J Cancer 64:425–427

Griffiths JR, Cady E, Edwards RHT, McCready VR, Wilkie DR, Wiltshaw E (1983) 31P-NMR studies of a human tumour in situ. Lancet 1:1435–1436

Grischke EM, Kaufmann M, Eberlein-Gonska M, Mattfeld T, Sohn Ch, Bastert G (1994) Angiogenesis as a diagnostic factor in primary breast cancer: Microvessel quantitation by stereological methods and correlation with color Doppler sonography. Onkologie 17:35–42

Groebe K, Vaupel P (1988) Evaluation of oxygen diffusion distances in human breast cancer xenografts using tumor-specific in vivo-data: Role of various mechanisms in the development of tumor hypoxia. Int J Radiat Oncol Biol Phys 15:691–697

Gullino PM (1970) Techniques for the study of tumor physiopathology. In: Busch H (ed) Methods in cancer research. Academic Press, New York, pp 45–91

Gullino PM (1975) Extracellular compartments of solid tumors, In: Becker EF (ed) Cancer, vol 3. Plenum, New York, pp 327–354

Gullino PM, Grantham FH, Smith SH, Haggerty AC (1965) Modifications of the acid-base status of the internal milieu of tumors. J Natl Cancer Inst 34:857–869

Gutmann R, Leunig M, Feyh J, Goetz AE, Messmer K, Kastenbauer E, Jain RK (1992) Interstitial hypertension in head and neck tumors in patients: correlation with tumor size. Cancer Res 52:1993–1995

Guyton AC, Hall JE (2006) Textbook of medical physiology, 11th edn. Elsevier, Philadelphia

Haider MA, Milosevic M, Fyles A, Sitartchouk I, Yeung I, Henderson E, Lockwood G, Lee TY, Roberts TPL (2005) Assessment of the tumor microenvironment in cervix cancer using dynamic contrast enhanced CT, interstitial fluid pressure and oxygen measurements. Int J Radiat Oncol Biol Phys 62:1100–1107

Hänsgen G, Krause U, Becker A, Stadler P, Lautenschläger C, Wohlrab W, Rath FW, Molls, M, Dunst J (2001) Tumor hypoxia, p53, and prognosis in cervical cancers. Int J Radiat Oncol Biol Phys 50:865–872

Harris AL (2002) Hypoxia—a key regulatory factor in tumour growth. Nat Rev Cancer 2:38–47

Heldin C-H, Rubin K, Pietras K, Östman A (2004) High interstitial fluid pressure—an obstacle in cancer therapy. Nature 4:806–813

Helmlinger G, Yuan F, Dellian M, Jain RK (1997) Interstitial pH and pO$_2$ gradients in solid tumors in vivo: high-resolution measurements reveal a lack of correlation. Nat Med 3:177–182

Hill SA, Pigott KH, Saunders MI, Powell MEB, Arnold S, Obeid A, Ward G, Leahy M, Hoskin PJ, Chaplin DJ (1996) Microregional blood flow in murine and human tumours assessed using laser Doppler microprobes. Br J Cancer 74 (Suppl):S260–S263

Hirst DG, Flitney FW (1997) The physiological importance and therapeutic potential of nitric oxide in the tumour-associated vasculature. In: Bicknell R, Lewis CE, Ferrara N (eds) Tumour angiogenesis. Oxford University Press, Oxford, pp 153–167

Höckel M, Knoop C, Schlenger K, Vorndran B, Baussmann E, Mitze M, Knapstein PG, Vaupel P (1993a) Intra-tumoral pO$_2$ predicts survival in advanced cancer of the uterine cervix. Radiother Oncol 26:45–50

Höckel M, Schlenger K, Aral B, Mitze M, Schäffer U, Vaupel P (1996a) Association between tumor hypoxia and malignant progression in advanced cancer of the uterine cervix. Cancer Res 56:4509–4515

Höckel M, Schlenger K, Höckel S, Aral B, Schäffer U, Vaupel P (1998) Tumor hypoxia in pelvic recurrences of cervical cancer. Int J Cancer 79:365–369

Höckel M, Schlenger K, Höckel S, Vaupel P (1999) Association between tumor hypoxia and malignant progression: The clinical evidence in cancer of the uterine cervix. In: Vaupel P, Kelleher DK (eds) Tumor hypoxia. Wissenschaftliche Verlagsgesellschaft, Stuttgart, pp 65–74

Höckel M, Schlenger K, Knoop C, Vaupel P (1991) Oxygenation of carcinomas of the uterine cervix: Evaluation of computerized O$_2$ tension measurements. Cancer Res 51:6098–6102

Höckel M, Schlenger K, Mitze M, Schäffer U, Vaupel P (1996b) Hypoxia and radiation response in human tumors. Semin Radiat Oncol 6:3–9

Höckel M, Vaupel P (2001a) Tumor hypoxia: Definitions and current clinical, biologic and molecular aspects. J Natl Cancer Inst 93:266–276

Höckel M, Vaupel P (2001b) Prognostic significance of tissue hypoxia in cervical cancer. CME J Gynecol Oncol 6:216–225

Höckel M, Vaupel P (2003) Oxygenation of cervix cancers: Impact of clinical and pathological parameters. Adv Exp Med Biol 510:31–35

Höckel M, Vorndran B, Schlenger K, Baussmann E, Knapstein PG (1993b) Tumor oxygenation: A new predictive parameter in locally advanced cancer of the uterine cervix. Gynecol Oncol 51:141–149

Hohenberger P, Felgner C, Haensch W, Schlag PM (1998) Tumor oxygenation correlates with molecular growth determinants in breast cancer. Breast Cancer Res Treat 48:97–106

Hossmann K-A, Mies G, Paschen W, Szabo L, Dolan E, Wechsler W (1986) Regional metabolism of experimental brain tumors. Acta Neuropathol 69:139–147

Hossmann KA, Niebuhr I, Tamura M (1982) Local cerebral blood flow and glucose consumption of rats with experimental gliomas. J Cerebral Blood Flow Metab 2:25–32

Jain RK (1994) Barrieren in Tumoren gegen Therapeutika. Spektrum der Wissenschaft. Septemberheft, pp 48–55

Jones EL, Prosnitz LR, Dewhirst MW, Marcom PK, Hardenbergh PH, Marks LB, Brizel DM, Vujaskovic Z (2004) Thermoradiotherapy improves oxygenation in locally advanced breast cancer. Clin Cancer Res 10:4287–4293

Kallinowski F, Buhr HJ (1995a) Can the oxygenation status of rectal carcinomas be improved by hypoxia? In: Vaupel P, Kelleher DK, Günderoth M (eds) Tumor oxygenation. Fischer, Stuttgart, Jena, New York, pp 291–296

Kallinowski F, Buhr HJ (1995b) Tissue oxygenation of primary, metastatic and xenografted rectal cancers. In: Vaupel P, Kelleher DK, Günderoth M (eds) Tumor oxygenation. Fischer, Stuttgart, Jena, New York, pp 205–209

Kallinowski F, Vaupel P (1988) pH distributions in spontaneous and isotransplanted rat tumors. Br J Cancer 58:314–321

Kayama T, Yoshimoto T, Fujimoto S, Sakurai Y (1991) Intratumoural oxygen pressure in malignant brain tumour. J Neurosurg 74:55–59

Kim CY, Tsai MH, Osmanian C, Graeber TG, Lee JE, Giffard RG, DiPaolo JA, Peehl DM, Giaccia AJ (1997) Selection of human cervical epithelial cells that possess reduced apoptotic potential to low oxygen conditions. Cancer Res 57:4200–4204

Kimura H, Braun RD, Ong ET, Hsu R, Secomb TW, Papahadjopoulos D, Hong K, Dewhirst M (1996) Fluctuations in red cell flux in tumor microvessels can lead to transient hypoxia and reoxygenation in tumor parenchyma. Cancer Res 56:5522–5528

Knisely JPS, Rockwell S (2002) Importance of hypoxia in the biology and treatment of brain tumors. Neuroimag Clin N Am 12:525–536

Knocke TH, Weitmann HD, Feldmann HJ, Selzer E, Pötter R (1999) Intratumoral pO_2-measurements as predictive assay in the treatment of carcinoma of the uterine cervix. Radiother Oncol 53:99–104

Kondo A, Safaei R, Mishima M, Niedner H, Lin Y, Howell SB (2001) Hypoxia-induced enrichment and mutagenesis of cells that have lost DNA mismatch repair. Cancer Res 61:7603–7607

Konerding MA, Fait E, Gaumann A (2001) 3D microvascular architecture of pre-cancerous lesions and invasive carcinomas of the colon. Br J Cancer 84:1354–1362

Koong AC, Mehta VK, Le QT, Fisher GA, Terris DJ, Brown JM, Bastidas AJ, Vierra M (2000) Pancreatic tumors show high levels of hypoxia. Int J Radiat Oncol Biol Phys 48:919–922

Lally BE, Rockwell S, Fischer DB, Collingridge DR, Piepmeier JM, Knisely JP (2004) The interactions of polarographic measurements of oxygen tension and histological grade in human glioma and surrounding peritumoral brain tissue. Int J Radiat Oncol 60:S194

Lartigau E, Randrianarivelo H, Avril M-F, Margulis A, Spatz A, Eschwege F, Guichard M (1997) Intratumoral oxygen tension in metastatic melanoma. Melanoma Res 7:400–406

Lartigau E, Haie-Meder C, Cosset MF, Delapierre M, Gerbaulet A, Eschwege F, Guichard M (1992a) Feasibility of measuring oxygen tension in uterine cervix carcinoma. Eur J Cancer 28A:1354–1357

Lartigau E, Le Ridant A-M, Lambin P, Weeger P, Martin L, Sigal R, Lusinchi A, Luboinski B, Eschwege F, Guichard M (1993) Oxygenation of head and neck tumors. Cancer 71:2319–2325

Lartigau E, Lusinchi A, Eschwege F, Guichard M (1999) Tumor oxygenation: The Gustave Roussy experience. In: Vaupel P, Kelleher DK (eds) Tumor hypoxia. Wissenschaftliche Verlagsgesellschaft, Stuttgart, pp 47–52

Lartigau E, Lusinchi A, Weeger P, Wibault P, Luboinski B, Eschwege F, Guichard M (1998) Variations in tumour oxygen tension (pO_2) during accelerated radiotherapy of head and neck carcinoma. Eur J Cancer 34:856–861

Lartigau E, Martin L, Lambin P, Haie-Meder C, Gerbaulet A, Eschwege F, Guichard M (1992b) Mesure de la pression partielle en oxygène dans des tumeurs du col utérin. Bull Cancer/Radiother 79:199–206

Lartigau E, Randrianarivelo H, Martin L, Stern S, Thomas CD, Guichard M, Weeger P, Le Ridant A-M, Luboinski B, Nguyen T, Ortoli J-C, Grange F, Avril M-F, Lusinchi A, Wibault P, Haie-Meder C, Gerbaulet A, Eschwege F (1994) Oxygen tension measurements in human tumors: The Institut Gustave-Roussy experience. Radiat Oncol Invest 1:285–291

Lawrentschuk N, Poon AMT, Foo SS, Johns Putra LG, Murone C, Davis ID, Bolton DM, Scott AM (2005) Assessing regional hypoxia in human renal tumours using ^{18}F-fluoromisonidazole positron emission tomography. BJU Int 96:540–546

Le QT, Chen E, Salim A, Cao Hongbin, Kong CS, Whyte R, Donington J, Cannon W, Wakelee H, Tibshirani R, Mitchell JD, Richardson D, O'Byrne KJ, Koong AC, Giaccia AJ (2006) An evaluation of tumor oxygenation and gene expression in patients with early stage non-small cell lung cancers. Clin Cancer Res 12:1507–1514

Le QT, Kovacs MS, Dorie MJ, Koong A, Terris DJ, Pinto HA, Goffinet DR, Nowels K, Bloch D, Brown JM (2003) Comparison of the comet assay and the oxygen microelectrode for measuring tumor oxygenation in head-and-neck cancer patients. Int J Radiat Oncol Biol Phys 56:375–383

Leo C, Giaccia AJ, Denko NC (2004) The hypoxic tumor microenvironment and gene expression. Semin Radiat Oncol 14:207–214

Leo C, Richter C, Horn L-C, Schütz A, Pilch H, Höckel M (2005) Expression of Apaf-1 in cervical cancer correlates with lymph node metastasis but not with intratumoral hypoxia. Gynecol Oncol 97:602–606

Less JR, Posner MC, Boucher Y, Borochovitz D, Wolmark N, Jain RK (1992) Interstitial hypertension in human breast and colorectal tumors. Cancer Res 52:6371–6374

Liotta LA, Kohn EC (2001) The microenvironment of the tumour-host interface. Nature 411:375–379

Ljungkvist ASE, Bussink J, Kaanders JHAM, Rijken PFJW, Begg AC, Raleigh JA, van der Kogel AJ (2005) Hypoxic cell turnover in different solid tumor lines. Int J Radiat Oncol Biol Phys 62:1157–1168

Lunt SJ, Kalliomaki TMK, Brown A, Yang VX, Milosevic M, Hill RP (2008) Interstitial fluid pressure, vascularity and metastasis in ectopic, orthotopic and spontaneous tumours. BMC Cancer 8:2

Lyng H, Sundfør K, Tanum G, Rofstad EK (1997) Oxygen tension in primary tumours of the uterine cervix and lymph node metastases of the head and neck. Adv Exp Med Biol 428:55–60

Lyng H, Sundfør K, Trope C, Rofstad EK (2000) Disease control of uterine cervical cancer: relationships to tumor oxygen tension, vascular density, cell density, and frequency of mitosis and apoptosis measured before treatment and during radiotherapy. Clin Cancer Res 6:1104–1112

Lyng H, Vorren AO, Sundfør K, Taksdal I, Lien HH, Kaalhus O, Rofstad EK (2001) Intra- and intertumor heterogeneity in blood perfusion of human cervical cancer before treatment and after radiotherapy. Int J Cancer Radiat Oncol Invest 96:182–190

Magagnin MG, Sergeant K, van den Beucken T, Rouschop KM, Jutten B, Seigneuric R, Lambin P, Devreese B, Koritzinsky M, Wouters BG (2007) Proteomic analysis of gene expression following hypoxia and reoxygenation reveals proteins involved in the recovery from endoplasmic reticulum and oxidative stress. Radiother Oncol 83:340–345

Martin L, Lartigau E, Weeger P, Lambin P, Le Ridant AM, Lusinchi A, Wibault P, Eschwege F, Luboinski B, Guichard M (1993) Changes in the oxygenation of head and neck tumors during carbogen breathing. Radiother Oncol 27:123–130

Mattern J, Kallinowski F, Herfarth C, Volm M (1996) Association of resistance-related protein expression with poor vascularization and low levels of oxygen in human rectal cancer. Int J Cancer 67:20–23

Mayer A, Höckel M, Vaupel P (2006) Endogenous hypoxia markers in locally advanced cancers of the uterine cervix: Reality or wishful thinking? Strahlenther Onkol 182:501–510

Mayer A, Höckel M, Wree A, Leo C, Horn L-C, Vaupel P (2008) Lack of hypoxic response in uterine leiomyomas despite severe tissue hypoxia. Cancer Res 68:4719–4726

Milosevic M, Fyles A, Haider M, Hedley D, Hill R (2004) The human tumor microenvironment: invasive (needle) measurement of oxygen and interstitial fluid pressure (IFP). Sem Radiat Oncol 14:249–258

Milosevic M, Fyles A, Hedley D, Pintilie M, Levin W, Manchul L, Hill R (2001a) Interstitial fluid pressure predicts survival in patients with cervic cancer independent of clinical prognostic factors and tumor oxygen measurements. Cancer Res 61:6400–6405

Milosevic M, Quirt I, Levin W, Fyles A, Manchul L, Chapman W (2001b) Intratumoral sickling in patient with cervix cancer and sickle trait: Effect on blood flow and oxygenation. Gynecol Oncol 83:428–431

Milosevic MF, Fyles AW, Wong R, Pintilie M, Kavanagh M-C, Levin W, Manchul LA, Keane TJ, Hill RP (1998) Interstitial fluid pressure in cervical carcinoma. Cancer 82:2418–2426

Molls M, Feldmann HJ, Füller J (1994) Oxygenation of locally advanced recurrent rectal cancer soft tissue sarcoma and breast cancer. Adv Exp Med Biol 345:459–463

Molls M, Vaupel P (eds) (2000) Blood perfusion and microenvironment of human tumors. Springer, Berlin, Heidelberg, New York

Moringlane JR (1994) Measurement of oxygen partial pressure in brain tumors under stereotactic conditions. Adv Exp Med Biol 345:471–477

Movsas B, Chapman JD, Greenberg RE, Hanlon AL, Horwitz EM, Pinover WH, Stobbe C, Hanks GE (2000) Increasing levels of hypoxia in prostate carcinoma correlate significantly with increasing clinical stage and patient age. Cancer 89:2018–2024

Movsas B, Chapman JD, Hanlon AL, Horwitz EM, Greenberg RE, Stobbe C, Hanks GE, Pollack A (2002) Hypoxic prostate/muscle pO_2 ratio predicts for biochemical failure in patients with prostate cancer: Preliminary findings. Urology 60:634–639

Movsas B, Chapman JD, Horwitz EM, Pinover WH, Greenberg RE, Hanlon AL, Iyer R, Hanks GE (1999) Hypoxic regions exist in human prostate carcinoma. Urology 53:11–18

Mueller MM, Fusenig NE (2004) Friends or foes—bipolar effects of the tumour stroma in cancer. Nat Rev Cancer 4:839–849

Mueller-Klieser W, Walenta S (1993) Geographical mapping of metabolites in biological tissue with quantitative bioluminescence and single photon imaging. Histochem J 25:407–420

Mueller-Klieser W, Walenta S, Paschen W, Kallinowski F, Vaupel P (1988) Metabolic imaging in microregions of tumors and normal tissues with bioluminescence and photon counting. J Natl Cancer Inst 80:842–848

Nathanson SD, Nelson L (1994) Interstitial fluid pressure in breast cancer, benign breast conditions, and breast parenchyma. Ann Surg Oncol 1:333–338

Negendank W (1992) Studies of human tumors by MRS: A review. NMR Biomed 5:303–324

Netti PA, Baxter LT, Boucher Y, Skalak R, Jain RK (1995) Time-dependent behavior of interstitial fluid pressure in solid tumors: Implication for drug delivery. Cancer Res 55:5451–5458

Newell K, Franchi A, Pouyssegur J, Tannock I (1993) Studies with glycolysis-deficient cells suggest that production of lactic acid is not the only cause of tumor acidity. Proc Natl Acad Sci USA 90:1127–1131

Newell K, Tannock I (1991) Regulation of intracellular pH and viability of tumor cells. Funktionsanal Biol Syst 20:219–234

Nordsmark M, Alsner J, Keller J, Nielsen OS, Jensen OM, Horsman MR, Overgaard J (2001) Hypoxia in human soft tissue sarcomas: Adverse impact on survival and no association with p53 mutations. Br J Cancer 84:1070–1075

Nordsmark M, Bentzen SM, Overgaard J (1994) Measurement of human tumour oxygenation status by a polarographic needle electrode. An analysis of inter- and intratumour heterogeneity. Acta Oncol 33:383–389

Nordsmark M, Bentzen SM, Rudat V, Brizel D, Lartigau E, Stadler P, Becker A, Adam M, Molls M, Dunst J, Terris DJ, Overgaard J (2005) Prognostic value of tumor oxygenation in 397 head and neck tumors after primary radiation therapy. An international multi-center study. Radiother Oncol 77:18–24

Nordsmark M, Hover M, Keller J, Nielsen OS, Jensen OM, Overgaard J (1996a) The relationship between tumor oxygenation and cell proliferation in human soft tissue sarcomas. Int J Radiat Oncol Biol Phys 35:701–708

Nordsmark M, Keller J, Nielsen OS, Lundorf E, Overgaard J (1997) Tumour oxygenation assessed by polarographic needle electrodes and bioenergetic status measured by ^{31}P magnetic resonance spectroscopy in human soft tissue tumours. Acta Oncol 36:565–571

Nordsmark M, Loncaster J, Aquino-Parsons C, Chou SC, Ladekarl M, Havsteen H, Lindegaard JC, Davidson SE, Varia M, West C, Hunter R, Overgaard J, Raleigh JA (2003) Measurements of hypoxia using pimonidazole and polarographic oxygen-sensitive electrodes in human cervix carcinomas. Radiother Oncol 67:35–44

Nordsmark M, Overgaard J (2000) A confirmatory prognostic study on oxygenation status and loco-regional control in advanced head and neck squamous cell carcinoma treated by radiation therapy. Radiother Oncol 57:39–43

Nordsmark M, Overgaard J (2004) Tumor hypoxia is independent of hemoglobin and prognostic for loco-regional tumor control after primary radiotherapy in advanced head and neck cancer. Acta Oncol 43:396–403

Nordsmark M, Overgaard M, Overgaard J (1996b) Pretreatment oxygenation predicts radiation response in advanced squamous cell carcinoma of the head and neck. Radiother Oncol 41:31–39

Park CC, Bissell MJ, Barcellos-Hoff MH (2000) The influence of the microenvironment on the malignant phenotype. Mol Med Today 6:324–329

Parker C, Milosevic M, Toi A, Sweet J, Panzarella T, Bristow R, Catton C, Catton P, Crook J, Gospodarowicz M, McLean M, Warde P, Hill RP (2004) Polarographic electrode study of tumor oxygenation in clinically localized prostate cancer. Int J Radiat Oncol Biol Phys 58:750–757

Paschen W (1985) Regional quantitative determination of lactate in brain sections. A bioluminescent approach. J Cerebral Blood Flow Metab 5:609–612

Paschen W, Djuricic B, Mies G, Schmidt-Kastner R, Linn F (1987) Lactate and pH in the brain: Association and dissociation in different pathophysiological states. J Neurochem 48:154–159

Pigott KH, Hill SA, Chaplin DJ, Saunders MI (1996) Microregional fluctuations in perfusion within human tumours detected using laser Doppler flowmetry. Radiother Oncol 40:45–50

Pitson G, Fyles A, Milosevic M, Wylie J, Pintilie M, Hill R (2001) Tumor size and oxygenation are independent predictors of nodal disease in patients with cervix cancer. Int J Radiat Oncol Biol Phys 51:699–703

Powell MEB, Collingridge DR, Saunders MI, Hoskin PJ, Hill SA, Chaplin DJ (1999) Improvement in human tumour oxygenation with carbogen of varying carbon dioxide concentrations. Radiother Oncol 50:167–171

Raab GH, Auer F, Scheich D, Molls M, Eiermann W (2002) Pretreatment intratumoral oxygen tension (pO₂) is not predictive for response to primary systemic chemotherapy (PSC) in operable T2 breast cancer. ASCO-Meeting 2002, Abstract no. 1806

Rampling R, Cruickshank G, Lewis AD, Fitzsimmons SA, Workman P (1994) Direct measurement of pO₂ distribution and bioreductive enzymes in human malignant brain tumors. Int J Radiat Oncol Biol Phys 29:427–431

Reinhold HS (1971) Improved microcirculation in irradiated tumours. Eur J Cancer 7:273–280

Reinhold HS (1987) Tumour microcirculation. In: Field SB, Franconi C (eds) Physics and technology of hyperthermia. Martinus Nijhoff Publishers, Dordrecht, Boston, Lancaster, pp 448–457

Reinhold HS, van den Berg-Blok A (1983) Vascularization of experimental tumours. Ciba Found Symp 100:100–119

Reinhold HS, van den Berg-Blok AE (1987) Circulation physiology of tumors. In: Kallman RF (ed) Rodent tumor models in experimental cancer therapy. Pergamon Press, New York, pp 39–42

Reynolds TY, Rockwell S, Glazer PM (1996) Genetic instability induced by the tumor microenvironment. Cancer Res 56:5754–5757

Ribatti D, Vacca A, Dammacco F (2003) New non-angiogenesis dependent pathways for tumour growth. Eur J Cancer 39:1835–1841

Rofstad EK, Galappathi K, Mathiesen B, Ruud EB (2007) Fluctuating and diffusion-limited hypoxia in hypoxia-induced metastasis. Clin Cancer Res 13:1971–1978

Rofstad EK, Sundfør K, Lyng H, Trope CG (2000) Hypoxia-induced treatment failure in advanced squamous cell carcinoma of the uterine cervix is primarily due to hxpoxia-induced radiation resistance rather than hypoxia induced metastasis. Br J Cancer 83:354–359

Roh HD, Boucher Y, Kalnicki S, Buchsbaum R, Bloomer WD, Jain RK (1991) Interstitial hypertension in carcinoma of uterine cervix patients: Possible correlation with tumor oxygenation and radiation response. Cancer Res 51:6695–6698

Rudat V, Stadler P, Becker A, Vanselow B, Dietz A, Wannenmacher M, Molls M, Dunst J, Feldmann HJ (2001) Predictive value of the tumor oxygenation by means of pO₂ histography in patients with advanced head and neck cancer. Strahlenther Onkol 177:462–468

Rudat V, Vanselow B, Wollensack P, Bettscheider C, Osman-Ahmet S, Eble MJ, Dietz A (2000) Repeatability and prognostic impact of the pretreatment pO₂ histography in patients with advanced head and neck cancer. Radiother Oncol 57:31–37

Runkel S, Wischnik A, Teubner E, Kaven E, Gaa J, Melchert F (1994) Oxygenation of mammary tumors as evaluated by ultrasound-guided computerized pO₂ histography. Adv Exp Med Biol 345:451–458

Saumweber DM, Kau RJ, Arnold W (1995) Tumor tissue oxygenation in primary squamous cell carcinomas of the head and neck—Preliminary results. In: Vaupel P, Kelleher DK, Günderoth M (eds) Tumor oxygenation. Fischer, Stuttgart, Jena, New York, pp 313–318

Scholbach T, Scholbach J, Krombach GA, Gagel B, Maneschi P, Di Martino E (2005) New method of dynamic color Doppler signal quantification in metastatic lymph nodes compared to direct polarographic measurements of tissue oxygenation. Int J Cancer 114:957–996

Semenza GL (2000) Hypoxia, clonal selection, and the role of HIF-1 in tumor progression. Crit Rev Biochem Mol Biol 35:71–103

Semenza GL (2002a) Involvement of hypoxia-inducible factor 1 in human cancer. Internal Med 41:79–83

Semenza GL (2002b) HIF-1 and tumor progression: Pathophysiology and therapeutics. Trends Mol Med 8:S62–S67

Semenza GL (2003) Targeting HIF-1 for cancer therapy. Nat Rev Cancer 3:721–732

Sevick EM, Jain RK (1989) Viscous resistance to blood flow in solid tumors: Effect of hematocrit on intratumor blood viscosity. Cancer Res 49:3513–3519

Shchors K, Evan G (2007) Tumor angiogenesis: Cause or consequence of cancer? Cancer Res 67:7059–7061

Sivridis E, Giatromanolaki A, Koukourakis MI (2003) The vascular network of tumours—what is it not for? J Pathol 201:173–180

Song CW, Lyons JC, Luo Y (1993) Intra- and extracellular pH in solid tumors: Influence on therapeutic response. In: Teicher BA (ed) Drug resistance in oncology. Marcel Dekker, New York, Basel, Hong Kong, pp 25–51

Song CW, Park H, Ross BD (1999) Intra- and extracellular pH in solid tumors. In: Teicher BA (ed) Antiangiogenic agents in cancer therapy. Humana Press Inc, Totowa, pp 51–64

Stadler P, Becker A, Feldmann HJ, Hänsgen G, Dunst J, Würschmidt F, Molls M (1999) Influence of the hypoxic subvolume on the survival of patients with head and neck cancer. Int J Radiat Oncol Biol Phys 44:749–754

Stadler P, Feldmann HJ, Creighton C, Kau R, Molls M (1998) Changes in tumor oxygenation during combined treatment with split-course radiotherapy and chemotherapy in patients with head and neck cancer. Radiother Oncol 48:57–164

Stohrer M, Boucher Y, Stangassinger M, Jain RK (2000) Oncotic pressure in solid tumors is elevated. Cancer Res 60:4251–4255

Stone HB, Brown JM, Phillips TL, Sutherland RM (1993) Oxygen in human tumors: correlations between methods of measurement and response to therapy. Radiat Res 136:422–434

Stone JE, Parker R, Gilks CB, Stanbridge EJ, Liao SY, Aquino-Parsons (2005) Intratumoral oxygenation of invasive squamous cell carcinoma of the vulva is not correlated with regional lymph node metastasis. Eur J Gynaecol Oncol 26:31–35

Strnad V, Keilholz L, Kirschner M, Meyer M, Sauer R (1997) Sauerstoffdruckverteilung in Lymphknotenmetastasen und die Veränderungen während akuter respiratorischer Hypoxie. Strahlenther Onkol 173:267–271

Stubbs M (1999) Application of magnetic resonance techniques for imaging tumour physiology. Acta Oncol 38:845–853

Stubbs M, Bhujwalla ZM, Tozer GM, Rodrigues LM, Maxwell RJ, Morgan R, Howe FA, Griffiths JR (1992) An assessment of ³¹P-MRS as a method of measuring pH in rat tumours. NMR Biomed 5:351–359

Stubbs M, Griffiths JR (1999) Monitoring cancer by magnetic resonance. Br J Cancer 80 (Suppl 1):86–94

Stubbs M, McSheehy PMJ, Griffiths JR, Bashford CL (2000) Causes and consequences of tumour acidity and implications for treatment. Mol Med Today 6:15–19

Sundfør K, Lyng H, Kongsgard U, Tropé C, Rofstad EK (1997) Polarographic measurement of pO₂ in cervix carcinoma. Gynecol Oncol 64:230–236

Sundfør K, Lyng H, Rofstad EK (1998a) Oxygen tension and vascular density in adenocarcinoma and squamous cell carcinoma of the uterine cervix. Acta Oncol 37:665–670

Sundfør K, Lyng H, Rofstad EK (1998b) Tumour hypoxia and vascular density as predictors of metastasis in squamous cell carcinoma of the uterine cervix. Br J Cancer 78:822–827

Sundfør K, Lyng H, Trope CG, Rofstad EK (2000) Treatment outcome in advanced squamous cell carcinoma of the uterine cervix: relationships to pretreatment tumor oxygenation and vascularization. Radiother Oncol 54:101–107

Sutherland RM (1988) Cell and environment interactions in tumor microregions: The multicell spheroid model. Science 240:177–184

Tannock IF, Rotin D (1989) Acid pH in tumors and its potential for therapeutic exploitation. Cancer Res 49:4373–4384

Terris DJ (2000) Head and neck cancer: The importance of oxygen. Laryngoscope 110:697–707

Thistlethwaite AJ, Leeper DB, Moylan DJ, Nerlinger RE (1985) pH distribution in human tumors. Int J Radiat Oncol Biol Phys 11:1647–1652

Toffoli S, Michiels C (2008) Intermittent hypoxia is a key regulator of cancer cell and endothelial cell interplay in tumours. FEBS J 275:2991–3002

Trédan O, Galmarini CM, Patel K, Tannock IF (2007) Drug resistance and the solid tumor microenvironment. J Natl Cancer Inst 99:1441–1454

Unger M, Weaver VM (2003) The tissue microenvironment as an epigenetic tumor modifier. Methods Mol Biol 223:315–347

van den Berg AP (1991) Tissue pH of human tumors and its variation upon therapy. Funktionsanal Biol Syst 20:235–255

van den Berg AP, Wike-Hooley JL, van den Berg-Blok AE, van der Zee J, Reinhold HS (1982) Tumour pH in human mammary carcinoma. Eur J Cancer Clin Oncol 18:457–462

Vaupel P (1990) Oxygenation of human tumors. Strahlenther Onkol 166:377–386

Vaupel P (1992) Physiological properties of malignant tumours. NMR Biomed 5:220–225

Vaupel P (1993) Oxygenation of solid tumors. In: Teicher BA (ed) Drug resistance in oncology. Marcel Dekker, New York, pp 53–85

Vaupel P (1994a) Blood flow, oxygenation, tissue pH distribution and bioenergetic status of tumors. Berlin: Ernst Schering Research Foundation, Lecture 23

Vaupel P (1994b) Blood flow and metabolic microenvironment of brain tumors. J Neuro-Oncol 22:261–267

Vaupel P (1998) Tumor blood flow. In: Molls M, Vaupel P (eds) Medical radiology—Diagnostic imaging and radiation oncology. Blood perfusion and microenvironment of human tumors. Springer, Berlin, Heidelberg, New York, pp 41–45

Vaupel P (2001) Durchblutung und Oxygenierungsstatus von Kopf-Hals-Tumoren. In: Böttcher HD, Wendt TG, Henke M (eds) Klinik des Rezidivtumors im Kopf-Hals-Bereich. Zuckschwerdt, München, pp 7–23

Vaupel P (2002) Durchblutung, Sauerstoffversorgung, Glukoseaufnahme und pH-Gradienten in Hirntumoren. In: Böttcher HD, Seifert V, Henke M, Mose St (eds) Klinik der hirneigenen Tumoren und Metastasen—Grundlagen, Diagnostik, Therapie. Zuckschwerdt, München, pp 34–49

Vaupel P (2004a) The role of hypoxia-induced factors in tumor progression. Oncologist 9 (Suppl. 5):10–17

Vaupel P (2004b) Tumor microenvironmental physiology and its implications for radiation oncology. Semin Radiat Oncol 14:198–206

Vaupel P (2006) Abnormal microvasculature and defective microcirculatory function in solid tumors. In: Siemann DW (ed) Vascular-targeted therapies in oncology. John Wiley & Sons, Chichester, UK, pp 9–29

Vaupel P (2008) Strikingly high respiratory quotients: A further characteristic of the tumor pathophysiome. Adv Exp Med Biol 614:121–125

Vaupel P, Briest S, Höckel M (2002a) Hypoxia in breast cancer: Pathogenesis, characterization and biological/therapeutic implications. Wien Med Wschr 152:334–342

Vaupel P, Dunst J, Engert A, Fandrey J, Feyer P, Freund M, Jelkmann W (2005) Effects of recombinant human erthropoietin (rHuEPO) on tumor control in patients with cancer-induced anemia. Onkologie 28: 216–221

Vaupel P, Grunewald WA, Manz R, Sowa W (1978) Intracapillary HbO_2 saturation in tumor tissue of DS-carcinosarcoma during normoxia. Adv Exp Med Biol 94:367–375

Vaupel P, Harrison L (2004) Tumor hypoxia: Causative factors, compensatory mechanisms, and cellular response. Oncologist 9 (Suppl. 5):4–9

Vaupel P, Höckel M (1999) Oxygenation status of breast cancer: The Mainz experience. In: Vaupel P, Kelleher DK (eds) Tumor hypoxia. Wissenschaftliche Verlagsgesellschaft, Stuttgart, pp 1–11

Vaupel P, Höckel M (2000) Blood supply, oxygenation status and metabolic micromilieu of breast cancers: Characterization and therapeutic relevance. Int J Oncol 17:869–879

Vaupel P, Höckel M (2001) Hypoxie beim Zervixkarzinom: Pathogenese, Charakterisierung und biologische/klinische Konsequenzen. Zentralbl Gynäkol 123: 192–197

Vaupel P, Höckel M (2004) Durchblutung, Oxygenierungsstatus und metabolisches Mikromilieu des Mammakarzinoms. Pathomechanismen, Charakterisierung und biologische/therapeutische Relevanz. In: Untch M, Sittek H, Bauerfeind I, Reiser M, Hepp H (eds) Diagnostik und Therapie des Mammakarzinoms—State of the Art. Zuckschwerdt, München, pp 347–367

Vaupel P, Höckel M, Mayer A (2007) Detection and characterization of tumor hypoxia using pO_2 histography. Antioxid Redox Signal 9:1221–1235

Vaupel P, Jain RK (eds) (1991) Tumor blood supply and metabolic microenvironment. Characterization and implications for therapy. Gustav Fischer, Stuttgart, New York

Vaupel P, Kallinowski F (1987) Hemoconcentration of blood flowing through human tumor xenografts. Int J Microcirc Clin Exp 6:72

Vaupel P, Kallinowski F, Groebe K (1988) Evaluation of oxygen diffusion distances in human breast cancer using inherent in vivo-data: Role of various pathogenetic mechanisms in the development of tumor hypoxia. Adv Exp Med Biol 222:719–726

Vaupel P, Kallinowski F, Okunieff P (1989) Blood flow, oxygen and nutrient supply, and metabolic microenvironment of human tumors: A review. Cancer Res 49:6449–6465

Vaupel P, Kelleher DK (eds) (1999) Tumor hypoxia. Wissenschaftliche Verlagsgesellschaft, Stuttgart

Vaupel P, Kelleher DK, Engel T (1994b) Stable bioenergetic status despite substantial changes in blood flow and tissue oxygenation. Br J Cancer 69:46–49

Vaupel P, Mayer A (2004) Erythropoietin to treat anaemia in patients with head and neck cancer. Lancet 363:992

Vaupel P, Mayer A (2005) Effects of anaemia and hypoxia on tumour biology. In: Bokemeyer C, Ludwig H (eds) Anaemia in Cancer, 2nd edn. Elsevier, Edinburgh, London, pp 47–66

Vaupel P, Mayer A, Briest S, Höckel M (2003a) Oxygenation gain factor: A novel parameter characterizing the association between hemoglobin level and the oxygenation status of breast cancers. Cancer Res 63:7634–7637

Vaupel P, Mayer A, Höckel M (2006a) Impact of hemoglobin levels on tumor oxygenation: the higher, the better? Strahlenther Onkol 182:63–71

Vaupel P, Mayer A, Höckel M (2006b) Oxygenation status of primary and recurrent squamous cell carcinomas of the vulva. Eur J Gynaecol Oncol 27:142–146

Vaupel P, Mueller-Klieser W (1983) Interstitieller Raum und Mikromilieu in malignen Tumoren. Mikrozirk Forsch Klin 2:78–90

Vaupel P, Schaefer C, Okunieff P (1994a) Intracellular acidosis in murine fibrosarcomas coincides with ATP depletion, hypoxia, and high levels of lactate and total P_i. NMR Biomed 7:128–136

Vaupel P, Schlenger K, Knoop M, Hoeckel M (1991) Oxygenation of human tumors: Evaluation of tissue oxygen distribution in breast cancers by computerized O_2 tension measurements. Cancer Res 51:3316–3322

Vaupel P, Thews O, Höckel M (1997) Durchblutung, Oxygenierung, pH-Verteilung und bioenergetischer Status maligner Tumoren. Arzneimitteltherapie 15:319–327

Vaupel P, Thews O, Hoeckel M (2001) Treatment resistance of solid tumors: Role of hypoxia and anemia. Med Oncol 18:243–259

Vaupel P, Thews O, Kelleher DK, Hoeckel M (1998) Current status of knowledge and critical issues in tumor oxygenation. Adv Exp Med Biol 454:591–602

Vaupel P, Thews O, Kelleher DK, Konerding MA (2003b) O_2 extraction is a key parameter determining the oxygenation status of malignant tumors and normal tissues. Int J Oncol 22:795–798

Vaupel P, Thews O, Mayer A, Höckel S, Höckel M (2002b) Oxygenation status of gynecologic tumors: What is the optimal hemoglobin level? Strahlenther Onkol 178:727–731

Vaupel, P, Mayer A, Höckel M (2004) Tumor hypoxia and malignant progression. Methods Enzymol 381:335–354

Vordermark D, Brown JM (2003) Endogenous markers of tumor hypoxia predictors of clinical radiation resistance? Strahlenther Onkol 179:801–811

Vujaskovic Z, Rosen EL, Blackwell KL, Jones EL, Brizel DM, Prosnitz LR, Samulski TV, Dewhirst MW (2003) Ultrasound guided pO_2 measurement of breast cancer reoxygenation after neoadjuvant chemotherapy and hyperthermia treatment. Int J Hyperthermia 19:498–506

Walenta S, Chau T-V, Schroeder T, Lehr H-A, Kunz-Schughart LA, Fuerst A, Mueller-Klieser W (2003) Metabolic classification of human rectal adenocarcinomas: a novel guideline for clinical oncologists? J Cancer Res Clin Oncol 129:321–326

Walenta S, Mueller-Klieser WF (2004) Lactate: Mirror and motor of tumor malignancy. Sem Radiat Oncol 14:267–274

Walenta S, Salameh A, Lyng H, Evensen JF, Mitze M, Rofstad EK, Mueller-Klieser W (1997) Correlation of high lactate levels in head and neck tumors with incidence of metastasis. Am J Pathol 150:409–415

Walenta S, Wetterling M, Lehrke M, Schwickert G, Sundfør K, Rofstad EK, Mueller-Klieser W (2000) High lactate levels predict likelihood of metastases, tumor recurrence, and restricted patient survival in human cervical cancers. Cancer Res 60:916–921

Warburg O (1925) Über den Stoffwechsel der Carcinomzelle. Klin Wschr 4:534–536

Warburg O (1930) The metabolism of tumours. A. Constable, London

Weinberg RA (2008) Coevolution in the tumor microenvironment. Nat Genetics 40:494–495

Weinmann M, Jendrossek V, Güner D, Goecke B, Belka C (2004) Cyclic exposure to hypoxia and reoxygenation selects for tumor cells with defects in mitochondrial apoptotic pathways. FASEB J 18:1906–1908

Weiss L, Hultborn R, Tveit E (1979) Blood flow characteristics in induced rat mammary neoplasia. Microvasc Res 17:S119

Weitmann HD, Gustorff B, Vaupel P, Knocke TH, Pötter R (2003) Oxygenation status of cervical carcinomas before and during spinal anesthesia for application of brachytherapy. Strahlenther Onkol 179:633–640

Wheeler RH, Ziessman HA, Medvec BR, Juni JE, Thrall JH, Keyes JW, Pitt SR, Baker SR (1986) Tumor blood flow and systemic shunting in patients receiving intraarterial chemotherapy for head and neck cancer. Cancer Res 46:4200–4204

Wike-Hooley JL, Haveman J, Reinhold HS (1984) The relevance of tumour pH to the treatment of malignant disease. Radiother Oncol 2:343–366

Wike-Hooley JL, van den Berg AP, van der Zee J, Reinhold HS (1985) Human tumour pH and its variation. Eur J Cancer Clin Oncol 21:785–791

Wilson CBJH, Lammertsma AA, McKenzie CG, Sikora K, Jones T (1992) Measurements of blood flow and exchanging water space in breast tumors using positron emission tomography: a rapid and noninvasive dynamic method. Cancer Res 52:1592–1597

Witz IP, Levy-Nissenbaum O (2006) The tumor microenvironment in the post-PAGET era. Cancer Lett 242:1–10

Wong RK, Fyles A, Milosevic M, Pintilie M, Hill RP (1997) Heterogeneity of polarographic oxygen tension measurements in cervix cancer: an evaluation of within and between tumor variability, probe position, and track depth. Int J Radiat Oncol Biol Phys 39:405–412

Young JS, Lumsden CE, Stalker AL (1950) The significance of the tissue pressure of normal testicular and of neoplastic (Brown-Pearce carcinoma) tissue in the rabbit. J Pathol Bacteriol 62:313–333

Yuan J, Narayanan L, Rockwell S, Glazer PM (2000) Diminished DNA repair and elevated mutagenesis in mammalian cells exposed to hypoxia and low pH. Cancer Res 60:4372–4376

Adhesion, Invasion, Integrins, and Beyond

Nils Cordes, Stephanie Hehlgans, and Iris Eke

CONTENTS

N. Cordes, MD, PhD
OncoRay-Center for Radiation Research in Oncology, Medical
Faculty Carl Gustav Carus, Dresden University of Technology,
Fetscherstraße 74, 01307 Dresden, Germany

S. Hehlgans, PhD
OncoRay-Center for Radiation Research in Oncology, Medical
Faculty Carl Gustav Carus, Dresden University of Technology,
Fetscherstraße 74, 01307 Dresden, Germany

I. Eke, MD
OncoRay-Center for Radiation Research in Oncology, Medical
Faculty Carl Gustav Carus, Dresden University of Technology,
Fetscherstraße 74, 01307 Dresden, Germany

KEY POINTS

- A precise and concerted interplay between both the cellular components, i.e., the cells and their mutations, and the acellular components, i.e., the tumor microenvironment, drives tumor growth and spread beyond physiological boundaries as well as promotes cellular resistance to conventional radiotherapy and chemotherapy.

- One of the prominent microenvironmental modulators of the sensitivity of tumor tissue and tumor-associated normal tissue to therapy is the interaction of cells with the extracellular matrix. Besides serving as structural support for the cells in a tissue, the extracellular matrix participates in the regulation of essential cell functions such as survival, proliferation, differentiation, adhesion, and migration.

- Adhesion and invasion are controlled by integrin receptors and are frequently dysregulated in cancer, with disastrous consequences such as local destruction of normal tissue, metastases, and ineffective local tumor control by anticancer therapeutics. Particularly compromised local tumor control evolves from the combination of genetic alterations and changes in the tumor microenvironment.

- Integrins and their associated signaling molecules are attractive target molecules to be inhibited by pharmacological small molecules aiming at optimization of conventional radio- and chemotherapy.

- Unraveling the intra- and extracellular networks a tumor cell exploits for its growth and spreading capability in more depth may foster the diagnosis of early-stage cancer, the development of novel drugs, and eventually improved patient survival.

Abstract

The importance of the tumor microenvironment for tumor development and progression becomes increasingly evident. A precise and concerted interplay between both the cellular components, i.e., the cells and their mutations, and the acellular components, i.e., the tumor microenvironment, drives tumor growth and spread beyond physiological boundaries as well as promotes cellular resistance to conventional radiotherapy and chemotherapy. One of the prominent microenvironmental modulators of the sensitivity of tumor tissue and tumor-associated normal tissue to therapy is the interaction of cells with the extracellular matrix. Besides serving as structural support for the cells in a tissue, the extracellular matrix participates in the regulation of essential cell functions such as survival, proliferation, differentiation, adhesion, and migration. In this chapter, the overarching function of the tumor-related extracellular matrix is depicted and summarized with regard to the molecular, pathophysiological, and radiobiological aspects associated with tumor biology, radiation, and chemoresistance in the context of cell adhesion molecule families, their interactions with other types of cell surface receptors, and the downstream network of signal transducers.

5.1 Introduction

A large body of evidence illustrates the complexity of tumor biology on both a cellular and an acellular level. Examples for cellular factors are the variety of genetic gain-of-function or loss-of-function mutations in key molecules involved in proliferation, multidrug resistance, and apoptosis, which are concertedly responsible for the commonly recognized "hallmarks of cancer" (CROCE 2008; HALAZONETIS et al. 2008; VARMUS et al. 2005).

Beyond these cellular factors, the acellular elements complementing the tumor as complex, autonomous tissues are increasingly identified as critical and potent carcinogenic promoters and modulators of tumor cell sensitivity to conventional radiation and chemotherapies. The panel of acellular elements comprises, among others, soluble growth factors, oxygen, metabolites, and the proteins of the extracellular matrix (ECM) (CORDES and PARK 2007; DURAND 1994; KIM et al. 2006; PETERSEN et al. 2003; TANNOCK 1996; VAUPEL and MAYER 2005; WEDGWOOD and YOUNES 2006).

The distinguishable parameter between a normal cell and a malignant cell is the acquisition of an autonomous positive feedback loop from those extracellular signals by the malignant cell. Most importantly, this process must not necessarily be associated with independence from extracellular signals as misleadingly reported. Uncoordinated reactions and the intracellular channeling and execution of these signals into action on extracellular growth signals integrate into perpetual mitosis of both the tumor cells themselves and of the normal cell types, which are overflowed with tumor cell-derived soluble growth factors. Similar to growth factors, tumor cells synthesize and secret proteins of the extracellular matrix and tissue-remodeling matrix-metalloproteinases to construct their own unique and progrowth microenvironment (CHANG and WERB 2001; CHUNG et al. 1992; LOPEZ-OTIN and MATRISIAN 2007; LYNCH and MATRISIAN 2002). Within this environment, specific niches provide a microenvironment that confers resistance to therapy with ionizing radiation and/or chemotherapeutics (DALTON 2003; DIAZ-MONTERO and MCINTYRE 2003; HEHLGANS et al. 2007b; HODKINSONS et al. 2007; LI and DALTON 2006; PASZEK and WEAVER 2004; WEAVER et al. 2002; ZAHIR and WEAVER 2004). Moreover, remodeling of the extracellular matrix generates migratory avenues for local tumor cell invasion and metastasis. Particularly the latter as limiting factor for patient's survival challenges systemic anticancer strategies and fosters the development of more targeted approaches against the primary tumor (BOARD and VALLE 2007; COCHRAN et al. 2008; LJUNGBERG 2007; MORABITO et al. 2007).

In addition to the intrinsic insensitivity of the majority of tumor cells to antigrowth signals, it can be hypothesized that some tumor cells grow in the before mentioned microenvironmental insensitivity-conferring niche or represent one of the tumor-initiating cells characterized by a great self-renewal potency and a slow doubling time.

Owing to an overarching function of the microenvironmental component called the extracellular matrix, this chapter depicts and summarizes the molecular, pathophysiological, and radiobiological aspects associated with tumor biology, radiation, and chemoresistance in the context of the cell adhesion molecule families, their interactions with other types of cell surface receptors and the downstream network of signal transducers.

Extracellular Matrix, Cell–Matrix Interactions, and Cell–Cell Interactions

The extracellular matrix represents the structural support for the cells in a tissue and further serves in regulating essential cell functions via cell surface receptors and as depot for growth factors. In connective tissues, the extracellular matrix either is between cells as interstitial matrix or organized as basement membrane providing anchorage for epithelial or endothelial cells (Alberts et al. 2002; Lodish et al. 2004). Either type of cell-matrix interaction can be found in all tissues and is mediated by different cell adhesion molecules (CAMs) mostly as transmembrane proteins (Hynes 2004). In general, the features mechanical stability and integrity of signal transduction in a tissue are also conducted by interactions between neighboring cells. These kinds of interactions are similarly accomplished by transmembrane proteins. Some of them are CAMs; others form, for example, intercellular tubes called gap junctions, which allow cell–cell communication via passage of molecules with a molecular weight below 1,000 kDa (Rousset 1996). To date, it is clear that all of these processes contribute to the proper regulation of normal tissue function and homeostasis as well as of malignant tissue in a differential and complex manner determined by the cumulated diversity of cellular alterations during the development of an individual tumor.

5.2.1
Extracellular Matrix

The presence of the extracellular matrix is essential for a large number of processes such as survival, proliferation, differentiation, adhesion, migration, and tissue integrity (Alavi and Stupack 2007; Blaschke et al. 1994; LaBarge et al. 2007; Petersen et al. 1998). The composition of the ECM based on the distribution of different molecules, as detailed below, depends on the tissue with its unique functions and its role in separating one tissue/organ from another.

An aspect of utmost importance is the direct impact of the ECM on the cell's dynamic in terms of cell shape, tissue tension, and motility resulting from membrane-spanning outside-in and inside-out signal transduction (Giancotti and Ruoslahti 1999; Hynes 2002). Signals are transduced by both CAMs and growth factor receptors, and their intracellularly converging cascades. Regarding growth factors, the ECM sequesters a wide range of cellular growth factors (Vlodavsky et al. 1990, 1991). On changes of the microenvironmental conditions, a set of proteases is able to release these deposited molecules to expeditiously act locally via their cognate transmembrane growth factor receptors. In this case, no de novo synthesis is required.

The molecular components assembling the ECM are produced and secreted by resident cells like fibroblasts (Hay 1989; Sugrue and Hay 1981). Subsequent to secretion, these components aggregate with the existent network of hydrophilic glycosaminoglycans and fibrillar and elastic proteins.

5.2.1.1
Proteoglycan Components

Glycosaminoglycans (GAGs) are carbohydrate polymers, which are usually attached to ECM proteins to form proteoglycans (Alberts et al. 2002; Bolender et al. 1981). Being molecules with a net negative charge, proteoglycans are hydrophilic, thus, attracting water molecules. This hydration characterizes the gel-like consistency of the ECM essential for the hydration of cells and as basis for the fibrillar and elastic proteins. Proteoglycans found in the ECM are outlined in the following:

1. *Keratan sulfate proteoglycans.* Keratan sulfate has variable sulfate content but does not contain uronic acid. Present in, e.g., cartilage, bone.
2. *Heparan sulfate proteoglycans.* Heparan sulfate, as linear polysaccharide, is ubiquitously expressed in human tissues. Its proteoglycanic form binds to various protein ligands/receptors to participate in the regulation of biological functions like embryonic development and metastasis.
3. *Chondroitin sulfate proteoglycans.* Chondroitin sulfate contributes to the elastic capacity and strength of tendons, ligaments, and cartilage.

5.2.1.2
Hyaluronic Acid

Hyaluronic acid is a polysaccharide consisting of alternative residues of D-glucuronic acid and N-acetylglucosamine. Hyaluronic acid, as major compound of the ECM and thus of the hydrophilic gel, realizes a high degree of absorbability to protect specific tissues against compression. Furthermore, hyaluronic acid contributes to the regulation of embryonic development, healing processes, inflammation, and tumor development

(ADAMIA et al. 2005; NAGANO and SAYA 2004). Its specific cognate transmembrane receptor is CD44.

5.2.1.3
Fibronectin

Fibronectin, a high-molecular-weight glycoprotein, contains ~5% carbohydrate that facilitates adhesion to the CAM family of integrins as well as other ECM proteins such as collagen and heparan sulfate (CZIROK et al. 2006; GOSPODAROWICZ et al. 1979; RUOSLAHTI 1999). On binding of fibronectin, the cellular cytoskeleton is reorganized allowing, e.g., cell movement along ECM structures. This process is particularly important for wound healing and blood clotting. In cancer, fibronectin has been suggested to support tumor development and to mediate resistance to chemo- and radiotherapy as a consequence of an increased expression (CORDES and PARK 2007; DAMIANO 1999, 2002; HEHLGANS et al. 2007b).

5.2.1.4
Collagen

The most abundant matrix proteins in the ECM are collagens (ALBERTS et al. 2002; RAMACHANDRAN and KARTHA 1954). These fibrillar proteins are mainly responsible for the structural support essential for many cell functions of the resident cells. Upon synthesis of procollagen, packaging of procollagen in the Golgi apparatus, and exocytosis, procollagen is cleaved at specific peptide sites by procollagen peptidases. The evolved tropocollagen units are organized into fibrils, which subsequently assembled in collagen fibers. The fibers then attach to cell membranes through diverse types of proteins such as fibronectin and integrins. To date, 28 types of collagens have been reported. The majority—over 90%—are the collagens I, II, III, and IV. Subgroups of collagens are fibrillar (types I, II, III, V, XI), fibril-associated collagens with interrupted triple helices (FACITs) (types IX, XII, XIV), short chains (type VIII, X), basement membrane (type IV), and others (type VI, VII, XIII). Several diseases have been ascribed to genetic defects in collagen-encoding genes. A few examples are osteogenesis imperfecta (collagen I) and scurvy, which results from defective collagen due to the lack of Vitamin C. In this case, Vitamin C is an essential enzyme for a posttranslational modification process of the collagen molecule.

5.2.1.5
Laminin

Laminins represent the major noncollagenous scaffolding molecules particularly of basal laminae (JOHNSON 1980). The members of this glycoprotein family are secreted and then integrated into existent ECM. In contrast to the collagenic fiber formation, laminins are organized as web-like networks, which effectively maintain a great capacity of tension force. Each laminin molecule is a heterotrimer assembled from alpha, beta, and gamma chains. Identified are the following chains: alpha chains (LAMA1, LAMA2, LAMA3, LAMA4, LAMA5), beta chains (LAMB1, LAMB2, LAMB3, LAMB4), and gamma chains (LAMC1, LAMC2, LAMC3). In summary, 15 different laminin heterotrimers are known. Laminins bind, for example, collagens and entactins.

5.2.1.6
Elastin

Elastin is synthesized by fibroblasts and smooth muscle cells. Elasticity in the tissue is given by elastin (ARDELT 1964). Tissues dependent on a great degree of elasticity are, e.g., blood vessels, lung, elastic ligaments, bladder, and skin.

The understanding of ECM structure, composition, and function is critical in comprehending the altered responsiveness of cancer cells upon irradiation and chemotherapy as well as the complex dynamics of local tumor cell invasion and distant metastasis. In the following, the variety of molecules involved in cell–matrix interactions and cell–cell contact are described in a more thorough manner.

5.2.2
Cell–Matrix Interactions

Interactions between cells and the ECM are facilitated through specifically organized areas of the cell membrane. Two well-known types of these interactions are the focal adhesions and the hemidesmosomes (Fig. 5.1; Table 5.1) (BROUSSARD et al. 2008; BURRIDGE et al. 1990; MARTIN et al. 2002).

The common feature of these adhesion-mediating sites is the presence of transmembrane integrin receptors forming an ECM-cytoskeleton nexus (see Sect. 5.3.1). In addition, many adapter proteins and signaling molecules congregate to build up a multiprotein complex at the cytoplasmic face of the cell membrane,

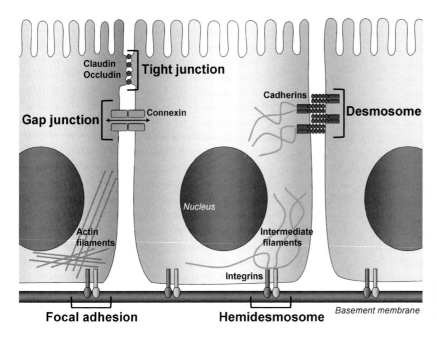

Fig. 5.1. Schematic delineation of cell–ECM and cell–cell interactions

Table 5.1. Different types of cell–ECM interactions

	Function	CAM	Occurrence
Focal adhesions	Anchorage	Integrins	E.g., cell migration, muscle–tendon connection
Hemidesmosomes	Anchorage	$\alpha_6\beta_4$ integrin	E.g., epithelium

termed a focal adhesion (Lo and Chen 1994). Courses of assembling and disassembling take place in remodeling tissues, during cell migration and self-renewal in turnover tissues. More stable focal adhesions are formed, e.g., in muscle cells anchored to their tendons. Hemidesmosomes, molecularly organized similarly to focal adhesions, play an important role in epithelial tissue mediating anchorage of epithelial cells to the basement membrane. The terminus hemidesmosome evolved from the terminus desmosome (i.e., macula adherents [Latin for "adhering spot"]; see Sect. 5.2.3), which represents a spot-like cell structure specialized for cell–cell contact on the lateral side of an epithelial cell. As hemidesmosomes are also integrin dependent, the $\alpha_6\beta_4$ integrin, as common example, facilitates a cytoplasmic connection between the anchor protein plectin to keratin intermediate filaments. This composition helps to compensate tensile or shearing forces and contributes therefore to tissue integrity.

Concerning focal adhesions in epithelial cells, these sites of adhesion connect the ECM to actin filaments via transmembrane integrin receptors (Hynes 2002).

To note, intermediate filaments are cytoskeletal structures that are formed by different members of a family of related, highly conserved proteins (Godsel et al. 2008). Most types of intermediate filaments are located in the cytoplasm. The nuclearly localized intermediate filaments are called lamins. Categorization of intermediate filaments into six groups has been done on the basis of similarities in amino acid sequence and protein structure. Types I and II intermediate filaments are acidic and basic keratins, namely epithelial keratins and trichocytic keratins (e.g., in hair and horns). Type III intermediate filaments are, e.g., vimentin (widely expressed in fibroblasts), Type IV intermediate filaments are, e.g., neurofilaments, type V intermediate filaments are nuclear lamins, type VI intermediate filaments are nestin. A well-known disease resulting from gene mutations in keratin 5 or keratin 14 intermediate filament genes is, e.g., epidermolysis bullosa simplex (FINE and GRIFFITH 1985; ISHIDA-YAMAMOTO et al. 1991).

Actin is one of the most highly conserved proteins and the monomeric subunit of microfilaments (ALBERTS et al. 2002; PERRY and COTTERILL 1965). Microfilaments belong to one of the three major components of the cytoskeleton. Actin is also a component of thin filaments managing contractility in muscle cells. Overall, actin serves in a variety of critical cellular mechanisms such as cell division, motility and shape, vesicle movement, signal transduction, and assembly and maintenance of cell junctions.

5.2.3
Cell–Cell Interactions

Desmosomes (macula adherents) are the subcellular correlates clenching neighboring cells together in simple/monolayer and stratified/multilayer epithelia and in muscle cells (Fig. 5.1; Table 5.2) (GREEN et al. 2007). These button-like attachment sites are located at the lateral side of a cell and contain transmembrane adhesion molecules of the cadherin family as well as different anchor proteins linking to the intracellular keratin cytoskeletal filaments. The extracellular portion of a cadherin, including five domains with calcium-binding motifs, binds to an identical cadherin on an adjacent cell for mediating cell–cell contact (PETTITT 2005). According to their structural composition, desmosomes fulfill different functions.

Tight junctions (zonula occludens), as second type of cell–cell contacts, serve as diffusion barrier to prevent the leakage of molecules and fluids through the intercellular space (Fig. 5.1, Table 5.2) (NIESSEN 2007; NIESSEN and GOTTARDI 2008). The barrier function is conferred by a branching network of independently sealing strands to result in a linkage of the cytoskeletons of neighboring cells. Multiple proteins, claudins and occludins representing the majority of components, crosslink the opposing cell membrane strands. Hence, the efficacy of tight junctions in preventing diffusion exponentially increases with the number of strands. In general, tight junctions achieve (1) attachment of cell to adjacent cells, (2) blocking of molecule diffusion between cells, and (3) preserving cellular polarity by preventing the motion of integral membrane proteins between the apical and basolateral surfaces of the cell. This includes the preservation and control of effective active transcellular transport or passive diffusion through the cell. They prevent the passage of molecules and ions through the space between cells. Tissues critically dependent on proper tight junction function are the epithelial tissue of the intestine, the epithelial tissue of the urinary tract and the endothelium of the brain, i.e., blood–brain barrier.

As third type of cell–cell contacts, gap junctions are composed of connexin monomers (Fig. 5.1; Table 5.2) (MESE et al. 2007; WANG and MEHTA 1995). Six monomers form a connexon hexamer, which serves as a hemichannel. When two hemichannels of adjacent cells associate, they establish a gap junction. This intercellular communication tunnel allows different molecules and ions, mostly small intracellular signaling molecules (intracellular mediators), with a molecular weight below 1,000 kDa to pass freely between cells (ROUSSET 1996). This type of cell–cell interaction is localized, for example, in the heart muscle, where it enables coordinated contraction.

Table 5.2. Different types of cell–cell interactions

	Function	CAM	Occurrence
Desmosomes	Anchorage	Cadherins	E.g., epithelium, heart muscle
Tight junctions	Occlusion	Claudins, occludins	E.g., intestine, urinary tract
Gap junctions	Communication	Connexin	E.g., heart, nervous system, bones

5.3
Cell Adhesion Molecules

5.3.1
Integrins

As outlined under Sect. 5.2.2, the CAMs of the integrin family present the main cell surface receptors for binding of cells to ECM proteins like fibronectin, collagen, or laminin (Table 5.3) (Hynes 2002; Martin et al. 2002; Schmidt et al. 1993; Schwartz 2001). Moreover, integrins also serve as adhesion molecules for cell–cell interactions, especially on blood cells. Integrins are composed of two different transmembrane glycoproteins, known as α and β subunits, which bind noncovalently to form an αβ heterodimer (Fig. 5.2). To date, 24 different integrin receptors have been identified (Hynes 2002). The ligand binding specificity of the heterodimers is influenced by the subunit combination and by cell-type specific factors. The binding of integrins to ECM proteins is accomplished by short amino acid sequences located at the large extracellular domain. Motifs for such integrin-binding sequences are RGD (arginine–glycine–aspartate), found in fibronectin or laminin or DGEA (aspartate–glycine–glutamic acid–alanine),

and GFOGER (glycine–phenylalanine–glycine–glutamic acid–arginine) found in collagen (Calderwood et al. 1995, 1997; Evans and Calderwood 2007; Liu et al. 2000; Ruoslahti 2003). Inside the cells, adapter proteins like talin, α-actinin, and vinculin bridge the gap between the cytoplasmic integrin domain and the cytoskeleton. This multiprotein complex forms the structural basis for an association with a large set of signal transduction molecules like focal adhesion kinase (FAK) and the Rous sarcoma oncogene (Src), eventually assembling a focal adhesion (Brakebusch and Fassler 2003). The signaling works in opposite directions. While ligand binding to the integrin extracellular domain leads to activation of numerous intracellular signaling pathways (outside-in signaling), certain intracellular processes stimulated by, e.g., docking of growth factors to their cognate transmembrane receptor alter the binding affinity and avidity of integrins (inside-out signaling) (Hynes 2002). These mechanisms are poorly understood, but may be due to conformational changes of the receptor. Because integrin function is independent from de novo synthesis and/or degradation, the integrin-related adhesion response in both directions can proceed within seconds. For example, this allows platelets to circulate unimpeded in the blood until damage of the vascular wall activates the integrins in the

Table 5.3. Families of cell adhesion molecules assigned to morphological, functional, and molecular characteristics

Characteristics	Integrins	Cadherins	Ig CAMs	Selectins
Ligands	ECM proteins, Ig CAMs	Cadherins	Ig CAMs, integrins, ECM proteins	Carbohydrates
Binding	Heterophilic	Homophilic	Homophilic, heterophilic	Heterophilic
Adhesion sites	Focal adhesions, hemidesmosomes, nonjunctional adhesion	Desmosomes, adherens junctions	Nonjunctional adhesion	Nonjunctional adhesion
Main function	Cell–matrix interactions	Cell–cell interactions	Cell–cell interactions	Cell–cell interactions
Tumor overexpression	E.g., HNSCC, breast cancer		E.g., neuroblastomas, SCLC	
Tumor downregulation		E.g., breast cancer, gastric cancer	E.g., gastrointestinal tumors	

HNSCC head and neck small cell cancer, *SCLC* small cell lung cancer

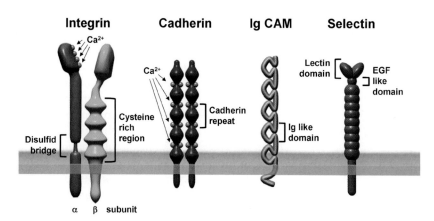

Fig. 5.2. The four families of cell adhesion molecules. Depiction of their heterodimeric, homodimeric or single chain structure, important functional domains, and Ca^{2+}-dependent sites in each one of the receptor types

platelet membrane enhancing the affinity for fibrinogen (MOROI and JUNG 1998). The fibrinogen connects the platelets to a clot and prevents bleeding. This switch in binding activity is also important for lymphogenic or hematogenic metastasis of cancer cells when entering and leaving the vessel. Regarding integrin function, interactions between these CAM and transmembrane growth factor receptors build the basis for optimized and most efficient intracellular signaling and regulation of all types of cellular mechanisms (PORTER and HOGG 1998). Whether this mutual and cooperative interrelation is caused by transactivation mediated by a panel of membrane-associated cytoplasmic signaling molecules or through direct interactions remains to be solved.

In cancer, integrins fulfill the same functions as they do in normal tissue (CHUNG et al. 2008; DANEN 2005; MOCHIZUKI and OKADA 2007; RAMSAY et al. 2007). Although widely examined, the most common feature in various human tumor entities including breast cancer or squamous cell carcinomas is an abnormal integrin expression relative to the corresponding normal tissue. However, the expression can differ within one single tumor and between tumors of the same entity.

Despite this diversity and unclear pathophysiological consequences of an altered integrin expression, recent findings suggest an association of β_1 integrin expression and overall survival of patients with invasive-ductal breast carcinomas (YAO et al. 2007). Accordingly, in vitro experiments showed a reversion of the trans-formed phenotype to a morphological and functional normal phenotype in breast cancer cells concomitant to a reduced tumor formation capability in vivo upon β_1 integrin inhibition (PARK et al. 2006). These observations indicate a strong contribution of integrins to oncogenic transformation.

Besides the expression of integrins, malignant cells acquire the ability to grow anchorage independent as a result of gain-of-function mutations in oncogenes localized within integrin-associated signaling pathways. In contrast, normal cells usually undergoing apoptosis upon detachment from ECM, a mechanism called anoikis. In vitro studies have shown that $\alpha_v\beta_6$ but not $\alpha_v\beta_5$ expression leads to reduced anoikis in squamous cell carcinoma cells (JANES and WATT 2004). This could be an explanation, why upregulation of $\alpha_v\beta_6$ seems to be a prognostic factor in human squamous cell carcinomas.

Another impact of integrins in cancer comes from gene mutation analyses. The poorly differentiated cell line SCC4, which originates from a human carcinoma of the tongue, is heterozygous for the point mutation T188I (T, threonine; I, isoleucine) in the β_1 integrin subunit (EVANS et al. 2004). This modification leads to constitutively active ligand binding independent from the type of associated β subunit. After transfection with wild-type β_1 integrin, the SCC4 cells begin to differentiate, indicating that this mutation may contribute to the neoplastic phenotype. Although these findings are remarkable because they show that alterations of integrin activation can influence the malignancy of cancer cells without changing the level of integrin expression, mutations in the β_1 integrin gene are rare. Screening of 124 human oral squamous cell carcinomas revealed six nucleotide changes, all of which could be also found in normal tissue of the patients (EVANS et al. 2004). Only one mutation resulted in an altered amino acid sequence of β_1 integrin. Analysis of the predicted structure suggests that this sequence variation does not interfere with the function of the heterodimeric receptor. Whether mutations of β_1 integrin or other integrin subunits play a general role in tumor development with respect to other cancer entities remains to be examined in further studies.

There are many ways how integrins can modulate the malignant characteristics of tumors including a modulation of the behavior of the primary tumor in terms of invasion as well as a modulation of the tumor's metastatic abilities. In addition to cadherins (see Sect. 5.3.2), the invasiveness of tumors depends on integrins (HOOD and CHERESH 2002; RAMSAY et al. 2007). Cell migration representing one part of the complex process of cell invasion is a highly dynamic sequence of focal adhesion assembly and focal adhesion disassembly. Starting with smaller focal adhesions at the leading edge of a migrating cell, called focal complexes, the assembly of a focal complex into a larger, stable focal adhesion progresses through the recruitment of additional proteins (SMALL and RESCH 2005). These stable focal adhesions remain stationary, providing the cells an anchor from which to move in any direction. During the course of migration, the focal adhesions move from the front to the rear of the cells in a caterpillar, traction-like manner. Focal adhesions reaching the rear edge are disassembled. Referring to the frequent increased migratory potential of tumor cells, upregulation, e.g., of the basement membrane integrin receptor $\alpha_6\beta_4$ correlates with poor prognosis in a variety of different cancers not only due to promoted tumor progression, but also particularly due to enhanced invasiveness (LIPSCOMB and MERCURIO 2005). In glioblastoma cell lines, for example, inhibition of either β_1 integrin or β_3 integrin with specific inhibitory monoclonal antibodies strongly impairs cell invasion into basement membrane (CORDES et al. 2003). This effect yielded from an integrin-dependent alteration of the proteolytic activity of matrix metalloproteinases (MMPs), which represent key enzymes to degrade the ECM and enable cells to invade. Correspondingly, it has been shown that $\alpha_v\beta_3$ integrin modulates MMP activity directly in endothelium and melanoma cells in vivo (BROOKS et al. 1996).

5.3.2
Cadherins

Cadherins are the main receptors for calcium-dependent cell–cell adhesion in most solid tissues (ALBERTS et al. 2002). Besides being responsible for the mechanical stability, they coordinate the integration of cells in functional structures like the epithelium and control cell movement in tissue development and organization, especially during embryogenesis (Table 5.3). Classical cadherins are transmembrane glycoproteins, which bind almost exclusively to the same type of receptor expressed on the other cell in a homophilic manner (Fig. 5.2). The intracellular domain is connected to the cytoskeleton via a group of anchor proteins known as catenins (PETTITT 2005; REYNOLDS 2007). This link-

age is essential for strong adhesive activity. Disassembly of this functional complex and therefore disruption of cell–cell contact can be caused by tyrosine phosphorylation of either cadherin or catenin by a variety of receptor tyrosine kinases (RTK) like epidermal growth factor receptor (EGFR) or insulin-like growth factor-1 receptor (IGF-1R). Contrariwise, cadherins are able to modulate RTK signaling, consequently interfering with many critical cellular processes (PETTITT 2005). Epithelial cadherin (E-cadherin)-mediated adhesion, for example, has been reported to reduce ligand-dependent EGFR activation, which results in decreased DNA synthesis and inhibition of cell growth (QIAN et al. 2004).

Considering these effects, it is not astonishing that cadherins are discussed to play a major role in tumorigenesis. E-cadherin especially is deemed a tumor suppressor (COWIN et al. 2005; REYNOLDS 2007). Many types of epithelial cancers show an inverse correlation of E-cadherin expression and patient outcome. According to the results of several studies, it has been postulated that the downregulation of E-cadherin is necessary for tumor cell invasion and formation of distant metastasis, and that reconstitution of the functional cadherin/catenin complex might lead to reduced malignancy (REYNOLDS 2007). The loss of cadherin-mediated cell–cell adhesion in cancer cells can be due to transcriptional mechanisms or increased proteolytic degradation by matrix metalloproteinases. For example, overexpression of dysadherin, a cancer-associated membrane protein, inactivates E-cadherin in a posttranscriptional manner, which induces experimental metastasis (INO et al. 2002). Mutations of the E-cadherin gene resulting in expression of a nonfunctional receptor have been found in lobular breast cancers, diffuse gastric cancers, and gynecological cancers (CHAN 2006; COWIN et al. 2005). Such mutations arise either de novo or can be inherited, which is the case with patients suffering from familiar diffuse gastric cancer.

5.3.3
Immunoglobulin Superfamily

The immunoglobulin-like (Ig-like) CAMs are widely expressed in different cell types including neurons, leukocytes, endothelial, and epithelial cells (Table 5.3) (ALBERTS et al. 2002). Although mediating mainly cell–cell adhesion, Ig-like CAMs are also capable of binding to ECM proteins (ACHESON et al. 1991). In contrast to integrins or cadherins, their binding affinity is much weaker and not dependent on the presence of divalent cations like Ca^{2+} or Mg^{2+}. Therefore, Ig-like CAMs are regarded to be responsible for the fine-adjustment mechanisms of adhesive processes and tissue organization. All members of this family have in common that the extracellular part contains one or more Ig-like domains, which are typical for antibodies (Fig. 5.2). Either the receptor can be tied to the membrane by a glycosylphosphatidylinositol anchor, or it can interact with intracellular signaling molecules via a transmembrane/cytoplasmic tail (Hemperly et al. 1990; Pollerberg et al. 1987).

The neural CAM (NCAM) is among the best-studied members of this group critical for brain development and memory formation (Mileusnic et al. 1999). It is expressed not only in neural cells, but also in a variety of other tissues like epithelium, colon, and pancreas. Interestingly, in numerous tumors, an altered NCAM expression pattern correlates with poor prognosis. Studies with transgenic mice have shown that loss of NCAM function increases lymphatic metastasis of pancreatic cancer by induction of vascular endothelial growth factor (VEGF) and tumor lymphangiogenesis (Crnic et al. 2004). Accordingly, downregulation of NCAM was found to be associated with enhanced malignancy and reduced survival of patients with colorectal, gastric, or pancreatic carcinomas (Fogar et al. 1997; Roesler et al. 1997; Tascilar et al. 2007). But there exist also contrary observations. NCAM overexpression in neuroblastomas and small cell lung cancer, for example, correlates with advanced stage and fatal course of disease and is used as prognostic marker (Gluer et al. 1998; Miyahara et al. 2001). Overall, the biological significance of NCAM for tumor development and progression is unclear to date and depends strongly on the tumor entity.

5.3.4
Selectins

Selectins are cell–cell adhesion molecules, which play a critical role in leukocyte diapedesis through the vascular wall due to inflammation or tissue injury (Table 5.3) (Alberts et al. 2002). The three closely related family members mainly expressed by leukocytes (L-selectin), platelets (P-selectin), and endothelial cells (E- and P-selectin) contain a characteristic extracellular lectin-domain that binds to carbohydrate ligands (Fig. 5.2). In contrast to other CAMs like cadherins or integrins, selectin function is confined to the vascular system.

Several studies have indicated that selectins also recognize cancer cells and therefore facilitate hematogenic metastasis. Overexpression of E-selectin in the liver of transgenic mice leads to redirection of melanoma cells in this organ (Biancone et al. 1996). Specific targeting E-selectin with antibodies has been shown to significantly decrease the number of experimental metastasis in vivo (Brodt et al. 1997). Not only E-selectin, but also other members of the selectin family are suggested to promote metastasis. P-selectin-deficient as well as L-selectin-deficient mice show a reduction of tumor metastasis in different mouse models. Another therapeutic approach uses the anticoagulant heparin for potentially blocking selectin-mediated adhesion of tumor cells to endothelium (Borsig et al. 2002). Taking into account the prominent impact of normal cells on tumor progression and tumor microenvironment, L-selectins on leukocytes have been hypothesized to contribute to cancer development and progression (Coussens and Werb 2002).

5.4
Integrin Signaling Molecules

Integrins, together with a range of structural molecules and signaling molecules, provide a connection between the outside and the inside of the cell (Brakebusch and Fassler 2003; Chung and Kim 2008; Hehlgans et al. 2007b; Hynes 2002; Schwartz 2001). This specific cell membrane area is called focal adhesion. It is characterized by specific types of macromolecular protein assemblies transmitting mechanical force and regulatory signals over the cell membrane. Effective regulation of an adequate cell behavior results from the interactions of cells with their surrounding ECM. Furthermore, integrin- and receptor tyrosine kinase-mediated signaling are connected to control the cellular fate, e.g., survival, cell cycle progression, proliferation, adhesion, migration, differentiation, and apoptosis (Fig. 5.3) (Schwartz 2001; Watt 2002).

One of the molecules, which plays a major role in the above-mentioned processes and also holds a central position in the growth factor receptor-integrin network, is the putative serine–threonine kinase integrin-linked kinase (ILK). ILK is bound to the cytoplasmic tail of β-integrin subunits through its C-terminal kinase domain (Figs. 5.3, 5.4a) (Hannigan et al. 1996). Downstream, ILK has been reported to phosphorylate the prosurvival protein kinase Akt on serine 473 and glycogen synthase kinase-3β (GSK3β) on serine 9 in a phosphatidylinositol-3 kinase (PI3K)-dependent manner (Delcommenne et al. 1998; Lynch et al. 1999). More recent findings suggest ILK to be a pseudokinase (Boudeau et al. 2006) and the RICTOR-mammalian target of rapamycin (mTOR) complex to be responsible for phosphorylation of Akt on serine 473 (Sarbassov et al. 2005). Pseudokinases are proteins that lack at least one of the highly conserved catalytic residues/motifs

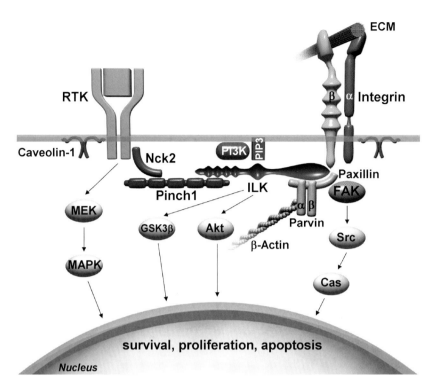

Fig. 5.3. Scheme of transmembrane integrins and selected integrin signaling mediators. Cooperative and mutual signal transduction between integrins and receptor tyrosine kinases optimally control critical cell functions like survival, proliferation, and apoptosis. *Akt* v-akt murine thymoma viral oncogene homolog 1, *ECM* extracellular matrix, *FAK* focal adhesion kinase, *GSK3β* glycogen synthase kinase-3β, *ILK* integrin-linked kinase, *Nck* non-catalytic (region of) tyrosine kinase adaptor protein, *Cas* (p130Cas), Crk-associated substrate, *Pinch1* particularly interesting new cysteine-histidine rich protein, *PI3K* phosphatidylinositol-3-kinase, *RTK* receptor tyrosine kinase, *MEK* mitogen-activated protein kinase kinase, *MAPK* mitogen-activated protein kinase, *PIP3* phosphatidylinositol (3,4,5)-triphosphate, *Src* Rous sarcoma oncogene

in the kinase-like domain. This event suggests these proteins to be inactive in terms of regular protein kinases. Phosphatidylinositol 3,4,5-triphosphate (PIP3) being a phospholipid component in the cytosolic side of cell membranes, seems to activate ILK through interaction with the central pleckstrin homology ([PH] PH domains facilitate protein recruitment to membranes, cellular compartments or enable protein-protein interactions) domain of ILK (Delcommenne et al. 1998). The N-terminal ankyrin repeat domain contains four ankyrin (ANK) repeats and is responsible for binding to the particularly interesting new cysteine-histidine-rich protein 1 (Pinch1). Ankyrins are important for attachment processes between integral membrane proteins and the cytoskeleton.

Pinch1 and its homologue Pinch2 are so-called LIM-only proteins, each consisting of five LIM domains (Braun et al. 2003; Dougherty et al. 2005; Stanchi et al. 2005). The name LIM derives from the initials of the three first described proteins containing LIM domains: *LIN-11, ISL1,* and *MEC-3*. LIM domains mediate protein–protein interactions and are composed of two cysteine-rich zinc finger structures. The first N-terminal LIM domain 1 of Pinch1 is essential for binding to the N-terminal ankyrin repeat domain of ILK (Figs. 5.3, 5.4b) (Tu et al. 1999; Velyvis et al. 2001). Moreover, Pinch1 serves as an important structural component in the RTK-integrin connective network by forming a ternary complex with ILK and Nck2, a Src homology (SH)2/SH3 adaptor protein (Tu et al. 1998; Vaynberg et al. 2005). Responsible for this interaction is the fourth LIM domain of Pinch1 and the third SH3 domain of Nck2. Nck2 itself binds to growth factor receptors like epidermal growth factor receptor or platelet-derived growth factor receptor β (PDGFRβ) with its C-terminal SH2 domain (Fig. 5.3, 5.4c) (Tu et al. 1998).

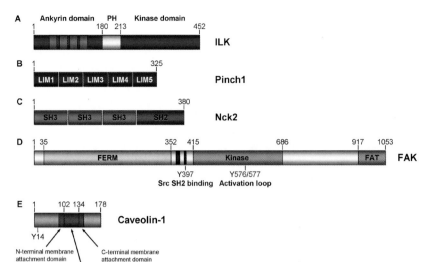

Fig. 5.4a–e. Essential transducers and modulators of integrin signals. Important functional domains and phosphorylation sites

A second important mediator of integrin signals is the 125-kDa protein focal adhesion kinase (Fig. 5.3) (Parsons 2003; Tachibana et al. 1995). FAK is a nonreceptor tyrosine kinase, which transmits signals from both integrins and RTKs to regulate cell shape, growth, survival, motility, adhesion, and migration. FAK activation, for example by adhesion, leads to autophosphorylation on tyrosine 397, which is then followed by recruitment of a signaling complex consisting of phosphorylated p130 Crk-associated substrate (p130Cas) on tyrosine 410, Src and phosphorylated paxillin on tyrosine 31 and 118 (Fig. 5.4d) (Calalb et al. 1995; Mitra et al. 2005; Parsons 2003). Once phosphorylated, FAK signals to mitogen-activated protein kinase (MAPK) and calpain-2 or recruits c-*Jun* N-terminal kinase (JNK) to focal adhesion sites to influence cell proliferation, migration, and apoptosis. FAK consists of 1,053 amino acids and contains an amino terminal region, which displays sequence homology to band 4.1 and ezrin/radixin/moesin (ERM) membrane-cytoskeletal linker proteins (Figs. 5.3, 5.4d) (Girault et al. 1999). This approximately 300–amino acid region, called FERM, is found in a number of membrane-targeted proteins (Chishti et al. 1998). FERM domains mediate interactions with cytoplasmic regions of transmembrane receptors and with phosphoinositides to efficiently localize FERM domain-containing proteins to membranes (Barret et al. 2000; Bompard et al. 2003; Hirao et al. 1996). The central FAK kinase domain spans approximately amino acids 415 to 618 and contains tyrosine 576/577 phosphorylation sites within

the activation loop of FAK (Nowakowski et al. 2002). Within the linker region between the FERM and kinase segment lies the tyrosine 397 phosphorylation site, which is not strictly an autophosphorylation site but is also activated by Src SH2 binding (Mitra et al. 2005; Siesser and Hanks 2006). This phosphorylation further stimulates FAK activity through phosphorylation of other phosphorylation sites, including tyrosine 576/577 residues (Caron-Lormier and Berry 2005). A second element in this linker region is the Src SH3-binding motif (Ceccarelli et al. 2006). The C-terminal focal adhesion targeting (FAT) domain is responsible for binding to paxillin and talin, an integrin-associated protein, and for localization of the protein to focal adhesions (Hayashi et al. 2002; Schlaepfer et al. 2004).

Another protein that has been lately discovered to be associated with integrin signaling is the integral membrane protein Caveolin-1 (Fig. 5.3, 5.4e). Caveolin proteins are major components of caveolae, invaginations of the cell membrane, which participate in important physiological functions of the cell including endocytosis, membrane trafficking, lipid homeostasis, and a number of signaling events (Anderson 1998; Fielding and Fielding 2003; Salanueva et al. 2007). So far, three Caveolin proteins, named Caveolin-1, -2, and -3, have been described. Caveolin-1 and -2 are mostly coexpressed with high expression levels in differentiated cells like endothelial, epithelial and smooth muscle cells, fibroblasts, adipocytes, and pneumocytes. Caveolin-2 is primarily expressed in muscle tissue-types (Song et al. 1996; Tang et al. 1996). All Caveolin isoforms contain a central transmembrane domain and cytosolic carboxy- and amino-terminal domains. The C-terminal membrane attachment domain contains three palmitoylation sites for anchoring of the protein to the membrane. The N-terminal membrane-proximal oligomerization domain mediates also interaction with other proteins for regulation of their activity (Couet et al. 1997; Li et al. 1996). Pathophysiological functions have been described for Caveolin-1, which is also involved in tumorigenesis, tumor suppression, differentiation, and oncogenic transformation (Carver and Schnitzer 2003; Galbiati et al. 1998; Williams and Lisanti 2005). Tyrosine 14–phosphorylated Caveolin-1 seems to accumulate at focal adhesion sites where it triggers extracellular signals (Lee et al. 2000; Mettouchi et al. 2001). Direct inhibition of Src and EGFR as well as direct activation of the insulin receptor by Caveolin-1 has been reported (Okamoto et al. 1998; Yamamoto et al. 1998). Caveolin-1 also interacts with β1 integrins and promotes Fyn-dependent Shc phosphorylation and MAPK activation (Wary et al. 1998; Wei et al. 1999).

5.5

Matrix Metalloproteinases

Matrix metalloproteinases are required for degradation of the extracellular matrix and therefore have important functions in tissue remodeling (Alberts et al. 2002). Tissue remodeling takes place not only under several physiological conditions like embryogenesis, angiogenesis, and wound healing, but also during pathological processes, namely tumor invasion, metastasis, and arthritis (Ra and Parks 2007).

On the cellular basis, MMPs are involved in all events requiring a change in ECM composition forming an optimized microenvironment for a cell to adhere, migrate, proliferate, apoptose, or differentiate. To date, 28 different MMPs have been identified, at first on the basis of genomic screening, from which 24 MMP proteins can be found tissue specifically in humans (Greenlee et al. 2007). In contrast to other endopeptidases, MMPs require a zinc ion as cofactor for their catalytic activity. They can be functionally classified in dependence on their substrate specificity in collagenases, gelatinases, stromelysins, and membrane-type MMPs (MT-MMPs) (Table 5.4).

Additionally, there are a number of MMPs, which do not fit exactly in this classification but are ordered with regard to structural similarities, evolutionary classification, or differential expression (Chang and Werb 2001; Ra and Parks 2007).

For tight regulation of function, MMPs are initially synthesized as inactive zymogens (i.e., a proenzyme or an inactive enzyme precursor) (Chang and Werb 2001). Responsible for this inactive state is a highly conserved prodomain consisting of the amino acids PRCGxPD (proline–arginine–cysteine–glycine–x–proline–aspartate), which inhibits enzymatic function of the protein by covering the catalytic site through direct interaction of the cysteine residue with the zinc ion in the active site. This event prevents substrate binding and cleavage resulting in the active form of a MMP. As well known mediator of MMP cleavage, urokinase-type plasminogen activator (uPA) and tissue-type plasminogen activator (tPA) have been assigned critical roles in cancer progression and metastasis development (Blasi and Carmeliet 2002; Kucharewicz et al. 2003; Sternlicht and Werb 2001). Other proteases involved in activation of MMPs are chymotrypsin, trypsin, and MMPs itself. Apart from the membrane bound MT-MMPs, which contain a transmembrane domain and are intracellularly activated once inserted into the cell membrane, MMPs are secreted into the extracellular space as inactive proenzyme (Hernandez-Barrantes et al. 2002; Nagase 1997). The second conserved domain is the catalytic domain with the structural metal binding 106 to 119 residues. The zinc-binding active site within this domain consists of 52 to 58 amino ac-

Table 5.4. Types of ECM-degrading MMPs

Family	MMP type	Substrate
Collagenase	1, 8, 13, 18	Triple-helical fibrillar collagens
Gelatinase	2, 9	Type IV collagen and gelatin
Stromelysin	3, 10, 11	Variety of ECM proteins but not collagens
Membrane type	14, 15, 16, 17	Variety of ECM proteins

ids. A conserved sequence HExxHxxGxxH (histidine–glutamic acid–xx–histidine–xx–glycine–xx–histidine) forms the zinc-binding motif, and three histidine residues mediate direct interaction with the zinc ion (Massova et al. 1998). The catalytic domain is linked to the third conserved domain, represented by a C-terminal hemopexin-like domain expressing a variable hinge region of up to 75 amino acids. The hemopexin domain seems to determine substrate specificity of the MMPs and serves as binding domain for tissue inhibitors of matrix metalloproteinases (TIMPs).

Beside the above-described intramolecular inhibition of catalytic function, TIMPs provide another regulatory mechanism controlling proper MMP function (Gomez et al. 1997; Sternlicht and Werb 2001). Four members of this family are known, TIMP-1 to -4. These inhibitors are also expressed in a tissue-specific way. They either inactivate active MMPs or inhibit the activation process. Gelatinases such as the well known MMP-2 and MMP-9 possess an additional gelatin-binding region within their catalytic domain before the zinc-binding motif. Membrane-type furin-activated MMPs contain a furin cleavage site within their prodomain and a C-terminal transmembrane domain.

In adults, the activity of MMPs is very low due to tight inhibitory regulation. This fragile balance is somehow perturbed during invasive tumor progression due to mutations in encoding MMP genes as well as inhibition and reduced expression of TIMPs. Overall, MMPs pronouncedly contribute to local tumor cell invasion and metastasis (Guo and Giancotti 2004; Sternlicht and Werb 2001).

In a variety of human cancers, the expression of different MMPs is elevated and responsible for metastatic events limiting the success of anticancer therapy (Erler et al. 2006; Jinga et al. 2006). In general, former and current efforts in targeting MMP expression and activity failed to show significant improvement or resulted in just slightly improved tumor control.

5.6
Migration and Metastasis

Elucidating the process of metastasis in the context of this chapter in more detail, clarification about the different molecules and steps involved is necessary. The set of molecular actors expressed by both tumor cells and tumor-associated normal cells like endothelial cells and fibroblasts is large and their activity is likely to depend in majority on paracrine effects. The complexity

of events responsible for the intrinsic pressure driving tumor cell outgrowth and settling at distant organ sites is unclear to date. Likely, a mutual combination of autonomous cellular factors such as constitutive activation of migration-related molecules and life-threatening microenvironmental changes in oxygen and metabolite levels triggers the tumor cells to search for better survival conditions.

For the execution of the metastatic circuit of actions, a tumor cell requires a range of prerequisites of which integrins, matrix metalloproteinases, and signal transduction are crucial (Friedl and Brocker 2000; Hood and Cheresh 2002; Munshi and Stack 2006). During the course of events, cells must detach from the ECM and neighboring cells, migrate while degrading the extracellular matrix, penetrate the basement membrane, a thin ECM structure that segregates tissue compartments, invade the bloodstream, a process called intravasation, survive the shear stress in the vasculature, exit the bloodstream in the target organ (extravasation), attach, and proliferate in their new surrounding (Guo and Giancotti 2004; Hood and Cheresh 2002). These different processes depend on dysregulation of integrin and receptor tyrosine kinase signaling in metastatic cells due to activating mutations in oncogenes and loss-of-function mutations in tumor suppressor genes (Bissell and Radisky 2001; Giancotti and Ruoslahti 1999; Hynes 2003). Additionally, upregulation of integrin expression in tumor cells has been shown to enhance migration, invasion, and tumor progression (Albelda et al. 1990; Guo and Giancotti 2004; Mercurio and Rabinovitz 2001; Plantefaber and Hynes 1989). For the transition from adenoma to invasive carcinoma, cells undergo a process, which involves a modification of integrin-mediated cell–ECM interactions (see Sect. 5.3.1) and E-cadherin-mediated cell–cell contacts (see Sect. 5.3.2).

Migration events, both in normal and malignant cells, are initiated by polarization of the cell, followed by actin polymerization at the leading edge of the cell and lamellipodium formation (Raucher and Sheetz 2000). Integrins and integrin-associated proteins accumulate at the leading edge of the cell to stimulate adhesion processes and signaling in response to new contact sites (Kiosses et al. 2001; Schmidt et al. 1993). The focal contact sites at the rear end of the cell are detached by cleavage of focal adhesion proteins or modulation of integrin affinity to ECM proteins (Franco and Huttenlocher 2005; Shiraha et al. 1999). Finally, the cell moves forward due to contractile forces (Lauffenburger and Horwitz 1996). FAK is essential for migration by interaction with cytosolic part of integrin subunits and growth factor receptors. Additional molecules involved are p130Cas, Src, Crk, and Rho-GTPases such as Rac controlling actin organization (KLEMKE et al. 1998). A second FAK-mediated promigratory pathway is the Grb2/SOS/Ras/ERK pathway (VAN NIMWEGEN and VAN DE WATER 2007). Integrins also participate in regulating proteases, for example MMP-2 and -9, that degrade the basement membrane, composed of ECM proteins like collagens type IV, laminins, and proteoglycans. An example for integrin–MMP interaction is the recruitment of MMP-2 by integrins on the outside of the cell, where MMP-2 degrades ECM components to facilitate migration and invasion of the cell (BROOKS et al. 1996). Furthermore, integrins can associate with uPA receptors (CHAPMAN and Wei 2001).

Conclusively, migratory and metastatic events result from concerted and complex actions that provide optimal avenues for cells to traverse from one point to another, in case of metastasis, beyond physiological borders and the intravascular phase.

5.7
Radiation and Chemoresistance of Tumor Cells Through Cell–Matrix Interactions

A current hypothesis is that malignant tumors, in general, develop areas, so-called niches (different from the "cancer stem cell" niche), which confer a high degree of resistance against ionizing irradiation or cytotoxic drugs to the tumor cells. The molecular characterization of these specific areas is ongoing but surely involves the binding of cells to the ECM as well as the binding of cells to other cells, regardless if malignant or normal.

As obvious from literature search, cell–cell contacts have been a focus of interest in cancer research for many years (RUCH and TROSKO 2001; TROSKO and RUCH 1998). Recently, the impact of cell–matrix interactions on tumor cell resistance was evidently demonstrated in several cell lines from different solid and hematologic tumor entities in vitro. Dependent on the characteristics, the phenomena were called "cell adhesion–mediated radiation resistance" (CAM-RR) or "cell adhesion–mediated drug resistance" (CAM-DR) (CORDES and MEINEKE 2003; DALTON 2003; DAMIANO et al. 1999). Most relevant for in vitro cancer research, this effect can easily be observed when comparing the radio- or chemosensitivity of cells plated on a conventional plastic culture dish with cells plated on different matrix proteins like fibronectin, collagen, or laminin. The contact with ECM proteins and the alterations in signaling caused by these interactions strongly support the cell to survive the treatment. A further increase in resistance can be achieved by placing the cells in a three-dimensional matrix, simulating more physiological growth conditions. There are ongoing efforts to reveal the underlying mechanisms and identify the cellular proteins involved in CAM-RR and CAM-DR, with the hope that this knowledge can add useful and successful novel therapeutic agents to cancer treatment.

It has been discovered early that integrins, the main receptors for ECM proteins, participate in the cellular response to geno- and cytotoxic stress. Irradiation, for example, leads to a dose-dependent upregulation of several integrin subunits or of specific heterodimeric integrin receptors (CORDES et al. 2003; WILD-BODE et al. 2001), while knockdown of integrin expression with small interfering RNA (siRNA) radiosensitizes numerous normal or neoplastic cells (CORDES et al. 2006, 2007; ESTRUGO et al. 2007). Experiments with mouse fibroblasts expressing a signaling-incompetent mutant of β_1 integrin demonstrated that not only integrin expression, but also integrin function is essential for cell survival after genotoxic injury (CORDES et al. 2006).

Unraveling the underlying molecular mechanism contributing to CAM-RR and CAM-DR, it was found that cell adhesion to fibronectin leads to an increase and prolongation of the radiation-induced G2-phase arrest in lung carcinoma cells, providing time for DNA damage repair thereby ensuring genome integrity (CORDES and VAN BEUNINGEN 2003). Similar effects were found in prostate epithelial cells after irradiation (KREMER et al. 2006).

Besides the modulation of cell cycle transition and DNA repair, integrins also seem in control of drug- and radiation-induced apoptotic cell death. Small cell lung cancer cells adherent to laminin, fibronectin, or collagen type IV undergo less apoptosis after treatment with different cytotoxic drugs than cells grown on a nonspecific control substrate (Sethi et al. 1999). Subsequent to inhibition of β_1 integrin, using a function-blocking β_1 integrin antibody, this prosurvival effect of matrix proteins was pronouncedly diminished. It was further confirmed in leukemia cells that integrins play a critical role for the regulation of apoptosis. While downregulation of β_1 integrin resulted in elevated caspase-3, -9, and -8 cleavage and enhanced radiation-induced apoptotic death, treatment with β_1 integrin stimulatory antibodies had the opposite effect and reduced significantly the rate of apoptosis (ESTRUGO et al. 2007). Eventually, Estrugo et al. delineated a novel mechanistic model showing fibronectin-ligated β_1 integrins to efficiently block caspases-8 cleavage upon radiation via recruitment and stimulation of Akt.

In addition to resistance against irradiation and classical cytotoxic drugs, integrin-mediated cell–ECM interactions reduce the efficacy of novel molecular therapeutics. Recently, Eke et al. (2006) showed that adhesion to fibronectin attenuates the anti-proliferative effect of a potent pharmacological EGFR tyrosine kinase inhibitor in human squamous cell carcinoma cells of the head and neck. An explanation for the antagonistic effects by cell adhesion lies in the concept of receptor transactivation where integrin–fibronectin binding cross-activates EGFR and vice versa. Moreover, as reviewed in Sect. 5.4, cytoplasmic signaling is rather organized like a network than as straight pathways of canonical order. Ongoing studies testing other molecular therapeutics are currently characterizing the more general aspects of this phenomenon, which would at least in part explain the low efficacy of targeting drugs like Erbitux (cetuximab, EGFR antibody), Iressa (gefitinib, EGFR tyrosine kinase inhibitor), or Avastin (bevacizumab, VEGF antibody) (Baumann et al. 2008; Krause et al. 2008; Zips et al. 2005).

But not only integrin-mediated cell adhesion modulates cellular radio- or chemosensitivity. Integrin downstream molecules such as ILK and FAK or integrin-associated proteins like Caveolin-1 have been reported to alter resistance against cyto- and genotoxic injury (Fig. 5.5) (Cordes et al. 2007; Eke et al. 2006, 2007; Hehlgans et al. 2007a, 2008; Kasahara et al. 2002). Most interestingly, ILK confers opposite survival effects upon irradiation as expected from the literature on drug sensitivity and ILK (Duxbury et al. 2005; Edwards et al. 2005; Persad et al. 2000). Human lung carcinoma cells, which are transfected with a constitutive active ILK mutant, are more sensitive to irradiation with X-rays than is the ILK wild type and control cells (Cordes 2004). These data could be confirmed in human squamous cell carcinoma cells of the head and neck (Eke et al. 2006, 2007). Consistent with these observations, reduction of ILK protein levels with siRNA confers radioresistance. Not only in solid tumors, but also in leukemia cells, ILK has shown antisurvival effects (Hess et al. 2007). ILK–overexpressing cells are highly sensitive to radiation-induced apoptosis, while downregulation of ILK results in radioprotection of the cells. These effects seem to be due to an interaction between ILK and different caspases. Interestingly, in mouse fibroblasts but not in tumor cells the radiosensitizing effect of ILK is antagonized when cells interact with different extracellular matrix proteins (Hehlgans et al. 2008) indicating that ILK modulates the radiation response of normal fibroblasts and cancer

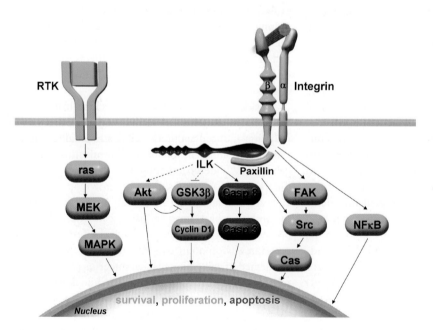

Fig. 5.5. A summary of our current knowledge how integrin signaling critically modifies certain cellular response pathways upon radiation- or drug-induced cytotoxic stress. Cascades in *green* mediate prosurvival signals from transmembrane located β integrins and RTKs via Ras/MEK/MAPK, Akt, or FAK/Src/Cas in a cell type- and/or context-dependent manner. The cascade in *red* transduces anti-survival signals via ILK, caspase-8 and caspase-3 to promote apoptosis

cells in a differential manner. Recent additional data provided evidence that ILK is strongly associated with differentiation in normal tissues as well as with redifferentiation in tumor tissues (HAASE et al. 2008).

In contrast to ILK, overexpression of the prosurvival integrin signaling mediator FAK protects leukemia cells from radiation- and chemo-induced apoptosis (KASAHARA et al. 2002). Silencing of FAK protein expression with siRNA mediated knockdown increases the radiosensitivity of different tumor cell lines originating from pancreatic cancer (CORDES et al. 2007), breast cancer, and colorectal cancer (MCLEAN et al. 2005). Others have shown that human melanoma cells become more sensitive to the chemotherapeutic agent 5-fluorouracil when FAK expression is downregulated (SMITH et al. 2005).

Besides the critical role of proximal integrin signaling proteins, the integral membrane protein Caveolin-1, essential for endo- and exocytosis and linking of integrins with growth factor receptors, is a critical modulator of cellular radiation sensitivity. Recently, CORDES et al.

(2007) showed that Caveolin-1 expression as well as the number of Caveolin-1-positive caveolae is induced by ionizing irradiation. In reference to this chapter, Caveolin-1-overexpression in pancreatic carcinoma cells leads to a significant reduction in radiosensitivity in comparison with control cells. Consistent with these results, a knockdown of Caveolin-1 enhanced the cellular radiosensitivity. These effects are partially channeled by a strong growth delay with a concomitant rise in G1-phase cells but may be also caused by activity changes in important prosurvival signaling pathways such as the Akt cascade (CORDES et al. 2007).

5.8
Summary and Perspective

Adhesion and invasion are controlled by integrin receptors and are frequently dysregulated in cancer with disastrous consequences such as local destruction of

Table 5.5. Therapeutic agents against integrins. Data summary of approved agents and agents currently evaluated in clinical trials

Active agent	Brand name	Target	Indications (approved)	Indications (in clinical trials)
Antibodies				
Natalizumab	Tysabri	$\alpha_4\beta_7$	Multiple sclerosis, Crohn's disease	
Abciximab	ReoPro	GPIIb/IIIa	Angioplasty	
Volociximab (M200)		$\alpha_5\beta_1$		Renal cell carcinoma, melanoma
Vitaxin (MEDI-522)		$\alpha_v\beta_3$		Melanoma, colorectal carcinoma, prostate cancer, rheumatoid arthritis, psoriasis
CNTO 95		α_v		Prostate cancer, melanoma
Peptides				
Cilengitide (EMD 121974)		$\alpha_v\beta_3,$ $\alpha_v\beta_5$		Glioblastoma, melanoma, lymphoma, renal cell carcinoma, colon carcinoma
Eptifibatide	Integrilin	$\alpha_2\beta_3$	Small heart attacks, angioplasty	
JSM6427		$\alpha_5\beta_1$		Macular degeneration
Non-peptides				
Tirofiban	Aggrastat	GPIIb/IIIa	Instable angina pectoris	
E7820		α_2		Colorectal carcinoma, lymphoma

Data obtained from http://www.clinicaltrials.gov and http://www.fda.gov

normal tissue, metastases, and ineffective local tumor control by anticancer therapeutics. In particular, aggravated local tumor control evolves from the combination of genetic alterations and changes in the tumor micromilieu. Being widely neglected for decades, the myriad micromilieu factors such as oxygen, lactate, and extracellular matrix are increasingly recognized as potent modulators of therapy resistance in cancer.

With respect to the content of this chapter, Table 5.5 summarizes the integrin targeting compounds current in clinical trials. Many of them are administrated in inflammatory diseases but others are given as monotherapy in a variety of human cancers. Speculatively not curative by themselves, anti-integrin agents might be potent when applied in combination with conventional radio- and chemotherapy as well as in a combination with other molecular drugs. Solving the intra- and extracellular networks a tumor cell exploits for its growth and spreading benefits in more depth may foster the diagnosis of early-stage cancer, the development of novel drugs, and eventually increased patient survival.

References

Acheson A, Sunshine JL, Rutishauser U (1991) NCAM polysialic acid can regulate both cell–cell and cell-substrate interactions. J Cell Biol 114:143–153

Adamia S, Maxwell CA, Pilarski LM (2005) Hyaluronan and hyaluronan synthases: potential therapeutic targets in cancer. Curr Drug Targets Cardiovasc Haematol Disord 5:3–14

Alavi A, Stupack DG (2007) Cell survival in a three-dimensional matrix. Methods Enzymol 426:85–101

Albelda SM, Mette SA, Elder DE et al (1990) Integrin distribution in malignant melanoma: association of the beta 3 subunit with tumor progression. Cancer Res 50:6757–6764

Alberts B, Johnson A, Lewis J et al (2002) Molecular biology of the cell, 4th edn. Garland Science, New York

Anderson RG (1998) The caveolae membrane system. Annu Rev Biochem 67:199–225

Ardelt W (1964) [Elastin, elastase, elastolysis.] (In Polish) Postepy Biochem 10:245–264

Barret C, Roy C, Montcourrier P et al (2000) Mutagenesis of the phosphatidylinositol 4,5-bisphosphate (PIP₂) binding site in the NH₂-terminal domain of ezrin correlates with its altered cellular distribution. J Cell Biol 151:1067–1080

Baumann M, Krause M, Hill R (2008) Exploring the role of cancer stem cells in radioresistance. Nat Rev Cancer 8:545–554

Biancone L, Araki M, Araki K et al (1996) Redirection of tumor metastasis by expression of E-selectin in vivo. J Exp Med 183:581–587

Bissell MJ, Radisky D (2001) Putting tumours in context. Nat Rev Cancer 1:46–54

Blaschke RJ, Howlett AR, Desprez PY et al (1994) Cell differentiation by extracellular matrix components. Methods Enzymol 245:535–556

Blasi F, Carmeliet P (2002) uPAR: a versatile signalling orchestrator. Nat Rev Mol Cell Biol 3:932–43

Board RE, Valle JW (2007) Metastatic colorectal cancer: current systemic treatment options. Drugs 67:1851–1867

Bolender DL, Seliger WG, Markwald RR et al (1981) Structural analysis of extracellular matrix prior to the migration of cephalic neural crest cells. Scan Electron Microsc (Pt 2):285–296

Bompard G, Martin M, Roy C et al (2003) Membrane targeting of protein tyrosine phosphatase PTPL1 through its FERM domain via binding to phosphatidylinositol 4,5-biphosphate. J Cell Sci 116 (Pt 12):2519–2530

Borsig L, Wong R, Hynes RO et al (2002) Synergistic effects of L- and P-selectin in facilitating tumor metastasis can involve non-mucin ligands and implicate leukocytes as enhancers of metastasis. Proc Natl Acad Sci USA 99:2193–2198

Boudeau J, Miranda-Saavedra D, Barton GJ et al (2006) Emerging roles of pseudokinases. Trends Cell Biol 16:443–452

Brakebusch C, Fassler R (2003) The integrin-actin connection, an eternal love affair. EMBO J 22:2324–2333

Braun A, Bordoy R, Stanchi F et al (2003) PINCH2 is a new five LIM domain protein, homologous to PINCH and localized to focal adhesions. Exp Cell Res 284:239–250

Brodt P, Fallavollita L, Bresalier RS et al (1997) Liver endothelial E-selectin mediates carcinoma cell adhesion and promotes liver metastasis. Int J Cancer 71:612–619

Brooks PC, Stromblad S, Sanders LC et al (1996) Localization of matrix metalloproteinase MMP-2 to the surface of invasive cells by interaction with integrin alpha v beta 3. Cell 85:683–693

Broussard JA, Webb DJ, Kaverina I (2008) Asymmetric focal adhesion disassembly in motile cells. Curr Opin Cell Biol 20:85–90

Burridge K, Nuckolls G, Otey C et al (1990) Actin-membrane interaction in focal adhesions. Cell Differ Dev 32:337–342

Calalb MB, Polte TR, Hanks SK (1995) Tyrosine phosphorylation of focal adhesion kinase at sites in the catalytic domain regulates kinase activity: a role for Src family kinases. Mol Cell Biol 15:954–963

Calderwood DA, Tuckwell DS, Humphries MJ (1995) Specificity of integrin I-domain-ligand binding. Biochem Soc Trans 23:504S

Calderwood DA, Tuckwell DS, Eble J et al (1997) The integrin alpha1 A-domain is a ligand binding site for collagens and laminin. J Biol Chem 272:12311–12317

Caron-Lormier G, Berry H (2005) Amplification and oscillations in the FAK/Src kinase system during integrin signaling. J Theor Biol 232:235–248

Carver LA, Schnitzer JE (2003) Caveolae: mining little caves for new cancer targets. Nat Rev Cancer 3:571–581

Ceccarelli DF, Song HK, Poy F et al (2006) Crystal structure of the FERM domain of focal adhesion kinase. J Biol Chem 281:252–259

Chan AO (2006) E-cadherin in gastric cancer. World J Gastroenterol 12:199–203

Chang C, Werb Z (2001) The many faces of metalloproteases: cell growth, invasion, angiogenesis and metastasis. Trends Cell Biol 11:S37–S43

Chapman HA, Wei Y (2001) Protease crosstalk with integrins: the urokinase receptor paradigm. Thromb Haemost 86:124–129

Chishti AH, Kim AC, Marfatia SM et al (1998) The FERM domain: a unique module involved in the linkage of cytoplasmic proteins to the membrane. Trends Biochem Sci 23:281–282

Chung J, Kim TH (2008) Integrin-dependent translational control: Implication in cancer progression. Microsc Res Tech 71:380–386

Chung LW, Li W, Gleave ME et al (1992) Human prostate cancer model: roles of growth factors and extracellular matrices. J Cell Biochem Suppl 16H:99–105

Cochran AJ, Ohsie SJ, Binder SW (2008) Pathobiology of the sentinel node. Curr Opin Oncol 20:190–195

Cordes N (2004) Overexpression of hyperactive integrin-linked kinase leads to increased cellular radiosensitivity. Cancer Res 64:5683–56892

Cordes N, Meineke V (2003) Cell adhesion-mediated radioresistance (CAM-RR). Extracellular matrix-dependent improvement of cell survival in human tumor and normal cells in vitro. Strahlenther Onkol 179:337–344

Cordes N, Park CC (2007) beta1 integrin as a molecular therapeutic target. Int J Radiat Biol 83 (11–12):753–760

Cordes N, van Beuningen D (2003) Cell adhesion to the extracellular matrix protein fibronectin modulates radiation-dependent G2 phase arrest involving integrin-linked kinase (ILK) and glycogen synthase kinase-3beta (GSK-3beta) in vitro. Br J Cancer 88:1470–1479

Cordes N, Hansmeier B, Beinke C et al (2003) Irradiation differentially affects substratum-dependent survival, adhesion, and invasion of glioblastoma cell lines. Br J Cancer 89:2122–2132

Cordes N, Seidler J, Durzok R et al (2006) beta1-integrin-mediated signaling essentially contributes to cell survival after radiation-induced genotoxic injury. Oncogene 25:1378–1390

Cordes N, Frick S, Brunner TB et al (2007) Human pancreatic tumor cells are sensitized to ionizing radiation by knockdown of caveolin-1. Oncogene 26:6851–6862

Couet J, Sargiacomo M, Lisanti MP (1997) Interaction of a receptor tyrosine kinase, EGF-R, with caveolins. Caveolin binding negatively regulates tyrosine and serine/threonine kinase activities. J Biol Chem 272:30429–30438

Coussens LM, Werb Z (2002) Inflammation and cancer. Nature 420:860–867

Cowin P, Rowlands TM, Hatsell SJ (2005) Cadherins and catenins in breast cancer. Curr Opin Cell Biol 17:499–508

Crnic I, Strittmatter K, Cavallaro U et al (2004) Loss of neural cell adhesion molecule induces tumor metastasis by upregulating lymphangiogenesis. Cancer Res 64:8630–8638

Croce CM (2008) Oncogenes and cancer. N Engl J Med 358:502–511

Czirok A, Zamir EA, Filla MB et al (2006) Extracellular matrix macroassembly dynamics in early vertebrate embryos. Curr Top Dev Biol 73:237–258

Dalton WS (2003) The tumor microenvironment: focus on myeloma. Cancer Treat Rev 29 Suppl 1:11–19

Damiano JS (2002) Integrins as novel drug targets for overcoming innate drug resistance. Curr Cancer Drug Targets 2:37–43

Damiano JS, Cress AE, Hazlehurst LA et al (1999) Cell adhesion mediated drug resistance (CAM-DR): role of integrins and resistance to apoptosis in human myeloma cell lines. Blood 93:1658–1667

Danen EH (2005) Integrins: regulators of tissue function and cancer progression. Curr Pharm Des 11:881–891

Delcommenne M, Tan C, Gray V et al (1998) Phosphoinositide-3-OH kinase-dependent regulation of glycogen synthase kinase 3 and protein kinase B/AKT by the integrin-linked kinase. Proc Natl Acad Sci USA 95:11211–1126

Diaz-Montero CM, McIntyre BW (2003) Acquisition of anoikis resistance in human osteosarcoma cells. Eur J Cancer 39:2395–2402

Dougherty GW, Chopp T, Qi SM et al (2005) The Ras suppressor Rsu-1 binds to the LIM 5 domain of the adaptor protein PINCH1 and participates in adhesion-related functions. Exp Cell Res 306:168–179

Durand RE (1994) The influence of microenvironmental factors during cancer therapy. In Vivo 8:691–702

Duxbury MS, Ito H, Benoit E et al (2005) RNA interference demonstrates a novel role for integrin-linked kinase as a determinant of pancreatic adenocarcinoma cell gemcitabine chemoresistance. Clin Cancer Res 11:3433–3438

Edwards LA, Thiessen B, Dragowska WH et al (2005) Inhibition of ILK in PTEN-mutant human glioblastomas inhibits PKB/Akt activation, induces apoptosis, and delays tumor growth. Oncogene 24:3596–35605

Eke I, Sandfort V, Mischkus A et al (2006) Antiproliferative effects of EGFR tyrosine kinase inhibition and radiation-induced genotoxic injury are attenuated by adhesion to fibronectin. Radiother Oncol 80:178–184

Eke I, Sandfort V, Storch K et al (2007) Pharmacological inhibition of EGFR tyrosine kinase affects ILK-mediated cellular radiosensitization in vitro. Int J Radiat Biol 83:793–802

Erler JT, Bennewith KL, Nicolau M et al (2006) Lysyl oxidase is essential for hypoxia-induced metastasis. Nature 440 (7088):1222–1226

Estrugo D, Fischer A, Hess F et al (2007) Ligand bound beta1 integrins inhibit procaspase-8 for mediating cell adhesion-mediated drug and radiation resistance in human leukemia cells. PLoS ONE 2:e269

Evans EA, Calderwood DA (2007) Forces and bond dynamics in cell adhesion. Science 316:1148–1153

Evans RD, Jones J, Taylor C et al (2004) Sequence variation in the I-like domain of the beta1 integrin subunit in human oral squamous cell carcinomas. Cancer Lett 213:189–194

Fielding CJ, Fielding PE (2003) Relationship between cholesterol trafficking and signaling in rafts and caveolae. Biochim Biophys Acta 1610:219–228

Fine JD, Griffith RD (1985) A specific defect in glycosylation of epidermal cell membranes. Definition in skin from patients with epidermolysis bullosa simplex. Arch Dermatol 121:1292–1296

Fogar P, Basso D, Pasquali C et al (1997) Neural cell adhesion molecule (N-CAM) in gastrointestinal neoplasias. Anticancer Res 17:1227–1230

Franco SJ, Huttenlocher A (2005) Regulating cell migration: calpains make the cut. J Cell Sci 118:3829–3838

Friedl P, Brocker EB (2000) The biology of cell locomotion within three-dimensional extracellular matrix. Cell Mol Life Sci 57:41–64

Galbiati F, Volonte D, Engelman JA et al (1998) Targeted downregulation of caveolin-1 is sufficient to drive cell transformation and hyperactivate the p42/44 MAP kinase cascade. EMBO J 17:6633–6648

Giancotti FG, Ruoslahti E (1999) Integrin signaling. Science 285:1028–1032

Girault JA, Labesse G, Mornon JP et al (1999) The N-termini of FAK and JAKs contain divergent band 4.1 domains. Trends Biochem Sci 24:54–57

Gluer S, Wunder MA, Schelp C et al (1998) Polysialylated neural cell adhesion molecule serum levels in normal children. Pediatr Res 44:915–919

Godsel LM, Hobbs RP, Green KJ (2008) Intermediate filament assembly: dynamics to disease. Trends Cell Biol 18:28–37

Gomez DE, Alonso DF, Yoshiji H et al (1997) Tissue inhibitors of metalloproteinases: structure, regulation and biological functions. Eur J Cell Biol 74:111–122

Gospodarowicz D, Greenburg G, Vlodavsky I et al (1979) The identification and localization of fibronectin in cultured corneal endothelial cells: cell surface polarity and physiological implications. Exp Eye Res 29:485–509

Green KJ, Simpson CL (2007) Desmosomes: new perspectives on a classic. J Invest Dermatol 127:2499–2515

Greenlee KJ, Werb Z, Kheradmand F (2007) Matrix metalloproteinases in lung: multiple, multifarious, and multifaceted. Physiol Rev 87:69–98

Guo W, Giancotti FG (2004) Integrin signalling during tumour progression. Nat Rev Mol Cell Biol 5:816–826

Haase M, Gmach CC, Eke I et al (2008) Expression of integrin-linked kinase is increased in differentiated cells. J Histochem Cytochem (in press)

Halazonetis TD, Gorgoulis VG, Bartek J (2008) An oncogene-induced DNA damage model for cancer development. Science 319:1352–1355

Hannigan GE, Leung-Hagesteijn C, Fitz-Gibbon L et al (1996) Regulation of cell adhesion and anchorage-dependent growth by a new beta 1-integrin-linked protein kinase. Nature 379:91–96

Hay ED (1989) Extracellular matrix, cell skeletons, and embryonic development. Am J Med Genet 34:14–29

Hayashi I, Vuori K, Liddington RC (2002) The focal adhesion targeting (FAT) region of focal adhesion kinase is a four-helix bundle that binds paxillin. Nat Struct Biol 9:101–106

Hehlgans S, Eke I, Cordes N (2007a) An essential role of integrin-linked kinase in the cellular radiosensitivity of normal fibroblasts during the process of cell adhesion and spreading. Int J Radiat Biol 83:769–779

Hehlgans S, Haase M, Cordes N (2007b) Signalling via integrins: implications for cell survival and anticancer strategies. Biochim Biophys Acta 1775:163–180

Hehlgans S, Eke I, Deuse Y et al (2008) Integrin-linked kinase: Dispensable for radiation survival of three-dimensionally cultured fibroblasts. Radiother Oncol 86:329–335

Hemperly JJ, DeGuglielmo JK, Reid RA (1990) Characterization of cDNA clones defining variant forms of human neural cell adhesion molecule N-CAM. J Mol Neurosci 2:71–78

Hernandez-Barrantes S, Bernardo M, Toth M et al (2002) Regulation of membrane type-matrix metalloproteinases. Semin Cancer Biol 12:131–138

Hess F, Estrugo D, Fischer A et al (2007) Integrin-linked kinase interacts with caspase-9 and -8 in an adhesion-dependent manner for promoting radiation-induced apoptosis in human leukemia cells. Oncogene 26:1372–1384

Hirao M, Sato N, Kondo T et al (1996) Regulation mechanism of ERM (ezrin/radixin/moesin) protein/plasma membrane association: possible involvement of phosphatidylinositol turnover and Rho-dependent signaling pathway. J Cell Biol 135:37–51

Hodkinson PS, Mackinnon AC, Sethi T (2007) Extracellular matrix regulation of drug resistance in small-cell lung cancer. Int J Radiat Biol 83:733–741

Hood JD, Cheresh DA (2002) Role of integrins in cell invasion and migration. Nat Rev Cancer 2:91–100

Hynes RO (2002) Integrins: bidirectional, allosteric signaling machines. Cell 110:673–687

Hynes RO (2003) Metastatic potential: generic predisposition of the primary tumor or rare, metastatic variants – or both? Cell 113:821–823

Hynes RO (2004) The emergence of integrins: a personal and historical perspective. Matrix Biol 23:333–340

Ino Y, Gotoh M, Sakamoto M et al (2002) Dysadherin, a cancer-associated cell membrane glycoprotein, down-regulates E-cadherin and promotes metastasis. Proc Natl Acad Sci USA 99:365–370

Ishida-Yamamoto A, McGrath JA, Chapman SJ et al (1991) Epidermolysis bullosa simplex (Dowling-Meara type) is a genetic disease characterized by an abnormal keratin-filament network involving keratins K5 and K14. J Invest Dermatol 97:959–968

Janes SM, Watt FM (2004) Switch from alphavbeta5 to alphavbeta6 integrin expression protects squamous cell carcinomas from anoikis. J Cell Biol 166:419–431

Jinga DC, Blidaru A, Condrea I et al (2006) MMP-9 and MMP-2 gelatinases and TIMP-1 and TIMP-2 inhibitors in breast cancer: correlations with prognostic factors. J Cell Mol Med 10:499–510

Johnson LD (1980) The biochemical properties of basement membrane components in health and disease. Clin Biochem 13:204–208

Kasahara T, Koguchi E, Funakoshi M et al (2002) Antiapoptotic action of focal adhesion kinase (FAK) against ionizing radiation. Antioxid Redox Signal 4:491–499

Kim DW, Huamani J, Fu A et al (2006) Molecular strategies targeting the host component of cancer to enhance tumor response to radiation therapy. Int J Radiat Oncol Biol Phys 64:38–46

Kiosses WB, Shattil SJ, Pampori N et al (2001) Rac recruits high-affinity integrin alphavbeta3 to lamellipodia in endothelial cell migration. Nat Cell Biol 3:316–320

Klemke RL, Leng J, Molander R et al (1998) CAS/Crk coupling serves as a "molecular switch" for induction of cell migration. J Cell Biol 140:961–972

Krause M, Baumann M (2008) Clinical biomarkers of kinase activity: examples from EGFR inhibition trials. Cancer Metastasis Rev 27:387–402

Kremer CL, Schmelz M, Cress AE (2006) Integrin-dependent amplification of the G2 arrest induced by ionizing radiation. Prostate 66:88–96

Kucharewicz I, Kowal K, Buczko W et al (2003) The plasmin system in airway remodeling. Thromb Res 112:1–7

LaBarge MA, Petersen OW, Bissell MJ (2007) Of microenvironments and mammary stem cells. Stem Cell Rev 3:137–146

Lauffenburger DA, Horwitz AF (1996) Cell migration: a physically integrated molecular process. Cell 84:359–369

Lee H, Volonte D, Galbiati F et al (2000) Constitutive and growth factor-regulated phosphorylation of caveolin-1 occurs at the same site (Tyr-14) in vivo: identification of a c-Src/Cav-1/Grb7 signaling cassette. Mol Endocrinol 14:1750–1775

Li S, Couet J, Lisanti MP (1996) Src tyrosine kinases, alpha subunits, and H-Ras share a common membrane-anchored scaffolding protein, caveolin. Caveolin binding negatively regulates the auto-activation of Src tyrosine kinases. J Biol Chem 271:29182–29190

Li ZW, Dalton WS (2006) Tumor microenvironment and drug resistance in hematologic malignancies. Blood Rev 20:333–342

Lipscomb EA, Mercurio AM (2005) Mobilization and activation of a signaling competent alpha6beta4integrin underlies its contribution to carcinoma progression. Cancer Metastasis Rev 24:413–423

Liu S, Calderwood DA, Ginsberg MH (2000) Integrin cytoplasmic domain-binding proteins. J Cell Sci 113 (Pt 20):3563–3571

Ljungberg B (2007) Prognostic markers in renal cell carcinoma. Curr Opin Urol 17:303–308

Lo SH, Chen LB (1994) Focal adhesion as a signal transduction organelle. Cancer Metastasis Rev 13:9–24

Lodish H, Berk A, Matsudaira P et al (2004) Molecular cell biology, 5th edn. Freeman, New York

Lopez-Otin C, Matrisian LM (2007) Emerging roles of proteases in tumour suppression. Nat Rev Cancer 7:800–808

Lynch CC, Matrisian LM (2002) Matrix metalloproteinases in tumor-host cell communication. Differentiation 70:561–573

Lynch DK, Ellis CA, Edwards PA et al (1999) Integrin-linked kinase regulates phosphorylation of serine 473 of protein kinase B by an indirect mechanism. Oncogene 18:8024–8032

Martin KH, Slack JK, Boerner SA et al (2002) Integrin connections map: to infinity and beyond. Science 296:1652–1653

Massova I, Kotra LP, Fridman R et al (1998) Matrix metalloproteinases: structures, evolution, and diversification. FASEB J 12:1075–1095

McLean GW, Carragher NO, Avizienyte E et al (2005) The role of focal-adhesion kinase in cancer—a new therapeutic opportunity. Nat Rev Cancer 5:505–415

Mercurio AM, Rabinovitz I (2001) Towards a mechanistic understanding of tumor invasion—lessons from the alpha-6beta 4 integrin. Semin Cancer Biol 11:129–141

Mese G, Richard G, White TW (2007) Gap junctions: basic structure and function. J Invest Dermatol 127:2516–2524

Mettouchi A, Klein S, Guo W et al (2001) Integrin-specific activation of Rac controls progression through the G(1) phase of the cell cycle. Mol Cell 8:115–127

Mileusnic R, Lancashire C, Rose SP (1999) Sequence-specific impairment of memory formation by NCAM antisense oligonucleotides. Learn Mem 6:120–127

Mitra SK, Hanson DA, Schlaepfer DD (2005) Focal adhesion kinase: in command and control of cell motility. Nat Rev Mol Cell Biol 6:56–68

Miyahara R, Tanaka F, Nakagawa T et al (2001) Expression of neural cell adhesion molecules (polysialylated form of neural cell adhesion molecule and L1-cell adhesion molecule) on resected small cell lung cancer specimens: in relation to proliferation state. J Surg Oncol 77:49–54

Mochizuki S, Okada Y (2007) ADAMs in cancer cell proliferation and progression. Cancer Sci 98:621–628

Morabito A, Piccirillo MC, Monaco K et al (2007) First-line chemotherapy for HER-2 negative metastatic breast cancer patients who received anthracyclines as adjuvant treatment. Oncologist 12:1288–1298

Moroi M, Jung SM (1998) Integrin-mediated platelet adhesion. Front Biosci 3:d719–d728

Munshi HG, Stack MS (2006) Reciprocal interactions between adhesion receptor signaling and MMP regulation. Cancer Metastasis Rev 25:45–56

Nagano O, Saya H (2004) Mechanism and biological significance of CD44 cleavage. Cancer Sci 95:930–935

Nagase H (1997) Activation mechanisms of matrix metalloproteinases. Biol Chem 378:151–560

Niessen CM (2007) Tight junctions/adherens junctions: basic structure and function. J Invest Dermatol 127:2525–2532

Niessen CM, Gottardi CJ (2008) Molecular components of the adherens junction. Biochim Biophys Acta 1778:562–571

Nimwegen MJ van, van de Water B (2007) Focal adhesion kinase: a potential target in cancer therapy. Biochem Pharmacol 73:597–609

Nowakowski J, Cronin CN, McRee DE et al (2002) Structures of the cancer-related Aurora-A, FAK, and EphA2 protein kinases from nanovolume crystallography. Structure 10:1659–1667

Okamoto T, Schlegel A, Scherer PE et al (1998) Caveolins, a family of scaffolding proteins for organizing "preassembled signaling complexes" at the plasma membrane. J Biol Chem 273:5419–5422

Park CC, Zhang H, Pallavicini M et al (2006) Beta1 integrin inhibitory antibody induces apoptosis of breast cancer cells, inhibits growth, and distinguishes malignant from normal phenotype in three dimensional cultures and in vivo. Cancer Res 66:1526–1535

Parsons JT (2003) Focal adhesion kinase: the first ten years. J Cell Sci 116:1409–1416

Paszek MJ, Weaver VM (2004) The tension mounts: mechanics meets morphogenesis and malignancy. J Mammary Gland Biol Neoplasia 9:325–3242

Perry SV, Cotterill J (1965) Interaction of actin and myosin. Nature 206:161–163

Persad S, Attwell S, Gray V et al (2000) Inhibition of integrin-linked kinase (ILK) suppresses activation of protein kinase B/Akt and induces cell cycle arrest and apoptosis of PTEN-mutant prostate cancer cells. Proc Natl Acad Sci USA 97:3207–3212

Petersen C, Eicheler W, Frommel A et al (2003) Proliferation and micromilieu during fractionated irradiation of human FaDu squamous cell carcinoma in nude mice. Int J Radiat Biol 79:469–477

Petersen OW, Ronnov-Jessen L, Weaver VM et al (1998) Differentiation and cancer in the mammary gland: shedding light on an old dichotomy. Adv Cancer Res 75:135–161

Pettitt J (2005) The cadherin superfamily. WormBook 29:1–9

Plantefaber LC, Hynes RO (1989) Changes in integrin receptors on oncogenically transformed cells. Cell 56:281–290

Pollerberg GE, Burridge K, Krebs KE et al (1987) The 180-kD component of the neural cell adhesion molecule N-CAM is involved in cell–cell contacts and cytoskeleton–membrane interactions. Cell Tissue Res 250:227–236

Porter JC, Hogg N (1998) Integrins take partners: cross-talk between integrins and other membrane receptors. Trends Cell Biol 8:390–396

Qian X, Karpova T, Sheppard AM et al (2004) E-cadherin-mediated adhesion inhibits ligand-dependent activation of diverse receptor tyrosine kinases. EMBO J 23:1739–1748

Ra HJ, Parks WC (2007) Control of matrix metalloproteinase catalytic activity. Matrix Biol 26:587–596

Ramachandran GN, Kartha G (1954) Structure of collagen. Nature 174 (4423):269–270

Ramsay AG, Marshall JF, Hart IR (2007) Integrin trafficking and its role in cancer metastasis. Cancer Metastasis Rev 26:567–578

Raucher D, Sheetz MP (2000) Cell spreading and lamellipodial extension rate is regulated by membrane tension. J Cell Biol 148:127–136

Reynolds AB (2007) p120-catenin: past and present. Biochim Biophys Acta 1773:2–7

Roesler J, Srivatsan E, Moatamed F et al (1997) Tumor suppressor activity of neural cell adhesion molecule in colon carcinoma. Am J Surg 174:251–257

Rousset B (1996) [Introduction to the structure and functions of junction communications or gap junctions]. (In French) Ann Endocrinol (Paris) 57:476–480

Ruch RJ, Trosko JE (2001) Gap-junction communication in chemical carcinogenesis. Drug Metab Rev 33:117–124

Ruoslahti E (1999) Fibronectin and its integrin receptors in cancer. Adv Cancer Res 76:1–20

Ruoslahti E (2003) The RGD story: a personal account. Matrix Biol 22:459–465

Salanueva IJ, Cerezo A, Guadamillas MC et al (2007) Integrin regulation of caveolin function. J Cell Mol Med 11:969–980

Sarbassov DD, Guertin DA, Ali SM et al (2005) Phosphorylation and regulation of Akt/PKB by the rictor-mTOR complex. Science 307:1098–1101

Schlaepfer DD, Mitra SK, Ilic D (2004) Control of motile and invasive cell phenotypes by focal adhesion kinase. Biochim Biophys Acta 1692:77–102

Schmidt CE, Horwitz AF, Lauffenburger DA et al (1993) Integrin-cytoskeletal interactions in migrating fibroblasts are dynamic, asymmetric, and regulated. J Cell Biol 123:977–991

Schwartz MA (2001) Integrin signaling revisited. Trends Cell Biol 11:466–470

Sethi T, Rintoul RC, Moore SM et al (1999) Extracellular matrix proteins protect small cell lung cancer cells against apoptosis: a mechanism for small cell lung cancer growth and drug resistance in vivo. Nat Med 5:662–668

Shiraha H, Glading A, Gupta K et al (1999) IP-10 inhibits epidermal growth factor-induced motility by decreasing epidermal growth factor receptor-mediated calpain activity. J Cell Biol 146:243–254

Siesser PM, Hanks SK (2006) The signaling and biological implications of FAK overexpression in cancer. Clin Cancer Res 12:3233–3237

Small JV, Resch GP (2005) The comings and goings of actin: coupling protrusion and retraction in cell motility. Curr Opin Cell Biol 17:517–523

Smith CS, Golubovskaya VM, Peck E et al (2005) Effect of focal adhesion kinase (FAK) downregulation with FAK antisense oligonucleotides and 5-fluorouracil on the viability of melanoma cell lines. Melanoma Res 15:357–362

Song KS, Scherer PE, Tang Z et al (1996) Expression of caveolin-3 in skeletal, cardiac, and smooth muscle cells. Caveolin-3 is a component of the sarcolemma and cofractionates with dystrophin and dystrophin-associated glycoproteins. J Biol Chem 271:15160–15165

Stanchi F, Bordoy R, Kudlacek O et al (2005) Consequences of loss of PINCH2 expression in mice. J Cell Sci 118:5899–5910

Sternlicht MD, Werb Z (2001) How matrix metalloproteinases regulate cell behavior. Annu Rev Cell Dev Biol 17:463–516

Sugrue SP, Hay ED (1981) Response of basal epithelial cell surface and Cytoskeleton to solubilized extracellular matrix molecules. J Cell Biol 91:45–54

Tachibana K, Sato T, D'Avirro N et al (1995) Direct association of pp125FAK with paxillin, the focal adhesion-targeting mechanism of pp125FAK. J Exp Med 182:1089–1099

Tang Z, Scherer PE, Okamoto T et al (1996) Molecular cloning of caveolin-3, a novel member of the caveolin gene family expressed predominantly in muscle. J Biol Chem 271:2255–22561

Tannock IF (1996) Treatment of cancer with radiation and drugs. J Clin Oncol 14:3156–3174

Tascilar O, Cakmak GK, Tekin IO et al (2007) Neural cell adhesion molecule-180 expression as a prognostic criterion in colorectal carcinoma: feasible or not? World J Gastroenterol 13:5476–5480

Trosko JE, Ruch RJ (1998) Cell–cell communication in carcinogenesis. Front Biosci 3:d208–d236

Tu Y, Li F, Wu C (1998) Nck-2, a novel Src homology2/3-containing adaptor protein that interacts with the LIM-only protein PINCH and components of growth factor receptor kinase-signaling pathways. Mol Biol Cell 9:3367–3382

Tu Y, Li F, Goicoechea S et al (1999) The LIM-only protein PINCH directly interacts with integrin-linked kinase and is recruited to integrin-rich sites in spreading cells. Mol Cell Biol 19:2425–2434

Varmus H, Pao W, Politi K et al (2005) Oncogenes come of age. Cold Spring Harb Symp Quant Biol 70:1–9

Vaupel P, Mayer A (2005) Hypoxia and anemia: effects on tumor biology and treatment resistance. Transfus Clin Biol 12:5–10

Vaynberg J, Fukuda T, Chen K et al (2005) Structure of an ultraweak protein–protein complex and its crucial role in regulation of cell morphology and motility. Mol Cell 17:513–523

Velyvis A, Yang Y, Wu C et al (2001) Solution structure of the focal adhesion adaptor PINCH LIM1 domain and characterization of its interaction with the integrin-linked kinase ankyrin repeat domain. J Biol Chem 276:4932–4939

Vlodavsky I, Korner G, Ishai-Michaeli R et al (1990) Extracellular matrix-resident growth factors and enzymes: possible involvement in tumor metastasis and angiogenesis. Cancer Metastasis Rev 9:203–226

Vlodavsky I, Fuks Z, Ishai-Michaeli R et al (1991) Extracellular matrix-resident basic fibroblast growth factor: implication for the control of angiogenesis. J Cell Biochem 45:167–176

Wang Y, Mehta PP (1995) Facilitation of gap-junctional communication and gap-junction formation in mammalian cells by inhibition of glycosylation. Eur J Cell Biol 67:285–296

Wary KK, Mariotti A, Zurzolo C et al (1998) A requirement for caveolin-1 and associated kinase Fyn in integrin signaling and anchorage-dependent cell growth. Cell 94:625–634

Watt FM (2002) Role of integrins in regulating epidermal adhesion, growth and differentiation. Embo J 21:3919–3926

Weaver VM, Lelievre S, Lakins JN et al (2002) beta4 integrin-dependent formation of polarized three-dimensional architecture confers resistance to apoptosis in normal and malignant mammary epithelium. Cancer Cell 2:205–216

Wedgwood A, Younes A (2006) Targeting lymphoma cells and their microenvironment with novel antibodies. Clin Lymphoma Myeloma 7(Suppl):S33–S40

Wei Y, Yang X, Liu Q et al (1999) A role for caveolin and the urokinase receptor in integrin-mediated adhesion and signaling. J Cell Biol 144:1285–1294

Wild-Bode C, Weller M, Rimner A et al (2001) Sublethal irradiation promotes migration and invasiveness of glioma cells: implications for radiotherapy of human glioblastoma. Cancer Res 61:2744–2750

Williams TM, Lisanti MP (2005) Caveolin-1 in oncogenic transformation, cancer, and metastasis. Am J Physiol 288:C494–C506

Yamamoto M, Toya Y, Schwencke C et al (1998) Caveolin is an activator of insulin receptor signaling. J Biol Chem 273:26962–26968

Yao ES, Zhang H, Chen YY et al (2007) Increased beta1 integrin is associated with decreased survival in invasive breast cancer. Cancer Res 67:659–664

Zahir N, Weaver VM (2004) Death in the third dimension: apoptosis regulation and tissue architecture. Curr Opin Genet Dev 14:71–80

Zips D, Eicheler W, Geyer P et al (2005) Enhanced susceptibility of irradiated tumor vessels to vascular endothelial growth factor receptor tyrosine kinase inhibition. Cancer Res 65:5374–5379

The Biology of Cancer Metastasis

6

Miodrag Gužvić and Christoph A. Klein

CONTENTS

KEY POINTS

- For at least one century, the prevailing view has considered metastasis as a late and final step in cancer progression. Also, supportive experimental data have been gathered, such as somatic genetic changes accumulating during local cancer progression—many of which can also be identified in metastases.
- More recent genetic data suggested that the metastatic potential cannot be acquired late in local progression in rare variant cells, but that dissemination of tumour cells begins very early after transformation. Primary tumours may often be poor surrogate markers for the genetics of disseminated tumour cells (DTCs) and thereby for response to adjuvant therapies.
- The cancer stem cell (CSC) hypothesis adds as a further complication a hierarchy of tumour cells, generated by non-genetic mechanisms, to the progression puzzle. This hypothesis assumes that only rare subpopulations of tumour cells, derived from organ-specific stem or progenitor cells, are driving the growth and spread of malignant cancers.
- Cytokeratins are the most specific and currently also the most sensitive markers to detect single DTCs in bone marrow, while the epithelial cell adhesion molecule (EpCAM; CD326) is favoured for the analysis of DTCs in lymph nodes, and for the detection of circulating tumour cells (CTC) in the blood stream several markers are in use.

M. Gužvić, MSc
Division of Oncogenomics, Department of Pathology, University of Regensburg, Franz-Josef-Strauss-Allee 11, 93053 Regensburg, Germany

C. A. Klein, MD
Professor, Division of Oncogenomics, Department of Pathology, University of Regensburg, Franz-Josef-Strauss-Allee 11, 93053 Regensburg, Germany

- Several lines of evidence suggest that DTCs evolve largely independently from the primary tumour, and that they accumulate genetic alterations until they eventually grow out.
- We suggest using the term *dissemination* for the processes of leaving the primary lesion and homing to and surviving in the new environment, and the term *metastasis* for the successful growth of a cancer cell to a clinically detectable, distant colony. Thereby, dissemination is necessary but not sufficient for lethal manifestation of metastasis, and metastatic growth can occur years after successful homing to a distant site, possibly triggered by intrinsic and extrinsic factors that were not present at the time of dissemination.
- The progression of a micrometastasis to a clinically manifest metastasis depends at least partially on its ability to induce a blood supply. As a consequence of the angiogenic switch, the dormant micrometastasis downregulates inhibitors of angiogenesis and starts to express angiogenic proteins.
- There is growing evidence that cellular senescence in aging tissues is associated with a secretory phenotype of the microenvironment that may stimulate neoplastic growth of epithelial cells.

Abstract

This chapter summarizes current concepts of dissemination (the processes of leaving the primary lesion and homing to and surviving in a new environment) and metastasis (the successful growth of a cancer cell to a clinically detectable, distant colony) and the role of microenvironmental as well as systemically acting factors in these processes. We review recent research on genotypes and phenotypes of early disseminated cancer cells and discuss the role of tumour dormancy, angiogenesis, and genetic background, aging and the immune system in metastasis.

6.1
Introduction

In most cancer literature metastasis is referred to as the 'major cause of cancer mortality', while the process of metastatic spread and the mechanisms involved are rarely addressed. In fact, very few research groups have been focusing on the genetics and epigenetics of disseminating cancer cells, the role of the microenvironment for homing, survival and colonization, and the selection pressures acting on tumour cells that are leaving the primary tumour (Fig. 6.1). In contrast, metastasis was and still is often viewed as the inevitable consequence of tumours that have become just too large to persist as a local disease. During recent years, this popular opinion has been challenged by new and interesting data. It is the goal of this chapter, to introduce the emerging concepts to scientifically interested physicians, as they might stimulate innovative translational research.

6.2
Metastatic Dissemination of Tumour Cells

6.2.1
Clinical Courses and Experimental Data from Primary Tumours and Metastases Do Not Enable a Coherent Understanding of Metastatic Progression

For at least one century, the prevailing view has considered metastasis as a late and final step in cancer progression. There are indeed good intuitive reasons for this opinion, such as that most cancer patients die from metastases and not from their primary disease or that early surgery is often the only chance to cure the patient. Also, supportive experimental data have been gathered, such as somatic genetic changes accumulating during local cancer progression—many of which can also be identified in metastases. The observed accumulation of genetic aberrations during local tumour growth (Fearon and Vogelstein 1990) was consequently extrapolated to systemic progression and, repeatedly, 'metastogenes' have been proposed, such as CD44v or PRL-3, thought to switch on a metastasiogenic program of invasion, dissemination, colonization and metastatic outgrowth (Saha et al. 2001; Zoller 1995). These data were consistent with another very influential observation. During transplantation experiments it was noted that only rare variant cells within the tumour will give rise to metastases (Fidler and Kripke 1977), so that a simple comparison between primary tumours and metastasis should enable the identification of those additional hits in the genome that transform a primary tumour cell into a metastatic cell. However, a recent study could not convincingly demonstrate the existence of metastasis-specific genes despite almost complete

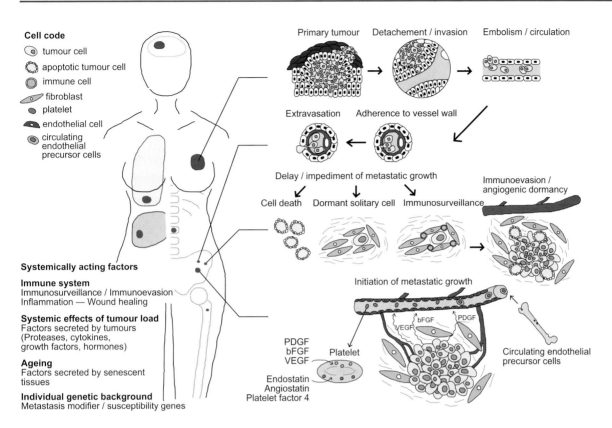

Cell code

- tumour cell
- apoptotic tumour cell
- immune cell
- fibroblast
- platelet
- endothelial cell
- circulating endothelial precursor cells

Systemically acting factors

Immune system
Immunosurveillance / Immunoevasion
Inflammation — Wound healing

Systemic effects of tumour load
Factors secreted by tumours
(Proteases, cytokines,
growth factors, hormones)

Ageing
Factors secreted by senescent
tissues

Individual genetic background
Metastasis modifier / susceptibility genes

Fig. 6.1. A holistic view of metastasis. *Left side* lists systemically acting factors that have been shown to influence the growth of metastases. *Right side* depicts the individual steps of metastatic spread. Tumour growth, invasion, intravasation and extravasation precede metastatic colonization at a distant site. Tumour cells may then undergo cell death or remain dormant for many years, either by the inability to leave the G_0 cell cycle state at all, by control of immune cells or, after collapse of the immunosurveillance, by an inability to induce angiogenesis. This dormancy period may be overcome when tumour cells accumulate advantageous genetic alterations that enable colonization. Tumours resuming metastatic growth have to induce angiogenesis in order to form a detectable metastasis via the secretion of cytokines. New endothelial cells do not all originate from neighbouring vessels. A few arrive as precursor bone-marrow-derived endothelial cells. Endothelial growth factors are not all delivered to the local endothelium directly from tumour cells. Some angiogenic regulatory proteins (both pro- and antiangiogenic) are scavenged by platelets, stored in alpha granules and seem to be released within the tumour vasculature. *PDGF* platelet-derived growth factor, *bFGF* basic fibroblast growth factor, *VEGF* vascular endothelial growth factor. (Figure modified from Aguirre-Ghiso 2007; Fidler 2003; Folkman 2007)

sequencing of the genomes of metastases and primary tumours (Jones et al. 2008).

It is not only the failure of large genome screens of advanced, highly aggressive tumours undertaken in the search for the 'metastogenes' that challenge the late-metastasis concept but also this view implies some fundamental inconsistencies. For example, it is well known by clinicians that metastases also develop in patients with small cancers or even in the absence of detectable primary tumours (so-called cancer of unknown primary, which ranks among the ten most frequent cancer diagnoses; Abbruzzese et al. 1994; van de Wouw et al. 2002). Furthermore, statistical evaluation of data from the Munich Tumour Registry comprising more than 12,000 breast cancer patients indicated that the process of metastasis might have already been initiated 5–7 years before clinical diagnosis of the primary tumour (Engel et al. 2003). Perhaps even better known is the successful prediction of the clinical outcome of a patient using gene expression profiling on microarrays. As the risk of metastatic disease within the first 5 years after surgery can be predicted with high accuracy from the gene expression profile of the primary tumour (Sotiriou and Piccart 2007), it was concluded that metastatic proclivity must be represented in the gene expression profile of the dominant cell clone. Thus, the metastatic potential cannot be acquired late in local progression in rare variant cells, but should be generated early (Bernards and Weinberg 2002).

6.2.2
Studying the Precursor Cells of Metastasis

It is relatively easy to generate lists of inconsistencies for every current model of metastasis, in particular as the concepts are now challenged by the cancer stem cell (CSC) hypothesis (Reya et al. 2001), which adds as a further complication a hierarchy of tumour cells, generated by non-genetic mechanisms, to the progression puzzle. The CSC hypothesis assumes that only rare subpopulations of tumour cells are driving the growth and spread of malignant cancers. These tumour cells are thought to be derived from organ-specific stem or progenitor cells and therefore are phenotypically and functionally defined. As the genetics of the CSCs in comparison to more differentiated and supposedly less relevant tumour cell populations have not yet been determined, concepts based on genetic data cannot yet be linked to this new paradigm. For all of these reasons, it is necessary to bridge the gap between primary tumours and metastases by analysing metastatic progenitor cells. To detect such cells from epithelial malignancies, various epithelial markers have been used in organs comprising only cells of mesenchymal origin, such as blood, bone marrow or lymph nodes. Cytokeratins are the most specific and currently also the most sensitive markers to detect single disseminated tumour cells (DTCs) in bone marrow, while the epithelial cell adhesion molecule (EpCAM; CD326) is favoured for the analysis of DTCs in lymph nodes, and for the detection of circulating tumour cells (CTC) in the blood stream several markers are in use (Pantel et al. 2008). When cell-based detection systems are used, DTCs can be isolated and analysed.

So far, mostly genetic data have been generated and current knowledge about the phenotype of DTCs is very circumstantial. There are three reasons for this:

1. Disseminated tumour cells are extremely rare. In patients without clinically manifest metastases, only 1–2 marker-positive cells are detected in bone marrow or histopathologically tumour-free lymph nodes per one million bone marrow or lymph node cells.
2. Initially, it was of the utmost importance to establish the malignant origin of the cytokeratin- or EpCAM-positive cells by genetic proof.
3. Phenotypic analysis of DTCs was restricted to double-staining approaches and therefore did not

enable comprehensive assessment of expressed genes. The genomic analysis confirmed the malignant origin of EpCAM- and cytokeratin-positive cells and provided conceptually very important insights.

6.2.3
Dissemination Can Be an Early Event in Malignant Cancers

A very puzzling observation in breast cancer patients without metastasis was the finding that DTCs from bone marrow generally display lower numbers of chromosomal aberrations than the matched primary tumours (Schardt et al. 2005; Schmidt-Kittler et al. 2003). This finding was in obvious conflict with the Fearon and Vogelstein model predicting: (1) genetic changes in addition to those in the primary tumour and (2) metastases as being derived from the most advanced and dominant clone of the primary tumour. The conflict with the second prediction arose from the fact that when patients receive curative surgery and cytokeratin-positive DTCs are detected in bone marrow the patients are at high risk for relapse (Braun et al. 2005). Thus, the survival data pointed to a high relevance of DTCs and made it difficult to dismiss the genetically less advanced cells as irrelevant. The failure to identify DTCs displaying the genetic changes of the dominant clone in the primary tumour indicated that either rare cells from the primary tumour disseminate or that the DTCs are derived from earlier stages of cancer development. The latter reasoning was supported by the observation that in some cases DTCs displayed completely normal karyotypes, although chromosomal aberrations emerge already in premalignant lesions. Even in these cells genetic analyses with higher resolution proved the malignant origin and uncovered in some cases clonal aberrations shared with the primary tumours (Schardt et al. 2005). The genetic data therefore indicated that dissemination of tumour cells begins very early after transformation, a hypothesis that could recently be confirmed in mouse models and ductal carcinoma in situ (DCIS) patients (Husemann et al. 2008).

6.2.4
Genetic Heterogeneity During Minimal Residual Disease

Patients without metastasis at diagnosis will eventually die from systemic cancer in 20–95% of cases, depending on the tumour type, although the primary tumours have been completely resected. This high rate of treatment failure has put adjuvant systemic therapies into the centre of clinical attention. However, while aiming at the prevention of lethal metastasis by early eradication of DTCs, these systemic therapies are administered generally in a blind way. In current clinical practice there is no effort to directly analyse the target cells of adjuvant therapies for selection of the therapeutic regimen. In contrast, it is assumed that the cells will somehow respond like the primary tumour cells (in drug response assays, using cultured primary tumour cells) or at least that molecular targets are identically expressed in DTCs as in primary tumours. The latter rationale underlies the *HER2* analysis of primary tumours to identify patients suitable for anti-*HER2*-based (e.g. trastuzumab) therapies (PICCART-GEBHART et al. 2005; ROMOND et al. 2005). However, only 50% of the patients with *HER2* amplification respond to adjuvant trastuzumab and the predictive power of primary tumour analysis is currently unclear. In fact, primary tumours as surrogate markers for therapy prediction are questionable for several reasons:

1. As stated above, primary tumours and DTCs diverge genetically, not only for the number of aberrations, but also for their specific nature. This has been shown for copy number changes (SCHMIDT-KITTLER et al. 2003; STOECKLEIN et al. 2008) and point mutations (KLEIN et al. 2002).

2. During minimal residual disease, DTCs of an individual patient are genetically very heterogeneous, at least in breast cancer (KLEIN et al. 2002).

3. Disseminated tumour cells diverge not only from the primary tumour but also when taken from different organs. A genetic comparison of DTCs from lymph nodes and from bone marrow in oesophageal cancer patients revealed selection of different genetic changes depending on the organ from which the cells were isolated (STOECKLEIN et al. 2008).

4. The same genetic defect (e.g. *HER2* amplification) had different prognostic impact when identified in primary tumours and DTCs. In DTCs of oesophageal cancer patients, amplification of *HER2* was a strong predictor of poor outcome, while no prognostic role in the primary tumours could be established. Moreover, the presence of *HER2* amplification in the primary tumours was not associated with its presence in DTCs (STOECKLEIN et al. 2008). From these data it can be concluded that primary tumours may often be poor surrogate markers for the genetics of DTCs and thereby for response to adjuvant therapies.

6.2.5
Clonal Expansion of Disseminated Tumour Cells Occurs Shortly Before Manifestation of Metastasis

All these findings suggest that dissemination of tumour cells often occurs early after transformation, that the DTCs evolve largely independently from the primary tumour, and that they accumulate genetic alterations until they eventually grow out. In this context, it is interesting that metastases display similar percentages of specific copy number changes as primary tumours. Although some genetic alterations are more frequently found in metastases than in primary tumours, no copy number changes have been found so far specific for metastasis in any type of cancer. On the other hand, each type of cancer is characterized by a typical set of karyotypic abnormalities (HEIM and MITELMAN 1995) and consequently one would expect that metastases display similar chromosomal aberrations as primary tumours, although in paired analyses of primary lesions and metastases, genetic differences are often striking (KUUKASJARVI et al. 1997; WALCH et al. 2000). Thus, to date it has not been finally clarified whether chromosomal aberrations shared between primary tumours and metastases indicate convergent evolution or true clonal descent. Interestingly, when bone marrow samples of patients with metastatic disease (e.g. breast cancer; KLEIN et al. 2002) or in the stage of minimal residual disease of very aggressive cancers (e.g. oesophageal cancer; STOECKLEIN et al. 2008) are analysed, several individually isolated DTCs display very similar chromosomal aberrations, suggesting that shortly before manifestation of metastasis clonal expansion of aggressive DTCs is taking place and eventually killing the patient.

6.3
Mechanisms of Metastasis

The findings that tumour cell dissemination is an early step in systemic cancer progression and thus often takes place years before clinical manifestation of metastases and that DTCs may need additional genetic hits for further progression indicate that dissemination and metastasis must be differentiated. We suggest using the term *dissemination* for the processes of leaving the primary lesion and homing to and surviving in the new environment, and the term *metastasis* for the successful growth of a cancer cell to a clinically detectable, distant colony. Thereby, dissemination is necessary but not sufficient for lethal manifestation of metastasis, and metastatic growth can occur years after successful homing to a distant site, possibly triggered by intrinsic and extrinsic factors that were not present at the time of dissemination. We will therefore summarize some insights into mechanisms involved at early and late stages of metastatic progression.

6.3.1
Homing and Survival of Tumour Cells at Ectopic Sites

6.3.1.1
Paget's "Seed-and-Soil" and Ewing's "Hemodynamic" Paradigm

One of the earliest observations made by scientists, who were studying metastatic progression in the eighteenth and nineteenth centuries, was the non-random pattern of target organ involvement (Table 6.1). Different primary cancers showed a more or less organ-specific pattern of metastasis. From these early discoveries eventually two concepts emerged that are still debated today: Stephen Paget's 'seed-and-soil' hypothesis and James Ewing's 'hemodynamic' hypothesis (FIDLER 2003; RIBATTI et al. 2006; WEISS 2000).

In 1889, Paget published his landmark paper where he proposed the 'seed-and-soil' hypothesis (PAGET 1889). Paget examined hundreds of autopsy records of women with breast cancer. His analysis revealed a non-random pattern of metastasis in visceral organs and

Table 6.1. Preferential sites of metastasis for different types of carcinoma (NGUYEN and MASSAGUE 2007)

Tumour type	Preferred metastatic sites
Breast (ER+)	Bone
Breast (ER−)	Visceral organs
Lung (SCLC)	Different organs
Lung (NSCLC)	Contralateral lung, brain, liver, bones, adrenals
Prostate	Bone
Pancreas	Liver
Colon	Liver, lungs, peritoneal cavity
Ovarian	Peritoneal cavity

ER oestrogen receptor, *SCLC* small cell lung carcinoma, *NSCLC* non-small cell lung carcinoma

bones. Neither random scattering throughout the body nor dispersal through the general circulation sufficiently explained the observed frequencies of metastatic growth at the various sites. He therefore proposed that certain tumour cells (which he termed the 'seed') had specific affinity for the environment of certain organs (which he termed the 'soil'). He concluded that metastases formed only when the seed finds compatible soil.

Thirty years later, James Ewing challenged Paget's 'seed-and-soil' hypothesis, and proposed that the non-random patterns of metastasis are the consequence of the anatomy of the vascular system (EWING 1928). In his concept, cancer cells growing at a primary site will enter the draining circulatory vessels and will subsequently be arrested with much higher chance in those secondary organs that are perfused by these blood or lymph vessels. Interestingly, both Paget and Ewing addressed the alternative explanation. While Paget was critical about the 'hemodynamic' hypothesis, dismissing that 'remote organs … are equally ready to receive and nourish any particle of the primary growth', Ewing stated that 'the predilection of metastases for particular organs may be due to special nutritional requirements dependent on the varying cell metabolism', and thereby acknowledged specific microenvironmental needs of different types of tumours (WEISS 2000).

The fact that two distinct but not mutually exclusive (see below) hypotheses were proposed based on the non-random distribution of metastases suggests that there are supporting and non-supporting findings for each hypothesis (WEISS 2000). For example, many autopsy studies concur with the observation that the number of metastases is often in proportion to the blood flow from the primary site to the secondary organ. However, one cannot neglect the cases where either more or fewer metastases are detected at a distant site than suggested by blood flow alone, indicating that determinants of the microenvironment are relevant (WEISS 1992). Certain tissues, such as brain, bone or adrenals, are served by a very small fraction of the circulatory system, but they are frequent sites of metastasis for certain cancers. Other organs, such as muscle, skin or kidneys, receive a considerable supply of blood while being only sporadically colonized by cancers (RIBATTI et al. 2006). However, the strong tendency of colon cancer cells to metastasize to liver may be the consequence of the fact that cancer cells enter the portal vein, which drains the lower gastrointestinal tract and perfuses the liver. Even if circulating colon cancer cells colonize the liver with low efficiency only, the high number of cancer cells trapped in the capillary beds of the liver may ensure over time that some of them will start to grow into metastases (WEINBERG 2007). Additional challenges for the 'hemodynamic' concept of Ewing included some cases of lymphatic metastasis that needed to be explained by 'retrograde lymphatic embolism', a reversal of lymphatic flow, due to obstruction of lymphatic vessels. Likewise, circulating cancer cells are often not trapped in capillaries of the first encountered organ, but appeared elsewhere. Here, the existence of arterial–venous shunts, large-bore direct connections between two parts of the circulatory system, was used as an explanation. Finally, it was recognized that it is not easy to discriminate whether the delivery of cells into the target organ occurred through veins or arteries.

On the other hand, the 'seed-and-soil' hypothesis is in need of an adequate explanation as to why contralateral metastases in paired organs, e.g. in breast or kidney cancer, are unusually rare. One would expect that the best suited 'soil' for metastasizing breast or renal carcinoma cells is the contralateral mammary or renal tissue, respectively. Thus, to rescue the 'seed-and–soil' concept in the absence of contralateral metastases one has to postulate that the normal organ does not provide an optimal soil for cancer cells. Consequently, it has been suggested that the microenvironment of cancer cells at the primary lesion is different from that of the originating tissue and that the tumour cells that grow in this changed microenvironment develop the phenotype, which enables them to survive (Weinberg 2007). Moreover, migratory, 'metastatic' cancer cells may be unsuited to survive in the healthy environment of their tissue of orgin, in addition to not being suited to survive in the changed environment of the primary site.

While the rate of perfusion of an organ was relatively easy to assess and thereby Ewing's hypothesis perfectly testable, seed and soil factors have remained unknown for a long time. Recently, chemotactic factors secreted by target organs, molecules mediating adhesion between cancer cells and target-organ cells, and cellular interactions between cancer cells and endothelial cells in target organs were identified as critical determinants (Muller et al. 2001; Weinberg 2007). It has also been shown that endothelial cells in different tissues express tissue-specific molecules on their luminal surfaces, which may interact with binding partners at the surface of circulating tumour cells (Pasqualini and Ruoslahti 1996). Interestingly, cancer cells seem to favour inflammatory sites and it is very possible that sites of chronic inflammation within the body are hospitable sites for metastatic cells (Weinberg 2007).

The availability of large-scale gene expression profiling has enabled further molecular insights into site-specific metastasis. Repeated rounds of tumour cell injection into mice and subsequent isolation of metastases from bone and lung selected patterns of expressed genes that supported site predilection in this model. Tumour cells expressing the 'lung-colonizing' signature did not home to the bone, and vice versa (Kang et al. 2003; Minn et al. 2005). Genes upregulated in bone-colonizing cells included interleukin-11, chemokine receptor CXCR4, connective tissue-derived growth factor and matrix metalloproteinase/MMP1 (collagenase 1), while the, and lung-colonizing cells characteristically expressed epidermal-growth-factor family member epiregulin, the chemokine GRO1/CXCL1, the matrix metalloproteinases MMP1 (collagenase 1) and MMP2 (gelatinase A), the cell adhesion molecule SPARC, the interleukin-13 decoy receptor IL13Rα2 and the cell adhesion receptor VCAM1. While the signatures can also be detected in some primary tumours, it is currently unclear whether they are indeed functionally relevant during the homing or outgrowth of DTCs of breast cancer patients. It will be interesting to see whether DTCs from bone marrow express the identified bone signature genes.

In summary, both Paget and Ewing identified fundamental principles that govern the probability of metastasis at a distant site, which depends on the frequency with which circulating cancer cells are mechanically arrested in an organ as well as the ease with which they are able to colonize it (Weinberg 2007).

6.3.2
Tumour Dormancy

A major difference between mouse models of metastasis and the clinical course of patients is the speed at which metastasis manifests. In xenotransplantation experiments, only a few days to weeks span the time between tumour cell injection and metastasis; in transgenic animals this period may be extended to months. In patients, tumour cell dissemination may often occur early after transformation of the primary lesion and therefore the time from homing to a distant site to manifestation of metastasis may, in most cases, be measured in years. Traditionally, a latency period after curative removal of the primary growth until clinical detection of metastasis that lasts longer than 5–6 years is termed tumour dormancy (Hadfield 1954; Willis 1952). Therefore, even if the metastasis-founder cell disseminates the day before surgical removal of the primary tumour, it is clear that human tumour cells usually do not initiate metastatic growth immediately after arrival but rest there for various periods of time. Our knowledge of the mechanisms regulating this dark stage of cancer progression is currently very limited but a better understanding may pave ways for innovative therapeutic approaches.

Until recently, the fact that single DTCs and micro-metastases are difficult to detect and are extremely rare has hampered the study of dormancy. Therefore, current thinking is derived from experimental models and extrapolation of clinical observations. Once disseminating tumour cells arrive at the distant site they may experience one of three fates: they may die, they may remain viable but quiescent or they may proliferate to form micrometastases (Fig. 6.1). The progression of a micrometastasis to a clinically manifest metastasis depends at least partially on its ability to induce a blood supply. So, the net result of dormancy on a clinical level derives from the inability to start proliferation at a rate that exceeds apoptosis or from the failure to induce angiogenesis (HOLMGREN et al. 1995). Immune reactions have been proposed to control the outgrowth of DTCs. However, experimental evidence for tumour surveillance regulating the latency period of systemic cancer is sparse (AGUIRRE-GHISO 2007), although it was shown that patients with DTCs in their bone marrow had more memory CD4 T cells and more CD56(+) CD8 T cells than patients with tumour cell-negative bone marrow (FEUERER et al. 2001).

One explanation for prolonged latency periods after homing to a distant site may be provided by the genetics of DTCs. As mentioned before, tumour cells do not disseminate in a state of full malignancy but have to acquire additional genetic hits (KLEIN and HOLZEL 2006). The time needed to acquire such genetic hits may be relatively long as the majority of DTCs does not seem to be in the cell cycle (PANTEL et al. 1993). Microenvironmental factors are likely to influence the progression of DTCs. Upon lodging in a non-orthotopic distant site DTCs must interpret the new environment, but very little is known about these first cellular interactions and it can only be speculated whether DTCs home to specific niches. However, there is first experimental evidence that primary tumours secrete factors [such as vascular endothelial growth factor (VEGF) or placental growth factor (PlGF)] that mobilize hematopoietic progenitor cells to various metastatic sites. These hematopoietic progenitor cells express VEGF receptor 1, preferentially localize to areas of increased fibronectin (synthesized by resident fibroblasts) and alter the local microenvironment, which leads to the activation of integrins and chemokines, such as SDF-1, which eventually promote attachment, survival and growth of circulating tumour cells (KAPLAN et al. 2005). Such premetastatic niches are thought to promote tumour progression. However, it has also been suggested that the microenvironment forces DTCs into a more differentiated state (AGUIRRE-GHISO 2007) and thereby induces dormancy.

6.3.3
Tumour Growth at Ectopic Sites

6.3.3.1
The Need for Angiogenesis

Angiogenesis is a prerequisite for the progression of a metastatic colony to a manifest metastasis. As the metastasis exceeds a certain size, the supply of nutrients and oxygen is hampered, and the end products of metabolism cannot diffuse out of colony easily. It is well-accepted that a primary tumour or metastasis can grow to a size of approximately 1 mm^3 and obtain sufficient supply of oxygen and nutrients by diffusion. Tumour growth beyond this size demands vascularization by means of angiogenesis (BOHLE and KALTHOFF 1999). The development of a vascular supply is a critical step that has been termed the 'angiogenic switch' (HANAHAN and FOLKMAN 1996). As a consequence of the angiogenic switch, the dormant micrometastasis downregulates inhibitors of angiogenesis (such as thrombospondin I) and starts to express angiogenic proteins [e.g. basic fibroblast growth factor (bFGF) and VEGF] (NAUMOV et al. 2006).

In order to create capillary sprouts, endothelial cells must proliferate, migrate and penetrate stroma, usually attracted by factors secreted by the growing micrometastasis (BOHLE and KALTHOFF 1999). In some cases, endothelial progenitor cells are recruited from bone marrow (NAUMOV et al. 2006) and the newly formed capillaries differ in cellular composition, permeability, stability, and regulation of growth from normal blood vessels (BOHLE and KALTHOFF 1999; SCHULZ 2005). The induction of angiogenesis is mediated by promoting and inhibiting molecules secreted by both tumour and cells from the microenvironment (Fig. 6.1). The balance of these secreted factors will determine whether angiogenesis will occur. During expansion of the tumour mass, some cells will lose oxygen supply and become hypoxic. Hypoxia will lead to an increase of hypoxia inducible factor (HIF) that will upregulate synthesis of proangiogenic proteins (NAUMOV et al. 2006). The switch of the tumour cell into the angiogenic phenotype leads to overexpression of angiogenic promoters that will enable recruitment of extracellular matrix and endothelial and other cells needed for angiogenesis. The most potent proangiogenic factor is VEGF, which is upregulated in the majority of human cancers and is a negative predictor of patients' prognosis (BOHLE and KALTHOFF 1999). Other proangiogenic factors are platelet-derived growth factor (PDGF), bFGF and nitric oxide synthase (NOS) (BOHLE and KALTHOFF 1999; NAUMOV et al. 2006). The often observed peritumoral inflammatory reaction also promotes angiogenesis through cytokines secreted by leukocytes (BOHLE and KALTHOFF 1999).

Since angiogenesis is important for the transition of an indolent to a malignant systemic disease, it is an attractive target for anticancer therapy. Therefore, a number of angiogenesis inhibitors and antibodies have been developed and are either introduced in clinical practice or are undergoing clinical trials. Examples include bevacizumab, an antibody that neutralizes VEGF and was approved by the FDA for treatment of colorectal cancer, or endostatin, a broad-spectrum angiogenesis inhibitor targeting several positive and negative regulators of angiogenesis (ABDOLLAHI et al. 2004). Currently more than 40 new drugs whose central mode of action is thought to be inhibition of angiogenesis are in clinical testing (FOLKMAN 2007) and we will soon know how effective and how robust this therapeutic approach will be.

6.4
Systemically Acting Factors: Genetic Background, Aging and the Immune System

Perhaps the major lesson that has been learned during recent years is that metastasis is not a consequence of seeding of fully autonomous cells. There is rarely such thing as a fully malignant cell ready to start growing independently at the distant site upon arrival. The ability of a tumour to form a metastasis is influenced by many interacting factors and is not only a function of somatic events in the tumour cells, but also of the constitutional genetic differences between individuals, affecting the gene expression of tumour cells in transit and at secondary sites. Thus, our view on metastasis must become more holistic and not surprisingly there are already data showing that metastasis is influenced by systemically acting factors (Fig. 6.1).

6.4.1
Metastasis and Genetic Background

Paget proposed from early on that metastasis is the result of characteristics of the seed *and* the soil. Clearly, the genetic background of each patient comprises information on tumour cell-intrinsic and microenvironmental factors influencing the manifestation of metastasis. Therefore, it is not surprising that there is a rapidly growing literature linking germ line polymorphisms to the emergence of metastasis. In a landmark experiment, it was shown that the same aggressive oncogene (polyoma middle T-antigen under control of a mammary specific promoter) in different mouse strains results in different rates of tumour growth and metastasis-free survival of the animals (LIFSTED et al. 1998). Moreover, a frequently used metastasis predictive gene signature (RAMASWAMY et al. 2003) is differentially expressed between *normal* mammary tissue of mice with metastasis-prone and metastasis-reduced genetic background (YANG et al. 2005), indicating that many if not all of the prognostic gene expression signatures may reflect more the response of a genetic background to malignant transformation than the consequence of specific somatic mutations. In humans, genetic polymorphisms and haplotypes are increasingly found to be associated with a propensity to systemic progression that potentially influence various metastatic mechanisms such as invasion (SUN et al. 2006), angiogenesis and stress response (MENENDEZ et al. 2006), and the interaction with the microenvironment (CRAWFORD et al. 2008). Whether systematic searches for metastasis susceptibility genes will have an impact on cancer screening and preventive measures has to be awaited.

6.4.2
Metastasis, Immune System and Ageing

Individual differences in the ability of the immune system to protect against or promote cancerous transformation or metastasis could likewise be a genetic trait. Currently, little is known about the role of the immune system in protecting specifically against systemic cancer spread (see above). However, for colorectal cancer, it was recently shown that the immune reaction at the tumour site determined clinical outcome regardless of the local extent and spread of the tumour. A weak adaptive immune reaction correlated with a very poor prognosis even in patients with minimal tumour invasion. Conversely, a high density of adaptive immune cells correlated with a highly favourable prognosis whatever the local extent of the tumour and the invasion of regional lymph nodes (GALON et al. 2006). As the study included a high number of patients representing a large fraction of the genetic heterogeneity of colorectal cancers, it is unlikely that the protective action of the immune system was limited to a subset of patients with specific oncogenic mutations. Rather, as in colorectal cancer no molecular marker has ever been shown to outperform the TNM staging system in a similar way, the data apparently demonstrate the amazing capability of the individual immune response of some patients to keep genetically instable tumours in check. Despite the phenomenon of immunoediting, i.e. selection of tumour cells with reduced immunogenicity (DUNN et al. 2002), the beneficial effect of the adaptive immunity appeared to persist throughout tumour progression from stage I disease to stage III disease. The data provide an interesting example of the coevolution of cancer and protective defence mechanisms, both being strongly determined by the individual's genetic constitution.

Finally, while this chapter cannot address external influences, such as carcinogens, cancer-promoting agents, infections, irradiation and systemic cytotoxic therapies, on carcinogenesis and specifically on metastasis, it should not end without mentioning one additional systemically acting factor that is likely to be the subject of scientific scrutiny in the coming years: ageing. While cancer incidence increases with age, it has also been noted that growth rates of breast cancers are often slower in older patients. This seems to be associated with a significant reduction of axillary lymph node metastases, vascular invasion and lymphoplasmacytic stromal reaction with increasing age (FISHER et al. 1997). In a comparison of metastatic efficiency of B16 melanoma cells injected into young, old and parabiotic (i.e. surgically unified old and young) mice, it was possible to directly measure the effect of age on the outgrowth of lung metastases. In unpaired mice, the number of metastatic colonies in the lungs was ten times higher in young than in old mice. However, in parabiotic mice, the number of metastases in young mice was almost comparable with that of unpaired young mice, while the number of metastases in old mice approached the level of young mice. Although the number remained stable in young parabiotic mice, their size was reduced. In old parabiotic mice, almost exclusively small colonies were observed as in unpaired old mice. The authors concluded that in these experiments the implantation of early metastatic colonies in the lung depends on systemic humoral factors while their growth is mainly dependent on local factors in the microenvironment and that both effects are modulated by age (HIRAYAMA et al. 1993). As there is growing evidence that cellular senescence in aging tissues is associated with a secretory phenotype of the microenvironment that may stimulate neoplastic growth of epithelial cells (CAMPISI 2005), upcoming studies have to unravel the molecular changes of the aging host and their influence on the manifestation of metastatic disease in patients.

References

Abbruzzese JL, Abbruzzese MC, Hess KR, Raber MN, Lenzi R, Frost P (1994) Unknown primary carcinoma: natural history and prognostic factors in 657 consecutive patients. J Clin Oncol 12:1272–1280

Abdollahi A, Hahnfeldt P, Maercker C, Grone HJ, Debus J, Ansorge W, Folkman J, Hlatky L, Huber PE (2004) Endostatin's antiangiogenic signaling network. Mol Cell 13:649–663

Aguirre-Ghiso JA (2007) Models, mechanisms and clinical evidence for cancer dormancy. Nat Rev Cancer 7:834–846

Bernards R, Weinberg RA (2002) A progression puzzle. Nature 418:823

Bohle AS, Kalthoff H (1999) Molecular mechanisms of tumor metastasis and angiogenesis. Langenbecks Arch Surg 384:133–140

Braun S, Vogl FD, Naume B, Janni W, Osborne MP, Coombes RC, Schlimok G, Diel IJ, Gerber B, Gebauer G, et al (2005) A pooled analysis of bone marrow micrometastasis in breast cancer. N Engl J Med 353:793–802

Campisi J (2005) Senescent cells, tumor suppression, and organismal aging: good citizens, bad neighbors. Cell 120:513–522

Crawford NP, Alsarraj J, Lukes L, Walker RC, Officewala JS, Yang HH, Lee MP, Ozato K, Hunter KW (2008) Bromodomain 4 activation predicts breast cancer survival. Proc Natl Acad Sci U S A 105:6380–6385

Dunn GP, Bruce AT, Ikeda H, Old LJ, Schreiber RD (2002) Cancer immunoediting: from immunosurveillance to tumor escape. Nat Immunol 3:991–998

Engel J, Eckel R, Kerr J, Schmidt M, Furstenberger G, Richter R, Sauer H, Senn HJ, Holzel D (2003) The process of metastasisation for breast cancer. Eur J Cancer 39:1794–1806

Ewing J (1928) Neoplastic diseases, 6th edn. Saunders, Philadelphia

Fearon ER, Vogelstein B (1990) A genetic model for colorectal tumorigenesis. Cell 61:759–767

Feuerer M, Rocha M, Bai L, Umansky V, Solomayer EF, Bastert G, Diel IJ, Schirrmacher V (2001) Enrichment of memory T cells and other profound immunological changes in the bone marrow from untreated breast cancer patients. Int J Cancer 92:96–105

Fidler IJ (2003) The pathogenesis of cancer metastasis: the 'seed and soil' hypothesis revisited. Nat Rev Cancer 3:453–458

Fidler IJ, Kripke ML (1977) Metastasis results from preexisting variant cells within a malignant tumor. Science 197:893–895

Fisher CJ, Egan MK, Smith P, Wicks K, Millis RR, Fentiman IS (1997) Histopathology of breast cancer in relation to age. Br J Cancer 75:593–596

Folkman J (2007) Angiogenesis: an organizing principle for drug discovery? Nat Rev Drug Discov 6:273–286

Galon J, Costes A, Sanchez-Cabo F, Kirilovsky A, Mlecnik B, Lagorce-Pages C, Tosolini M, Camus M, Berger A, Wind P, et al (2006) Type, density, and location of immune cells within human colorectal tumors predict clinical outcome. Science 313:1960–1964

Hadfield G (1954) The dormant cancer cell. BMJ 4888:607–610

Hanahan D, Folkman J (1996) Patterns and emerging mechanisms of the angiogenic switch during tumorigenesis. Cell 86:353–364

Heim S, Mitelman F (1995) Cancer cytogenetics, 2nd edn. Wiley-Liss, New York

Hirayama R, Takemura K, Nihei Z, Ichikawa W Takagi Y, Mishima Y, Utsuyama M, Hirokawa K (1993) Differential effect of host microenvironment and systemic humoral factors on the implantation and the growth rate of metastatic tumor in parabiotic mice constructed between young and old mice. Mech Ageing Dev 71:213–221

Holmgren L, O'Reilly MS, Folkman J (1995) Dormancy of micrometastases: balanced proliferation and apoptosis in the presence of angiogenesis suppression. Nat Med 1:149–153

Husemann Y, Geigl JB, Schubert F, Musiani P, Meyer M, Burghart E, Forni G, Eils R, Fehm T, Riethmuller G, et al (2008) Systemic spread is an early step in breast cancer. Cancer Cell 13:58–68

Jones S, Chen WD, Parmigiani G, Diehl F, Beerenwinkel N, Antal T, Traulsen A, Nowak MA, Siegel C, Velculescu VE, et al (2008) Comparative lesion sequencing provides insights into tumor evolution. Proc Natl Acad Sci U S A 105:4283–4288

Kang Y, Siegel PM, Shu W, Drobnjak M, Kakonen SM, Cordon-Cardo C, Guise TA, Massague J (2003) A multigenic program mediating breast cancer metastasis to bone. Cancer Cell 3:537–549

Kaplan RN, Riba RD, Zacharoulis S, Bramley AH, Vincent L, Costa C, MacDonald DD, Jin DK, Shido K, Kerns SA, et al (2005) VEGFR1-positive haematopoietic bone marrow progenitors initiate the pre-metastatic niche. Nature 438:820–827

Klein CA, Holzel D (2006) Systemic cancer progression and tumor dormancy: mathematical models meet single cell genomics. Cell Cycle 5:1788–1798

Klein CA, Blankenstein TJ, Schmidt-Kittler O, Petronio M, Polzer B, Stoecklein NH, Riethmuller G (2002) Genetic heterogeneity of single disseminated tumour cells in minimal residual cancer. Lancet 360:683–689

Kuukasjarvi T, Karhu R, Tanner M, Kahkonen M, Schaffer A, Nupponen N, Pennanen S, Kallioniemi A, Kallioniemi OP, Isola J (1997) Genetic heterogeneity and clonal evolution underlying development of asynchronous metastasis in human breast cancer. Cancer Res 57:1597–1604

Lifsted T, Le Voyer T, Williams M, Muller W, Klein-Szanto A, Buetow KH, Hunter KW (1998) Identification of inbred mouse strains harboring genetic modifiers of mammary tumor age of onset and metastatic progression. Int J Cancer 77:640–644

Menendez D, Krysiak O, Inga A, Krysiak B, Resnick MA, Schonfelder G (2006) A SNP in the flt-1 promoter integrates the VEGF system into the p53 transcriptional network. Proc Natl Acad Sci U S A 103:1406–1411

Minn AJ, Gupta GP, Siegel PM, Bos PD, Shu W, Giri DD, Viale A, Olshen AB, Gerald WL, Massague J (2005) Genes that mediate breast cancer metastasis to lung. Nature 436:518–524

Muller A, Homey B, Soto H, Ge N, Catron D, Buchanan ME, McClanahan T, Murphy E, Yuan W, Wagner SN, et al (2001) Involvement of chemokine receptors in breast cancer metastasis. Nature 410:50–56

Naumov GN, Akslen LA, Folkman J (2006) Role of angiogenesis in human tumor dormancy: animal models of the angiogenic switch. Cell Cycle 5:1779–1787

Nguyen DX, Massague J (2007) Genetic determinants of cancer metastasis. Nat Rev Genet 8:341–352

Paget S (1889) The distribution of secondary growths in cancer of the breast. Lancet 1:571–573

Pantel K, Braun S, Kutter D, Lindemann F, Schaller G, Funke I, Izbicki JR, Riethmüller G (1993) Differential expression of proliferation-associated molecules in individual micrometastatic carcinoma cells. J Natl Cancer Inst 85:1419–1424

Pantel K, Brakenhoff RH, Brandt B (2008) Detection, clinical relevance and specific biological properties of disseminating tumour cells. Nat Rev Cancer 8:329–340

Pasqualini R, Ruoslahti E (1996) Organ targeting in vivo using phage display peptide libraries. Nature 380:364–366

Piccart-Gebhart MJ, Procter M, Leyland-Jones B, Goldhirsch A, Untch M, Smith I, Gianni L, Baselga J, Bell R, Jackisch C, et al (2005) Trastuzumab after adjuvant chemotherapy in HER2-positive breast cancer. N Engl J Med 353:1659–1672

Ramaswamy S, Ross KN, Lander ES, Golub TR (2003) A molecular signature of metastasis in primary solid tumors. Nat Genet 33:49–54

Reya T, Morrison SJ, Clarke MF, Weissman IL (2001) Stem cells, cancer, and cancer stem cells. Nature 414:105–111

Ribatti D, Mangialardi G, Vacca A (2006) Stephen Paget and the 'seed and soil' theory of metastatic dissemination. Clin Exp Med 6:145–149

Romond EH, Perez EA, Bryant J, Suman VJ, Geyer CE Jr, Davidson NE, Tan-Chiu E, Martino S, Paik S, Kaufman PA, et al (2005) Trastuzumab plus adjuvant chemotherapy for operable HER2-positive breast cancer. N Engl J Med 353:1673–1684

Saha S, Bardelli A, Buckhaults P, Velculescu VE, Rago C, St Croix B, Romans KE, Choti MA, Lengauer C, Kinzler KW, et al (2001) A phosphatase associated with metastasis of colorectal cancer. Science 294:1343–1346

Schardt JA, Meyer M, Hartmann CH, Schubert F, Schmidt-Kittler O, Fuhrmann C, Polzer B, Petronio M, Eils R, Klein CA (2005) Genomic analysis of single cytokeratin-positive cells from bone marrow reveals early mutational events in breast cancer. Cancer Cell 8:227–239

Schmidt-Kittler O, Ragg T, Daskalakis A, Granzow M, Ahr A, Blankenstein TJ, Kaufmann M, Diebold J, Arnholdt H, Muller P, et al (2003) From latent disseminated cells to overt metastasis: genetic analysis of systemic breast cancer progression. Proc Natl Acad Sci U S A 100:7737–7742

Schulz W (2005) Molecular biology of human cancers. Springer, Netherlands

Sotiriou C, Piccart MJ (2007) Taking gene-expression profiling to the clinic: when will molecular signatures become relevant to patient care? Nat Rev Cancer 7:545–553

Stoecklein NH, Hosch SB, Bezler M, Stern F, Hartmann CH, Vay C, Siegmund A, Scheunemann P, Schurr P, Knoefel WT, et al (2008) Direct genetic analysis of single disseminated cancer cells for prediction of outcome and therapy selection in esophageal cancer. Cancer Cell 13:441–453

Sun T, Gao Y, Tan W, Ma S, Zhang X, Wang Y, Zhang Q, Guo Y, Zhao D, Zeng C, et al (2006) Haplotypes in matrix metalloproteinase gene cluster on chromosome 11q22 contribute to the risk of lung cancer development and progression. Clin Cancer Res 12:7009–7017

van de Wouw AJ, Janssen-Heijnen ML, Coebergh JW, Hillen HF (2002) Epidemiology of unknown primary tumours: incidence and population-based survival of 1285 patients in Southeast Netherlands, 1984–1992. Eur J Cancer 38:409–413

Walch AK, Zitzelsberger HF, Bink K, Hutzler P, Bruch J, Braselmann H, Aubele MM, Mueller J, Stein H, Siewert JR, et al (2000) Molecular genetic changes in metastatic primary Barrett's adenocarcinoma and related lymph node metastases: comparison with nonmetastatic Barrett's adenocarcinoma. Mod Pathol 13:814–824

Weinberg RA (2007) The biology of cancer, Garland Science, New York

Weiss L (1992) Comments on hematogenous metastatic patterns in humans as revealed by autopsy. Clin Exp Metastasis 10:191–199

Weiss L (2000) Metastasis of cancer: a conceptual history from antiquity to the 1990s. Cancer Metastasis Rev 19:I–XI, 193–383

Willis RA (1952) The spread of tumours in the human body. Butterworth, London

Yang H, Crawford N, Lukes L, Finney R, Lancaster M, Hunter KW (2005) Metastasis predictive signature profiles pre-exist in normal tissues. Clin Exp Metastasis 22:593–603

Zoller M (1995) CD44: physiological expression of distinct isoforms as evidence for organ-specific metastasis formation. J Mol Med 73:425–438

Role of the Immune System in Cancer Development and Therapeutic Implications

7

Gabriele Multhoff and Sabrina T. Astner

CONTENTS

G. Multhoff, PhD
Klinik und Poliklinik für Strahlentherapie und Radiologische Onkologie, Klinikum rechts der Isar der TU München, Ismaninger Straße 22, 81675 München, Germany

S. T. Astner, MD
Klinikum rechts der Isar der TU München, Klinik und Poliklinik für Strahlentherapie und Radiologische Onkologie und Helmholtz Zentrum München, Deutsches Forschungszentrum für Gesundheit und Umwelt (GmbH), Ismaningerstraße 22, 81675 München, Germany

KEY POINTS

- The humoral as well as the cellular immune system play important roles in the control of cancer.
- Therapeutic efficacy of immunological approaches is limited by a restricted availability of tumor-specific antigens. Presently cancer/testis (CT), activation markers, differentiation, amplification, mutational antigens, and danger signals serve as tumor-associated target structures.
- The efficacy of cytokine therapies and cell-based approaches (T cells, dendritic cells, natural killer [NK] cells) is presently tested in preclinical and in clinical trials.
- Presently, several monoclonal antibodies have been approved by the US Food and Drug Administration (FDA) for the treatment of cancer. The target structures of these antibodies include CD20 for non-Hodgkin's lymphoma (NHL) and B-NHL; CD33 for CD33 positive acute myeloid leukemia, epithelial cell-adhesion molecule (EpCam) (expired 2000), vascular endothelial growth factor (VEGF) and epidermal growth factor receptor (EGFR) for colorectal cancer, ErbB2 (human epidermal growth factor receptor 2 [HER2]) for breast cancer, and CD52 for B-cell chronic lymphocytic leukemia (B-CLL). Numerous other antibodies are currently being tested in clinical trials.

Abstract

This chapter elucidates immunological aspects in cancer therapy. For many years, the impact of the immune system in cancer immunity was a matter of debate. Nowadays, it is generally accepted that an active immune system can monitor, edit, and destroy malignantly transformed cells in vitro and in established tumor mouse models. However, the capacity of the immune system to fight human tumors is limited, as human tumors are highly individual, complex, and dynamic systems that have the capacity to modulate anticancer immune responses and to affect the tumor microenvironment. Here, we describe the development of innovative immunological strategies from a preclinical stage to clinical application. In the last decade, especially humanized monoclonal antibodies (mAb) have emerged as promising pharmaceutical tools ("magic bullet") for the treatment of cancer in combination with radio- and/or chemotherapy.

7.1
Introduction

Immune homeostasis is a fine balance between the induction of immune responses that defend against foreign pathogens and the suppression of immune responses for the maintenance of self-tolerance to prevent autoimmune diseases. Since tumor cells develop from the host's own tissue they might be considered as being "self" by the immune system, and this makes the generation of an efficient immune defense against cancer difficult. However, Rudolf Virchow (1863) succeeded in detecting infiltrating leukocytes in tumor tissues (overview in Mantovani et al. 1992). A few years later, William Coley (1890) associated the presence of fatal bacterial infections with the induction of antitumor immune responses in patients with partially resected tumors (Coley 1893). Based on these earlier findings, Paul Ehrlich postulated the "virulent capacity of tumors" in 1909.

The substantial progress that has been made in the treatment of cancer using radio- and chemotherapy led to reduced attention about the involvement of the immune system in the control of cancer for several decades. However, with an increase in the understanding of the molecular mechanisms of immune recognition and regulation came accumulating evidence that the immune system plays a crucial role in the control of cancer. Nowadays, it is generally accepted that an active immune system can monitor, edit, and destroy ma-

lignantly transformed cells in vitro and in established tumor mouse models (Smyth et al. 2001; Dunn et al. 2002). However, the capacity of the immune system to fight against cancer in humans is limited, as human tumors are highly individual, complex, and dynamic systems, which have the capacity to modulate anticancer immune responses and to affect the tumor microenvironment.

Nevertheless, correlative relationships between altered immune function, tumor development, and antitumor immune responses (Dunn et al. 2002, 2004) have been observed in spontaneous human tumors.

Spontaneous remission is defined as a complete or partial, temporary, or permanent disappearance of all or at least some relevant tumor parameters in the absence of any proven medical intervention. For a variety of different cancer entities such as colon cancer (Beechey et al. 1986), mammary carcinomas (Larsen et al. 1999), malignant melanoma (Mackensen et al. 1994), acute myeloid leukemia (AML) (Tzankov et al. 2001), and liver metastases of a non-small cell lung (NSCLC) carcinoma (Kappauf et al. 1997), spontaneous remissions have been documented. Furthermore, immunocompromised individuals such as those with human immunodeficiency virus (HIV) infection are more susceptible to lymphomas and Karposi's sarcomas (Boshoff and Weiss 2002). Together with promising results derived from xenograft and syngeneic tumor mouse models, which have demonstrated the capacity of humoral (antibody) and cellular immune responses to eradicate established tumors, these findings further support the concept of cancer immunosurveillance or immunoediting (Dunn et al. 2004).

7.2
Immune System

The ability of the immune system to effectively respond to tumors is dependent on the following assumptions:
- Tumor cells differ from normal cells.
- The immune system can recognize these differences.
- The immune system is in an active state and capable in generating an effective and protective immune response.

These prerequisites indicate that cancer immunoediting is a dynamic process that involves both the tumor as well as the immunocompetent effector system. The efficient eradication of tumors in a living organism requires crosstalk between leukocytes of the innate and adaptive arms of the immune system, which reside in different immunological compartments. It has been shown that the cytokine interferon-gamma (IFN-γ), and the cytolytic effector molecules perforin and granzyme are secreted by cells of the innate and adaptive immune system, which contribute to the host's immune defense against cancer. Following uptake into tumor cells, intracellular located granzyme B initiates apoptosis via the activation of procaspases 3, 7, 10 inactive cytosolic inhibitor of caspase-activated DNase (ICAD), and the disruption of the membrane potential of mitochondria, which causes the release of cytochrome c into the cytosol. The situation of the host's immune defense is complicated by the fact that throughout evolution, tumors have adopted strategies to interfere with and to overcome the immune system. These immune escape mechanisms involve the downregulation of major histocompatibility complex class I (MHC I) and costimulatory molecules, the loss of tumor-specific antigens, the stimulation of inhibitory receptors expressed on effector cells, the stimulation of the growth of inhibitory CD4/CD25 double-positive regulatory T cells (T_{regs}), and the secretion of inhibitory molecules such as serpin-protease inhibitors, which interfere with the apoptosis cascade. For example, about 60% of metastases express significantly reduced levels of MHC class I on their cell surfaces. These findings indicate that a better understanding of the interaction between immune cells, tumor cells, and the tumor microenvironment and their consequences will guide the development of more effective approaches for controlling and successfully treating cancer.

7.3
Tumor Markers

As mentioned earlier, a key barrier to the generation of protective anticancer immune responses is that, in contrast to pathogens, tumors are not typically seen as being "foreign" by the host's immune system. It is therefore essential to identify and characterize tumor-specific antigens/peptides that can be used for the development of innovative immunotherapeutic strategies. Recent approaches include the serological analysis of recombinant cDNA expression libraries (SEREX) (CHEN et al. 1997), differential gene expression analysis, and T-cell epitope cloning (TEPIC), using samples obtained from patients with cancer (BOON and VAN DER BRUGGEN 1996; VAN DEN EYNDE AND BOON 1997). These methods have identified antigens that can be grouped into various categories including cancer/testis, activation, differentia-

tion, amplification, mutational antigens, danger signals such as membrane-bound heat shock proteins (HSPs), and pathogens (Table 7.1).

7.3.1
Cancer/Testis Antigens

The expression pattern of cancer/testis (CT) antigens in healthy human individuals is restricted to germline tissues such as testis and placenta. Nevertheless, a high proportion of melanoma, bladder cancer, lung, esophageal, and ovarian tumors show a surface positive phenotype in a lineage nonspecific fashion (BOON et al. 1997; VAN DEN EYNDE and BOON 1997; OLD and CHEN 1998). The expression of these antigens frequently maps to genes on the X chromosome. The CT antigens are also linked to the unique class of differentiation antigens that have the capacity to elicit a cellular and humoral immune response. Representative CT antigen members that belong to multigene families are summarized in Table 7.1.

7.3.2
Activation Antigens

Mucins (MUC-1, 2, 3, 4, 11, 12, 13) are a family of highly glycosylated proteins that can be grouped into the activation antigens. They are predominantly found on mammary, ovarian, and pancreatic carcinomas (BOON and VAN DER BRUGGEN 1996). Weakly glycosylated members of this protein family are expressed on healthy epithelial cells. Membrane location of MUC-1 and MUC-4 is achieved through a hydrophobic membrane-spanning domain that mediates plasma membrane retention (SINGH et al. 2004). A mouse monoclonal antibody (mAb) directed against CD227 is able to detect the membrane-bound form of MUC-1.

7.3.3
Differentiation Antigens

The following members of the differentiation antigens including tyrosinase, gp100, and Melan-A/Mart-1 are expressed on normal melanocytes. Prostate-specific antigen (PSA) is found on the cell surface of healthy prostate tissue. Compared with normal tissues, the expression density of these and other antigens including carcino-embryogenic antigen (CEA), alpha-1-fetoprotein, and epithelial cell-adhesion molecule (EpCam) in tumors is highly increased. Due to the lack of tumor-specificity of these antigens, it is important to note that

Table 7.1. Categories of tumor-associated antigens

Antigen category	Antigens
CT	Melanoma associated antigen (MAGE-1, -2, -3) (Boon and van der Bruggen 1996) NY-ESO-1 = LAGE-1 (esophageal cancer, ovarian cancer) (Odunsi et al. 2003; Jager et al.1999) B-melanoma antigen (BAGE)
Activation	MUC-1, 2, 3, 4, 11, 12, 13
Differentiation	CEA α-1-Fetoprotein EpCam Tyrosinase (Brichard et al. 1993) Melan-A/Mart-1 (Coulie et al. 1994) Glycoprotein (gp100) (Kawakami 1995) PSA
Amplification	Her2/neu proto-oncogen (c-erb-B2; Cheever et al. 1995) p53 (Scanlan et al. 1998) Preferentially expressed antigen in melanoma (PRAME) Aldolase A
Mutational	Human leukocyte antigen allele type A2 (HLA-A2) CDK4 (Wolfel et al. 1995) β-Catenin (Robbins et al. 1996) Caspase 8 (Mandruzzato et al. 1997) Melanoma-ubiquitous mutated (MUM-1) Mutated p53 (Gnjatic et al. 1998)
Damage signals	HSP70, HSP 72, HSP 90 Gp 96
Pathogens	Human papilloma virus (HPV) types 16 and 18 (Tindle 1996) Epstein-Barr virus (EBV) (Lennette et al. 1995) Human T-cell lymphotropic virus type I (HTLV-1; leukemia) HHV-8 *Helicobacter pylori* bacteria (chronic gastritis and stomach carcinoma)

an efficient immune response against these tissue-specific antigens can also affect normal tissues. One well-known example is the destruction of normal melanocytes by cytotoxic Melan-A–specific T cells, which can cause vitiligo in the healthy skin of melanoma patients. A list of differentiation antigens with a high expression on tumors is shown in Table 7.1.

7.3.4
Amplification Antigens

This group of antigens is ubiquitously and widely expressed in normal tissues but highly overexpressed in tumor cells. Important representatives of this group are Her-2/neu, which is predominantly overexpressed on adenocarcinoma of the colon, mammary, ovarian,

pancreatic, and lung carcinomas and p53, PRAME, and aldolase A, which are overexpressed in lung carcinomas (Coulie et al. 1999; Gure et al. 2000).

7.3.5
Mutational Antigens

Although this group of antigens—mostly peptides—are ubiquitously expressed in normal tissues, they are expressed in a mutated form in many tumors. In general, each tumor exhibits an individual pattern of mutation, and the resultant antigenic profile is therefore considered as being tumor-specific and unique (Wang and Rosenberg 1999; Renkvist et al. 2001). Most mutations are point mutations that are translated into individually mutated proteins. Since these mutations cause severe changes in the activity of the encoded proteins, these antigens affect the oncogenic potential of the tumor. Examples of mutational antigens that are found in a variety of different tumor entities are listed in Table 7.1.

7.3.6
HSPs

HSPs were firstly discovered in 1962 (Ritossa 1962) as a set of evolutionary conserved molecules whose expression is highly inducible not only by a variety of different stress stimuli such as elevated temperatures, irradiation, heavy metals, cytostatic drugs, amino acid analogue, glucose deprivation, oxidative stress, but also by inflammation or viral and bacterial infections. Under physiological conditions, HSPs are required for cell differentiation and antigen processing for proper protein folding of nascent polypeptides, for transport of proteins along membranes, and for prevention of protein aggregation (Morimoto 1991; Pierce 1994). In contrast to normal tissues, malignantly transformed cells such as tumors have been found to overexpress HSPs in the cytosol, which might cause the translocation of them into the plasma membrane and into the extracellular milieu. Members of the HSP70 and HSP90 families are present on the plasma membranes of a number of different tumor entities (Multhoff et al. 1997; Shin et al. 2003) where they act as danger signals for the innate (Schmitt et al. 2007) and adaptive cellular immune system. T cells have been found to recognize HSP-chaperoned immunogenic peptides that are cross-presented by antigen-presenting cells (APCs) (Srivastava et al. 1998). In contrast, natural killer (NK) cells have the capacity to recognize membrane-bound Hsp70 on tumors, even in the absence of immunogenic peptides. Since the corresponding normal tissues lack an HSP membrane expression, the presence of HSPs on the plasma membrane is considered as a tumor-specific antigen (unpublished observation). HSPs that are predominantly found on tumor cell surfaces and in the extracellular space are Hsp70, Hsp72, and a major stress inducible member of the HSP70 family, Gp96 (glucose-related protein 96), an endoplasmic reticulum (ER)-residing member of the HSP90 family.

7.3.7
Pathogens

A small proportion of tumors (2–5%) are initiated by viral infections, which causes a transformation of human cells (Coulie et al. 1999). Human papilloma virus type 16 and 18 are associated with cervical carcinomas (Bontkes et al. 2000; Youde et al. 2000, Rudolf et al. 2001), Epstein-Barr virus infections with Burkitt's lymphomas, human T-lymphotropic virus (HTLV-1) with T-cell lymphomas, and human herpes virus 8 (HHV-8) infections with Karposi's sarcoma. A chronic bacterial infection of the stomach with *Helicobacter pylori* has been associated with gastritis and with gastric tumors.

7.4
Preclinical Immunotherapeutic Approaches

A better understanding of the molecular basis of the immune homeostasis and its regulatory mechanisms has re-attracted many researchers to the concept of augmenting the antitumor responses. An emerging number of newly identified tumor-associated antigens (TAA) including differentiation, mutational, amplification, CT, danger signals that have been identified using expression libraries, differential gene expression analysis (Chen et al. 1997), T-cell epitope cloning (Boon and van der Bruggen 1996), and bioinformatics (Scanlan et al. 2000) have also advanced this field. The following section aims to summarize immunoediting and immunotherapeutic concepts including nonspecific cytokine therapies, specific antibody, and cell-based concepts that have been tested successfully in animal models. The proof of principle and the in vivo efficacy of some of these have already been demonstrated in first human clinical trials.

7.4.1
Cytokines

Cytokines, also termed as interleukins, lymphokines, or chemokines, are small (8–30 kDa) signaling proteins and glycoproteins that are predominantly produced by hematopoietic cells. Their main function is to recruit and stimulate the immune system against pathogens and to support differentiation and developmental processes during embryogenesis. Cytokine-based immunostimulation is believed to have the potential to treat established primary tumors and distant metastases. One of the earlier immunological approaches aimed on the broad, nonspecific stimulation of the adaptive (T lymphocytes) and innate (NK cells) immune system by the administration of high doses of recombinant interleukin 2 (IL-2) (Rosenberg 1986). Large-scale production of interferons, using recombinant DNA technology in 1983 enabled the first systematical evaluation of appropriate dose, route, and schedule for application in humans. Meanwhile, cytokines have an established role in therapy of malignant melanoma and renal cell carcinoma as described later in this chapter.

7.4.2
Antibodies

The development of the technology for producing mAb from hybridoma cells (KOHLER and MILSTEIN 1975), for which Kohler, Jerne, and Milstein were awarded the Nobel Prize in Physiology and Medicine in 1984, led to the hypothesis that the "magic bullet" against cancer has been found. Despite their high degree of specificity and affinity, the development of clinically applicable antibodies for the treatment of cancer has proven to be more complex than was originally anticipated. Patients that had been treated with the first generation of murine mAb developed a human–anti-mouse antibody response (HAMA) against the therapeutic agent, and this drastically limited the therapeutic success. Nowadays, therapeutic antibodies are humanized either by grafting CDR (complimentarity-determining regions) onto human antibodies, or by creating chimeric antibodies by transferring the murine Fab antigen–binding variable region onto a human constant Fc portion. Approval has already been achieved for the clinical application of humanized monoclonal antibodies, which are directed against CD20 (Rituxan, MabThera, Zenapax, Zevalin, Bexxar) for the treatment of non-Hodgkin's and cutaneous B-cell (KERL et al. 2006) lymphomas, CD33

(Mylotarg) for the treatment of CD33-positive myeloid leukemia, CD52 (Campath, Mabcampath) for the treatment of B-cell chronic lymphocytic leukemia (B-CLL), EpCam (Panorex) for the treatment of colorectal cancer, ErbB2 (Herceptin) for Her-2 overexpressing breast cancer, and vascular endothelial growth factor (VEGF) (Avastin) and epidermal growth factor receptor (EGFR) (Erbitux, Vectibix) for the treatment of colon carcinoma.

Naked, unconjugated antibodies kill their tumor targets by different mechanisms including antibody dependent cell-mediated cytotoxicity (ADCC) (STEPLEWSKI et al. 1985), complement-dependent cytotoxicity (CDC) (HOUGHTON et al. 1983), and by the direct induction of apoptosis via death receptor targeting (CONTASSOT et al. 2007). Alterations of signal transduction (TRAUTH et al. 1989), blocking of ligand-receptor interactions (YANG et al. 1999), and the prevention of the enzymatic cleavage of cell surface proteins (BASELGA et al. 2001) can also be involved. The antibody Apomab, which is directed against the death receptor DR5, augments apoptosis of colorectal, NSCLC, and pancreatic model tumor cell lines by clustering of DR5 at the cell surface and thus stimulating a death-inducing signaling pathway involving caspase 8 and Fas-associated cell death (ADAMS et al. 2008). Effector cells of the innate immune system (NK cells, monocytes, macrophages) expressing Fc-gamma (Fc-γ) receptors such as low (CD16)-, intermediate (CD32)-, and high (CD64)-affinity Fc receptors can mediate ADCC after antibody binding to the tumor targets. Another possibility is to use antibodies as vehicles to more specifically deliver toxic compounds such

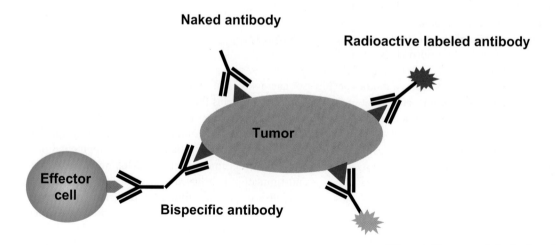

Fig. 7.1. Principles of tumor cell kill by antibodies: bispecific antibody-mediating effector-tumor cell interaction, naked antibody mediating antibody dependent cellular cytotoxicity (ADCC), radioactive labeled antibody mediating targeted internalization of radionuclides, and chemotherapy-labeled antibody-mediating targeted internalization of cytostatic drugs

as radionuclides and/or chemotherapeutics directly to the tumors. The principles of antibody-mediated tumor kill are schematically illustrated in Fig. 7.1.

Despite these promising strategies, the clinical outcome of antibody-based therapies is still limited by a number of factors including their relatively short in vivo half-life and clearance from the host's body, the insufficient degree of glycosylation of humanized antibodies, variations in the affinity and avidity of the humanized antibodies, and the low amount of tumor-specific or tumor-associated antigens.

7.4.3
Cell-Based Therapies

Adoptive cell-transfer therapies have developed into potent treatments for patients with highly immunogenic tumors including metastatic melanoma (DUDLEY and ROSENBERG 2007). Current studies are aimed at improving GMP (good manufacturer practice) methods for generating and administering appropriate lymphocyte populations in future clinical trials and improving the resilience of antitumor immunity in tumor patients.

7.4.3.1
Dendritic Cells

Dendritic cells (DCs) can be subdivided in two developmental lineages, the myeloid and the lymphoid (STEINMAN and INABA 1999). DCs control the activity of B lymphocytes, T lymphocytes, and NK cells (BANCHEREAU and STEINMAN 1998). As professional APCs, their primary task is to capture foreign antigens from the periphery, process and maturate them into peptides, and present them on MHC molecules to naïve T cells. In the absence of essential costimulatory signals that are concomitantly delivered, T-cell activation is insufficient. Apart from their activating function, DCs are also able to tolerize the immune system against self-antigens in order to avoid autoimmune reactions (TURLEY 2002). The migratory capacity of DCs is regulated by chemokines. The expression of the chemokine receptor CCR7 promotes the migration of immature DCs to inflamed tissues and that of mature DCs to the draining lymph nodes, where the antigen is presented to naïve T cells (SALLUSTRO and LANZAVECCHIA 2000).

Although lymphodepletion by chemotherapy and total body irradiation can reduce the absolute number of APCs, it also has been shown to promote their maturation into an active state, as indicated by an upregulation of CD86 and MHC class II antigens in

a mouse model (ZHANG et al. 2002). Irradiation has also been found to stimulate secretion of the inflammatory cytokine IL-12 by DCs, which subsequently activates T cells and NK cells. The maturation of DCs and their capacity for antigen cross-presentation is also enhanced by the secretion of tumor-necrosis factor (TNF), IL-1, and IL-4 and by the presence of "danger signals" such as lipopolysaccharide (LPS) and/or HSPs (ASEA and STEIN-STREILEIN 1998). DCs pulsed with tumor lysates (NAIR et al. 1997), tumor protein extracts (ASHLEY et al. 1997), and/or synthetic peptides can generate protective immunity to subsequent tumor challenge in tumor mouse models. The requirements for GMP-grade production of the cell products presently limit the applicability of this therapeutic approach in human patients.

7.4.3.2
T Cells

The term *immunosurveillance*, which characterizes the important role of T cells in generating an antitumor immune response, was established in 1967 by Burnet. Generally, T lymphocytes can be grouped roughly into CD4 T helper and CD8 cytotoxic T cells. T cells, composing between 60 and 80% of the peripheral blood lymphocyte (PBL) pool, recognize their targets via the T-cell receptors (TCRs), but only after primary stimulation by APCs such as monocytes, macrophages, or DCs (LANZAVECCHIA and SALLUSTO 2001). The enormous heterogenicity of TCRs is obtained by variable-diversity-joining gene recombination and crossover events. APCs present processed foreign peptides to CD8 T cells in the context of MHC class I and to CD4 T cells in the context of MHC class II molecules. As indicated above, an effective, long-lasting T-cell stimulation requires concomitant costimulation via interactions between essential costimulatory molecules such as B7 on APCs and CD28 on responding T cells.

Tumor-specific cytotoxic lymphocytes (CTL) play a crucial role in the immunotherapy of cancer (GATTINONI et al. 2006) by directly targeting and killing tumor cells that express appropriate antigens for which they are specific, whereas CD4 T cells provide help for these events via the secretion of pro-inflammatory cytokines such as IL-2. Although IL-2 is a growth factor for T and NK cells, which promotes expansion and cytotoxic function of effector cells, it is also essential for the maintenance of peripheral self-tolerance (FURTADO et al. 2002). Non-mutated self-antigens expressed by tumors primarily serve as target antigens for CD8 CTLs. Adoptive cell transfer therapies involve ex vivo activation and expansion of tumor-reactive T-cell populations that are then transferred into patients. Although the immunoreconstitution with ex vivo expanded tumor-infiltrating lymphocytes (TILs) (WANG and ROSENBERG 1999) has shown some success, more recent data indicate that the adoptive transfer of TILs after non-myeloablative, but lymphodepleting systemic chemotherapy is superior with respect to tumor regression. It thus appears that the removal of the host's immune system increases the efficacy of the adaptive cell transfer. One explanation for this might be that the depletion reduces the number and activity of endogenous immunoregulatory T-cell populations such as CD4/CD25 double-positive T_{regs} (NI and REDMOND 2006). These cells might compete with CD8 T cells for activating cytokines and/or the availability of APCs and thereby suppress antitumor immune responses. T_{regs} are characterized by an upregulated expression of the transcription factor fork-head box P3 (FoxP3) protein and by a constitutively high expression of the IL-2 receptor alpha chain (CD25), the glucocorticoid-induced TNF-receptor related protein (GITR), the cytotoxic T-lymphocyte associated antigen 4 (CTLA-4), and in the case of humans, low levels of CD127. A number of studies suggest that T_{regs} are involved in the control of antitumor immune responses, and these cells have been shown to accumulate in tumor lesions, where they inhibit the function of tumor infiltrating cytotoxic T cells (ANTONY et al. 2005). However, in addition to T_{regs} (ZHANG et al. 2005), CD11b$^+$Gr1$^+$ myeloid suppressor cells (MSCs), NK cells, and natural killer T (NKT) cells (KRONENBERG 2005) have been found to exert immunosuppressive functions. Apart from the arginine metabolism, the exact mechanisms of action of these cells have yet to be elucidated (BRONTE and ZANOVELLO 2005). Another reason could be that homing of lymphocytes is improved following depletion of the host's immune cells.

7.4.3.3
NK Cells

NK cells, also formerly termed large granular lymphocytes (LGLs), are specialized cells of the innate immune system that exert their function against pathogen-infected and tumor cells as a first line of defense. NK cells, which compose about 5 to 20% of circulating lymphocytes (TRINCHIERI 1989), can stimulate the immune system indirectly by the release of high amounts of IFN-γ, or mediate a direct cytotoxic response via the secretion of perforin and granzymes or via FAS–FAS ligand interaction. The discrimination of self and non-self by

NK cells is regulated by a fine balance of activating (short intracellular immunoreceptor tyrosine-based activation motifs [ITAM]) and inhibiting (long intracellular immunoreceptor tyrosine-based inhibition motifs [ITIM]) receptors. These receptors can be grouped into the following main receptor families: immunoglobulin like receptors with specificity for *HLA* alleles; C-type lectin receptors NKG2D, CD94, NKG2A, NKG2C; and natural cytotoxicity receptors (NCRs) NKp30, NKp44, NKp46. The cytokines IL-2 and IL-15 are crucial to the survival, expansion, and differentiation of NK cells (KOKA et al. 2003). NK cells play key roles in the crosstalk between the innate and adaptive immunity (DEGLI-ESPOSTI et al. 2005; PULENDRAN and AHMED 2006). Knockout mice for recombinant activating gene 2 (*RAG-2*), perforin, interferon gamma, or STAT-1 or NK deficient mice are more susceptible to the development of tumors than their wild-type counterparts (DUNN et al. 2004; SMYTH et al. 2001 b). NK cells kill their susceptible targets by releasing cytotoxic granules containing granzymes and/or perforin via interactions with death-inducing ligands (TRAIL, FAS ligand) through the secretion of inflammatory cytokines (IFN-γ, TNF-α), and T-cell recruiting chemokines such as RANTES, MIP1-α, MIP1-β), and via antibody dependent cellular cytotoxicity (ADCC) (SMYTH et al. 2001a; ROBERTSON 2002). In contrast, cytokines such as IL-2, IL-12, IL-15, IL-18, IL-21, IL-23, and IL-27 augment NK cell–mediated tumor activities (MA et al. 2006a; SMYTH et al. 2004). Remarkably, alloreactive NK cells have been shown to prevent graft versus host disease (GvHD) by eliminating the recipient antigen-specific DCs in a mouse acute myelogenous leukemia (AML) model system (RUGGERI et al. 2002; MILLER et al. 2005).

7.4.4
mAbs

mAbs, targeting tumor-specific antigens, can initiate ADCC via their Fc part and with the help of activated NK cells, macrophages, granulocytes, and the complement system. Experimentally, mAbs such as trastuzumab, rituximab, and anti-EGF receptor have been shown to induce ADCC. Macrophages and granulocytes express both activating and inhibitory Fc receptors, whereas NK cells present only the low affinity activating Fc-γ receptor (CD16). The interaction of NK cells with Fc-γ ligand initiates the release of IFN-γ, TNF-α, and T-cell-recruiting chemokines. This release can be enhanced by the addition of pro-inflammatory cytokines such as IL-2 and IL-15 (PARIHAR et al. 2002).

Other approaches for enhancing antibody-mediated NK cell activity involve the use of oligodeoxynucleotides (ODN) containing unmethylated CpG motifs, which mimic bacterial DNA. The Toll-like receptor 9 (TLR-9) has been identified as the receptor for CpGs by TLR-9 knockout mouse systems. The use of bacillus Calmette-Guerin (BCG) (Brandau et al. 2001; Suttmann et al. 2006) as an adjuvant is another method for a nonspecific stimulation of NK cells via the secretion of IL-12 and IFN-γ by monocytes. More recently, defensins, a family of cysteine-rich cationic polypeptides that are constitutively expressed by epithelial cells, have been found to attract immature DCs and thus induce signaling through TLR-4. The presence of NK cells and CD8-positive T cells is a prerequisite for their antitumor activity (Ma et al. 2006b). Last, but not least, HSP70 or peptides derived thereof, acting as classical danger signals, have been found to activate NK cells against Hsp70 membrane–positive cancer cells in vitro (Gastpar et al. 2005), in tumor mouse models (Stangl et al. 2006), and in a clinical phase I trial (Krause et al. 2003). The mechanism of tumor cell lysis has been characterized as a perforin-independent, granzyme B-mediated apoptosis (Gross et al. 2003).

7.5
Role of Immunotherapy in Clinical Practice

From the large pool of potential immunotherapeutics until today, only a few have made their way to clinical application. This section summarizes the clinically relevant immunotherapies in their typical fields of application.

7.5.1
Malignant Melanoma

Immunotherapy has a long history in malignant melanoma, which is considered a highly immunogenic tumor. However, two large trials testing the efficacy of adjuvant IFN-γ showed no advantage for patients with high-risk primary tumors or lymph node metastases (Southwest Oncology Group [Meyskens et al. 1990]; European Organization for Research and the Treatment of Cancer, unpublished). A phase II study on IFN-β as an adjuvant for melanoma demonstrated possible advantages and led to the initiation of a randomized study whose results have not been published so far. IFN-α is the first substance that has shown a significant advantage in prospective randomized trials. IFN-α2a and IFN-α2b differ by two amino acids and can be regarded as equivalent on the basis of their effectiveness. Low-dose IFN-α (3 million IU subcutaneously, three times weekly for 18–24 months) should be offered all patients with primary melanoma thicker than 1.5 mm and no indication of lymph node involvement, on the basis of three studies that showed a significant increase in the recurrence-free survival time (Grob et al. 1998; Pehamberger et al. 1998; Cameron et al. 2001).

A variety of randomized studies with different IFN-α dosages as an adjuvant has been conducted in patients with lymph node metastases. The clearest results are available for IFN-α2b, using a high-dose regimen (initiation: 20 million IU/m^2 intravenously daily day one to five every week for 4 weeks, maintenance: 10 million IU/m^2 subcutaneously three times weekly for 11 months). The first prospective randomized study showed an incidence in the recurrence-free survival prolonging disease free and overall survival (Kirkwood et al. 1996).

Table 7.2. IFN-α in malignant melanoma

Treatment concept	Tumor extension	Scheme	Effect
Adjuvant	Primary tumor >1.5 mm thickness, no lymph node involvement, R0 resection	Low dose	Prolonged RFS
	Positive lymph nodes, R0 resection	High dose	Prolonged RFS Prolonged DFS Prolonged OS
Palliative	Inoperable recurrent tumor Metastasized tumor (stage IV)	IFN-α combined with chemotherapy	Objective response Unchanged OS

RFS recurrence free survival, *DFS* disease free survival, *OS* overall survival

A follow-up confirmatory trial testing high-dose IFN vs. lower-dose IFN vs. observation was not able to confirm the earlier results (KIRKWOOD et al 2000). A third trial comparing high-dose IFN vs. a vaccine was terminated early because a clear disease-free and survival advantage for the IFN arm was evident early. On the other hand, IFN treatment was associated with higher toxicity compared with the vaccine arm (KIRKWOOD et al. 2000).

Based on these studies, IFN-α was introduced as standard adjuvant therapy for stage III resected melanoma. However, toxicity remains an issue. Flu-like syndromes including fever, chills, headache, malaise, myalgias, arthralgias, and fatigue acutely occur during therapy with interferons and diminish over time with continued daily or alternate daily administration. Vigorous hydration is essential, as patients tend to become dehydrated.

Inoperable recurrent tumors, inoperable regional metastases, and distant metastases (stage IV) are the major indications for systemic chemotherapy and chemoimmunotherapy in malignant melanoma. Many studies have evaluated the effectiveness of cytokine monotherapy in patients with advanced disease. Both IFN-α as well as IL-2 can achieve remission rates comparable with that of cytostatic agents (KEILHOLZ et al. 1997). Treatment with IL-2 resulted in prolonged complete remissions in 5% of patients (DILLMAN et al. 1997). The combination of cytostatic agents and cytokines leads to an increase in the objective response rate similar to polychemotherapy, but no improvement of overall survival (FALKSON et al. 1998; BAJETTA et al. 1994; SMITH et al. 1992). The tolerability of chemotherapy is reduced by IFN-α as well as by IL-2. As treatment in such situations is primarily palliative, the effect of any regimen on the quality of life must be carefully considered. As a first-line treatment, single-agent therapy is recommended, as polychemotherapy or biochemotherapy do not show significant advantages for prolongation of survival and are more toxic (Table 2.2).

Peptide immunization, vaccination with dendritic cells and hybrid vaccines, adoptive transfer of T cells, and immunization with naked and packaged DNA have been tested in phase I studies only and should only be used in clinical trials (GARBE et al. 2008).

7.5.2
Renal Cell Carcinoma

Metastatic renal cell carcinoma (RCC) has been notoriously resistant to conventional chemotherapy. In the early 1980s, the observation of spontaneous remissions in RCC led to a search for therapeutic agents with potential to improve the immunologic response against RCC tumor cells. Early trials used in vitro stimulation of T cells with IL-2 to produce lymphokine-activated killer (LAK) cells that were co-administered with high-dose IL-2. However, it was later recognized that the therapeutic effect resided predominantly with high-dose IL-2, and the use of LAK cells was abandoned (ROSENBERG et al. 1993). However, the utility of high dose IL-2 is limited by its toxicity. Side effects include fever, chills, lethargy, diarrhea, nausea, anemia, thrombocytopenia, eosinophilia, diffuse erythroderma, hepatic dysfunction, confusion, and in approximately 5% of patients, myocarditis. IL-2 can lead to a capillary leak syndrome, leading to fluid retention, hypotension, and respiratory distress syndrome. Early high-dose studies were associated with 2–4% mortality. These patients require intensive supportive care. Mortality rates could be decreased to less than 1% in experienced treatment centers.

In spite of toxicity, the response to high-dose IL-2 treatment in metastatic RCC may be spectacular with long-lasting CRs in individual cases. However, overall responses are achievable in only about 20% of patients, and complete long-lasting responses occur in only about 5% (FYFE et al. 1995). In a National Institutes of Health trial that randomized patients to receive high-dose IL-2 or a dose that was 10 times lower, a significantly higher response rate with high-dose IL-2 than with low-dose intravenous IL-2 (21 versus 13%) was seen, but no overall survival difference and a higher morbidity as anticipated were found (YANG et al. 2003). This was confirmed in a multi-institutional phase III trial testing intravenous high-dose IL-2 or low-dose subcutaneous IL-2 plus IFN-α (response rates were 23.2 vs. 9.9%), while there was no significant difference in overall survival (17 vs. 13 months). As expected, there were more grade 3 and 4 toxicities in the high-dose IL-2 arm (MCDERMOTT et al. 2005). It can be concluded that high-dose IL-2 is an acceptable therapy for patients with little or no comorbidities and excellent performance status, for whom the possibility of long-term CR is worth the complexity, risk, and acute toxicity of the treatment. How to best sequence or combine IL-2 with newer drugs is unknown. In phase II studies, recombinant IFN-α was reported to induce response in RCC in up to 29% of cases. However, in contrast to IL-2, IFN-α alone has no curative potential, and CRs are rare and of short duration. In a randomized trial comparing IFN-α with medroxyprogesterone acetate, IFN-α treatment was associated with a longer survival time, although the benefit was minimal (median survival time, 8.5 versus 6 months), and patients treated with IFN-α had a lower quality of life (MEDICAL RESEARCH COUNCIL 1999).

A large study of 425 patients evaluated the activity of low-dose IL-2 in combination with IFN-α, as well as each agent alone. IFN-α or IL-2 alone had low response rates, but the response rate for the combination was significantly higher ($p < 0.01$), with significantly improved 1-year event-free survival ($p = 0.01$). However, no difference in overall survival was seen (NEGRIER et al. 1998).

In the future, new biologic agents might play a more important role than unspecific immunomodolators in RCC. Seventy-five percent of all RCC are clear-cell RCC. These are characteristically associated with loss of function of the von Hippel-Lindau (*VHL*) gene, resembling a constitutively activated hypoxic response resulting from upregulation of the hypoxia factor (HIF). HIF activation results in upregulation of genes encoding VEGF, transforming growth factor (TGF), Met, stromal cell-derived factor (SDF)-1 and chemokine receptor CXCR4, among others.

Small-molecule multikinase inhibitors that target VEGF receptors (sunitinib and sorafenib) have a favorable toxicity profile and can prolong time to progression and preserve quality of life when used in newly diagnosed or previously treated patients. Lately, sunitinib malate has been shown to be more effective than IFN-α in a large multicenter phase III trial (median progression-free survival 11 vs. 5 months) (MOTZER et al. 2007).

IFN-α does not improve survival or relapse-free survival as an adjuvant. A phase III study treating patients with pT3-4a and/or node-positive RCC was not able to show a benefit of low dose IFN-α given daily for 5 days every 3 weeks for up to 12 cycles compared with postoperative observation (median survival 7.4 years in the observation arm and 5.1 years in the treatment arm, median recurrence-free survival 3.0 years in the observation arm and 2.2 years in the interferon arm) (MESSING et al. 2003). Also, a similar study using high dose IFN-α showed no benefit (CLARK et al. 2003). Those results were confirmed in a prospectively randomized clinical trial to investigate the role of adjuvant immunochemotherapy in high-risk patients with RCC. Two hundred and three RCC patients were stratified into three risk groups: patients with tumor extending into renal vein/vena cava or invading beyond Gerota's fascia (pT3b/c pN0 or pT4 pN0), patients with locoregional lymph node infiltration (pN[+]), and patients after complete resection of tumor relapse or solitary metastasis (R0). There was no relapse-free survival benefit, and the overall survival was inferior with an adjuvant 8-week-outpatient, sc-rIL-2/sc-rIFN-α2a/iv-5-fluorouracil (5-FU)–based immunochemotherapy compared with observation (ATZPODIEN et al. 2005). In summary, there is no role for immunomodolators in the adjuvant treatment of RCC.

7.5.3
Hematologic Malignancies

IFN is an effective treatment in hairy cell leukemia (QUESADA et al. 1986). Nine complete and 17 partial responses were documented by bone marrow core biopsies. Peripheral blood hematologic indices improved or normalized in all patients. Previously untreated patients showed significantly higher complete remission rates than did patients who had undergone splenectomy. Therapy was well tolerated, and most patients experiencing tumor remission also reported an improved quality of life. Another study found similar results in a small population of patients, with an overall response rate of 93% (FOON et al. 1986). On IFN treatment, peripheral blood counts returned to normal levels. This study also assessed NK cell activity and immunologic surface markers, and noted normalization of both parameters after therapy. Today, new nucleoside analogs show better results. Yet, IFN-α is still the first option in recurrences or if there are contraindication against nucleoside analogs.

A significant survival benefit of more than 89 months in a phase II trial in patients with chronic myelogenous leukemia suggests that IFN is effective in this disease as well (ALLAN et al. 1995; OHNISHI et al. 1995). This survival advantage was independent of cytogenetic improvement with IFN, which was also noted. 7 to 8% of the patients showed complete remission with IFN-α monotherapy. GUILHOT et al. (1997) were able to show better results with combinations of IFN-α and cytosinarabinoside.

In non-Hodgkin's lymphoma (NHL), post–stem cell transplant IL-2 has shown activity. Low-dose IL-2 was also evaluated in combination with histamine, but no differences in response were observed compared with IL-2 alone.

7.6
Clinical Use of mAbs

7.6.1
Naked Antibodies

More than 200 mAbs have been tested in clinical studies, but the number of clinically relevant antibodies remains limited (Table 2.3). The first mAb that received US Food and Drug Administration (FDA) approval is rituximab, which is a chimeric antibody directed against the surface antigen CD20 on B lymphocytes, expressed on most B-cell NHL and subtypes of acute lymphatic leukemias (ALL). In combination with poly-chemotherapy, rituximab is used for primary therapy of follicular NHL and diffuse large B-cell NHL as well as for maintenance therapy in recurrent follicular B-NHL after successful induction chemotherapy. Chemoimmunotherapy with rituximab is standard in therapy of primary and recurrent mantle cell lymphoma (TOBINAI et al. 2006; TOBINAI 2007). Rituximab might also be successful in combination with chemotherapy in CLL and in Burkitt's lymphoma, improving progression-free and overall survival.

Alemtuzumab is a humanized antibody directed against CD52 on B and T lymphocytes, and monocytes, macrophages, eosinophilic granulocytes, and NK cells. It is approved for clinical application in fludarabine-refractory CLL. In those patients, remission rates of 40% can be achieved. Interestingly, alemtuzumab has been shown to be especially effective for bone marrow manifestations of CLL. The role of alemtuzumab in primary therapy of CLL is not yet clear. Further studies will evaluate whether the efficacy of alemtuzumab in recurrences can be enhanced. Promising results were seen with alemtuzumab-chemoimmunotherapy in periphery T-cell lymphoma (RAVANDI and O'BRIEN 2006). In contrast to rituximab, therapy with alemtuzumab is accompanied by heavier infusion-associated complications such as fever, shivering, dyspnea, or exanthema, and a higher rate of infectious complications.

Metastasized human epidermal growth factor receptor 2 (HER2)-expressing breast cancer treatment was the first indication for trastuzumab, a HER2-specific humanized monoclonal antibody. HER2 is a receptor tyrosine kinase of the EGFR family that is overexpressed in 25–30% of all breast cancer patients. Overexpression of HER2 leads to enhanced cell proliferation. A phase III study combining trastuzumab with first-line chemotherapy showed prolonged progression-free and overall survival (LIN and RUGO 2007). It has also been approved as monotherapy for chemotherapy refractory metastasized breast cancer (LIGIBEL and WINER 2002). In addition, efficacy of adjuvant chemotherapy can be significantly enhanced by trastuzumab (COLOMER 2005).

The chimeric mAb cetuximab is directed against EGFR. EGFR plays an important role in pathogenesis and progression of solid tumors such as colorectal cancer, NSCLC, and head and neck tumors. Binding of cetuximab to EGFR hinders the activation of intracellular tyrosine kinases and the following signal transduction pathway. The antibody also induces direct lysis of the tumor cells. A multicenter phase II study (BOND-1) was able to show that combination of irinotecan with cetuximab could overcome irinotecan resistance. In 23% of the patients, tumor remission, and in 30% stable disease was reached (SALTZ 2005). Cetuximab is now used for therapy of metastasized colorectal carcinoma in combination with irinotecan after progression with irinotecan monotherapy. In a phase III study of locally advanced head and neck tumors, the combination of cetuximab with radiotherapy significantly prolonged survival (BONNER et al. 2007). In metastasized NSCLC, a phase II study showed that combination of cisplatin, vinorelbin, and cetuximab leads to a significant survival benefit compared with chemotherapy with cisplatin and vinorelbin alone (LILENBAUM 2006).

Bevacizumab is a VEGF-specific humanized mAb. Binding to VEGF inhibits tumor angiogenesis. It is ap-

Table 7.3. mAbs in clinical use

Generic name	Target antigen	Structure	Application
Rituximab	CD20	Chimeric IgG-1κ	B-NHL Mantle cell lymphoma CLL B-precursor ALL
Alemtuzumab	CD52	Humanized IgG-1 κ	CLL Peripheral T-cell lymphomas
Trastuzumab	HER2	Humanized IgG-1 κ	Breast cancer
Cetuximab	EGFR	Chimeric IgG-1 κ	Head and neck cancer Colorectal carcinoma NSCLC
Bevacizumab	VEGF	Humanized IgG-1 κ	Colorectal carcinoma NSCLC

IgG immunoglobulin G

proved in combination with irinotecan and 5-FU for first-line therapy of metastasized colorectal carcinoma. Patients with contraindications for irinotecan can be successfully treated with 5-FU and bevacizumab. In primary therapy of advanced NSCLC, the addition of bevacizumab to carboplatin and paclitaxel leads to enhanced progression-free and overall survival (Sandler et al. 2006; Lyseng-Williamson and Robinson 2006). Contraindications are squamous cell histology and brain metastases because of enhanced risk of heavy bleeding.

7.6.2
Radioimmunoconjugates

With the help of immunoconjugates, cytotoxic substances such as radioisotopes, cytokines, enzymes, or toxins can specifically be targeted to the tumor cells by the monoclonal antibody. Only two radioimmunoconjugates have approval for therapy, ^{90}Y–ibritumomab tiuxetan and ^{131}I-tositumomab. Both are directed against CD20 and are used for recurrent or refractory follicular B-NHL after therapy with rituximab. The radioimmunoconjugates might also be successful in therapy of transformed follicular NHL and primary diffuse large cell B-NHL.

References

Adams C, Totpal K, Lawrence D, Marsters S, Pitti R, Yee S, Ross S, Deforge L, Koeppen H, Sagolla M, Compaan D, Lowman H, Hymowitz S, Ashkenazi A (2008) Structural and functional analysis of the interaction between the agonistic monoclonal antibody Apomab and the proapoptotic receptor DR5. Cell Death Differ 15:751–761

Allan NC, Richards SM, Shepherd PC (1995) UK Medical Research Council randomized, multicenter trial of interferon alfa n1 for chronic myeloid leukaemia: improved survival irrespective of cytogenetic response. Lancet 345:1392–1397

Antony PA, Piccirillo CA, Akpinarli A, Finkelstein SE, Speiss PJ, Surman DR, Palmer DC, Chan CC, Klebanoff CA, Overwijk WW, Rosenberg SA, Restifo NP (2005) CD8$^+$ T cell immunity against a tumor/self-antigen is augmented by CD4$^+$ T helper cells and hindered by naturally occurring T regulatory cells. J Immunol 174:2591–2601

Asea A, Stein-Streilein J (1998) Signalling through NK1.1 triggers NK cells to die but induces NK T cells to produce interleukin-4. Immunology 93:296–305

Ashley DM, Faiola B, Nair S, Hale LP, Bigner DD, Gilboa E (1997) Bone marrow-generated dendritic cells pulsed with tumor extracts or tumor RNA induce antitumor immunity against central nervous system tumors. J Exp Med 186:1177–1182

Atzpodien J, Schmitt E, Gertenbach U, Fornara P, Heynemann H, Maskow A et al., German Cooperative Renal Carcinoma Chemo-Immunotherapy Trials Group (DGCIN) (2005) Adjuvant treatment with interleukin-2- and interferon-alpha2a-based chemoimmunotherapy in renal cell carcinoma post tumor nephrectomy: results of a prospectively randomized trial of the German Cooperative Renal Carcinoma Chemoimmunotherapy Group (DGCIN). Br J Cancer 92:843–846

Bajetta E, Di Leo A, Zampino MG, Sertoli MR, Comella G, Bardugni M et al (1994) Multicenter randomized trial of dacarbazine alone or in combination with two different doses and schedules of interferon alfa-2a in the treatment of advanced melanoma. J Clin Oncol 12:806–811

Bancherau J, Steinman RM (1998) Dendritic cells and the control of immunity. Nature 392:245–252

Baselga J, Albanell J, Molina MA, Arribas J (2001) Mechanism of action of trastuzumab and scientific update. Semin Oncol 28:4–11

Beechey RT, Edwards BE, Kelland CH (1986) Adenocarcinoma of the colon: an unusual case. Med J Aust 144:211–213

Bonner JA, Harari PM, Giralt J, Azarnia N, Shin DM, Cohen RB, Jones CU, Sur R, Raben D, Jassem J, Ove R, Kies MS, Baselga J, Youssoufian H, Amellal N, Rowinsky EK, Ang KK (2006) Radiotherapy plus cetuximab for squamous-cell carcinoma of the head and neck. N Engl J Med 354:567–578

Bontkes HJ, de Gruijl TD, van den Muysenberg AJ, Verheijen RH, Stukart MJ, Meijer CJ, Scheper RJ, Stacey SN, Duggan-Keen MF, Stern PL, Man S, Borysiewicz LK, Walboomers JM (2000) Human papillomavirus type 16 E6/E7-specific cytotoxic T lymphocytes in women with cervical neoplasia. Int J Cancer 88:92–98

Boon T, van der Bruggen BP (1996) Human tumor antigens recognized by T lymphocytes. J Exp Med 183:725–729

Boon T, Coulie PG, van den Eynde B (1997) Tumor antigens recognized by T cells. Immunol Today 18:267–268

Boshoff C, Weiss R (2002) AIDS-related malignancies. Nat Rev Cancer 2:373–382

Brandau S, Riemensberger J, Jacobsen M, Kemp D, Zhao W, Zhao X, Jocham D, Ratliff TL, Bohle A (2001) NK cells are essential for effective BCG immunotherapy. Int J Cancer 92:697–702

Brichard V, Van Pel A, Wolfel T, Wolfel C, De Plaen E, Lethe B, Coulie P, Boon T (1993) The tyrosinase gene codes for an antigen recognized by autologous cytolytic T lymphocytes on HLA-A2 melanomas. J Exp Med 178:489–495

Bronte V, Zanovello P (2005) Regulation of immune responses by L-arginine metabolism. Nat Rev Immunol 5:641–654

Cameron DA, Cornbleet MC, MacKie RM, Hunter JA, Gore M, Hancock B, Smyth JF. (2001) Adjuvant interferon alpha 2b in high risk melanoma—the Scottish study. Br J Cancer 84:1146–1149

Cheever MA, Disis ML, Bernhard H, Gralow JR, Hand SL, Huseby ES, Qin HL, Takahashi M, Chen W (1995) Immunity to oncogenic proteins. Immunol Rev 145:33–59

Chen YT, Scanlan MJ, Sahin U, Tureci O, Gure AO, Tsang S, Williamson B, Stockert E, Pfreundschuh M, Old LJ (1997) A testicular antigen aberrantly expressed in human cancers detected by autologous antibody screening. Proc Natl Acad Sci USA 94:1914–1918

Clark JI, Atkins MB, Urba WJ, Creech S, Figlin RA, Dutcher JP et al (2003) Adjuvant high-dose bolus interleukin-2 for patients with high risk renal cell carcinoma: a cytokine working group randomized trial. J Clin Oncol 21:3133–3140

Coley WB (1893) II. Hawkins on tubercular peritonitis. Ann Surg 17:462–464

Colomer R (2005) What is the best schedule for administration of gemcitabine-taxane? Cancer Treat Rev 31:S23–S28

Contassot E, Gaide O, French LE (2007) Death receptors and apoptosis. Dermatol Clin 25:487–501, vii

Coulie PG, Brichard V, Van Pel A, Wolfel T, Schneider J, Traversari C, Mattei S, De Plaen E, Lurquin C, Szikora JP, Renauld JC, Boon T (1994) A new gene coding for a differentiation antigen recognized by autologous cytolytic T lymphocytes on HLA-A2 melanomas. J Exp Med 180:35–42

Coulie PG, Ikeda H, Baurain JF, Chiari R (1999) Antitumor immunity at work in a melanoma patient. Adv Cancer Res 76:213–242

Degli-Esposti MA, Smyth MJ (2005) Close encounters of different kinds: dendritic cells and NK cells take centre stage. Nat Rev Immunol 5:112–124

Dillman RO, Church C, Barth NM, Oldham RK, Wiemann MC (1997) Long-term survival after continuous infusion interleukin-2; Cancer Biother Radiopharm 12:243–248

Dudley ME, Rosenberg SA (2007) Adoptive cell transfer therapy. Semin Oncol 34:524–531

Dunn GP, Bruce AT, Ikeda H, Old LJ, Schreiber RD (2002) Cancer immunoediting: from immunosurveillance to tumor escape. Nat Immunol 3:991–998

Dunn GP, Old LJ, Schreiber RD (2004) The three Es of cancer immunoediting. Annu Rev Immunol 22:329–360

Falkson CI, Ibrahim J, Kirkwood JM, Coates AS, Atkins MB, Blum RH (1998) Phase III trial of dacarbazine versus dacarbazine with interferon alpha-2v versus dacarbazine with tamoxifen in patients with metastatic malignant melanoma: an Eastern Cooperative Oncology Group study. J Clin Oncol 16:1743–1751

Foon KA, Maluish AE, Abrams PG, et al. (1986) Recombinant leukocyte A interferon therapy for advanced hairy cell leukemia. Therapeutic and immunologic results. Am J Med. 80:351–356

Furtado GC, Curotto de Lafaille MA, Kutchukhidze N, Lafaille JJ (2002) Interleukin 2 signaling is required for CD4+ regulatory T cell function. J Exp Med 196:851–857

Fyfe G, Fisher RI, Rosenberg SA et al (1995) Results of treatment of 255 patients with metastatic renal cell carcinoma who received high-dose recombinant interleukin-2 therapy. J Clin Oncol 13:688–696

Garbe C, Hauschild A, Volkenandt M, Schadendorf D, Stolz W, Reinhold U, Kortmann RD, Kettelhack C, Frerich B, Keilholz U, Dummer R, Sebastian G, Tilgen W, Schuler G, Mackensen A, Kaufmann R (2008) Evidence-based and interdisciplinary consensus-based German guidelines: systemic medical treatment of melanoma in the adjuvant and palliative setting. Melanoma Res. Apr 18:152–160

Gastpar R, Gehrmann M, Bausero MA, Asea A, Gross C, Schroeder JA, Multhoff G (2005) Heat shock protein 70 surface-positive tumor exosomes stimulate migratory and cytolytic activity of natural killer cells. Cancer Res 65:5238–5247

Gattinoni L, Powell DJ, Jr., Rosenberg SA, Restifo NP (2006) Adoptive immunotherapy for cancer: building on success. Nat Rev Immunol 6:383–393

Gnjatic S, Cai Z, Viguier M, Chouaib S, Guillet JG, Choppin J (1998) Accumulation of the p53 protein allows recognition by human CTL of a wild-type p53 epitope presented by breast carcinomas and melanomas. J Immunol 160:328–333

Grob JJ, Dreno B, de la SP, Delaunay M, Cupissol D, Guillot B et al (1998) Randomized trial of interferon alpha-2a as adjuvant therapy in resected primary melanoma thicker than 1.5 mm without clinically detectable node metastases. French Cooperative Group on Melanoma. Lancet 351:1905–1910

Gross C, Koelch W, DeMaio A, Arispe N, Multhoff G (2003) Cell surface-bound heat shock protein 70 (Hsp70) mediates perforin-independent apoptosis by specific binding and uptake of granzyme B. J Biol Chem 278:41173–41181

Guilhot F, Chastang C, Michallet M, Guerci A, Harousseau JL, Maloisel F, Bouabdallah R, Guyotat D, Cheron N, Nicolini F, Abgrall JF, Tanzer J (1997) Interferon alpha-2b combined with cytarabine versus interferon alone in chronic myelogenous leukaemia. N Engl J Med 337:223–229

Gure AO, Stockert E, Scanlan MJ, Keresztes RS, Jager D, Altorki NK, Old LJ, Chen YT (2000) Serological identification of embryonic neural proteins as highly immunogenic tumor antigens in small cell lung cancer. Proc Natl Acad Sci USA 97:4198–4203

Houghton AN, Brooks H, Cote RJ, Taormina MC, Oettgen HF, Old LJ (1983) Detection of cell surface and intracellular antigens by human monoclonal antibodies. Hybrid cell lines derived from lymphocytes of patients with malignant melanoma. J Exp Med 158:53–65

Jager E, Stockert E, Zidianakis Z, Chen YT, Karbach J, Jager D, Arand M, Ritter G, Old LJ, Knuth A (1999) Humoral immune responses of cancer patients against "Cancer-Testis" antigen NY-ESO-1:correlation with clinical events. Int J Cancer 84:506–510

Kappauf H, Gallmeier WM, Wunsch PH, Mittelmeier HO, Birkmann J, Buschel G, Kaiser G, Kraus J (1997) Complete spontaneous remission in a patient with metastatic non-small-cell lung cancer. Case report, review of the literature, and discussion of possible biological pathways involved. Ann Oncol 8:1031–1039

Kawakami Y, Eliyahu S, Jennings C, Sakaguchi K, Kang X, Southwood S, Robbins PF, Sette A, Appella E, Rosenberg SA (1995) Recognition of multiple epitopes in the human melanoma antigen gp100 by tumor-infiltrating T lymphocytes associated with in vivo tumor regression. J Immunol 154:3961–3968

Keilholz U, Goey SH, Punt CJ, Proebstle TM, Salzmann R, Scheibenbgen C et al (1997) Interferon alfa-2a and interleukin-2 with or without cisplatin in metastatic melanoma: a randomized trial of the European Organization for Research and Treatment of Cancer Melanoma Cooperative Group. J Clin Oncol 15:2579–2588

Kerl K, Prins C, Saurat JH, French LE (2006) Intralesional and intravenous treatment of cutaneous B-cell lymphomas with the monoclonal anti-CD20 antibody rituximab: report and follow-up of eight cases. Br J Dermatol 155:1197–1200

Kirkwood JM, Strawderman MH, Ernstoff MS, Smith TJ, Borden EC, Blum RH (1996) Interferon alfa-2b adjuvant therapy of high-risk resected cutaneous melanoma: the Eastern Cooperative Oncology Group Trial EST 1684. J Clin Oncol 14:7–17

Kirkwood JM, Ibrahim JG, Sondak VK et al (2000) High and low-dose interferon alfa-2b in high risk melanoma: first analysis of intergroup trial E1690/S9111/C9190. J Clin Oncol 18:2444–2458

Kirkwood JM, Ibrahim JG, Sosman JA et al (2000) High-dose interferon alfa-2b significantly prolongs relapse-free and overall survival compared with GM2-KLH/QS-21 vaccine in patients with resected stage IIB-III melanoma: results of an intergroup trial E1694/S9512/C509801. J Clin Oncol 19:2370–2380

Kohler G, Milstein C (1975) Continuous cultures of fused cells secreting antibody of predefined specificity. Nature 256:495–497

Koka R, Burkett PR, Chien M, Chai S, Chan F, Lodolce JP, Boone DL, Ma A (2003) Interleukin (IL)-15Rα-deficient natural killer cells survive in normal but not IL-15Rα-deficient mice. J Exp Med 197:977–984

Krause SW, Rothe G, Gnad M, Reichle A, Andreesen R (2003) Blood leukocyte subsets and cytokine profile after autologous peripheral blood stem cell transplantation. Ann Hematol 82:628–636

Kronenberg M (2005) Toward an understanding of NKT cell biology: progress and paradoxes. Annu Rev Immunol 23:877–900

Lanzavecchia A, Sallusto F (2001) Antigen decoding by T lymphocytes: from synapses to fate determination. Nat Immunol 2:487–492

Larsen SS, Egeblad M, Jaattela M, Lykkesfeldt AE (1999) Acquired antiestrogen resistance in MCF-7 human breast cancer sublines is not accomplished by altered expression of receptors in the ErbB-family. Breast Cancer Res Treat 58:41–56

Lennette ET, Winberg G, Yadav M, Enblad G, Klein G (1995) Antibodies to LMP2A/2B in EBV-carrying malignancies. Eur J Cancer 31A: 1875–1878

Ligibel JA, Winer EP (2002) Trastuzumab/chemotherapy combinations in metastatic breast cancer. Semin Oncol 29:38–43

Lilenbaum RC (2006) The evolving role of cetuximab in non-small cell lung cancer. Clin Cancer Res 12:4432s-4435s

Lin A, Rugo HS (2007) The role of trastuzumab in early stage breast cancer: current data and treatment recommendations. Curr Treat Options Oncol 8:47–60

Lyseng-Williamson KA, Robinson DM (2006) Spotlight on bevacizumab in advanced colorectal cancer, breast cancer, and non-small cell lung cancer. BioDrugs 20:193–195

Ma A, Koka R, Burkett P (2006a) Diverse functions of IL-2, IL-15, and IL-7 in lymphoid homeostasis. Annu Rev Immunol 24:657–679

Ma XT, Xu B, An LL, Dong CY, Lin YM, Shi Y, Wu KF (2006b) Vaccine with beta-defensin 2-transduced leukemic cells activates innate and adaptive immunity to elicit potent antileukemia responses. Cancer Res 66:1169–1176

Mackensen A, Carcelain G, Viel S, Raynal MC, Michalaki H, Triebel F, Bosq J, Hercend T (1994) Direct evidence to support the immunosurveillance concept in a human regressive melanoma. J Clin Invest 93:1397–1402

Mandruzzato S, Brasseur F, Andry G, Boon T, van der BP (1997) A CASP-8 mutation recognized by cytolytic T lymphocytes on a human head and neck carcinoma. J Exp Med 186:785–793

Mantovani G, Proto E, Lai P, Turnu E, Sulis G, Puxeddu P, Del Giacco GS (1992) [Controlled trial of thymostimulin treatment of patients with primary carcinoma of the larynx resected surgically. Immunological and clinical evaluation and therapeutic prospects]. Recenti Prog Med 83:303–306

McDermott DF, Regan MM, Clark JI et al (2005) Randomized phase III trial of high-dose interleukin-2 versus subcutaneous interleukin-2 and interferon in patients with metastatic renal cell carcinoma. J Clin Oncol 23:133–141

Medical Research Council Renal Cancer Collaborators (1999) Interferon-alpha and survival in metastatic renal carcinoma: early results of a randomized controlled trial. Lancet 353:14–17

Messing EM, Manola J, Wilding G, Propert K, Fleischmann J, Crawford ED et al (2003) Eastern Cooperative Oncology Group/Intergroup trial. Phase III study of interferon alfa-NL as adjuvant treatment for resectable renal cell carcinoma: an Eastern Cooperative Oncology Group/Intergroup trial. J Clin Oncol 21:1214–1222

Meyskens FL Jr, Kopecky K, Samson M, Hersh E, Macdonald J, Jaffe H et al (1990) Recombinant human interferon gamma: adverse effects in high-risk sag I and II cutaneous malignant melanoma. J Natl Cancer Inst 82:1071

Miller JS, Soignier Y, Panoskaltsis-Mortari A, McNearney SA, Yun GH, Fautsch SK, McKenna D, Le C, Defor TE, Burns LJ, Orchard PJ, Blazar BR, Wagner JE, Slungaard A, Weisdorf DJ, Okazaki IJ, McGlave PB (2005) Successful adoptive transfer and in vivo expansion of human haploidentical NK cells in patients with cancer. Blood 105:3051–3057

Morimoto RI (1991) Heat shock: the role of transient inducible responses in cell damage, transformation, and differentiation. Cancer Cells 3:295–301

Motzer RJ, Hutson TE, Tomczak P, Michaelson MD, Bukowski RM, Rixe O et al. (2007) Sunitinib versus interferon alfa in metastatic renal-cell carcinoma. N Engl J Med 356:115–124

Multhoff G, Botzler C, Jennen L, Schmidt J, Ellwart J, Issels R (1997) Heat shock protein 72 on tumor cells: a recognition structure for natural killer cells. J Immunol 158:4341–4350

Nair SK, Snyder D, Rouse BT, Gilboa E (1997) Regression of tumors in mice vaccinated with professional antigen-presenting cells pulsed with tumor extracts. Int J Cancer 70:706–715

Negrier S, Escudier B, Lasset Ch, Doullard JY, Savary J, Chevreau Ch, Ravaud A, Mercatello A, Peny J, Mousseau M, Philip T, Tursz T (1998) Recombinant human interleukin-2, recombinant human interferon alpha-2a, or both in metastatic renal-cell carcinoma. N Engl J Med 338:1272–1278

Ni CN, Redmond HP (2006) Regulatory T-cells and autoimmunity. J Surg Res 130:124–135

Odunsi K, Jungbluth AA, Stockert E, Qian F, Gnjatic S, Tammela J, Intengan M, Beck A, Keitz B, Santiago D, Williamson B, Scanlan MJ, Ritter G, Chen YT, Driscoll D, Sood A, Lele S, Old LJ (2003) NY-ESO-1 and LAGE-1 cancer-testis antigens are potential targets for immunotherapy in epithelial ovarian cancer. Cancer Res 63:6076–6083

Old LJ, Chen YT (1998) New paths in human cancer serology. J Exp Med 187:1163–1167

Ohnishi K, Ohno R, Tomonaga M et al (1995) A randomized trial comparing interferon-alfa with busulfan for newly diagnosed chronic myelogenous leukemia in chronic phase. Blood. 86:906–916

Parihar R, Dierksheide J, Hu Y, Carson WE (2002) IL-12 enhances the natural killer cell cytokine response to Ab-coated tumor cells. J Clin Invest 110:983–992

Pehamberger H, Soyer HP, Steiner A, Kofler R, Binder M, Mischer P et al (1998) Adjuvant interferon alfa-2a treatment in resected primary stage II cutaneous melanoma. Austrian Malignant Melanoma Cooperative Group. J Clin Oncol 16:1425–1429

Pierce SK (1994) Molecular chaperones in the processing and presentation of antigen to helper T cells. Experientia 50:1026–1030

Pulendran B, Ahmed R (2006) Translating innate immunity into immunological memory: implications for vaccine development. Cell 124:849–863

Quesada JR, Hersh EM, Manning J et al (1986) Treatment of hairy cell leukemia with recombinant alfa-interferon. Blood. 68:493–497

Ravandi F, O'Brien S (2006) Alemtuzumab in CLL and other lymphoid neoplasms. Cancer Invest 24:718–725

Renkvist N, Castelli C, Robbins PF, Parmiani G (2001) A listing of human tumor antigens recognized by T cells. Cancer Immunol Immunother 50:3–15

Ritossa P (1962) [Problems of prophylactic vaccinations of infants.]. Riv Ist Sieroter Ital 37:79–108

Robbins PF, El Gamil M, Li YF, Kawakami Y, Loftus D, Appella E, Rosenberg SA (1996) A mutated beta-catenin gene encodes a melanoma-specific antigen recognized by tumor infiltrating lymphocytes. J Exp Med 183:1185–1192

Robertson MJ (2002) Role of chemokines in the biology of natural killer cells. J Leukoc Biol 71:173–183

Rosenberg SA (1986) Adoptive immunotherapy of cancer using lymphokine activated killer cells and recombinant interleukin-2. Important Adv Oncol 55–91

Rosenberg SA, Packard BS, Aebersold PM, Solomon D, Topalian SL, Toy ST, Simon P, Lotze MT, Yang JC, Seipp CA (1988) Use of tumor-infiltrating lymphocytes and interleukin-2 in the immunotherapy of patients with metastatic melanoma. A preliminary report. N Engl J Med 319:1676–1680

Rosenberg SA, Lotze MT, Yang JC et al. (1993) Prospective randomized trial of high-dose interleukin-2 alone or in conjunction with lymphokine-activated killer cells for the treatment of patients with advanced cancer. J Natl Cancer Inst 85:622–632

Rudolf MP, Man S, Melief CJ, Sette A, Kast WM (2001) Human T-cell responses to HLA-A-restricted high binding affinity peptides of human papillomavirus type 18 proteins E6 and E7. Clin Cancer Res 7:788s–795s

Ruggeri L, Capanni M, Tosti A, Urbani E, Posati S, Aversa F, Martelli MF, Velardi A (2002) Innate immunity against hematological malignancies. Cytotherapy 4:343–346

Sallusto F, Lanzavecchia A (2000) Understanding dendritic cell and T-lymphocyte traffic through the analysis of chemokine receptor expression. Immunol Rev 177:134–140

Saltz LB (2005) Metastatic colorectal cancer: is there one standard approach? Oncology (Williston Park) 19:1147–1154

Sandler A, Gray R, Perry MC, Brahmer J, Schiller JH, Dowlati A, Lilenbaum R, Johnson DH (2006) Paclitaxel-carboplatin alone or with bevacizumab for non-small-cell lung cancer. N Engl J Med 355:2542–2550

Scanlan MJ, Altorki NK, Gure AO, Williamson B, Jungbluth A, Chen YT, Old LJ (2000) Expression of cancer-testis antigens in lung cancer: definition of bromodomain testis-specific gene (BRDT) as a new CT gene, CT9. Cancer Lett 150:155–164

Scanlan MJ, Chen YT, Williamson B, Gure AO, Stockert E, Gordan JD, Tureci O, Sahin U, Pfreundschuh M, Old LJ (1998) Characterization of human colon cancer antigens recognized by autologous antibodies. Int J Cancer 76:652–658

Schmitt E, Parcellier A, Gurbuxani S, Cande C, Hammann A, Morales MC, Hunt CR, Dix DJ, Kroemer RT, Giordanetto F, Jaattela M, Penninger JM, Pance A, Kroemer G, Garrido C (2003) Chemosensitization by a non-apoptogenic heat shock protein 70-binding apoptosis-inducing factor mutant. Cancer Res 63:8233–8240

Schmitt E, Gehrmann M, Brunet M, Multhoff G, Garrido C (2007) Intracellular and extracellular functions of heat shock proteins: repercussions in cancer therapy. J Leukoc Biol 81:15–27

Shin BK, Wang H, Yim AM, Le Naour F, Brichory F, Jang JH, Zhao R, Puravs E, Tra J, Michael CW, Misek DE, Hanash SM (2003) Global profiling of the cell surface proteome of cancer cells uncovers an abundance of proteins with chaperone function. J Biol Chem 278:7607–7616

Singh AP, Moniaux N, Chauhan SC, Meza JL, Batra SK (2004) Inhibition of MUC4 expression suppresses pancreatic tumor cell growth and metastasis. Cancer Res 64:622–630

Smith KA, Green JA, Eccles JM (1992) Interferon alpha 2a and vindesin in the treatment of advanced malignant melanoma. Eur J Cancer 28:438–441

Smyth MJ, Trapani JA (2001) Lymphocyte-mediated immunosurveillance of epithelial cancers? Trends Immunol 22:409–411

Smyth MJ, Cretney E, Takeda K, Wiltrout RH, Sedger LM, Kayagaki N, Yagita H, Okumura K (2001a) Tumor necrosis factor-related apoptosis-inducing ligand (TRAIL) contributes to interferon gamma-dependent natural killer cell protection from tumor metastasis. J Exp Med 193:661–670

Smyth MJ, Crowe NY, Godfrey DI (2001b) NK cells and NKT cells collaborate in host protection from methylcholanthrene-induced fibrosarcoma. Int Immunol 13:459–463

Smyth MJ, Cretney E, Kershaw MH, Hayakawa Y (2004) Cytokines in cancer immunity and immunotherapy. Immunol Rev 202:275–293

Srivastava PK (1997) Purification of heat shock protein-peptide complexes for use in vaccination against cancers and intracellular pathogens. Methods 12:165–171

Srivastava PK, Menoret A, Basu S, Binder RJ, McQuade KL (1998) Heat shock proteins come of age: primitive functions acquire new roles in an adaptive world. Immunity 8:657–665

Stangl S, Wortmann A, Guertler U, Multhoff G (2006) Control of metastasized pancreatic carcinomas in SCID/beige mice with human IL-2/TKD-activated NK cells. J Immunol 176:6270–6276

Steinman RM, Inaba K (1999) Myeloid dendritic cells. J Leukoc Biol 66:205–208

Steplewski Z, Spira G, Blaszczyk M, Lubeck MD, Radbruch A, Illges H, Herlyn D, Rajewsky K, Scharff M (1985) Isolation and characterization of anti-monosialoganglioside monoclonal antibody 19–9 class-switch variants. Proc Natl Acad Sci USA 82:8653–8657

Suttmann H, Riemensberger J, Bentien G, Schmaltz D, Stockle M, Jocham D, Bohle A, Brandau S (2006) Neutrophil granulocytes are required for effective bacillus Calmette-Guerin immunotherapy of bladder cancer and orchestrate local immune responses. Cancer Res 66:8250–8257

Tindle RW (1996) Human papillomavirus vaccines for cervical cancer. Curr Opin Immunol 8:643–650

Tobinai K (2007) 4. Antibody therapy for malignant lymphoma. Intern Med 46:99–100

Tobinai K, Watanabe T, Ogura M, Morishima Y, Ogawa Y, Ishizawa K, Minami H, Utsunomiya A, Taniwaki M, Terauchi T, Nawano S, Matsusako M, Matsuno Y, Nakamura S, Mori S, Ohashi Y, Hayashi M, Seriu T, Hotta T (2006) Phase II study of oral fludarabine phosphate in relapsed indolent B-cell non-Hodgkin's lymphoma. J Clin Oncol 24:174–180

Trauth BC, Klas C, Peters AM, Matzku S, Moller P, Falk W, Debatin KM, Krammer PH (1989) Monoclonal antibody-mediated tumor regression by induction of apoptosis. Science 245:301–305

Trinchieri G (1989) Biology of natural killer cells. Adv Immunol 47:187–376

Turley SJ (2002) Dendritic cells: inciting and inhibiting autoimmunity. Curr Opin Immunol 14:765–770

Tzankov A, Ludescher C, Duba HC, Steinlechner M, Knapp R, Schmid T, Grunewald K, Gastl G, Stauder R (2001) Spontaneous remission in a secondary acute myelogenous leukaemia following invasive pulmonary aspergillosis. Ann Hematol 80:423–425

Van den Eynde BJ, Boon T (1997) Tumor antigens recognized by T lymphocytes. Int J Clin Lab Res 27:81–86

Van den Eynde BJ, van der Brugge BP (1997) T cell defined tumor antigens. Curr Opin Immunol 9:684–693

Wang RF, Rosenberg SA (1999) Human tumor antigens for cancer vaccine development. Immunol Rev 170:85–100

Wolfel T, Hauer M, Schneider J, Serrano M, Wolfel C, Klehmann-Hieb E, De Plaen E, Hankeln T, Meyer zum Buschenfelde KH, Beach D (1995) A p16INK4a-insensitive CDK4 mutant targeted by cytolytic T lymphocytes in a human melanoma. Science 269:1281–1284

Yang JC, Sherry RM, Steinberg SM et al. (2003) Randomized study of high-dose and low-dose interleukin-2 in patients with metastatic renal cancer. J Clin Oncol 21:3127–3132

Yang XD, Jia XC, Corvalan JR, Wang P, Davis CG, Jakobovits A (1999) Eradication of established tumors by a fully human monoclonal antibody to the epidermal growth factor receptor without concomitant chemotherapy. Cancer Res 59:1236–1243

Youde SJ, Dunbar PR, Evans EM, Fiander AN, Borysiewicz LK, Cerundolo V, Man S (2000) Use of fluorogenic histocompatibility leukocyte antigen-A*0201/HPV 16 E7 peptide complexes to isolate rare human cytotoxic T-lymphocyte-recognizing endogenous human papillomavirus antigens. Cancer Res 60:365–371

Zhang H, Chua KS, Guimond M, Kapoor V, Brown MV, Fleisher TA, Long LM, Bernstein D, Hill BJ, Douek DC, Berzofsky JA, Carter CS, Read EJ, Helman LJ, Mackall CL (2005) Lymphopenia and interleukin-2 therapy alter homeostasis of CD4+CD25+ regulatory T cells. Nat Med 11:1238–1243

Zhang Y, Louboutin JP, Zhu J, Rivera AJ, Emerson SG (2002) Preterminal host dendritic cells in irradiated mice prime CD8+ T cell-mediated acute graft-versus-host disease. J Clin Invest 109:13

Tumor Detection by Biological Markers

Carsten Nieder and Adam Pawinski

CONTENTS

KEY POINTS

- Screening, i.e., testing for a condition when the person has no recognized signs or symptoms of that condition, can only be justified if an increase in overall survival or other important endpoints related to disease complications and symptoms can be demonstrated. In addition, there must be a treatment for the disease that is more effective when applied to screening-detected cancers than clinically detected cancers. People with positive screening tests usually undergo confirmatory examinations to determine whether the condition is present.
- Physical examination and endoscopy, with or without cytology and biopsy, are still mainstays of cancer detection.
- The use of classical serum tumor markers, e.g., for screening of breast, lung, or bowel cancer, has largely failed. Unanswered questions still remain about the pros and cons of prostate-specific antigen measurements.
- Advances in proteomic technologies have created tremendous opportunities for biomarker discovery and biological studies of cancer. Early results are presented here.
- The paradigm of vaccination against virus-induced cancers or precancerous lesions has been corroborated in clinical trials, e.g., in cervical cancer.

C. Nieder, MD
Department of Medicine, Nordlandssykehuset HF, Prinsensgate 164, 8092 Bodø, Norway

A. Pawinski, MD
Department of Medicine, Nordlandssykehuset HF, Prinsensgate 164, 8092 Bodø, Norway

- One of the direct and indirect lessons learned from unsuccessful cancer prevention studies is that cancer biology is more complex than previously thought, and that the outcome of prevention trials might be less predictable than anticipated, both with regard to efficacy and toxicity of some of the agents studied so far. Whether different targets can be utilized to provide the right intervention for the appropriate high-risk group in a given type of cancer is currently being examined in the next generation of clinical trials.

8.1
Introduction

This chapter contains a brief discussion of cancer prevention and early detection strategies, and addresses some of the controversies around recent clinical trials. It is meant to provide a guide to more detailed reviews for the interested reader rather than summarizing these topics in a comprehensive fashion. As treatment of advanced malignant diseases still results in less satisfactory results than treatment of early-stage disease, the need for reducing the number of patients diagnosed in advanced or incurable stages is obvious. Also, in terms of aggressiveness of treatment, side effects, quality of life, and other aspects of cancer survivorship, less aggressive or intense treatment will result in many advantages. This will also impact on several economical aspects of treatment, even if the cost of cancer screening and/or prevention must be balanced against the cost reduction, i.e., the net health benefits must come at a reasonable cost. Other important aspects that often fuel the discussion include the potential harm and damage associated with, for example, cancer screening (false-positive results, treatment of biologically insignificant lesions that would never threaten the patient's life, and so on). This leads to the search for tailored strategies targeting populations that are at higher than average risk and resulting in improved health outcomes.

Reducing the number of patients diagnosed with malignant diseases and the number of cancer survivors that eventually develop second primary tumors after effective initial treatment is an important goal of current anticancer strategies (NG and TRAVIS 2008). This requires detailed knowledge about carcinogenesis and risk factors for cancer development and progression in

order to tailor effective prevention programs. Dietary interventions, smoking cessation, increased physical activity, and pharmacologic interventions based on rational targets are among the strategies studied so far (SHAIPANICH et al. 2006; PRENTICE et al. 2007; LANZA et al. 2007; THOMPSON et al. 2007; VAN ADELSBERG et al. 2007; WILT et al. 2008). In addition, achieving early diagnosis of curable tumors will reduce the need for more aggressive, but nevertheless less effective, treatment of advanced tumors. The potential implications, e.g., in terms of cost-reduction, quality of life, role functioning, and so forth, are obvious. It would, however, be naïve to believe that development of cancer prevention and early detection programs that try to target populations at higher than average risk, and spare the potential disadvantages to as many people as possible, is less complicated and time-consuming than development of more effective and less toxic therapeutic strategies. One must not forget that screening can only be justified if an increase in overall survival or other important endpoints related to disease complications and symptoms can be demonstrated (MYERS et al. 2007). In addition, there must be a treatment for the disease that is more effective when applied to screening-detected cancers than clinically detected cancers.

8.2
Some Issues Around Cancer Prevention

One of the first seminal papers that reported a clinical cancer prevention trial was published in 1981 (PETO et al. 1981). Since then, and based on current concepts of cancer initiation and progression, numerous nutritional and pharmacologic approaches have been studied, including radical scavengers, enzyme inhibitors, immune modulators, inflammation inhibitors, and DNA repair modulators. In addition, the paradigm of vaccination against virus-induced cancers or precancerous lesions has been corroborated in clinical trials, e.g., in cervical cancer (PAAVONEN et al. 2007; HERZOG et al. 2008; KOSHIOL et al. 2008; MYERS et al. 2008). *Helicobacter pylori* screening and treatment is a recommended gastric cancer risk-reduction strategy in high-risk populations (FOCK et al. 2008). One of the direct and indirect lessons learned from unsuccessful studies is that cancer biology is more complex than previously thought, and that the outcome of prevention trials might be less predictable than anticipated (ARBER and LEVIN 2008; BARDIA et al. 2008; ZHANG et al. 2008). No clear recommendation can be given for the use of statins or antioxidants at this time (BONOVAS et al. 2007, 2008; BARDIA et al. 2008), yet uncertainty exists as to whether previous studies were optimal with regard to dose and timing of the intervention. Nevertheless, important and relevant targets for cancer prevention continue to exist. Whether these targets can be utilized to provide the right intervention for the appropriate high-risk group in a given type of cancer is currently being examined in the next generation of clinical trials (e.g., dutasteride in prostate cancer, and various calcium or vitamin D studies). Such trials will also need to address the role of potential confounders, e.g., interactions of the test drug(s) with other concomitant medications as discussed in the recent report by DING et al. (2008).

8.3
Tumor Detection by Serum Markers

The use of classical tumor markers, such as carcinoembryonic antigen, squamous cell carcinoma antigen, and neuron-specific enolase, to name just a few, for screening and early detection of common malignant tumors, e.g., lung and breast cancer, has largely resulted in disappointing results. A helpful marker would separate the population, which has no recognized signs or symptoms of the malignant disease the test is supposed to detect, into two different groups either having or not having the disease, e.g., lung cancer. Ideally, false-negative or false-positive results would not exist. Such highly accurate results typically are not seen; thus, problems with over-diagnosis and overtreatment might be the consequence. In addition, common malignant diseases, such as lung or breast cancer, are tremendously heterogeneous both on a histologic and molecular level. It is not the aim of a test to detect a lesion that would never progress to a clinically meaningful condition, e.g., invasive cancer. Prostate-specific antigen (PSA) has increasingly been used for prostate cancer screening in recent years in addition to digital rectal examination (ROOBOL et al. 2007). The low positive predictive value of elevated PSA results in large numbers of unnecessary prostate biopsies (LILJA et al. 2008; MARGREITER et al. 2008); thus, the benefits of prostate cancer screening in average-risk men are not clear. Controversy exists also about screening in elderly men. Shared decision making, i.e., informing men of the pros and cons, is often recommended. In a cohort of 740 men in Göteborg, Sweden, undergoing biopsy during the first round of the European Randomized study of Screening for Prostate Cancer, a not-only-PSA-based approach was evaluated (VICKERS et al. 2008). It included additional kallikreins and suggests that multiple kallikrein forms measured in blood can predict the result of biopsy in previously unscreened men with elevated PSA. A multivariable model can determine which men should be advised to undergo biopsy and which might be advised to continue screening, but defer biopsy until there was stronger evidence of malignancy. The American Cancer Society guidelines have recently been published by SMITH et al. (2008). They also address screening for breast, colorectal, cervix, and endometrial cancer. Besides PSA, no other serum tumor marker is mentioned in the guidelines.

Advances in proteomic technologies have created tremendous opportunities for biomarker discovery and biological studies of cancer (GRÄNTZDÖRFFER et al. 2008; HANASH et al. 2008). The probability that proteomics will impact clinical practice is currently greater than ever, but there remain several obstacles in making this a reality. Yet, some encouraging preliminary experience has been reported. Proteomic expression profiling has, for example, recently been studied in breast cancer (DE NOO et al. 2006a). In a randomized block design pre-operative serum samples obtained from 78 breast cancer patients and 29 controls were used to generate high-resolution MALDI-TOF protein profiles. The spectra generated using C8 magnetic-beads-assisted mass spectrometry were smoothed, binned, and normalized after baseline correction. Linear discriminant analysis with double cross-validation, based on principal component analysis, was used to classify the protein profiles. A total recognition rate of 99%, a sensitivity of 100%, and a specificity of 97% for the detection of breast cancer were shown. The area under the curve of the classifier was 98%, which demonstrates the separation power of the classifier. Although preliminary, the high sensitivity and specificity indicate the potential usefulness of serum protein profiles for the detection of breast cancer. Almost identical results were found in a small group of patients with colorectal cancer (DE NOO et al. 2006b).

8.4
Tumor Detection by Other Tests

Physical examination and endoscopy are still mainstays of cancer detection, e.g., in the gastrointestinal (GI) tract, the skin, and the lower urogenital tract (GUPTA et al. 2008; PALKA et al. 2008; REX and EID 2008; SHIRODKAR and LOKESHWAR 2008). Screening for cervical cancer (and cervical intraepithelial neoplasia) with the Papanicolaou (Pap) test is a good example for this strategy. Newer techniques that employ liquid-based cytology have recently been developed. Endoscopic trimodal imaging incorporating white-light endoscopy, autofluorescence imaging, and narrow-band imaging is under evaluation in GI tumors (VAN DEN BROEK et al. 2008).

Quantification of circulating cell-free plasma DNA by real-time PCR may be a new tool for detection of breast cancer with a potential to clinical applicability together with other current methods (CATARINO et al. 2008). A recent review provides further information on measuring extracellular nucleic acids, both DNA and mRNA in different biological media, including serum, plasma, saliva, urine, and bronchial lavage (O'DRISCOLL 2007). SELDI and MALDI profiling are being used increasingly to search for biomarkers in both blood and urine. Both techniques provide information predominantly on the low molecular weight proteome (<15 kDa). There have been several reports that colorectal cancer is associated with changes in the serum proteome that are detectable by SELDI, and after that, proteomic changes have also been assessed in urine (WARD et al. 2008). These early data await confirmation by other groups. Metabolomics is the quantitative measurement of the metabolic response to pathophysiological stimuli. This analysis provides a metabolite pattern that can be characteristic of various benign and malignant conditions. ISSAQ et al. (2008) evaluated high performance liquid chromatography coupled online with a mass spectrometer metabolomic approach to differentiate urine samples from healthy individuals and patients with bladder cancer. This study with a limited number of patients also suggests that further evaluation of this approach is justified. Other approaches try to predict lung cancer employing volatile biomarkers in the breath (CHAN et al. 2008; PHILLIPS et al. 2008); thus, the hope to improve early detection of cancer with relatively simple, but accurate, tests based on examination of body fluids, breath, or mucosa specimens has not decreased despite several disappointing studies that failed to alter our clinical practice in the past. The role of imaging studies providing anatomical and/or physiological and functional information are discussed in greater detail in Chap. 9 of this volume. Regarding the specific roles of breast magnetic resonance imaging, magnetic resonance colonography, computed tomographic colonography, and lung computed tomography, the interested reader is referred to PETERS et al. (2008), WARNER et al. (2008), HALLIGAN and TAYLOR (2007), MULHALL et al. (2005), PURKAYASTHA et al. (2005), BLANCHON et al. (2007), and CRONIN et al. (2008).

References

Arber N, Levin B (2008) Chemoprevention of colorectal neoplasia: the potential for personalized medicine. Gastroenterology 134:1224–1237

Bardia A, Tleyjeh IM, Cerhan JR et al. (2008) Efficacy of antioxidant supplementation in reducing primary cancer incidence and mortality: systematic review and meta-analysis. Mayo Clin Proc 83:23–34

Blanchon T, Bréchot JM, Grenier PA et al. (2007) Baseline results of the Depiscan study: a French randomized pilot trial of lung cancer screening comparing low dose CT scan (LDCT) and chest X-ray (CXR). Lung Cancer 58:50–58

Bonovas S, Filioussi K, Flordellis CS et al. (2007) Statins and the risk of colorectal cancer: a meta-analysis of 18 studies involving more than 1.5 million patients. J Clin Oncol 25:3462–3468

Bonovas S, Filioussi K, Sitaras NM (2008) Statin use and the risk of prostate cancer: a metaanalysis of 6 randomized clinical trials and 13 observational studies. Int J Cancer 123:899–904

Catarino R, Ferreira MM, Rodrigues H et al. (2008) Quantification of free circulating tumor DNA as a diagnostic marker for breast cancer. DNA Cell Biol 27:415–421

Chan HP, Lewis C, Thomas PS (2008) Exhaled breath analysis: novel approach for early detection of lung cancer. Lung Cancer epub

Cronin P, Dwamena BA, Kelly AM et al. (2008) Solitary pulmonary nodules: meta-analytic comparison of cross-sectional imaging modalities for diagnosis of malignancy. Radiology 246:772–782

De Noo ME, Deelder A, van der Werff M et al. (2006a) MALDI-TOF serum protein profiling for the detection of breast cancer. Onkologie 29:501–506

De Noo ME, Mertens BJ, Ozalp A, et al. (2006b) Detection of colorectal cancer using MALDI-TOF serum protein profiling. Eur J Cancer 42:1068–1076

Ding EL, Mehta S, Fawzi WW et al. (2008) Interaction of estrogen therapy with calcium and vitamin D supplementation on colorectal cancer risk: reanalysis of Women's Health Initiative randomized trial. Int J Cancer 122:1690–1694

Fock KM, Talley N, Moayyedi P et al. (2008) Asia-Pacific consensus guidelines on gastric cancer prevention. J Gastroenterol Hepatol 23:351–365

Gräntzdörffer I, Carl-McGrath S, Ebert MP et al. (2008) Proteomics of pancreatic cancer. Pancreas 36:329–336

Gupta AK, Brenner DE, Turgeon DK (2008) Early detection of colon cancer: new tests on the horizon. Mol Diagn Ther 12:77–85

Halligan S, Taylor SA (2007) CT colonography: results and limitations. Eur J Radiol 61:400–408

Hanash SM, Pitteri SJ, Faca VM (2008) Mining the plasma proteome for cancer biomarkers. Nature 452:571–579

Herzog TJ, Huh WK, Downs LS (2008) Initial lessons learned in HPV vaccination. Gynecol Oncol 109:S4–S11

Issaq HJ, Nativ O, Waybright T et al. (2008) Detection of bladder cancer in human urine by metabolomic profiling using high performance liquid chromatography/mass spectrometry. J Urol 179:2422–2426

Koshiol J, Lindsay L, Pimenta JM et al. (2008) Persistent human papillomavirus infection and cervical neoplasia: a systematic review and meta-analysis. Am J Epidemiol 168:123–137

Lanza E, Yu B, Murphy G et al. (2007) The polyp prevention trial continued follow-up study: no effect of a low-fat, high-fiber, high-fruit, and -vegetable diet on adenoma recurrence eight years after randomization. Cancer Epidemiol Biomarkers Prev 16:1745–1752

Lilja H, Ulmert D, Vickers AJ (2008) Prostate-specific antigen and prostate cancer: prediction, detection and monitoring. Nat Rev Cancer 8:268–278. Erratum in: Nat Rev Cancer 8:403

Margreiter M, Stangelberger A, Valimberti E et al. (2008) Biomarkers for early prostate cancer detection. Minerva Urol Nefrol 60:51–60

Mulhall BP, Veerappan GR, Jackson JL (2005) Meta-analysis: computed tomographic colonography. Ann Intern Med 142:635–650

Myers RE, Sifri R, Hyslop T et al. (2007) A randomized controlled trial of the impact of targeted and tailored interventions on colorectal cancer screening. Cancer 110:2083–2091

Myers E, Huh WK, Wright JD et al. (2008) The current and future role of screening in the era of HPV vaccination. Gynecol Oncol 109:S31–S39. Erratum in: Gynecol Oncol 110:270

Ng AK, Travis LB (2008) Second primary cancers: an overview. Hematol Oncol Clin North Am 22:271–289

O'Driscoll L (2007) Extracellular nucleic acids and their potential as diagnostic, prognostic and predictive biomarkers. Anticancer Res 27:1257–1265

Paavonen J, Jenkins D, Bosch FX et al. (2007) Efficacy of a prophylactic adjuvanted bivalent L1 virus-like-particle vaccine against infection with human papillomavirus types 16 and 18 in young women: an interim analysis of a phase III double-blind, randomised controlled trial. Lancet 369:2161–2170. Erratum in: Lancet 370:1414

Palka KT, Slebos RJ, Chung CH (2008) Update on molecular diagnostic tests in head and neck cancer. Semin Oncol 35:198–210

Peters NH, Borel Rinkes IH, Zuithoff NP et al. (2008) Meta-analysis of MR imaging in the diagnosis of breast lesions. Radiology 246:116–124

Peto R, Doll R, Buckley JD et al. (1981) Can dietary beta-carotene materially reduce human cancer rates? Nature 290:201–208

Phillips M, Altorki N, Austin JH et al. (2008) Detection of lung cancer using weighted digital analysis of breath biomarkers. Clin Chim Acta 393:76–84

Prentice RL, Thomson CA, Caan B et al. (2007) Low-fat dietary pattern and cancer incidence in the Women's Health Initiative Dietary Modification Randomized Controlled Trial. J Natl Cancer Inst 99:1534–1543

Purkayastha S, Tekkis PP, Athanasiou T et al. (2005) Magnetic resonance colonography versus colonoscopy as a diagnostic investigation for colorectal cancer: a meta-analysis. Clin Radiol 60:980–989

Rex DK, Eid E (2008) Considerations regarding the present and future roles of colonoscopy in colorectal cancer prevention. Clin Gastroenterol Hepatol 6:506–514

Roobol MJ, Grenabo A, Schröder FH et al. (2007) Interval cancers in prostate cancer screening: comparing 2- and 4-year screening intervals in the European Randomized Study of Screening for Prostate Cancer, Gothenburg and Rotterdam. J Natl Cancer Inst 99:1296–1303

Shaipanich T, McWilliams A, Lam S (2006) Early detection and chemoprevention of lung cancer. Respirology 11:366–372

Shirodkar SP, Lokeshwar VB (2008) Bladder tumor markers: from hematuria to molecular diagnostics—Where do we stand? Expert Rev Anticancer Ther 8:1111–1123

Smith RA, Cokkinides V, Brawley OW (2008) Cancer screening in the United States, 2008: a review of current American Cancer Society guidelines and cancer screening issues. CA Cancer J Clin 58:161–179

Thompson IM, Pauler Ankerst D et al. (2007) Prediction of prostate cancer for patients receiving finasteride: results from the Prostate Cancer Prevention Trial. J Clin Oncol 25:3076–3081

Van Adelsberg J, Gann P, Ko AT et al. (2007) The VIOXX in Prostate Cancer Prevention study: cardiovascular events observed in the rofecoxib 25 mg and placebo treatment groups. Curr Med Res Opin 23:2063–2070

Van den Broek FJ, Fockens P, van Eeden S et al. (2008) Endoscopic tri-modal imaging for surveillance in ulcerative colitis: randomised comparison of high-resolution endoscopy and autofluorescence imaging for neoplasia detection; and evaluation of narrow-band imaging for classification of lesions. Gut 57:1083–1089

Vickers AJ, Cronin AM, Aus G et al. (2008) A panel of kallikrein markers can reduce unnecessary biopsy for prostate cancer: data from the European Randomized Study of Prostate Cancer Screening in Göteborg, Sweden. BMC Med 6:19

Ward DG, Nyangoma S, Joy H et al. (2008) Proteomic profiling of urine for the detection of colon cancer. Proteome Sci 6:19

Warner E, Messersmith H, Causer P et al. (2008) Systematic review: using magnetic resonance imaging to screen women at high risk for breast cancer. Ann Intern Med 148:671–679

Wilt TJ, MacDonald R, Hagerty K et al. (2008) Five-alpha-reductase inhibitors for prostate cancer prevention. Cochrane Database Syst Rev:CD007091

Zhang SM, Cook NR, Manson JE et al. (2008) Low-dose aspirin and breast cancer risk: results by tumour characteristics from a randomised trial. Br J Cancer 98:989–991

9

Tumor Imaging with Special Emphasis on the Role of Positron Emission Tomography in Radiation Treatment Planning

Anca-Ligia Grosu, Wolfgang A. Weber, and Ursula Nestle

CONTENTS

KEY POINTS

- Radiological imaging of malignant processes has evolved tremendously over recent decades. It not only provides better detection with superior anatomical resolution through rapid advances in CT and MRI technology, but it also provides functional and physiological information. For example, in lung cancer the diagnostic accuracy of FDG-PET is between 85% and 90%.
- In brain tumors, the sensitivity and specificity of MET-PET for tumor detection and tumor tissue extension are significantly higher in comparison to MRI, CT or FDG-PET.
- While CT-based three-dimensional (3-D) treatment planning already represented a major step compared to the 2-D era, integration of MRI and PET and refinement of image fusion techniques resulted in further significant improvements.
- The high percentage of changes in radiotherapy target volumes of lung cancer patients by FDG-PET reported in the literature is mainly caused by two factors: the ability to distinguish the tumor from collapsed lung tissue and the higher accuracy of FDG-PET in lymph node staging compared to CT.
- Problems include the low resolution of PET images, which is caused by physical factors (size of the detector crystals, positron range in matter, non-collinearity of annihilation gamma rays and detector scatter) and also by movement of the target during acquisition due to relatively long acquisition times, which leads to a blurred margin of the accumulating structure. Other problems include patient positioning and image coregistration.

A.-L. Grosu, MD
Department of Radiation Oncology, Universitätsklinikum Freiburg, Robert-Koch-Straße 3, 79106 Freiburg, Germany

W. A. Weber, MD
Department of Nuclear Medicine, Universitätsklinikum Freiburg, Robert-Koch-Straße 3, 79106 Freiburg, Germany

U. Nestle, MD
Department of Radiation Oncology, Universitätsklinikum Freiburg, Robert-Koch-Straße 3, 79106 Freiburg, Germany

- The possible impact of FDG-PET for target volume delineation in head and neck cancer has been investigated in several trials. All these studies showed that FDG-PET could have a significant impact on gross target volume (GTV) delineation in comparison to CT (or MRI) alone. Here, as in lung tumors, in about one third of cases FDG-PET led to an increase in GTV, whereas in another one third of cases the GTV became smaller, if based on FDG alone.
- In recent years, PET tracers have been developed that can visualize biological pathways with particular significance for tumor response to the treatment. These are, for example, hypoxia, cell proliferation, and angiogenesis.
- Ongoing clinical studies will provide important data on the added value of PET, dynamic MRI, diffusion tensor MRI, and other recently developed imaging methods regarding target volume delineation as well as response monitoring.

Abstract

Precise imaging of the primary tumor, the drainage lymph nodes, and possible sites of distant metastases is mandatory to stage a malignant disease, arrive at a treatment recommendation, and eventually define an accurate gross tumor and clinical target volume for radiotherapy. Better target definition and delineation on a daily basis is surely important in quality assurance for fractionated radiation therapy. The availability of metabolic images obtained by magnetic resonance (MR) spectroscopy, positron emission tomography (PET), and others impacts on staging, treatment planning, and response monitoring. A broad range of techniques, including dynamic magnetic resonance imaging (MRI), PET, and single-photon emission computed tomography (SPECT), provide measurements of various features of tumor blood flow and microvasculature. Using PET to measure glucose consumption enables visualization of tumor metabolism, and MR spectroscopy techniques provide complementary information on energy metabolism. Changes in protein and DNA synthesis can be assessed through uptake of labeled amino acids and nucleosides. Advanced imaging techniques can be used to assess tumor malignancy, extent, and infiltration, and might provide diagnostic clues to distinguish between

lesion types. For the detection of metastatic lymph nodes, lymphotropic nanoparticle-enhanced MRI using ultra-small superparamagnetic iron oxide particles has greater accuracy as compared with conventional techniques and has been instrumental in delineating the lymphatic drainage of the prostate gland. The focus of the present chapter is the impact of PET on radiation treatment planning.

9.1
Introduction

The first rationale for using positron emission tomography (PET) in target volume delineation for radiation treatment planning is the higher sensitivity and specificity of PET for tumor tissue, in comparison to computed tomography (CT) and magnetic resonance imaging (MRI), in some tumor entities. This has been demonstrated in many studies that compared the results of PET with the results of the radiological investigations and histology. The hypothesis tested in these studies was that using PET in addition to CT and/or MRI enables tumor tissue detection with a higher accuracy. The ideal PET tracer in this situation should be taken up homogenously from all the cells of the whole tumor and the intensity of the PET uptake should be directly proportional to the density of tumor cells.

The second rationale for integrating PET in the process of radiation treatment planning is the ability of PET to visualize biological pathways, which can be targeted by radiation therapy. The imaging of hypoxia, angiogenesis, proliferation, apoptosis, etc. leads to the identification of different areas within an inhomogeneous tumor mass, areas which can be individually targeted. For example, hypoxic areas can be treated with higher radiation doses than non-hypoxic areas.

The goal of this chapter is to discuss the use of PET for target delineation in the process of radiation treatment planning.

9.2
PET for Target Volume Delineation

The impact of PET for gross tumor volume (GTV) delineation will be discussed based on three examples: amino acids-PET in brain gliomas, fluorine-18-labeled glucose analog fluorodeoxyglucose (FDG)-PET in lung cancer, and FDG-PET in head and neck tumors.

9.2.1
Amino Acids-PET and Single-Photon Emission CT in Brain Tumors

[11]C-labeled methionine (MET), ^{123}I-labeled alpha-methyltyrosine (IMT), and ^{18}F-labeled O-(2-fluoroethyl)-L-tyrosine (FET) are the most important radiolabeled amino acids used in the diagnosis of brain tumors. These three tracers have shown a very similar uptake intensity and distribution in brain tumors (LANGEN et al. 1997; WEBER et al. 2000). Currently available amino acid-PET tracers are accumulated by L and A amino acid transporters. Tumor cells take up radiolabeled amino acids at a high rate, while there is only a relatively low uptake in normal cerebral tissue. At the level of the blood–brain barrier (BBB) they are independent from the BBB disturbance.

Summarizing the data of the literature based on a PubMed search (using the key words: methionine, PET, and brain tumors) we found 45 clinical trials published between 1983 and March 2007, including 1,721 patients. In 11 studies investigating 706 patients, the data were analyzed using MET-PET-guided stereotactic biopsies. The main message of the trials is that the sensitivity and the specificity of MET-PET for tumor detection and tumor tissue extension are significantly higher in comparison to MRI, CT, or FDG-PET (WEBER et al. 2008).

We evaluated the impact of MET-PET in target volume delineation for radiation treatment planning, compared to MRI, in 39 patients with brain gliomas after tumor resection (GROSU et al. 2003, 2005a). MET uptake corresponded to the gadolinium (Gd) enhancement in only 13% of the cases. In 74% of the patients MET volume extended beyond the contrast-enhancing regions, indicating residual tumor. In 69% of the cases Gd enhancement could be outlined beyond the volume of MET uptake, showing postoperative BBB disturbance. Similar results were also reported evaluating the impact of IMT-single-photon emission CT (SPECT) in target volume delineation in non-resected (GROSU et al. 2000) and resected (GROSU et al. 2002) patients with gliomas. Focal IMT uptake after tumor resection was highly correlated with poor survival, suggesting that amino acids are specific markers for residual tumor tissue (WEBER et al. 2001). The first study evaluating the value of MET-PET or IMT-SPECT for treatment outcome was performed in 44 patients with recurrent gliomas re-irradiated using stereotactic fractionated radiotherapy (SFR) (GROSU et al. 2005b). A prospective non-randomized trial has shown that in patients treated based on amino acids-PET or -SPECT, the median survival time was significant higher (9 months) in comparison to patients

treated based on CT/MRI alone (5 months, $p=0.03$). The results of this pilot study have yet to be verified in a randomized trial.

9.2.2
FDG-PET in Gross Tumor Volume Delineation of Lung Cancer

In lung cancer, the diagnostic accuracy of FDG-PET is between 85% and 90% (Figs. 9.1, 9.2) (DWAMENA et al. 1999; HELLWIG et al. 2001; MACMANUS et al. 2001). In the late 1990s this promising diagnostic performance led to the idea of integrating PET into radiotherapy planning (MUNLEY et al. 1999; NESTLE et al. 1999).

In earlier reviews (GROSU et al. 2005c; NESTLE et al. 2002, 2006) the literature about the integration of FDG-PET in radiotherapy planning of non-small cell lung cancer (NSCLC) has been surveyed. To date, over 20 studies in more than 600 patients have shown that the use of FDG-PET image data may lead to an advantage for the patient. The main sources of this possible advantage are the better coverage of the primary tumor and the protection of healthy tissue. In this context it is interesting that the FDG-based target volumes may be both smaller or larger compared to CT-based ones. The high percentage of changes in target volumes by FDG-PET (20–100%) reported in the literature concerning various parameters of the planning process (field sizes, GTV, clinical target volume [CTV], planning target volume [PTV], normal tissue complication probability [NTCP], etc.) is mainly caused by two factors: the ability to distinguish the tumor from collapsed lung tissue (atelectasis) and the higher accuracy of FDG-PET in lymph node staging compared to CT. However, because inflammation in the collapsed lung may also lead to FDG accumulation, PET does not help with GTV definition in these cases.

A significant parameter, especially in the context of collapsed lung tissue, is the reduction of interobserver variability (IOV) of the GTV delineation by FDG data integrated in the planning process. Here, several authors have shown clear improvements (CALDWELL et al. 2001; STEENBAKKERS et al. 2006; VAN DE STEENE et al. 2002). The Toronto group (CALDWELL et al. 2001) demonstrated a reduction of the IOV from 1:2.3 to 1:1.6 after adding FDG-PET information to CT images for GTV delineation of advanced NSCLC.

However, despite the improvement of the IOV, the gold standard method for the delineation of the GTV has not been set yet. The problem is the low resolution of PET images, which is caused by physical factors (size of the detector crystals, positron range in matter, non-

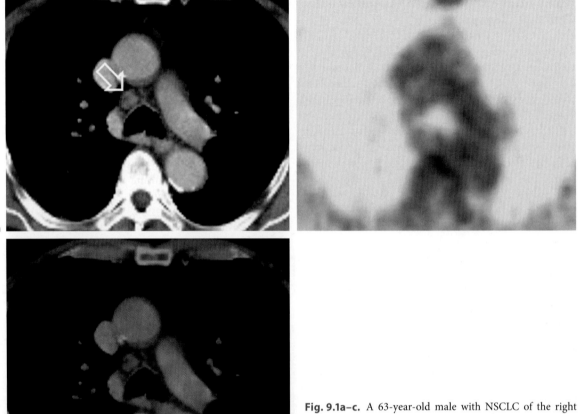

Fig. 9.1a–c. A 63-year-old male with NSCLC of the right upper pulmonary lobe. On CT N2 disease was suspected based on a pathologically enlarged lymph node in the mediastinum (*arrow* in **a**). FDG-PET (**b**) and FDG-PET/CT (**c**) demonstrate homogeneous tracer distribution without focally increased FDG uptake staging this patient as N0. Histopathology verified an N0 nodal status

collinearity of annihilation gamma rays, and detector scatter) (CHERRY 2006), and also by biological factors (movements of the target during acquisition due to relatively long acquisition times), which leads to a blurred margin of the accumulating structure (NESTLE et al. 2006).

Various methods are used for the delineation of FDG accumulations for GTV contouring. Easily applicable is the visual contouring by the physician, in analogy to the method used with CT-based contouring. However, a significant IOV remains (PÖTZSCH et al. 2006). To improve this IOV, clinical protocols have been applied (MACMANUS et al. 2007) and have succeeded in a significant convergence of FDG-based GTVs contoured by different observers. However, visual contouring remains observer dependent and by further distribution of the method into clinical practice, the varying experience of the radiotherapist with PET will influence

the quality of visual GTV contouring. Therefore other methods for automatic and/or semiautomatic threshold contouring of the—often high contrast—FDG accumulations have been reported. Easily applicable at most PET and/or radiotherapy planning systems is the use of a threshold of a fixed FDG concentration, expressed as standardized uptake value (SUV, i.e., decay-corrected tissue activity/tissue volume divided by injected activity/body weight). However, there are numerous technical and biological factors influencing the SUV. Furthermore, the FDG accumulation in normal tissues may vary, being even higher than the threshold values suggested in the literature (e.g., SUV=2.5). Therefore, other than for diagnostic purposes where the maximum SUV of a lesion may give an impression of the malignancy of the lesion, the use of a fixed SUV threshold is not suitable for GTV contouring. Also easily applicable at most systems is a threshold relative to

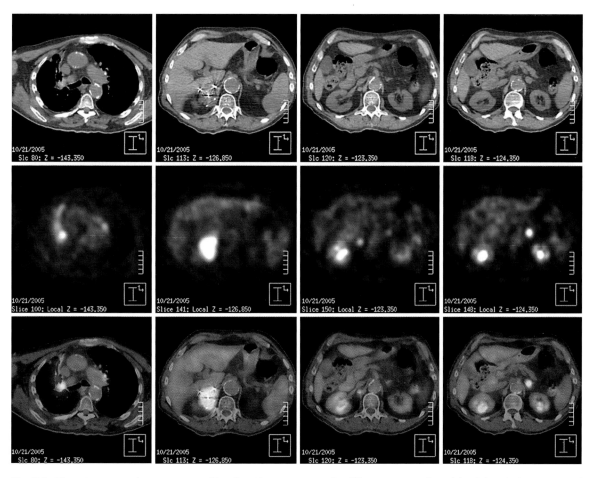

Fig. 9.2. These images are from a 70-year-old male with recurrent small-cell lung cancer evaluated for CyberKnife treatment of an isolated right adrenal lesion. PET/CT showed previously unsuspected mediastinal, left adrenal, and retroperitoneal disease

the maximum FDG accumulation of the lesion. This method is derived from the imaging of homogenous structures such as phantoms filled with radioactivity. In 1997, ERDI et al. used 40% of the maximum FDG accumulation for contouring 17 homogenous lung metastases leading to volumes that were comparable to those measured by CT. Thus, many groups have used this method since then. Meanwhile, it has been shown that ungated PET images may depict the probability of the presence of lung tumors over the whole breathing cycle (CALDWELL et al. 2003; YAREMKO et al. 2005), which means that the "true" volume of a lung lesion contoured in an FDG-PET dataset must be by the amount of breathing excursions larger than the volume measured in CT. Furthermore, lung tumors often show a relatively inhomogeneous FDG accumulation. Therefore, it has been shown that applied in primary lung tumors, thresholding by a percentage of the maximum

accumulation intensity may lead to insufficient coverage of lesions (NESTLE et al. 2005).

More promising is the use of contrast-dependent methods (SCHAEFER et al. 2008). These methods use the information on the accumulation intensity in the questionable lesion as well as in the neighboring background. An example of a relatively simple contrast-oriented method is the "Homburg algorithm" (SCHAEFER et al. 2008; NESTLE et al. 2005, 2007):

$$I_{threshold} = A \times I_{lesion} + B \times I_{background}$$

Here, I_{lesion} is the mean FDG accumulation (SUV or Intensity) of a 3-D isocontour of, for example, 70% of the maximum of the lesion, while $I_{background}$ is the mean FDG accumulation in the surrounding normal tissue. A and B are parameters that mainly depend on the imaging characteristics of the PET system, which has to be determined by phantom measurements (Schaefer et al. 2008). Other contrast-oriented algorithms lead to similar contouring results and also need a calibration by phantom measurements.

In our experience, other than absolute or relative SUVs, contrast-oriented algorithms are quite robust under clinical conditions. However, the calibration to the PET and radiotherapy planning system used is mandatory (Nestle et al. 2005, 2006, 2007). As technical factors like the methods of reconstruction, attenuation correction of PET images, and data transfer do influence PET imaging, they have to be defined before and kept constant after calibration.

Overall, it must be kept in mind that the choice of the method for GTV contouring may have a significant impact on the size of the GTV (Nestle et al. 2005) and that the most important factor in PET-based GTV delineation is the close collaboration of nuclear medicine and radiotherapy departments on the side of the medical as well as on the side of the physical and technical staff.

Crucial points in this context are patient positioning and image coregistration. It must be kept in mind that patient position may change, not only between acquisition on stand-alone PET and CT scanners, but also during PET/CT acquisition. Not correcting for the consequent differences in tumor localization leads to a geographical miss, if PET-derived GTVs are transmitted to CT datasets without critical evaluation of the quality of coregistration. This is best done by comparing anatomical landmarks detectable by both imaging techniques, such as carina tracheae, lung apices, spine, sternum, thoracic wall, and—with care due to breathing mobility—diaphragm. Although non-rigid coregistration algorithms may solve some of the positioning problems, at the moment, rigid coregistration algorithms are the method of choice. It may well be that the deformation of the image data caused by

non-rigid algorithms may result in geometrical inexactnesses or geographical misses, especially in tumors which are not clearly depicted by the morphological method. Unfortunately, these are the cases in which the integration of FDG-PET into radiotherapy planning is most helpful. Further research is needed to clarify this point.

The highest possible benefit for the patients from FDG-based radiotherapy planning can only be gained if, due to the exact depiction of tumor localization by PET, the irradiation of normal tissues can be omitted. In lung cancer, this would mean departing from the clinical concept of "elective nodal irradiation" (ENI) of large macroscopically normal parts of the mediastinum when defining the CTV (Kiricuta 2001). Omitting ENI could lead to a significant protection of highly radiosensitive normal tissues, for example lung, with the consequence of obtaining higher irradiation doses in the tumor. First clinical data with (De Ruysscher et al. 2005) and even without FDG-PET (Rosenzweig et al. 2007) have shown that the risk of "out of field" recurrences after targeting the macroscopic tumor alone is small, much smaller than the risk for local ("in field") tumor progression. However, prospective randomized clinical studies will have to show that this policy is safe and beneficial for the patients. The data from 26 patients with NSCLC treated with involved-field radiotherapy who had local failure and a post-radiotherapy PET scan were analyzed by Sura et al. (2008). The patterns of failure were visually scored and defined as follows: (1) within the GTV/PTV; (2) within the GTV, PTV, and outward; (3) within the PTV and outward; and (4) outside the PTV. Local failure was also evaluated as originating from nodal areas versus the primary tumor. All the patients had recurrence originating from their primary tumor. Of 8 primary tumors that had received a dose of <60 Gy, 6 (75%) had failure within the GTV and 2 (25%) at the GTV margin. At doses of ≥60 Gy,

▶ **Fig. 9.3a–d.** Central necrosis of metastatic lymph nodes. **a,b** Bilateral nodal metastases of oropharyngeal SCC. **a** Post-contrast CSE T1-weighted coronal image with FS shows three different metastatic nodal patterns: (1) an area of low signal intensity surrounded by an intensely contrast-enhanced rim (*black curved arrow*); (2) an area of intermediate signal intensity with a bright rim (*thin white arrow*); (3) an area of intermediate signal intensity partially "obscured" by an intensely "flashing" rim (*thick white arrow*). Fat is well suppressed at the level of the white star, but less satisfactorily so at the level of the white notch. **b** FSE T2-weighted coronal image without FS in a strictly similar slice location to 3a clearly reveals central necrosis as a very bright cystic area within the node display-

ing the lowest T1 signal intensity (*black curved arrow*), whereas the other nodes are not necrotic-cystic. **c,d** Close-ups of metastatic jugular nodes of an infiltrating SCC of the right vallecula (*white notch*). **c** Post-contrast CSE transverse T1-weighted image without FS. Necrotic areas within the nodes display very low signal intensity (*arrowheads*). A non-necrotic lymph node (*arrow*) and submandibular gland (*double arrows*) exhibit similar signal intensity. **d** FSE T2-weighted transverse image without FS in a similar slice location to that in 3c shows very bright signal intensity of the nodal necrotic-cystic areas. Signal intensities of the non-necrotic node and the submandibular gland are significantly different

6 (33%) of 18 had failure within the GTV, 11 (61%) at the GTV margin, and 1 (6%) was a marginal miss (*p*<0.05). The authors concluded that with lower doses, the pattern of recurrences was mostly within the GTV, suggesting that the dose might have been a factor for tumor control, whereas at greater doses, the treatment

failures were mostly at the margin of the GTV. They also mentioned that visual incorporation of PET data for GTV delineation might be inadequate, and more sophisticated approaches of PET registration should be evaluated.

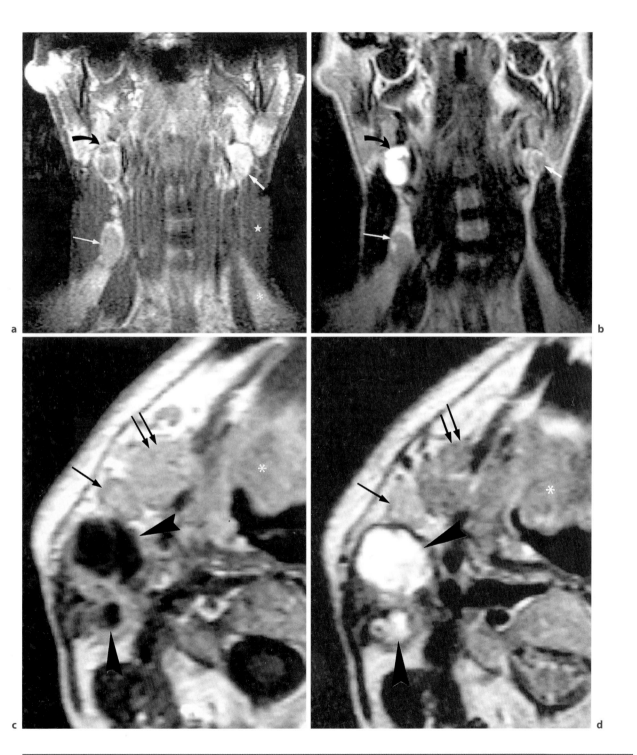

9.2.3
FDG-PET in Head and Neck Cancer

Anatomical imaging continues to provide important information on disease extent and prognostic factors, as illustrated in Fig. 9.3. However, other imaging methods are being used in addition to CT and MRI. GAMBHIR et al. (2001) summarized the data of eight studies (468 patients) that evaluated the impact of FDG-PET in staging of head and neck cancer: the average sensitivity and specificity for FDG-PET were 87% and 89%, respectively, whereas for CT were 62% and 73%, respectively. For tumor diagnosis the sensitivity and specificity of FDG-PET, assessed in seven trials incorporating 193 patient studies, were 93% and 70%, in comparison to CT with 66% and 56%, respectively. However, the standard diagnosis of tumor infiltration in head and neck cancer remains the histological evaluation.

Since this analysis was published, more advanced data have been reported: LIU et al. (2007) performed a systematic review of the performance of FDG-PET in head and neck cancer, namely about diagnosis of residual or recurrent nasopharyngeal carcinoma. In this thoroughly conducted analysis of data from 1,813 patients, FDG-PET compared to CT and MRI is by far the method with the best diagnostic performance: the overall sensitivity of PET being 0.95 and 0.9 versus 0.76 and 0.59 for CT and 0.78 and 0.76 for MRI.

Furthermore, the new technology of combined PET/CT has been brought into the clinic and was evaluated by several groups. Hybrid PET/CT enables a better correlation of FDG accumulations with anatomy, which is very helpful for the interpretation of PET scans in the topographically complex head and neck region. Overall, it has been shown that the diagnostic accuracy of PET/CT, especially concerning equivocal findings, is higher compared to that of PET alone (JEONG et al. 2002) and maintains the superiority of FDG-PET compared to CT (SCHWARTZ et al. 2005a) and to MRI (DRESEL et al. 2003).

However, as in lung cancer, the diagnostic accuracy of FDG-PET and/or PET/CT in head and neck cancer is not 100%. The main causes for false-negative findings are again the presence of micrometastatic disease in lymph nodes or very small primary lesions. False-negative PET results may also be caused by flat superficial growth, which is not uncommon in this area (DRESEL et al. 2003). In a group of 116 patients with mixed stage and site primary or recurrent head and neck tumors, DRESEL et al. (2003) diagnosed 86% of the tumors and 82% of the involved cervical lymph nodes correctly, translating to false-negative rates of 14–18%. In a highly preselected group of operated clinically N0 patients with oral cancer, with 9/142 histologically metastatic lymph node levels, SCHÖDER et al. (2006) described 3/9 false FDG-negative lymph node levels (1 directly adjacent to the primary tumor). Therefore, the rates of false-negative FDG-PET findings in head and neck patients seem to be higher than in lung cancer, although no meta-analysis on this topic has been performed yet. For the surgical treatment, however, it has been concluded that management of cervical lymph nodes should not be based on FDG-PET/CT alone.

False-positive FDG-PET findings, as was also seen in the Schöder group of patients and in many other diagnostic studies (CHAN et al. 2006; DRESEL et al. 2003; GOSHEN et al. 2006), may be caused by inflammation accounting for 6/133 false FDG-positive neck levels caused by inflammatory lymphoid hyperplasia in the Schöder data. False-positive FDG accumulations may furthermore be found in the metabolically active lymphoid tissues of the tonsils, the base of tongue, and the Waldeyer's ring, while a variable symmetric or asymmetric uptake may be seen in salivary glands and may also be variable in muscles, including the larynx, depending on the activities of the patient after injection of the FDG (ABOUZIED et al. 2005). By including the anatomical information of CT (NAKAMOTO et al. 2005), the rates of false-positive FDG-PET/CT findings appear lower than those reported in the earlier literature on FDG-PET alone (GOSHEN et al. 2006; ZIMNY et al. 2002).

There are two main technical problems in FDG-based definition of target volumes for patients with head and neck cancer: coregistration and GTV delineation:

1. Coregistration is a delicate problem in the head and neck area. Impreciseness in coregistration of some millimeters may soon lead to a significant geographical miss in the complex flexible anatomy with the structures of interest being relatively small. When using rigid coregistration algorithms, positioning aids like masks used for radiotherapy must be used for the PET acquisition, too. If these are not used, PET scans from this area of the body can not be rigidly registered to a planning CT or MRI with sufficient accuracy. Although non-rigid coregistration algorithms are advocated by some authors (IRELAND et al. 2007) to solve the positioning problem, it has not yet been proven that with non-rigid coregistration of image data the tumor structures are registered correctly to anatomical imaging. To our knowledge there is no method available to date that can take into account, for example, the different grades of rigidity of anatomical structures (e.g. bone, soft tissue, airways, etc.) in the head and neck area. Therefore, further research is needed at this point. Until then, thorough patient positioning for

PET, CT, and treatment application and rigid image coregistration is mandatory.

2. FDG-based delineation of the GTV is another challenging problem. The key feature in this context is that the structures of interest are relatively small compared to a voxel size of PET. Including one set of surrounding voxels more or less into the GTV may lead to significant changes of volume, and therefore of tumor covering on one side and normal tissue complications on the other side. As had been seen by FORD et al. (2006), who compared different percentages of the maximum intensity as thresholds, the Nijmegen group (SCHINAGL et al. 2007) also showed large differences in the resulting volumes between various methods applied for GTV contouring, which led to differences of nearly 100%. The Nijmegen group concluded that, as in lung cancer, a contrast-oriented method (source/background ratio) seems preferable. The Ghent group (DAISNE et al. 2003, 2004) showed that by contouring larynx cancers preoperatively by a contrast-oriented method the results in comparison to pathological specimens were more accurate than CT- and MRI-based GTV delineation. However, in a later planning trial on intensity-modulated radiotherapy (IMRT), the same group (GEETS et al. 2007) favored another, gradient-based method.

In a first clinical trial with 41 patients, the group of MADANI et al. (2007) performed an FDG-guided focal dose escalation using IMRT for patients with head and neck cancer. While applying conservative doses to elective lymph node levels, doses to GTVs defined by CT and FDG-PET were escalated up to a NID_{2Gy} of 78.2 Gy. However, in preliminary evaluation of the pattern of recurrence, 4/9 locoregional recurrences were located outside the PET-defined GTV and 1/9 at the border of the PET-defined GTV, although the above-mentioned contrast-oriented method for FDG-based GTV contouring was used, which had been verified by correlation with pathological specimens (DAISNE et al. 2004). Possible reasons for the relatively high rate of recurrences outside the PET-defined GTV are false FDG-negative nodal disease together with steep dose gradients in the IMRT plans and the fact that not all patients received concomitant chemotherapy. However, the other 4/9 locoregional recurrences appeared within the high-dose volumes showing the need for further dose escalation to the gross tumor while 9/14 relapsing patients had distant metastases, supporting the need for additional chemotherapy.

The possible impact of FDG-PET for target volume delineation for radiation treatment planning has mean-

while been investigated in nine trials (CIERNIK et al. 2003; CONNELL et al. 2007; DAISNE et al. 2004; GEETS et al. 2007; NISHIOKA et al. 2002; PAULINO et al. 2005; RAHN et al. 1998; SCARFONE et al. 2004; SCHWARTZ et al. 2005b) incorporating 248 patients with different tumor stages and locations. All these studies showed that FDG-PET could have a significant impact on GTV delineation in comparison to CT (or MRI) alone, the results ranging between 9% and 100% of the cases. Here, as in lung tumors, in each about one third of cases FDG-PET led to an increase of GTV, whereas in another one third of cases the GTV became smaller, if based on FDG alone. Therefore, an FDG-based radiotherapy of head and neck cancer patients might lead to a significant gain in normal tissue protection especially concerning the parotid gland, with a relevant improvement of quality of life.

Overall, the optimum method for GTV delineation in this area has not been defined yet. In the end, the results of further clinical trials will have to show if it is beneficial to use FDG-PET-based GTV reduction in the radiotherapy planning of head and neck tumors.

9.3
PET for Visualization of Tumor Biology

In recent years, PET tracers have been developed that can visualize biological pathways with particular significance for tumor response to the treatment. These are, for example, hypoxia, cell proliferation, and angiogenesis. The volumes defined by using images acquired after injection of these tracers may be used as subvolumes of the tumor, like a target within the GTV, which could be irradiated with a higher dose, for example by IMRT. This concept is called "dose painting," and is as yet a promising hypothesis waiting to be validated by clinical and experimental data (BENTZEN 2005; BRADLEY et al. 2004; BUCK et al. 2005; LING et al. 2000, 2004; TANDERUP et al. 2006).

9.3.1
Hypoxia

Hypoxia, i.e., an insufficient tissue oxygenation, is a well-known factor causing radioresistance of cells. Clinically, low tumor oxygenation, for example in patients with head and neck tumors, has been shown to be associated with a poor prognosis after radiotherapy (NORDSMARK et al. 2005). Although the underlying mechanisms of radioresistance are still subject to investigation (KORITZINSKY et al. 2005; TROOST et al. 2005; WILLIAMS et al. 2005; YAROMINA et al. 2005), it appears very interesting to image hypoxia in vivo in order to increase local doses to radioresistant regions. Several bioreductive substances have been evaluated as hypoxia tracers. The tracers investigated are mainly nitroimidazole compounds, for example [18F]-fluoromisonidazole ([18F]-FMISO), which was the first nitroimidazole compound developed for PET, [123I]-iodoazomycin arabinoside ([123I]-IAZA) and [18F]-azomycin arabinoside ([18F]-FAZA). With these tracers, the bioreductive molecule attracts a single electron leading to free radical metabolites that are further reduced and bound to cell constituents under hypoxic conditions. [60Cu]-labeled methylthiosemicarbazone ([60Cu]-ATSM) has also being proposed for hypoxia imaging.

The first data about the use of hypoxia PET for the visualization of a hypoxic subvolume were published by a group at the University of Washington (KOH et al. 1995; RASEY et al. 1996). Based on experimental and clinical data, they considered a tumor pixel with a tumor/blood [18F]-FMISO ratio ≥1.4 at the late image acquisition interval (120 min following injection) as indicative for the presence of hypoxia. Therefore, the percentage of pixels within the imaged volume that had a tumor/blood [18F]-FMISO ratio ≥1.4 were defined as fractional hypoxic volume (FHV). The authors assessed the dynamics of FHV during radiotherapy in 7 patients with NSCLC and showed that it decreased from the beginning to the end of the treatment (KOH et al. 1995). In a study published about 10 years later, the Tübingen group assessed the predictive value of [18F]-FMISO after radiation therapy in 14 patients with NSCLC and 26 patients with head and neck cancer (ESCHMANN et al. 2005). In the lung cancer group SUV measured 4 h after tracer injection did not correlate with the tumor recurrence after radiotherapy, whereas in the head and neck group for an SUV >2 the correlation was statistically significant. A tumor-to-mediastinum ratio >2 was a predictive factor for local recurrence in the lung cancer group. The authors performed qualitative analysis of time–activity curves and defined three curve types: rapid tracer washout, intermediate (delayed) washout, and a tracer accumulation curve. The tracer accumulation curve correlated with a higher incidence of local recurrence, while the rapid-washout curve was a predictive factor for better local tumor control.

[60Cu]-ATSM is a bioreductive molecule also being proposed for tumor hypoxia imaging. In a trial including 14 patients with NSCLC treated with radiation and/or chemotherapy it was shown that the mean tumor-to-muscle activity ratio before treatment was significantly

lower in responders (1.5±0.4) than in non-responders (3.4±0.8; $p=0.002$). The tumor/muscle ratio of 3 could discriminate the responders from non-responders. The mean SUV for [60Cu]-ATSM was not significantly different in responders versus non-responders (DEHDASHTI et al. 2003). GROSU et al. (2007) evaluated the distribution of hypoxia in 18 patients with head and neck tumors using FAZA-PET. The hypoxic subvolume was located in a single confluent area in 61% of patients, was diffusely dispersed in the whole tumor mass in 22%, and missing in 17%. Only patients with a confluent distribution of the tracer would be suitable for a dose painting approach based on hypoxia. However, such an approach could lead to a dose escalation to 105 Gy in tumor without exceeding the normal tissue tolerance (LEE et al. 2008).

The results of these studies could open new perspectives for radiation treatment planning. They demonstrated the feasibility of in vivo PET studies performed with tracers which in experimental models were closely related to tissue hypoxia. Furthermore, they showed, even in a small number of patients, a significant correlation between hypoxia-tracer uptake and treatment response. However, clinical trials analyzing the impact of FHV as a target for radiation treatment planning in lung cancer have not been done so far.

In the preparation of such trials, several issues have to be addressed. Firstly, the tracer used for radiotherapy application must be carefully chosen. It would ideally be captured specifically by hypoxic cells using an oxygen-specific retention mechanism, be sufficiently delivered in a perfusion-limited microenvironment, produce a low level of non-specific metabolites, and have no labeled metabolites of hypoxia tracers found in the circulation at the time of imaging. Secondly, the method of quantification must be sorted out. Considering the phenomena of perfusion, diffusion, and hypoxia-induced tracer retention and inspired by recent immunohistochemical investigations with the hypoxia tracer pimonidazole (BUSSINK et al. 2003), the Tübingen group proposed that the kinetic model is a more valid criterion to quantify hypoxia in vivo than a criterion based on static SUV at an early time point. However, depending on the tracer used, static imaging, which is much easier to implement in the planning process, may also be feasible. Thirdly, the method of application of radiotherapy must be chosen. To date, two IMRT models are proposed: The model of CHAO et al. (2001) is defined as a target in target, which by using IMRT is irradiated with a higher dose than the rest of the tumor. In a more sophisticated technique, ALBER et al. (2003) propose a method which allows the inclusion of biological imaging data in the optimization of IMRT to produce an image intensity based dose modulation, voxel by voxel.

An essential question, however, is how to account for setup variations and target movements. Due to the relatively low contrast of hypoxia-PET images, contouring hypoxia targets can be expected to pose more problems than [^{18}F]-FDG imaging already does. Furthermore, setup and target movement errors have to be applied when using these data for PTV delineation. Depending on the quality of immobilization, it may be necessary to apply margins to every voxel of the GTV with a defined dose prescription.

Another essential question addresses the reproducibility of the intratumoral distribution of hypoxia. In a recent study NEHMEH et al. (2008) evaluated the dynamics of the FMISO uptake in PET over 3 days in 14 patients with untreated head and neck tumors. The authors describe variability in spatial hypoxia tracer uptake. Only 6/13 patients had well-correlated intratumoral distributions of FMISO, suggestive of chronic hypoxia.

In the end, the results of such clinical trials will have to be awaited to find out about the clinical benefit from hypoxia-based dose intensification.

9.3.2
Proliferation

The proliferation of tumor cells is the basic mechanism for malignant growth. Therefore, it has been tried to image this parameter, which is thought to be more specific for malignancy compared to, for example, glucose consumption. [^{18}F]-fluorine-labeled thymidine analog 3'-deoxy-3'-[^{18}F]-fluorothymidine (FLT) is retained in the cell after phosphorylation by thymidine kinase 1, whose levels correlate with cell proliferation.

The FLT uptake in malignant tissue, measured by SUV, seems to be generally lower than the [^{18}F]-FDG uptake. The sensitivity seems to be higher for primary tumors than for lymph node metastases (BUCK et al. 2005). Furthermore, the specificity of the tracer is not 100%: proliferation of lymphocytes and non-specific increased accumulation due to increased perfusion and vascular permeability could lead to false-positive results (SHIELDS et al. 1998; YAP et al. 2006).

Until now, there are no trials analyzing the impact of FLT-PET on radiation treatment planning. However, it visualizes a biological pathway with a high impact in tumor treatment. Therefore, it could play an important role in the development of new image-based dose distributions and guide treatment fractionation strategies and deserves to be investigated in future clinical trials.

9.3.3
Angiogenesis

The $\alpha v \beta 3$ integrin is an important receptor for cell adhesion involved in tumor-induced angiogenesis and metastasis. It mediates migration of activated endothelial cells through the basement membrane during formation of new blood vessels. Particularly interesting is that this integrin is expressed only on the cell surface of tumor cells or activated endothelial cells, and not on normal endothelial cells of established vessels. HAUBNER et al. (2001) and BEER et al. (2007) described the noninvasive imaging of $\alpha v \beta 3$ integrin expression using F18-labeled RDG-containing glycopeptide and PET. In squamous cell carcinoma of head and neck, for example, $\alpha v \beta 3$ integrin seems to be expressed on the endothelial cells and not on the tumor cells. This suggests that RGD-PET could be used as a surrogate for the visualization and evaluation of tumor angiogenesis (BEER et al. 2007).

Conclusion

PET could improve the delineation of GTV in some tumor entities like brain tumors, lung cancer, and head and neck cancer. Therefore, its impact on the clinical outcome has to be evaluated in prospective trials. The role of PET for the visualization of tumor biology is unclear. However, this approach could open new perspectives in treatment planning and monitoring of solid tumors and has to be assessed in the future in experimental and clinical studies.

References

Abouzied MM, Crawford ES, Nabi HA (2005) 18F-FDG imaging: pitfalls and artifacts. J Nucl Med Technol 33:145–155

Alber M, Paulsen F, Eschmann SM, Machulla HJ (2003) On biologically conformal boost dose optimization. Phys Med Biol 48:N31–N35

Beer AJ, Grosu AL, Carlsen J, Kolk A, Sabria M, Stangier I, Watzlowik P, Wester HJ, Haubner R, Schwaiger M (2007) Feasibility of (18F)galacto-RGD PET for imaging of $\alpha v \beta 3$ expression on neovasculature in patients with squamous cell carcinoma of head and neck. Clin Cancer Res 13:6610–6616

Bentzen SM (2005) Radiation therapy: intensity modulated, image guided, biologically optimized and evidence based. Radiother Oncol 77:227–230

Bradley J, Thorstad WL, Mutic S, Miller TR, Dehdashti F, Siegel BA, Bosch W, Bertrand RJ (2004) Impact of FDG-PET on radiation therapy volume delineation in non-small-cell lung cancer. Int J Radiat Oncol Biol Phys 59:78–86

Buck AK, Hetzel M, Schirrmeister H, Halter G, Moller P, Kratochwil C, Wahl A, Glatting G, Mottaghy FM, Mattfeldt T, Neumaier B, Reske SN (2005) Clinical relevance of imaging proliferative activity in lung nodules. Eur J Nucl Med Mol Imaging 32:525–533

Bussink J, Kaanders JH, van der Kogel AJ (2003) Tumor hypoxia at the micro-regional level: clinical relevance and predictive value of exogenous and endogenous hypoxic cell markers. Radiother Oncol 67:3–15

Caldwell CB, Mah K, Ung YC, Danjoux CE, Balogh JM, Ganguli SN, Ehrlich LE (2001) Observer variation in contouring gross tumor volume in patients with poorly defined non-small-cell lung tumors on CT: the impact of 18FDG-hybrid PET fusion. Int J Radiat Oncol Biol Phys 51:923–931

Caldwell CB, Mah K, Skinner M, Danjoux CE (2003) Can PET provide the 3D extent of tumor motion for individualized internal target volumes? A phantom study of the limitations of CT and the promise of PET. Int J Radiat Oncol Biol Phys 55:1381–1393

Chan SC, Ng SH, Chang JT, Lin CY, Chen YC, Chang YC, Hsu CL, Wang HM, Liao CT, Yen TC (2006) Advantages and pitfalls of 18F-fluoro-2-deoxy-D-glucose positron emission tomography in detecting locally residual or recurrent nasopharyngeal carcinoma: comparison with magnetic resonance imaging. Eur J Nucl Med Mol Imaging 33:1032–1040

Chao KS, Bosch WR, Mutic S, Lewis JS, Dehdashti F, Mintun MA, Dempsey JF, Perez CA, Purdy JA, Welch MJ (2001) A novel approach to overcome hypoxic tumor resistance: Cu-ATSM-guided intensity-modulated radiation therapy. Int J Radiat Oncol Biol Phys 49:1171–1182

Cherry SR (2006) The 2006 Henry N. Wagner Lecture: Of mice and men (and positrons)–advances in PET imaging technology. J Nucl Med 47:1735–1745

Ciernik IF, Dizendorf E, Baumert BG, Reiner B, Burger C, Davis JB, Lutolf UM, Steinert HC, Von Schulthess GK (2003) Radiation treatment planning with an integrated positron emission and computer tomography (PET/CT): a feasibility study. Int J Radiat Oncol Biol Phys 57:853–863

Connell CA, Corry J, Milner AD, Hogg A, Hicks RJ, Rischin D, Peters LJ (2007) Clinical impact of, and prognostic stratification by, F-18 FDG PET/CT in head and neck mucosal squamous cell carcinoma Head Neck 29:986–995

Daisne JF, Sibomana M, Bol A, Doumont T, Lonneux M, Gregoire V (2003) Tri-dimensional automatic segmentation of PET volumes based on measured source-to-background ratios: influence of reconstruction algorithms. Radiother Oncol 69:247–250

Daisne JF, Duprez T, Weynand B, Lonneux M, Hamoir M, Reychler H, Gregoire V (2004) Tumor volume in pharyngolaryngeal squamous cell carcinoma: comparison of CT, MR imaging, and FDG PET and validation with surgical specimen. Radiology 233:93–100

Dehdashti F, Mintun MA, Lewis JS, Bradley J, Govindan R, Laforest R, Welch MJ, Siegel BA (2003) In vivo assessment of tumor hypoxia in lung cancer with 60Cu-ATSM. Eur J Nucl Med Mol Imaging 30:844–850

De Ruysscher D, Wanders S, van Haren E, Hochstenbag M, Geeraedts W, Utama I, Simons J, Dohmen J, Rhami A, Buell U, Thimister P, Snoep G, Boersma L, Verschueren T, van Baardwijk A, Minken A, Bentzen SM, Lambin P (2005) Selective mediastinal node irradiation based on FDG-PET scan data in patients with non-small-cell lung cancer: a prospective clinical study. Int J Radiat Oncol Biol Phys 62:988–994

Dresel S, Grammerstorff J, Schwenzer K, Brinkbaumer K, Schmid R, Pfluger T, Hahn K (2003) [18F]FDG imaging of head and neck tumours: comparison of hybrid PET and morphological methods. Eur J Nucl Med Mol Imaging 30:995–1003

Dwamena BA, Sonnad SS, Angobaldo JO, Wahl RL (1999) Metastases from non-small cell lung cancer: mediastinal staging in the 1990s–meta-analytic comparison of PET and CT. Radiology 213:530–536

Erdi YE, Mawlawi O, Larson SM, Imbriaco M, Yeung H, Finn R, Humm JL (1997) Segmentation of lung lesion volume by adaptive positron emission tomography image thresholding. Cancer 80:2505–2509

Eschmann SM, Paulsen F, Reimold M, Dittmann H, Welz S, Reischl G, Machulla HJ, Bares R (2005) Prognostic impact of hypoxia imaging with 18F-misonidazole PET in non-small cell lung cancer and head and neck cancer before radiotherapy. J Nucl Med 46:253–260

Ford EC, Kinahan PE, Hanlon L, Alessio A, Rajendran J, Schwartz DL, Phillips M (2006) Tumor delineation using PET in head and neck cancers: threshold contouring and lesion volumes. Med Phys 33:4280–4288

Gambhir SS, Czernin J, Schwimmer J, Silverman DH, Coleman RE, Phelps ME (2001) A tabulated summary of the FDG PET literature. J Nucl Med 42:1S–93S

Geets X, Lee JA, Bol A, Lonneux M, Gregoire V (2007) A gradient-based method for segmenting FDG-PET images: methodology and validation. Eur J Nucl Med Mol Imaging 34:1427–1438

Goshen E, Davidson T, Yahalom R, Talmi YP, Zwas ST (2006) PET/CT in the evaluation of patients with squamous cell cancer of the head and neck. Int J Oral Maxillofac Surg 35:332–336

Grosu AL, Weber W, Feldmann HJ, Wuttke B, Bartenstein P, Gross MW, Lumenta C, Schwaiger M, Molls M (2000) First experience with I-123-alpha-methyl-tyrosine SPECT in the 3-D radiation treatment planning of brain gliomas. Int J Radiat Oncol Biol Phys 47:517–526

Grosu AL, Feldmann H, Dick S, Dzewas B, Nieder C, Gumprecht H, Frank A, Schwaiger M, Molls M, Weber WA (2002) Implications of IMT-SPECT for postoperative radiotherapy planning in patients with gliomas. Int J Radiat Oncol Biol Phys 54:842–854

Grosu AL, Lachner R, Wiedenmann N, Stark S, Thamm R, Kneschaurek P, Schwaiger M, Molls M, Weber WA (2003) Validation of a method for automatic image fusion (Brain-LAB System) of CT data and 11C-methionine-PET data for stereotactic radiotherapy using a LINAC: first clinical experience. Int J Radiat Oncol Biol Phys 56:1450–1463

Grosu AL, Weber WA, Riedel E, Jeremic B, Nieder C, Franz M, Gumprecht H, Jaeger R, Schwaiger M, Molls M (2005a) L-(methyl-11C) methionine positron emission tomography for target delineation in resected high-grade gliomas before radiotherapy Int J Radiat Oncol Biol Phys 63:64–74

Grosu AL, Weber WA, Franz M, Stark S, Piert M, Thamm R, Gumprecht H, Schwaiger M, Molls M, Nieder C (2005b) Reirradiation of recurrent high-grade gliomas using amino acid PET (SPECT)/CT/MRI image fusion to determine gross tumor volume for stereotactic fractionated radiotherapy. Int J Radiat Oncol Biol Phys 63:511–519

Grosu AL, Piert M, Molls M (2005c) Experience of PET for target localisation in radiation oncology. Br J Radiol 78:18–32

Grosu AL, Souvatzoglou M, Roper B, Dobritz M, Wiedenmann N, Jacob V, Wester HJ, Reischl G, Machulla HJ, Schwaiger M, Molls M, Piert M (2007) Hypoxia imaging with FAZA-PET and theoretical considerations with regard to dose painting for individualization of radiotherapy in patients with head and neck cancer. Int J Radiat Oncol Biol Phys 69:541–551

Haubner R, Wester HJ, Weber WA (2001) Noninvasive imaging of alpha(v)beta3 integrin expression using 18F-labeled RGD-containing glycopeptide and positron emission tomography Cancer Res 61:1781–1785

Hellwig D, Ukena D, Paulsen F, Bamberg M, Kirsch CM (2001) Meta-analysis of the efficacy of positron emission tomography with F-18-fluorodeoxyglucose in lung tumors. Basis for discussion of the German Consensus Conference on PET in Oncology 2000. Pneumologie 55:367–377

Ireland RH, Dyker KE, Barber DC, Wood SM, Hanney MB, Tindale WB, Woodhouse N, Hoggard N, Conway J, Robinson MH (2007) Nonrigid image registration for head and neck cancer radiotherapy treatment planning with PET/CT. Int J Radiat Oncol Biol Phys 68:952–957

Jeong HJ, Min JJ, Park JM, Chung JK, Kim BT, Jeong JM, Lee DS, Lee MC, Han SK, Shim YS (2002) Determination of the prognostic value of [^{18}F]fluorodeoxyglucose uptake by using positron emission tomography in patients with non-small cell lung cancer. Nucl Med Commun 23:865–870

Kiricuta IC (2001) Selection and delineation of lymph node target volume for lung cancer conformal radiotherapy. Proposal for standardizing terminology based on surgical experience. Strahlenther Onkol 177:410–423

Koh WJ, Bergman KS, Rasey JS, Peterson LM, Evans ML, Graham MM, Grierson JR, Lindsley KL, Lewellen TK, Krohn KA (1995) Evaluation of oxygenation status during fractionated radiotherapy in human non-small cell lung cancers using [F-18]fluoromisonidazole positron emission tomography. Int J Radiat Oncol Biol Phys 33:391–398

Koritzinsky M, Seigneuric R, Magagnin MG, van den Beucken T, Lambin P, Wouters BG (2005) The hypoxic proteome is influenced by gene-specific changes in mRNA translation. Radiother Oncol 76:177–186

Langen KJ, Ziemons K, Kiwit JC, Herzog H, Kuwert T, Bock WJ, Stocklin G, Feinendegen LE, Muller-Gartner HW (1997) 3-[123I]iodo-alpha-methyltyrosine and [methyl-11C]-L-methionine uptake in cerebral gliomas: a comparative study using SPECT and PET. J Nucl Med 38:517–522

Lee NY, Mechalakos JG, Nehmeh S, Lin Z, Squire OD, Cai S, Chan K, Zanzonico PB, Greco C, Ling CC, Humm JL, Schöder H (2008) Fluorine-18-labeled fluoromisonidazole positron emission and computed tomography-guided intensity-modulated radiotherapy for head and neck cancer: a feasibility study. Int J Radiat Oncol Biol Phys 70:2–13

Ling CC, Humm J, Larson S, Amols H, Fuks Z, Leibel S, Koutcher JA (2000) Towards multidimensional radiotherapy (MD-CRT): biological imaging and biological conformality. Int J Radiat Oncol Biol Phys 47:551–560

Ling CC, Yorke E, Amols H, Mechalakos J, Erdi Y, Leibel S, Rosenzweig K, Jackson A (2004) High-tech will improve radiotherapy of NSCLC: a hypothesis waiting to be validated. Int J Radiat Oncol Biol Phys 60:3–7

Liu T, Xu W, Yan WL, Ye M, Bai YR, Huang G (2007) FDG-PET, CT, MRI for diagnosis of local residual or recurrent nasopharyngeal carcinoma, which one is the best? A systematic review. Radiother Oncol 85:327–335

MacManus MP, Hicks RJ, Matthews JP, Hogg A, McKenzie AF, Wirth A, Ware RE, Ball DL (2001) High rate of detection of unsuspected distant metastases by PET in apparent stage III non-small-cell lung cancer: implications for radical radiation therapy. Int J Radiat Oncol Biol Phys 50:287–293

MacManus MP, Bayne M, Fimmell N, Reynolds J, Everitt S, Ball D, Pitman A, Ware R, Lau E (2007) Reproducibility of "intelligent" contouring of gross tumor volume in non-small cell lung cancer on PET/CT images using a standardized visual method. Int J Radiat Oncol Biol Phys 69:S154–S155

Madani I, Duthoy W, Derie C, De Gersem W, Boterberg T, Saerens M, Jacobs F, Gregoire V, Lonneux M, Vakaet L, Vanderstraeten B, Bauters W, Bonte K, Thierens H, De Neve W (2007) Positron emission tomography-guided, focal-dose escalation using intensity-modulated radiotherapy for head and neck cancer. Int J Radiat Oncol Biol Phys 68:126–135

Munley MT, Marks LB, Scarfone C, Sibley GS, Patz EF Jr, Turkington TG, Jaszczak RJ, Gilland DR, Anscher MS, Coleman RE (1999) Multimodality nuclear medicine imaging in three-dimensional radiation treatment planning for lung cancer: challenges and prospects. Lung Cancer 23:105–114

Nakamoto Y, Tatsumi M, Hammoud D, Cohade C, Osman MM, Wahl RL (2005) Normal FDG distribution patterns in the head and neck: PET/CT evaluation. Radiology 234:879–885

Nehmeh SA, Lee NY, Schroder H, Squire O, Zanzonico PB, Erdi YE, Greco C, Mageras G, Pham HS, Larson SM, Ling CC, Humm JL (2008) Reproducibility of intratumor distribution of (18)F-fluoromisonidazole in head and neck cancer. Int J Radiat Oncol Biol Phys 70:235–242

Nestle U, Walter K, Schmidt S, Licht N, Nieder C, Motaref B, Hellwig D, Niewald M, Ukena D, Kirsch CM, Sybrecht GW, Schnabel K (1999) 18F-deoxyglucose positron emission tomography (FDG-PET) for the planning of radiotherapy in lung cancer: high impact in patients with atelectasis. Int J Radiat Oncol Biol Phys 44:593–597

Nestle U, Hellwig D, Schmidt S, Licht N, Walter K, Ukena D, Rübe C, Baumann M, Kirsch CM (2002) 2-Deoxy-2-[18F] fluoro-D-glucose positron emission tomography in target volume definition for radiotherapy of patients with non-small-cell lung cancer. Mol Imaging Biol 4:257–263

Nestle U, Kremp S, Schaefer-Schuler A, Sebastian-Welsch C, Hellwig D, Rübe C, Kirsch CM (2005) Comparison of different methods for delineation of 18F-FDG PET-positive tissue for target volume definition in radiotherapy of patients with non-small cell lung cancer. J Nucl Med 46:1342–1348

Nestle U, Kremp S, Grosu A (2006) Practical integration of [(18)F]-FDG-PET and PET-CT in the planning of radiotherapy for non-small cell lung cancer (NSCLC): the technical basis, ICRU-target volumes, problems, perspectives. Radiother Oncol 81:209–225

Nestle U, Schaefer-Schuler A, Kremp S, Groeschel A, Hellwig D, Rube C, Kirsch CM (2007) Target volume definition for (18)F-FDG PET-positive lymph nodes in radiotherapy of patients with non-small cell lung cancer. Eur J Nucl Med Mol Imaging 34:453–462

Nishioka T, Shiga T, Shirato H, Tsukamoto E, Tsuchiya K, Kato T, Ohmori K, Yamazaki A, Aoyama H, Hashimoto S, Chang TC, Miyasaka K (2002) Image fusion between 18FDG-PET and MRI/CT for radiotherapy planning of oropharyngeal and nasopharyngeal carcinomas. Int J Radiat Oncol Biol Phys 53:1051–1057

Nordsmark M, Bentzen SM, Rudat V, Brizel D, Lartigau E, Stadler P, Becker A, Adam M, Molls M, Dunst J, Terris DJ, Overgaard J (2005) Prognostic value of tumor oxygenation in 397 head and neck tumors after primary radiation therapy. An international multi-center study. Radiother Oncol 77:18–24

Paulino AC, Koshy M, Howell R, Schuster D, Davis LW (2005) Comparison of CT- and FDG-PET-defined gross tumor volume in intensity-modulated radiotherapy for head-and-neck cancer. Int J Radiat Oncol Biol Phys 61:1385–1392

Pötzsch C, Hofheinz F, van den Hoff J (2006) Vergleich der Inter-Observer-Variabilität bei manueller und automatischer Volumenbestimmung in der PET. Nuklearmedizin (German) 45:A42

Rahn AN, Baum RP, Adamietz IA, Adams S, Sengupta S, Mose S, Bormeth SB, Hor G, Bottcher HD (1998) Value of 18F fluorodeoxyglucose positron emission tomography in radiotherapy planning of head-neck tumors. Strahlenther Onkol 174:358–364

Rasey JS, Koh WJ, Evans ML, Peterson LM, Lewellen TK, Graham MM, Krohn KA (1996) Quantifying regional hypoxia in human tumors with positron emission tomography of [18F]fluoromisonidazole: a pretherapy study of 37 patients. Int J Radiat Oncol Biol Phys 36:417–428

Rosenzweig KE, Sura S, Jackson A, Yorke E (2007) Involved-field radiation therapy for inoperable non-small-cell lung cancer. J Clin Oncol 25:5557–5561

Scarfone C, Lavely WC, Cmelak AJ, Delbeke D, Martin WH, Billheimer D, Hallahan DE (2004) Prospective feasibility trial of radiotherapy target definition for head and neck cancer using 3-dimensional PET and CT imaging J Nucl Med 45:543–552

Schaefer A, Kremp S, Hellwig D, Ruebe C, Kirsch CM, Nestle U (2008) A contrast-oriented algorithm for FDG-PET-based delineation of tumour volumes for the radiotherapy of lung cancer: derivation from phantom measurements and validation in patient data. Eur J Nucl Med Mol Imaging 35: 1989–1999

Schinagl DA, Vogel WV, Hoffmann AL, van Dalen JA, Oyen WJ, Kaanders JH (2007) Comparison of five segmentation tools for 18F-fluoro-deoxy-glucose-positron emission tomography-based target volume definition in head and neck cancer. Int J Radiat Oncol Biol Phys 69:1282–1289

Schöder H, Carlson DL, Kraus DH, Stambuk HE, Gonen M, Erdi YE, Yeung HW, Huvos AG, Shah JP, Larson SM, Wong RJ (2006) 18F-FDG PET/CT for detecting nodal metastases in patients with oral cancer staged N0 by clinical examination and CT/MRI. J Nucl Med 47:755–762

Schwartz DL, Ford E, Rajendran J, Yueh B, Coltrera MD, Virgin J, Anzai Y, Haynor D, Lewellyn B, Mattes D, Meyer J, Phillips M, Leblanc M, Kinahan P, Krohn K, Eary J, Laramore GE (2005a) FDG-PET/CT imaging for preradiotherapy staging of head-and-neck squamous cell carcinoma. Int J Radiat Oncol Biol Phys 61:129–136

Schwartz DL, Ford EC, Rajendran J, Yueh B, Coltrera MD, Virgin J, Anzai Y, Haynor D, Lewellen B, Mattes D, Kinahan P, Meyer J, Phillips M, Leblanc M, Krohn K, Eary J, Laramore GE (2005b) FDG-PET/CT-guided intensity modulated head and neck radiotherapy: a pilot investigation. Head Neck 27:478–487

Shields AF, Grierson JR, Dohmen BM, Machulla HJ, Stayanoff JC, Lawhorn-Crews JM, Obradovich JE, Muzik O, Mangner TJ (1998) Imaging proliferation in vivo with [F-18]FLT and positron emission tomography. Nat Med 4:1334–1336

Steenbakkers RJ, Duppen JC, Fitton I, Deurloo KE, Zijp LJ, Comans EF, Uitterhoeve AL, Rodrigus PT, Kramer GW, Bussink J, De Jaeger K, Belderbos JS, Nowak PJ, van Herk M, Rasch CR (2006) Reduction of observer variation using matched CT-PET for lung cancer delineation: a three-dimensional analysis. Int J Radiat Oncol Biol Phys 64:435–448

Sura S, Greco C, Gelblum D, Yorke ED, Jackson A, Rosenzweig KE (2008) (18)F-fluorodeoxyglucose positron emission tomography-based assessment of local failure patterns in non-small-cell lung cancer treated with definitive radiotherapy. Int J Radiat Oncol Biol Phys 70:1397–1402

Tanderup K, Olsen DR, Grau C (2006) Dose painting: art or science? Radiother Oncol 79:245–248

Troost EG, Bussink J, Kaanders JH, van Eerd J, Peters JP, Rijken PF, Boerman OC, van der Kogel AJ (2005) Comparison of different methods of CAIX quantification in relation to hypoxia in three human head and neck tumor lines. Radiother Oncol 76:194–199

Van de Steene J, Linthout N, de Mey J, Vinh-Hung V, Claassens C, Noppen M, Bel A, Storme G (2002) Definition of gross tumor volume in lung cancer: inter-observer variability. Radiother Oncol 62:37–49

Weber WA, Wester HJ, Grosu AL, Herz M, Dzewas B, Feldmann HJ, Molls M, Stocklin G, Schwaiger M (2000) O-(2-[18F]fluoroethyl)-L-tyrosine and L-[methyl-11C] methionine uptake in brain tumours: initial results of a comparative study. Eur J Nucl Med 27:542–549

Weber WA, Dick S, Reidl G, Dzewas B, Busch R, Feldmann HJ, Molls M, Lumenta CB, Schwaiger M, Grosu AL (2001) Correlation between postoperative 3-[(123)I]iodo-L-alpha-methyltyrosine uptake and survival in patients with gliomas. J Nucl Med 42:1144–1150

Weber WA, Grosu AL, Czernin J (2008) Technology insight: advances in molecular imaging and an appraisal of PET/CT scanning. Nat Clin Pract Oncol 5:160–170

Williams KJ, Telfer BA, Xenaki D, Sheridan MR, Desbaillets I, Peters HJ, Honess D, Harris AL, Dachs GU, van der Kogel A, Stratford IJ (2005) Enhanced response to radiotherapy in tumours deficient in the function of hypoxia-inducible factor-1. Radiother Oncol 75:89–98

Yap CS, Czernin J, Fishbein MC, Cameron RB, Schiepers C, Phelps ME, Weber WA (2006) Evaluation of thoracic tumors with 18F-fluorothymidine and 18F-fluorodeoxyglucose-positron emission tomography Chest 129:393–401

Yaremko B, Riauka T, Robinson D, Murray B, Alexander A, McEwan A, Roa W (2005) Thresholding in PET images of static and moving targets. Phys Med Biol 50:5969–5982

Yaromina A, Holscher T, Eicheler W, Rosner A, Krause M, Hessel F, Petersen C, Thames HD, Baumann M, Zips D (2005) Does heterogeneity of pimonidazole labelling correspond to the heterogeneity of radiation-response of FaDu human squamous cell carcinoma? Radiother Oncol 76:206–212

Zimny M, Wildberger JE, Cremerius U, DiMartino E, Jaenicke S, Nowak B, Bull U (2002) Combined image interpretation of computed tomography and hybrid PET in head and neck cancer. Nuklearmedizin 41:14–21

Quantitative Cell Kill
of Radio- and Chemotherapy

10

Michael Molls, Carsten Nieder, Claus Belka, and Jan Norum

CONTENTS

KEY POINTS

- Many anticancer drugs are cell-cycle specific and therefore most active against cells that are proliferating. Thus, the non-proliferating fraction is difficult to eradicate. Tumor regrowth in between cycles of therapy (repopulation) also contributes to limited efficacy.
- Experimental evidence suggests that single radiation doses result in 1% or less cell survival compared with 10–50% with cytotoxic drugs. Although clinically impressive remissions of solid tumors might occur after chemotherapy, the underlying cell kill is often not larger than 1–2 log and pathological examination of tissue specimens reveals residual viable tumor cells.
- The two Stockholm breast cancer trials in women treated with modified radical mastectomy provide a comparison of postoperative radiotherapy and chemotherapy with a median follow-up of 18 years. Locoregional recurrence was observed in 14% after radiotherapy and 24% after chemotherapy in premenopausal patients (hazard ratio 0.67, $p = 0.048$) and in 12% after radiotherapy and 26% after chemotherapy in postmenopausal patients (hazard ratio 0.43, $p < 0.001$).

M. Molls, MD
Professor, Director, Clinic of Radiation Oncology, Klinikum rechts der Isar, Technische Universität München, Ismaninger Straße 22, 81675 Munich, Germany

C. Belka, MD
Professor, Director, Clinic of Radiation Oncology, Ludwigs-Maximilians-Universität München, Marchioninistraße 15, 81377 Munich, Germany

C. Nieder, MD
Professor, University of Tromsø, Department of Internal Medicine – Oncology, Nordlandssykehuset HF Hospital, Prinsensgate 164, 8092 Bodø, Norway

J. Norum, MD
Professor, Department of Oncology, University Hospital Tromsø, Postboks, 9038 Tromsø, Norway

- The curative potential of chemotherapy alone has remained low in most solid tumors. Obviously chemotherapy or medical treatment alone is unable to control definitively macroscopic solid tumors in adults (either metastases or primary tumors) with the exception of testicular carcinomas. As a result of the limited efficacy, current studies are trying to enrich the patient population that is likely to respond, based, for example, on gene signatures or different pathology features that might predict the outcome.

- The introduction of combined modality approaches was a highly significant step in the evolution of curative cancer treatment. The most pronounced increase in therapeutic gain was probably seen by combining surgery and/or radiation with chemotherapy. As recently suggested from the data of patients with glioblastoma, head and neck, and esophageal cancer who received radiotherapy alone or radio- and chemotherapy, the effect of the drugs in combined modality treatment corresponds to the equivalent of 9–12 Gy in 2-Gy fractions. In many clinical situations, radiation dose escalation by 9–12 Gy would result in increased late toxicity risks. Under these circumstances, combining radio- and chemotherapy increases the therapeutic window.

- In practice, the efficacy of radiotherapy might be reduced by limitations in imaging/detection of malignant cells (target volume definition), precision of treatment delivery (intra- and interfraction motion), and various factors related to tumor biology (oxygenation, cell cycle distribution, etc.).

- Both experimental and clinical observations have repeatedly confirmed the influence of initial tumor volume or cell number on local control and the need for administration of higher radiation doses in large-volume disease.

Abstract

This chapter contains a review of the potential of radio- and chemotherapy to eradicate tumor cells. With regard to the amount of quantitative cell kill, important differences exist between ionizing radiation and chemother-apy. In principle, radiation treatment can be designed to cover the whole tumor with a homogeneously distributed full radiation dose, capable of inactivation of all tumor cells. In contrast, pharmacotherapy is limited by the fact that the dose of the active, cell-killing form of the compound is variable within the tumor and its cells. This results from problems in the delivery of drugs (perfusion, interstitial fluid pressure, tissue pH, protein binding, etc.), cellular uptake, efflux, inactivation, and other mechanisms of resistance. In many instances, the agent does not reach the relevant therapeutic targets in the required concentration and for a sufficient time period. In fact, the pharmacokinetic profile of anticancer drugs is characterized by substantial interpatient variability where two- to threefold variation is not uncommon. These issues even gain complexity with simultaneous administration of two or more drugs. Such multiagent regimens with different modes of action might be valuable when each agent kills different tumor cells, which would not become inactivated by the other agent. Depending on variations in actual drug concentration, a fixed combination of two drugs might either show additivity or antagonism in the same tumor cells. Both preclinical and clinical data confirm that rationally designed drug combinations often lead to improved results. Several studies support the superior quantitative cell kill of radiotherapy and suggest that simultaneous application of radio- and chemotherapy is an important measure to increase the efficacy of non-surgical cancer treatment.

10.1
Introduction

10.1.1
Clinical Relevance
of Radio- and Chemotherapy

The curative potential of radiotherapy, for example, for limited-stage malignancies of the skin and other organs that could be treated to high doses with the technology available at that time, was explored very soon after the landmark discoveries by Wilhelm Conrad Roentgen and many other enthusiastic pioneers in the newly emerging field of radiation medicine. As early as 1912, the German journal *Strahlentherapie & Onkologie* was published for the first time. The elegant work on dose-effect relationships of, for example, Magnus Strandqvist, which was published in 1944, has been summarized in one of the early issues of the *Interna-*

tional Journal of Radiation Oncology Biology and Physics (DEL REGATO 1989). Driven by rapid progress in both machine development, discovery of new isotopes, and understanding of the basic biological principles, the number of indications and successful treatment strategies has increased tremendously during the twentieth century. Eventually, the basis for high-precision proton and heavy ion beam application has been established (LAWRENCE et al. 1963). Today, patients with early-stage solid tumors (T1, T2; N0; M0), such as prostate cancer or non-small cell lung cancer (NSCLC), are cured by linear accelerator photon radiation treatment alone [prostate: brachytherapy or intensity modulated radiation treatment (IMRT) (NGUYEN and ZIETMAN 2007); lung: stereotactic fractionated radiation treatment (ZIMMERMANN et al. 2006)].

Later during that century, the first encouraging efforts in systemic chemotherapy with cytotoxic drugs, in particular in patients with leukemias, malignant lymphomas, and testicular cancer, contributed to a continuous increase and refinement of cancer treatment approaches (BEN-ASHER 1949; SCOTT 1970). More and more specific drug targets have been discovered, rational drug combinations have been designed, and, thus, an unprecedented number of clinically established neoadjuvant, adjuvant, and palliative regimens have become available today. However, the curative potential of chemotherapy alone has remained low in most solid tumors. The introduction of combined modality approaches was a highly significant step in the evolution of curative cancer treatment. Parallel to refinements of each single modality, combined treatment has actively been investigated in recent decades in both preclinical and clinical studies around the world. When judged at this time, the most pronounced increase in therapeutic gain was probably seen by combining surgery and/or radiation with chemotherapy.

Meanwhile a huge body of evidence supports the use of combined modality approaches based on the combination of ionizing radiation with cytostatic and cytotoxic drugs. In this regard, several randomized phase III trials for many relevant cancer sites provide a sound basis for level-one evidence-based decisions. This holds true especially for glioblastoma multiforme (STUPP et al. 2005), head and neck cancers including nasopharyngeal cancer and laryngeal cancer (BRIZEL et al. 1998; FORASTIERE et al. 2003; BUDACH et al. 2005), esophageal cancer (MINSKY et al. 2002; SIEWERT et al. 2007), colorectal and anal cancer (BARTELINK et al. 1997; SAUER et al. 2004), cervical cancer (GREEN et al. 2001), as well as lung cancer (SCHAAKE-KONING et al. 1992).

10.2
Basic Considerations

10.2.1
Treatment Aims

The most important aim of curative cancer treatment is to eradicate all tumor cells. With regard to the amount of quantitative cell kill, it has to be emphasized that important differences exist between ionizing radiation and chemotherapy (Fig. 10.1). In principle, radiation treatment can be designed to cover the whole tumor with a homogeneously distributed full radiation dose, capable of inactivation of all tumor cells. In contrast, pharmacotherapy is limited by the fact that the dose of the active, cell-killing form of the compound is variable within the tumor and its cells (Fig. 10.2). This results from problems in the delivery of drugs (perfusion, interstitial fluid pressure, tissue pH, protein binding, etc.), cellular uptake, efflux, metabolization, inactivation, and other molecular and cellular mechanisms of resistance. In many instances, the agent does not reach the relevant therapeutic targets in the required concentration and for a sufficient time period (TANNOCK et al. 2002; PRIMEAU et al. 2005; MINCHINTON and TANNOCK 2006). In fact, the pharmacokinetic profile of anticancer drugs is characterized by substantial interpatient variability where two- to three-fold variation is not uncommon (BRUNSVIG et al. 2007). These issues even gain complexity with simultaneous administration of two or more drugs. Such multiagent regimens with different modes of action might be valuable when each agent kills different tumor cells, which would not become inactivated by the other agents; however, sometimes all agents might act on the same cell, causing much more damage than necessary for cell death. Depending on variations in actual drug concentration, a fixed combination of two drugs might either show additivity or antagonism in the same tumor cells (LEE et al. 2006). Cells surviving initial chemotherapy may upregulate active resistance mechanisms, which allows for growth despite therapy (TEICHER et al. 1990; GRAHAM et al. 1994). Furthermore, cells may survive until therapy cessation by downregulating metabolism/cycling, becoming temporarily quiescent (STEWART et al. 2007). Another factor that interferes with our ability to deliver tumor-eradicating treatment is toxicity/damage to normal tissues and organs. While such toxicity typically is limited to the tumor surroundings in the context of surgery and radiotherapy, more widespread effects limit the maximum tolerable doses of systemically administered agents (bone marrow toxicity, neuropathy, cardiac

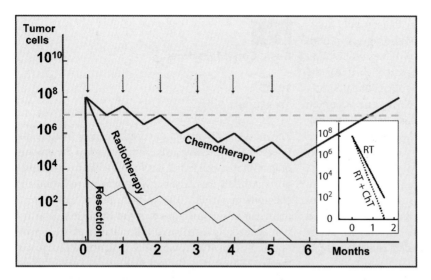

Fig. 10.1. Differences in quantitative cell kill and time course. Influence of different therapeutic modalities on number of tumor cells during a course of treatment, based on models
(Tannock 1989, 1992; Minchinton and Tannock 2006). The *dashed line* represents the
border between microscopic and macroscopic tumors, defined as a size of approximately
5 mm. Compared with surgical resection and fractionated radiotherapy, multiple courses of
chemotherapy (in this case six, indicated by *arrows*) are less efficient in cell kill. While microscopic disease might be eradicated (*lower chemotherapy curve*), clinical evidence suggests
that most macroscopic solid tumors (exception: more sensitive testicular cancers) will shrink
temporarily but eventually regrow from surviving residues (*upper chemotherapy curve*). As
shown in the *inset*, the strength of chemotherapy in combination with radiation treatment
(in addition to spatial cooperation) is the modification of the slope of the curve

Ionizing Radiation

Homogeneous dose distribution. Tumor cell
kill depends on intrinsic radiosensitivity, local
physiology and biochemical status of the tumor
subvolumes. In principle, the whole tumor can
be covered by the radiation dose required to
kill all tumor cells.

Pharmaceuticals

Inhomogeneous dose distribution. Tumor cell
kill depends on delivery of the drug, uptake in
tumor tissue and cells, local physiology,
biochemical status, multidrug resistance etc.
Often, subvolumes and relevant therapeutic
targets are not covered by the full drug dose

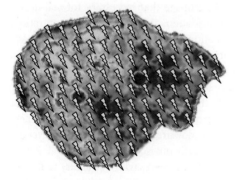
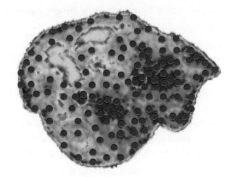

Fig. 10.2. Comparison between tumor dose distribution in radiation treatment and pharmaceutical treatment. Il-
lustrative tumor sections from a squamous cell carcinoma demonstrate biological heterogeneity, reflected by the
differently colored areas, within the tumor. Homogeneous radiation dose distribution within the tumor irrespective
of differences in biology, physiology, functional factors, structure, and morphology. Heterogeneous dose distribution
for drug treatment, related, for example, to regional differences in perfusion, pH, metabolism, etc. Drug molecules
are shown as *red circles*. (The histological section is courtesy of W. Müller-Klieser, Johannes Gutenberg University,
Mainz, Germany)

damage, kidney damage, infertility, etc.). Here it is also worth noting that in contrast to malignant tissues the normal tissue of the different organs does not develop resistance toward anticancer pharmaceuticals. Systemic radiotherapy such as radionuclides for the treatment of bone metastases or certain types of lymphomas will of course also be able to cause some of the systemic effects. This particular type of radiation treatment, however, will not be discussed in greater detail in this chapter.

10.2.2
Aspects Specific to Radiotherapy

As illustrated in Fig. 10.1, the quantitative cell kill of ionizing radiation is significantly larger than that of chemotherapy (Tannock 1992, 1998; Minchinton and Tannock 2006). The magnitude of the relatively low efficiency of chemotherapy might vary with cell type, culture conditions, drug, exposure time, etc. Experimental evidence suggests, however, that single radiation doses result in 1% or less cell survival compared with 10–50% with cytotoxic drugs (Epstein 1990; Kim et al. 1992; Simoens et al. 2003; Eliaz et al. 2004). Although clinically impressive remissions of solid tumors might occur after chemotherapy, the underlying cell kill is often not larger than 1–2 log and pathological examination of tissue specimens reveals residual viable tumor cells. From these cells local, regional, and distant failure can eventually emerge.

In practice, the efficacy of radiotherapy might be reduced by limitations in imaging/detection of malignant cells (target volume definition), precision of treatment delivery (intra- and interfraction motion), and various factors related to tumor biology, which will be discussed later in this chapter. However, the experience with image-guided high-precision radiotherapy based on combined biological and anatomical imaging suggests that the magnitude of such limitations is likely to diminish (Grosu et al. 2006).

Extensive discussion of radiobiological principles is beyond the scope of this chapter, yet a few definitions will be mentioned. The response of tumors to radiotherapy is determined by several factors such as repopulation, reoxygenation, number of clonogenic cells, and their intrinsic radiosensitivity. Since the introduction of mammalian cell survival curves, the parameters D_0 and N have been used as quantitative measures of inherent radiation sensitivity, as was the shoulder width Dq (Thames and Suit 1986). Today the ratio alpha/beta is the most common parameter for characterization of cell survival curves. It is also a measure of fractionation sensitivity.

When combining two treatment modalities, the resulting net effect on cell killing is mainly described by the terms "additivity, synergism, and subadditivity," which are derived from experimental investigations. They are not applicable to the clinical situation and do not reflect the results of clinical trials, where changes from radiation as a monotherapy to multimodal treatment usually do not result in extraordinarily favorable cure rates (or supra-additivity), although they have led to important gradual improvement. It appears prudent to refer to the term "enhancement of radiation effect" within a clinical context.

The smaller the tumor, the higher is the success rate of radiation treatment, as illustrated in the Japanese study of carbon ion therapy for stage I NSCLC (Miyamoto et al. 2007). For T1 disease, the local control rate was 98% at a median follow-up of 39 months, while it was 80% for T2 tumors. With the same modality, 97% of choroidal melanoma were locally controlled at 3 years (Tsuji et al. 2007). For skull base chondrosarcomas, local control was achieved in 90% of the cases at 4 years (Schulz-Ertner et al. 2007). In small early-stage NSCLC, comparable local control data were published for stereotactic radiosurgery with photon beams (Zimmermann et al. 2006; Hof et al. 2007). In early, stage Ib squamous cell carcinoma of the uterine cervix, radiation therapy alone resulted in 5-year survival of 93.5% and local control of 92% (Ota et al. 2007). Radiation doses that control early stage T1 prostate cancer result in less favorable outcome when administered to advanced T3 disease (Zelefsky et al. 2008). With higher doses and/or combined radiation and androgen ablation, however, high 5- and 10-year local control rates can be achieved even in T3 tumors (Zelefsky et al. 2008). Both experimental and clinical observations have repeatedly confirmed the influence of initial tumor volume or cell number on local control (Khalil et al. 1997; Zhao et al. 2007) and the need for administration of higher radiation doses in large-volume disease. The preclinical data of radiotherapy under hypoxic and ambient conditions also suggest that the dose-volume relationship is present under both conditions, i.e., not just related to increasing hypoxia in larger tumors.

Whether surgery and radiotherapy are equally effective in small-volume disease is difficult to judge as very few direct randomized comparisons with sufficient sample size have been published. One of the best examples is probably the French trial comparing 658 breast cancer patients with clinically uninvolved lymph nodes, which were treated with lumpectomy plus axillary dissection or axillary radiotherapy (Louis-Sylvestre et al. 2004). In the group with dissected axilla, 21% of the patients were node positive. The median follow-up was 180 months.

Recurrence in the axillary nodes was less frequent in the surgery arm (1% versus 3%, $p = 0.04$); however, distant metastases rates and overall survival were not significantly different, suggesting that the small difference in axillary control is not clinically meaningful. Different non-randomized studies, for example, in patients with inflammatory breast cancer initially treated with induction chemotherapy at the University of Texas M. D. Anderson Cancer Center in Houston, Texas, USA, also suggest that local treatment with either surgery or radiotherapy is equally effective (UENO et al. 1997). Comparing urological and radiotherapeutic literature one can state that in early prostate cancer (up to T2a category, cN0, cM0) the cure rates of radiation treatment and prostatectomy do not differ in a significant manner. A similar situation exists also for other tumor entities, especially, for example, for head and neck cancers.

10.2.3
Aspects Specific to Chemotherapy

Many anticancer drugs are cell-cycle specific and therefore most active against cells that are proliferating. Thus, the non-proliferating fraction is difficult to eradicate. Tumor regrowth (repopulation) in between cycles of therapy also contributes to limited efficacy. Typically, one tries to administer the highest possible dose of drugs in the shortest possible time intervals. Even the use of dose-dense regimens, high-dose treatment with bone marrow or hematopoietic stem cell transplantation, and the development of non-cross-resistant regimens has not yet resulted in cure of the most common solid tumors with chemotherapy.

In earlier studies of neoadjuvant chemotherapy for locally advanced breast cancer, pathological complete remission (pCR) at surgery was seen in 5–15% of patients (typically anthracycline-based regimens) and it was found that pCR patients had better long-term outcomes (FERRIERE et al. 1998; KARLSSON et al. 1998). Even with modern drug combinations, pCR after neoadjuvant chemotherapy (for breast cancer with or without trastuzumab) is seen in only 15–38% of breast cancer patients (DEO et al. 2003; SMITH et al. 2004; EVANS et al. 2005; REITSAMER et al. 2005; VON MINCKWITZ et al. 2005; ARDAVANIS et al. 2006; HURLEY et al. 2006; VEYRET et al. 2006; ARNOULD et al. 2007) and 9–20% of cervical cancer patients (BUDA et al. 2005; MODARRESS et al. 2005). In a randomized setting, the pCR rate in cervical cancer was much lower after neoadjuvant chemotherapy alone than after radiochemotherapy (10% versus 43%; $p < 0.05$; MODARRESS et al. 2005). The definitive cure rates with chemotherapy alone would certainly be

lower than the pCR rates, because some surviving clonogenic tumor cells, which are not readily detectable, are still present in the histopathological specimen. As mentioned above, the curves shown in Fig. 10.1 depend on several variables related to patient selection, tumor microenvironment and sensitivity, agent and dose, etc. They are meant to illustrate the principle; however, the results of some neoadjuvant chemotherapy trials demonstrate the variability in the steepness of these curves. As a result of the limited efficacy of chemotherapy, current studies are trying to enrich the patient population that is likely to respond, based, for example, on gene signatures or different pathology features that might predict the outcome (MINNA et al. 2007).

As recently demonstrated from an exploratory analysis of data from two parallel phase III chemotherapy studies in metastatic colorectal cancer, even non-responders, despite a poorer prognosis than responders, achieved extended progression-free and overall survival from more effective drug combinations, which were tested against older standards (GROTHEY et al. 2008). One of the trials examined IFL (irinotecan, 5-fluorouracil, leucovorin) versus IFL plus the angiogenesis inhibitor bevacizumab, and the other trial compared IFL to oxaliplatin, 5-fluorouracil, and leucovorin. The hazard ratios for the different study endpoints and drug regimens ranged from 0.63 to 0.76 in responders and non-responders. In a large analysis of 1,508 patients with advanced or metastatic colorectal cancer treated in a phase III study, 4% had complete remission after chemotherapy alone (DY et al. 2007). The three treatment arms of the study consisted of IFL, oxaliplatin plus 5-fluorouracil/leucovorin, and irinotecan plus oxaliplatin. The highest rate of complete remissions was 6%, observed in the oxaliplatin plus 5-fluorouracil/leucovorin arm. Size of the metastases significantly influenced the likelihood of complete remission. Of the patients with initial complete remission to chemotherapy, 84% developed progression within 5 years. The median time to progression was 15 months. With second-line chemotherapy, complete remission is even more unlikely in this disease.

10.3
Attempts to Compare the Efficacy of Radio- and Chemotherapy

10.3.1
Animal Studies

In this section, examples are discussed that are focused on the undifferentiated human hypopharyngeal cell line

FaDu. This cell line was first described in 1972 and has a doubling time in vitro of about 1.2–2.8 days. Extensive experiments by the group from Dresden, Germany, are summarized in Table 10.1 and compared to data from other groups. Among different, but equally sized human head and neck squamous cell carcinomas growing in nude mice, which received total body irradiation before tumor transplantation, the radiation dose to control 50% of the tumors (TCD$_{50}$) after a sufficient follow-up of 120 days varied tremendously (YAROMINA et al. 2007). After local radiation treatment with 30 fractions over 6 weeks, the TCD$_{50}$ was, for example, 45 Gy for UT-SCC-8 cells, 85 Gy for FaDu cells, and 127 Gy for SAS cells. Thus, FaDu represents a cell line that is neither particularly sensitive nor resistant. Another reason for focusing on this cell line is the number of data available for review. Some in vitro data from experiments with FaDu are shown in Table 10.2. Comparable variations in sensitivity across a panel of cell lines were made for different pharmacological agents and tumor cell lines, emphasizing the role of intrinsic sensitivity. As shown in Table 10.1, FaDu tumors can be controlled with clinically readily achievable doses of radiation, while the results of chemotherapy at the maximum tolerated dose vary tremendously. Some drug combinations achieve better results than the respective single treatments. As previously described by other authors, reduction of the tumor volume before the start of radiotherapy, in this example by the use of epidermal growth factor receptor-tyrosine kinase inhibition, failed to translate into improved local tumor control after sufficient follow-up (KRAUSE et al. 2007). All these observations question the value of clinical strategies where radiotherapy or simultaneous radiochemotherapy is preceded by induction chemotherapy or tyrosine kinase inhibitors. Summarizing this paragraph it is also very important to note that one has to be very cautious when transferring experimental in vitro and in vivo results into the clinical

Table 10.1. Overview of animal experiments with subcutaneously implanted FaDu tumor cells

Reference	Model	Treatment details	Results
SCHÜTZE et al. (2007a)	Nude mice having received 4 Gy TBI	Ambient conditions without anesthesia, air-breathing animals	Single dose 25 Gy controlled 29% at day 120 Single dose 35 Gy controlled 57% at day 120
KRAUSE et al. (2007)	Nude mice having received 4 Gy TBI	Ambient conditions without anesthesia, air-breathing animals	Total doses 8–60 Gy, 5 fractions in 5 days Evaluation of tumor control at day 120 Up to 32 Gy: <25% of tumors are controlled TCD$_{50}$=41 Gy TCD$_{100}$=60 Gy
CAO et al. (2005)	Nude mice	Maximum tolerable dose	10–20% cure with capecitabine or irinotecan 80–90% cure with combination of both agents
AZRAK et al. (2004)	Nude mice	Maximum tolerable dose	<30% cure with irinotecan 0% cure with 5-fluorouracil 60–100% cure with combination of both agents
JOSCHKO et al. (1997)	Nude mice having received 5 Gy TBI	Maximum tolerable dose	Daily gemcitabine results in a median time to regrowth to 200% of the initial volume of 5 days Once weekly gemcitabine results in a median time to regrowth to 200% of the initial volume of 13 days Twice weekly gemcitabine results in a median time to regrowth to 200% of the initial volume of 16 days
JOSCHKO et al. (1997)	Nude mice having received 5 Gy TBI	Ambient conditions without anesthesia, air-breathing animals	40 Gy in 20 fractions in 2 weeks results in a median time to regrowth to 200% of the initial volume of 43 days

TBI Total body irradiation

Note that the sensitivity to drug treatment might change with tumor location within the host animal, as described by (HOLDEN et al. 1997). In general, time to regrowth is a less valuable and accepted endpoint than local tumor control

Table 10.2. Overview of in vitro experiments with the FaDu cell line (cell culture conditions varied between the individual reports)

Agent	IC_{50} (µmol/l)	Resistance fraction	Radiation therapy parameters		Reference
Cisplatin	1.02 ± .15	5.3 ± 1.5			Lee et al. (2006)
5-Fluorouracil	7.59 ± 1.15	25.4 ± 1.1			
Paclitaxel	1.25 ± 0.57	11.8 ± 2.3			
			SF 0.1	4.1–4.5 Gy	Schütze et al. (2007b)
			SF 0.01	7.3–7.7 Gy	

IC_{50} Inhibitory concentration at 50% survival, *SF 0.1* radiation dose reducing the survival fraction to 1%

IC_{50} values for FaDu are within the range of those reported for other squamous cell carcinoma, for example, Raitanen et al. (2002)

IC_{50} values for different cell lines treated with the same agent are variable: 3–35 nM, for example, for paclitaxel (Gorodetsky et al. 1998) and 5–50 nM for docetaxel (Clarke and Rivory 1999)

situation. Often one must conclude that experimental treatments especially with pharmacological substances are highly efficient whereas with corresponding treatments in patients the efficiency cannot be reproduced.

10.3.2
Clinical Data

Direct randomized comparisons unfortunately are very rare. However, the two Stockholm breast cancer trials in women treated with modified radical mastectomy provide a comparison of postoperative radiotherapy and chemotherapy with a median follow-up of 18 years (Rutqvist and Johansson 2006). All patients had node-positive disease or a tumor diameter exceeding 30 mm. The radiation dose was 46 Gy in 2-Gy fractions to the chest wall, axilla, supraclavicular fossa, and the ipsilateral internal mammary nodes. Chemotherapy initially consisted of 12 cycles (later 6 cycles) of cyclophosphamide 100 mg/m² orally on days 1–14, methotrexate 40 mg/m² i.v. on days 1 and 8, and 5-fluorouracil 600 mg/m² i.v. on days 1 and 8 (CMF). In the trial that included premenopausal patients, 291 were allocated to CMF and 256 to radiotherapy. In each arm, 12% were node negative. Sixty-two and 64% were estrogen-receptor positive, respectively. Locoregional recurrence was observed in 14% after radiotherapy and 24% after chemotherapy (hazard ratio 0.67, $p = 0.048$). The absolute benefit increased with the number of positive lymph nodes. As might be expected, fewer patients developed distant recurrence after CMF and the eventual difference in breast cancer deaths was 50% versus 56%. This

difference in favor of CMF was not statistically significant ($p = 0.12$), but the sample size was very limited. In the trial that included postmenopausal patients, 182 were allocated to CMF and 148 to radiotherapy. Ten and 12% were node negative, respectively. Sixty-seven and 68% were estrogen-receptor positive, respectively. Locoregional recurrence was observed in 12% after radiotherapy and 26% after chemotherapy (hazard ratio 0.43, $p<0.001$). Again, distant recurrence was reduced by treatment with CMF, as were breast cancer deaths ($p = 0.07$). While treatment of breast cancer has changed to a greater extent after the initiation of these two trials, their results add to the evidence of increased local cell kill after radiotherapy compared to systemic chemotherapy. Data from a subgroup of patients from the Stockholm trials suggest that the magnitude of expression of certain DNA repair proteins (Mre11, Rad50, Nbs1) is associated with the favorable response to radiotherapy (Söderlund et al. 2007).

In an observational study in patients with metastatic melanoma, local treatment with fractionated radiotherapy, single-fraction radiosurgery, or hyperthermia each was superior to systemic treatment (dacarbazine, fotemustine, carboplatin, temozolomide) with regard to local response rates (Richtig et al. 2005). Another study describes the response rate and time to progression in patients with metastatic esophageal cancer treated with chemotherapy alone or combined chemo- and radiotherapy (Lee et al. 2007). All 74 patients initially received two cycles of capecitabine/cisplatin chemotherapy. Patients with distant lymph node metastases continued with lower doses of the same two drugs plus radiotherapy to 54 Gy, while patients with non-lymph node distant metastases continued on full-dose chemotherapy. Partial response to the first two cycles was observed in 20% and 15%, respectively (not significantly different). After treatment completion, a significant difference in favor of radiotherapy-containing treatment was observed (36% versus 63%). Median time to progression also was longer, 5.9 versus 8.4 months ($p = 0.03$).

Interesting data can also be derived from various recently published randomized studies in stage IIIB/IV NSCLC. Some of these studies used chemotherapy combinations, while one focused on palliative radiotherapy to the chest (different fractionation regimens) with only a few of the patients receiving additional chemotherapy (SUNDSTROM et al. 2004). With the lowest radiation dose of 17 Gy in 2 fractions, 2-year survival was 8%. With 15 fractions of 2.8 Gy, 13% was achieved. These figures are very close to those reported by the same group with carboplatin/vinorelbine or carboplatin/gemcitabine, i.e., 7% (HELBEKKMO et al. 2007), and those from studies of cisplatin/vinorelbine (YASUDA et al. 2006) or carboplatin/paclitaxel (PACCAGNELLA et al. 2006). Although various types of imbalances between the study populations might exist and some chemotherapy patients likely will also have received radiotherapy, the data are compatible with the hypothesis that the cell kill induced by commonly used cytostatic regimens can only be compared to that of palliative radiotherapy with low to moderate total doses.

While radiotherapy with or without androgen deprivation has long been accepted as the primary curative treatment modality in patients with prostate cancer, the limited experience with chemotherapy before prostatectomy (docetaxel or epirubicin) suggests that pCR is very unlikely. In fact, it was not observed at all in the studies by DREICER et al. (2004), FEBBO et al. (2005), and FRANCINI et al. (2008). Assuming that surviving cancer cells will ultimately result in treatment failure, current cytotoxic drugs are not suitable for curative treatment in this disease, although their palliative role in hormone-refractory disease clearly has been established in recent years (BERTHOLD et al. 2008).

In most clinical situations, chemotherapy augments the radiation-induced cell kill within the irradiated volume and may improve distant control. To maximize augmentation of cell kill, optimization of parameters of drug exposure is necessary. It has been shown, for example, that continuous infusion is better than bolus administration of 5-fluorouracil. The following example illustrates the efficacy of chemotherapy as a radiation enhancer. In the large randomized FFCD 9203 trial in rectal cancer preoperative radiotherapy (45 Gy in 25 fractions) resulted in a pCR in 4%, whereas the addition of 5-fluorouracil and folinic acid improved this figure to 12% (GERARD et al. 2005). As recently suggested from the data of patients with glioblastoma who received radiotherapy alone or radiotherapy plus temozolomide (STUPP et al. 2005), the effect of the drug in combined modality treatment corresponds to the equivalent of 9.1 Gy in 2-Gy fractions (JONES and SANGHERA 2007). In patients treated with neoadjuvant combined chemo- and radiotherapy for esophageal cancer (data from 26 trials combined), it was estimated that 1 g/m^2 of 5-fluorouracil was equivalent to a radiation dose of 1.9 Gy and that 100 mg/m^2 cisplatin was equivalent to a radiation dose of 7.2 Gy (GEH et al. 2006). A combined analysis of 14 head and neck cancer trials confirms these data (KASIBHATLA et al. 2007). With 2–3 cycles of cisplatin, carboplatin, and/or 5-fluorouracil containing radiochemotherapy regimens, the additional dose corresponds to 12 Gy in 2 Gy per fraction daily. In many clinical situations, radiation dose escalation by 9–12 Gy would result in increased late toxicity risks. Under these circumstances, combining radio- and chemotherapy increases the therapeutic window.

While radiation alone can be considered as a curative treatment in a variety of early-stage solid tumors (especially T1-2 N0 M0, for example, skin, anal, cervix, larynx, lung, and prostate cancers, see also above), long-term control with chemotherapy alone is rarely observed. Even in the adjuvant situation, chemotherapy often fails to control micrometastatic disease. Current concepts of cancer biology suggest that most traditional chemotherapy approaches fail to eradicate cancer stem cells, which are slow-cycling cells that often express multidrug resistance (MDR) proteins (MILLER et al. 2005). It has been proposed that approaches targeting this subpopulation of cancer cells might increase the efficacy of drug treatment (KORKAYA and WICHA 2007). Previous strategies of chemotherapy intensification, either by local delivery, systemic high-dose treatment, or simultaneous administration of several non-cross-resistant drugs, for example, 8-drugs-in-1-day, were mostly disappointing (FARQUHAR et al. 2005). Among newer concepts is the so-called metronomic chemotherapy, which refers to prolonged administration of comparatively low doses of cytotoxic drugs with minimal or no drug-free breaks. This strategy is thought to have an antiangiogenic basis and shows encouraging results in preclinical models (SHAKED et al. 2005). It is now also combined with maximum-tolerated dose chemotherapy and targeted agents in vivo (PIETRAS and HANAHAN 2005). Again we like to mention here that in summary one has to assume that especially in macroscopic but very often also in microscopic tumors the specific pathophysiology (vessel architecture, blood flow, interstitial pressure, etc.) is the predominant biological factor minimizing drug efficiency due to an inhomogeneous drug distribution within the tumor tissue and leaving tumor subvolumes with inefficient drug concentrations (MINCHINTON and TANNOCK 2006).

10.4
Interaction of Radiation and Chemotherapy

Therapeutic gain is defined by an increase of tumor control and finally survival without a parallel increase in the severity of specific side effects (Fig. 10.3). Only a few reports are available proving that the combination of radiation and chemotherapy actually results in an increased therapeutic gain. A very nice preclinical example is the comprehensive studies with cisplatin and 5-fluorouracil in different tumors transplanted into mice, which were reported by KALLMAN et al. (1992). In our opinion, this group has demonstrated in an excellent fashion how clinically relevant experiments of radiochemotherapy can be designed. Also worth mentioning is a clinical example, a randomized German phase III trial (BUDACH et al. 2005), where a total of 384 stage III and stage IV head and neck cancer patients were randomly assigned to receive either 30 Gy (2 Gy/day) followed by 1.4 Gy b.i.d. (2 fractions per day) to a total dose of 70.6 Gy concurrently with 5-fluorouracil

and mitomycin C (C-HART) or 14 Gy (2 Gy/day) followed by 1.4 Gy b.i.d. to a total dose of 77.6 Gy (HART). The overall treatment time was equal in both groups. At 5 years, the locoregional control and overall survival rates were significantly better in the radiochemotherapy arm compared with the radiation-only arm. Interestingly, the maximum acute reactions of mucositis, moist desquamation, and erythema were significantly lower in the radiochemotherapy arm compared with radiotherapy alone. No differences in late reactions and overall rates of secondary neoplasms were observed; thus, this trial impressively documents that the combination of radiotherapy with chemotherapy agents may effectively widen the therapeutic window; however, it is clear that although the specific toxicities may not be increased, new toxicities in terms of hemotoxicity will be added; thus, the net effect of radiochemotherapy results from a cooperation regarding tumor control and, in parallel, a diversification of toxicities. Independently of the term "therapeutic gain," the interaction of radiation with chemotherapy follows a precise nomenclature based on some groundbreaking theoretical considerations published in the late 1970s (STEEL 1979; STEEL and PECKHAM 1979). In every case of a scientific description and quantification of the effects of combined modality therapy in appropriate models, it is highly recommended to adhere to the proposed nomenclature. The complexity of effects increases with each step of investigation, i.e., from cell culture to tumor-bearing

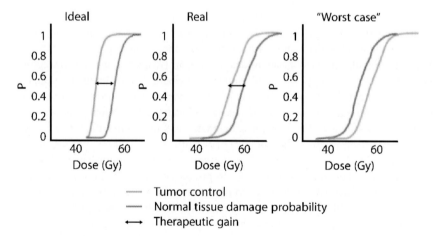

Fig. 10.3. Therapeutic gain. Therapeutic gain is defined as the resulting benefit when tumor control is weighted against the normal tissue damage. In an ideal setting (*left*) the probability of normal tissue damage is minimal at a dose level with a maximal probability of tumor control. More realistically (*middle*), doses required to achieve local control are associated with a certain, but low, probability of normal tissue damage. In situations where the doses required to control the tumor are continuously higher than the doses being toxic (*right*), treatment will be palliative in most cases ("worst case")

animal to cancer patient (WURSCHMIDT et al. 2000). A thorough examination of all possible treatment combinations and administration schedules for a given drug plus radiation is very challenging, as can be seen in the publication by KALLMAN et al. (1992), who studied in depth the radiosensitizing effects of cisplatin and other chemotherapeutic substances.

10.4.1
Spatial Interaction

On a large scale, chemotherapy and radiation may be effective on several levels. The concept of spatial interaction was devised to mean that chemotherapy and radiation act on spatially distinct compartments of the body, resulting in a net gain in tumor control. The concept of spatial interaction does not take into account any drug–radiation interaction on the level of the tumor itself, but rather assumes that radiation or chemotherapy would be active in different compartments, respectively. In a narrow sense, this concept describes the fact that chemotherapy would be employed for the sterilization of distant microscopic tumor seeding, whereas radiation

would achieve local control (Fig. 10.4). Obviously, this is a theoretical consideration only, since chemotherapy also increases local control and radiotherapy reduces distant metastasis via increased local control rates; thus, when integrating the concept of spatial interaction into a more complete view on combined modality, spatial cooperation is still of major importance. In a more narrow sense, the aspect of spatial interaction is of major importance when one attempts to adequately cover sanctuary sites during multimodality approaches for certain types of leukemia and lymphomas. Next to spatial effects, several other important mechanisms may increase the efficacy of a combined treatment approach. In this regard, inhibition of repopulation and effective killing of hypoxic radioresistant cells by medical substances may contribute to the efficacy of a combined treatment.

10.4.2
Role of Repopulation

The fractionated treatment of tumors with ionizing radiation is associated with the phenomenon of repopulation (KIM and TANNOCK 2005). Speaking simply, a cer-

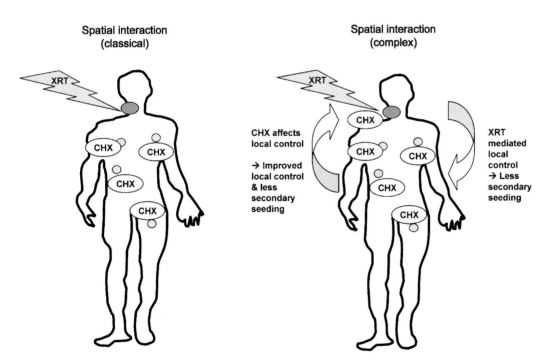

Fig. 10.4. Spatial interaction. In a classical interpretation (*left*) the term spatial interaction refers to the fact that chemotherapy (*CHX*) is effective on tumor compartments where radiation (*XRT*) has no efficacy, and vice versa, resulting in a generally increased control rate. In a more complex view (*right*), spatial interaction is relevant on multiple interacting levels: increased local control by radiation reduces the risk of a secondary seeding. Furthermore, the interaction of radiation with chemotherapy increases local control; thus, in addition to the classical spatial interaction, several levels of interacting feedback loops exist, which increase efficacy of spatial interactions

tain amount of tumor cells repair the induced damage in between two fractions and proliferate. Repopulation may neutralize around 0.5 Gy/day; however, the range of repopulation is considerably large and may reach higher levels (TROTT 1990; BAUMANN et al. 1994; BU-DACH et al. 1997). Based on these findings, radiation biologists advocated the use of accelerated radiation schedules; however, the acute and late effects of such approaches turned out to be more intense so that the final value of those approaches in terms of a real therapeutic gain remains unclear (BECK-BORNHOLDT et al. 1997; DISCHE et al. 1997; HORIOT et al. 1997). The phenomenon of repopulation must also be taken into account when trying to design combined modality regimens. In theoretical models, cell loss from neoadjuvant chemotherapy preceding fractionated radiation treatment might trigger accelerated repopulation (Fig. 10.5). Then, a certain percentage of the daily radiation dose is wasted to counteract increased tumor cell proliferation.

Under such conditions, despite a response to chemotherapy, cell survival after radiotherapy is no better than after the same course of radiotherapy alone (yet toxicity results from both modalities). Accelerated repopulation has also been described after treatment of murine breast tumors with sequential, weekly cycles of 5-fluorouracil and cyclophosphamide (WU and TANNOCK 2003).

The clinical observation that the simultaneous combination of 5-fluorouracil, mitomycin C, or cisplatin with radiation is of value in rapidly proliferating squamous cell cancers has led to the assumption that the addition of drugs may influence the potential of cancer cells to repopulate. At least for mitomycin C this effect was documented precisely using a xenograft model (BUDACH et al. 2002). In this model, transplanted tumors were treated with 11×4.5 Gy fractionated radiation under ambient conditions with or without mitomycin C followed by a graded top-up dose on days 16, 23, 30, or 37 given under hypoxic conditions. Repopula-

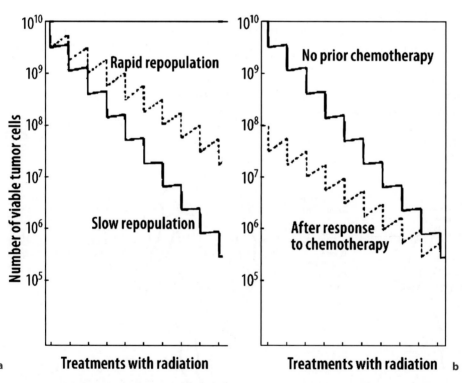

Fig. 10.5a,b. Influence of tumor cell repopulation on outcome. **a** Cell survival during a fractionated course of radiotherapy depends not only on the proportion of cells killed with each dose (which is equal for the two examples shown), but also on the rate of proliferation of surviving cells between the fractions, which differs between the two curves. **b** Hypothetical diagram to illustrate the number of surviving cells in a tumor during treatment with radiation alone, or during radiation treatment in a tumor that has responded to neoadjuvant chemotherapy (i.e., cell number reduced to 1% at start of radiotherapy) but where proliferation has been stimulated. Despite neoadjuvant chemotherapy, ultimate cell survival is similar. (From TANNOCK 1989, 1992)

tion in the interval between the fractionated treatment and the top-up dose accounted for 1.33 Gy top-up dose per day in animals not receiving mitomycin C, but only 0.68 Gy in animals receiving the drug; thus, at least mitomycin C may increase the efficacy of radiation by the inhibition of repopulation.

10.4.3
Role of Hypoxia

As known for years, radiation-induced cell kill is strongly dependent on the presence of adequate oxygen tensions. In larger tumors, for example, head and neck cancers, areas of hypoxia and even anoxia are present leading to an increased radiation resistance of clonogenic tumor cells within such areas (MOLLS and VAUPEL 1998; STADLER et al. 1999; NORDSMARK et al. 2005; WOUTERS et al. 2005). It has been speculated that chemotherapeutic agents, especially those killing even hypoxic cells, may overcome global radiation resistance simply by killing radioresistant hypoxic cells, thereby being of special value in highly hypoxic tumors (TEICHER et al. 1981; ROCKWELL 1982).

Comparing the effects of several cytostatic drugs in combination with radiation on the growth of a C3H mammary carcinoma, it turned out that cyclophosphamide, adriamycin, and mitomycin C had the most significant effect on the proportional cell kill of hypoxic cells. In contrast, bleomycin and cisplatin did not exert strong effects on hypoxic cells (GRAU and OVERGAARD 1988). In addition, it has clearly been shown that tumor blood flow in xenografts is increased after mitomycin C treatment (DURAND and LEPARD 1994). Using two different squamous cell carcinomas, the latter authors tested the drug's influence on the outcome of radiation treatment with or without hypoxia (DURAND and LEPARD 2000). The authors reported neither an increased killing of hypoxic cells by mitomycin C nor a consistent increase in tumor blood flow rates; however, mitomycin C in combination with radiation was associated with a slight increase in cell killing of hypoxic subpopulations of the xenograft system. Based on this observation it was concluded that the efficacy of a combined treatment with mitomycin C and radiation cannot be rationalized on either a complementary cytotoxicity or on drug-induced improvement in tumor oxygenation secondary to an increased blood flow.

In the case of paclitaxel it has been tested whether the enhanced killing by the combination of paclitaxel and radiation is connected to the presence of oxygen.

Using an MCA-4 xenograft system, the authors could show that in the absence of oxygen the paclitaxel-mediated change of the TCD_{50} value is strikingly less prominent (MILAS et al. 1994, 1995); thus, it can be concluded that at least in part the influence of paclitaxel on the radiation response is mediated via an optimized oxygenation. In a clinical trial of neoadjuvant chemotherapy in breast cancer, paclitaxel significantly decreased the mean interstitial fluid pressure and improved oxygenation, effects which were not observed in a randomized control group receiving doxorubicin (TAGHIAN et al. 2005).

In conclusion, several sets of data indicate that the efficacy of chemotherapy in combination with radiation may be related to an increased oxygenation of hypoxic tumors; however, it still remains speculative whether or to what amount the efficacy of a combined treatment is strictly related to specific influences on the hypoxic cell compartment (Fig. 10.6).

10.5
Molecular Interactions

10.5.1
DNA Damage

One of the underlying molecular aspects of the efficacy of the combination of radiation and chemotherapy, which has been understood in more detail, is the influence on DNA repair. The induction of DNA damage is probably one of the most crucial events after irradiation of cells. In this regard, ionizing radiation triggers a wide array of lesions including base damage, single-strand breaks, and notably, double-strand breaks (DSB). After irradiation, different molecular systems are involved in recognition and repair of the damage. Whereas most of the induced damage is quickly repaired, DSB repair is slow and unrepaired DSBs are considerably important for the final induction of cell death.

Many chemotherapeutic agents, especially those known to be of value in combination with radiation, also induce considerable DNA damage or interfere with effective DNA repair; therefore, two general patterns of interactions may be separated: (1) the combination of the drug with radiation directly leads to more damage and (2) the drug may interact with the DNA repair pathway thus increasing the level of DNA damage more indirectly; however, one has to assume that none of the potential mechanisms acts without the other in real settings.

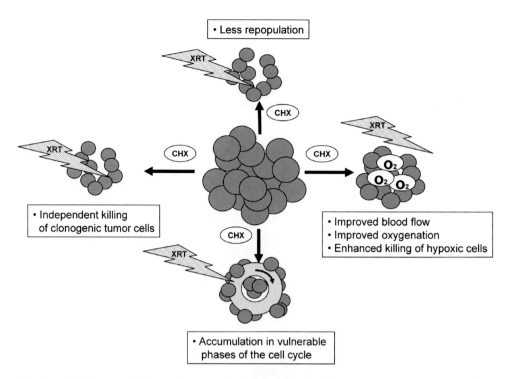

Fig. 10.6. Mechanisms of chemoradiation on a cellular level. At least four major mechanisms contribute to the efficacy of the combination of radiation with chemotherapy. In general, the addition of chemotherapy adds to the combined effect simply by an additional independent killing of clonogenic tumor cells. This mechanism is backed up by several other more interactive pathways: chemotherapy may induce a certain reassortment of tumor cells in more vulnerable phases of the cell cycle, chemotherapy may reduce the level of repopulation during a course of fractionated radiotherapy, and, finally, chemotherapy may partially overcome hypoxia-mediated radiation resistance

Cisplatin, for example, acts by complex formation with guanosine residues and subsequent adduct formation ultimately resulting in intra- and interstrand crosslinks. This type of damage is mostly removed by base excision repair and mismatch repair. Several sets of data suggest that single-strand damage induced by radiation in close vicinity to DNA damage triggered by cisplatin results in a mutual inhibition of the damage-specific repair system; thus, the amount of resulting damage leads to an increased net cell kill (BEGG 1990; YANG et al. 1995).

Similarly, etoposide, which is a strong topoisomerase IIa-directed toxin, induces DSBs mostly during the S-phase of the cell cycle (BERRIOS et al. 1985; EARNSHAW and HECK 1985). Again, several lines of evidence show that the combination of both agents results in a strongly increased level of damage (GIOCANTI et al. 1993; YU et al. 2000).

The biochemical pathways involved in DNA repair and DNA synthesis overlap in several regards; thus, drugs acting on the synthesis of DNA putatively also interfere with the repair of DNA damage after applica-

tion of ionizing radiation. Several prototypical radiation sensitizers may act via these mechanisms. Besides cisplatin, 5-fluorouracil is probably the most commonly employed drug in clinical combined modality settings. Basically, 5-fluorouracil inhibits thymidylate synthase thereby reducing the intracellular pool of nucleoside triphosphates (PINEDO and PETERS 1988; MILLER and KINSELLA 1992). In addition, the drug is integrated into DNA via fluorodeoxyuridine, also contributing to its antineoplastic effects. Several lines of evidence suggest that the amount of 5-fluorouracil integrated into DNA directly correlates with the radiosensitizing effect. In addition, the complementation of the cell culture medium with higher levels of thymidine reverses the effects of 5-fluorouracil on the radiation sensitivity (LAWRENCE et al. 1994; McGINN et al. 1996).

Gemcitabine, which is another radiation sensitizer, was also shown to deplete the pool of deoxynucleosides and is integrated into DNA. The drug is known to exert a pronounced radiosensitizing effect in squamous cancer cells, as well as adenocarcinoma cells from pancreatic cancer. In vitro this effect was especially pronounced during the S-phase passage (ROBERTSON et al. 1996; LAWRENCE et al. 1997; ROSIER et al. 1999). Although few data regarding the mechanistic basis of the interaction between radiation and gemcitabine are available, the exact mechanism remains elusive. The radiation-sensitizing effect was seen over a prolonged time period (~48 h) after incubation of HT29 cells with low doses of gemcitabine (100 nm). During the first 48 h the level of S-phase cells increased, whereas the amount of deoxynucleosides remained low even up to 72 h (SHEWACH et al. 1994; LAWRENCE et al. 1997); thus, it seems likely that the depletion of the deoxynucleoside pools in combination with an increased killing of cells in S-phase is a mechanism responsible for an enhanced radiation susceptibility mediated by gemcitabine.

10.5.2
Radiation Sensitization Via Cell Cycle Synchronization

The fact that striking differences in the radiation sensitivity occur as cells move through the different phases of the cell cycle has stimulated the speculation that the efficacy of a combined treatment may also be related to possible effects on the reassortment of cells in more vulnerable cell cycle phases.

Several experimental settings provide evidence that cell cycle effects are involved in the modulation of the efficacy of combined modality approaches. In this regard the use of a temperature-sensitive p53 mutant allows the analysis of cell cycle effects. The underlying hypothesis was that fluoropyrimidine-mediated radiosensitization occurs only in tumor cells that inappropriately enter S-phase in the presence of drug resulting in a subsequent repair defect of the radiation-induced damage. The use of the mutated p53 allowed p21-mediated arrest prior to S-phase entry when cells are grown under 32°C, in contrast to no arrest in cells grown at the non-permissive temperatures of 38°C. The radiation-sensitizing effect of fluoropyrimidine was directly connected to the lacking G1 arrest when cells were grown under non-permissive temperatures; thus, the fluoropyrimidine-mediated radiosensitization clearly requires progression into S-phase (NAIDA et al. 1998).

In an extension of these findings, NAIDA et al. (1998) analyzed the effects of fluorodeoxyuridine on the radiation sensitivity in HT29 and SW620 human colon cancer cells under nearly complete inhibition of thymidylate synthase (both cell lines harbor a similar p53 mutation). Interestingly, only the HT29 cells were sensitized. As an underlying feature, the authors found that

only the HT29 cells progressed into S-phase and demonstrated increased cyclin E-dependent kinase activity. In contrast, SW620 cells were found to be arrested just past the G1-S boundary and an increase in kinase activity was not detectable; thus, the findings underline the requirement of an S-phase transition for the efficacy of halogenated fluoropyrimidines in combination with radiation. These findings also highlight the role of molecules involved in cell cycle regulation as key players for the modulation of a combined modality approach (MCGINN et al. 1994; LAWRENCE et al. 1996a–c). In addition to the fact that the S-phase transition is required for the radiosensitization effect, it has also been shown that fluoropyrimidines under defined dosage conditions facilitate the accumulation of cells in S-phase (MILLER and KINSELLA 1992).

In addition to the findings on halogenated fluoropyrimidines, several other sets of data obtained with paclitaxel suggest that an increased radiation sensitivity occurred at the time of a taxane-induced G2-M block; however, the situation for taxane combinations is highly complex in so far as other data provide evidence that the mitotic arrest is not sufficient for the effects of paclitaxel (GEARD and JONES 1994; HENNEQUIN et al. 1996). The picture becomes even more complicated when taking into account that radiation was shown to decrease the net killing of taxanes (SUI et al. 2004). In this regard, it has been shown that the combination of paclitaxel and gamma radiation did not produce a synergistic or additive effect in a breast cancer and epidermoid cancer cell model. Instead, the overall cytotoxicity of the combination was lower than that of the drug treatment alone. In particular apoptosis induction was found to be strikingly reduced. A detailed analysis revealed that radiation resulted in cell cycle arrest at the G2 phase preventing the G1-M transition-dependent cytotoxic effects of paclitaxel. Furthermore, radiation inhibited paclitaxel-induced IκBα degradation and bcl-2 phosphorylation and increased the protein levels of cyclin B1 and inhibitory phosphorylation of p34(cdc2).

Taken together, the impact of chemotherapy-induced cell cycle alterations as a major mechanism for the efficacy of the combined action is still questionable. In clinical settings, the importance of an adequate cell cycle progression for the efficacy of radiochemotherapy approaches has been impressively documented. In the case of a neoadjuvant 5-fluorouracil-based radiochemotherapy for rectal cancer, it has been shown that a decrease of the cell cycle inhibitory protein p21 during neoadjuvant treatment is strongly associated with an improved disease-specific survival. This finding has been corroborated by the observation that a parallel increase of the expression level of the proliferation marker ki-67 is similarly associated with an improved outcome (RAU et al. 2003); thus, preclinical findings on the action of 5-fluorouracil in combination with radiation are clearly reflected by clinical observations.

10.6
Potential Influences on Programmed Cell Death Pathways

In order to inactivate a tumor cell, several distinct yet overlapping pathways may be activated. Besides the induction of pure apoptosis, other cell inactivation modalities, including programmed necrosis, mitotic catastrophe, senescence, or terminal differentiation, may be triggered (BELKA 2006). The influence of a combined modality treatment on any of these end points has never been analyzed in greater detail; thus, only very few data are available showing that the combination of paradigmatic radiation sensitizers with radiation quantitatively alters the induction of certain predefined mechanisms of cell death (Fig. 10.7).

In the case of gemcitabine, the efficacy of a combined treatment in terms of apoptosis induction has been analyzed in more detail using HT29 colon cancer cells, UMSCC-6 head and neck cancer cells, and A549 lung cancer cells. A key feature was that all cell systems differ substantially in the ability to undergo radiation-induced apoptosis, with HT29 being the most apoptosis-sensitive cell in this experimental setting. It turned out that the radiosensitization of HT29 cells was accompanied by an increase in apoptosis, whereas in UM-SCC-6 cells and A549 cells, the radiosensitizing effect was mediated via non-apoptotic mechanisms; thus, this effect is rather a cell-type-specific feature than a general property of the drug.

In the case of definitive treatment approaches in esophageal or rectal cancer, the importance of apoptosis signaling has been documented. Esophageal cancer patients with lack of the proapoptotic Bax molecule have significantly reduced outcome rates (STURM et al. 2001). Similar findings have been observed for neoadjuvant radiation or radiochemotherapy in patients with rectal tumors with a low expression of Bax (CHANG et al. 2005; NEHLS et al. 2005).

10.7
Effects of Protracted Drug Exposure

More than 30 years ago, in vitro studies demonstrated increased efficacy when tumor cells were exposed to mitomycin C or several other drugs for a prolonged time (SHIMOYAMA 1975). This finding was confirmed

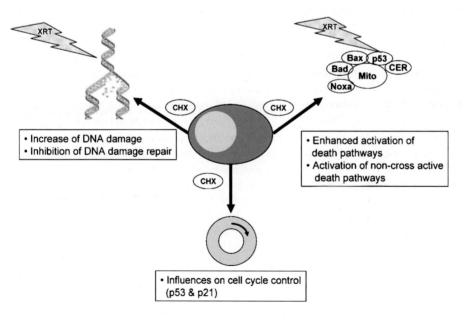

Fig. 10.7. Mechanisms of chemoradiation on a molecular level. The most prominent points of interaction of radiation with chemotherapy being of importance for the efficacy of a combined modality treatment are found on the level of DNA damage induction and repair, cell death induction, and cell cycle control

in clinical trials of continuous infusion versus bolus 5-fluorouracil (SEIFERT et al. 1975). Furthermore, and probably related to avoidance of peak concentrations, reduced normal tissue toxicity was observed. In principle, these divergent effects on tumor and normal tissues improve the therapeutic window. Considering tumors, longer exposure times of 5-fluorouracil result in enhanced cell killing also in the context of simultaneous radiation therapy (MOON et al. 2000). A combined analysis of more than 3,100 patients with rectal cancer treated with preoperative radiochemotherapy demonstrated that the pCR rate was significantly higher when continuous infusion 5-fluorouracil was used, as compared with other modes of delivery (HARTLEY et al. 2005). Protracted exposure is also currently being tested for other drugs such as temozolomide. Whether such regimens hold promise depends on the mode of action of the drug, cell-cycle specificity, pharmacokinetics, etc.

10.8
Conclusion

A large body of in vitro results and data from animal experiments and clinical trials show very clearly the high efficacy of radiotherapy and the fact that cell kill from chemotherapy is often comparable to that of rather low doses of radiation. The underlying principles are now better understood than in earlier decades. They provide the basis for development of improved methods of delivery, modification of blood flow and microenvironment, measures to counteract resistance and metabolization, and, maybe most importantly, rationally designed combination treatment. Compared with the relatively homogeneous models used for description of experimental end points, the clinical situation is complicated by a very complex tumor biology with changes in physiological and microenvironmental parameters over time, and even differences between the primary tumor itself and regional lymphatic metastases, which receive identical treatment. There has been a long-lasting interest in prediction of individual response, for example, by means of pretherapeutic ex vivo chemosensitivity testing in cell culture or determination of molecular marker genes (SHIMIZU et al. 2004; STAIB et al. 2005). More recently, treatment monitoring early during a course of chemotherapy or radiochemotherapy by means of positron emission tomography, diffusion magnetic resonance imaging, and other biological imaging methods has shown promising results (WEBER 2005). Nevertheless, treatment individualization, also with regard to nor-

mal tissue toxicity and drug metabolism, for example, based on single nucleotide polymorphisms (EFFERTH and VOLM 2005; ROBERT et al. 2005), continues to be an area of active investigation.

References

Ardavanis A, Scorilas A, Tryfonopoulos D, et al (2006) Multidisciplinary therapy of locally far-advanced or inflammatory breast cancer with fixed perioperative sequence of epirubicin, vinorelbine, and fluorouracil chemotherapy, surgery, and radiotherapy: long-term results. Oncologist 11:563–573

Arnould L, Arveux P, Couturier J, et al (2007) Pathologic complete response to trastuzumab-based neoadjuvant therapy is related to the level of HER-2 amplification. Clin Cancer Res 13:6404–6409

Azrak RG, Cao S, Slocum HK, et al (2004) Therapeutic synergy between irinotecan and 5-fluorouracil against human tumor xenografts. Clin Cancer Res 10:1121–1129

Bartelink H, Roelofsen F, Eschwege F, et al (1997) Concomitant radiotherapy and chemotherapy is superior to radiotherapy alone in the treatment of locally advanced anal cancer: results of a phase III randomized trial of the European Organization for Research and Treatment of Cancer Radiotherapy and Gastrointestinal Cooperative Groups. J Clin Oncol 15:2040–2049

Baumann M, Liertz C, Baisch H, et al (1994) Impact of overall treatment time of fractionated irradiation on local control of human FaDu squamous cell carcinoma in nude mice. Radiother Oncol 32:137–143

Beck-Bornholdt HP, Dubben HH, Liertz-Petersen C, Willers H (1997) Hyperfractionation: where do we stand? Radiother Oncol 43:1–21

Begg AC (1990) Cisplatin and radiation: interaction probabilities and therapeutic possibilities. Int J Radiat Oncol Biol Phys 19:1183–1189

Belka C (2006) The fate of irradiated tumor cells. Oncogene 25:969–971

Ben-Asher S (1949) Nitrogen mustard therapy: the use of methyl-bis(B-chloroethyl) amine hydrochloride in Hodgkin's disease, leukemia, lymphosarcoma and cancer of the lung. Am J Med Sci 217:162–168

Berrios M, Osheroff N, Fisher PA (1985) In situ localization of DNA topoisomerase II, a major polypeptide component of the Drosophila nuclear matrix fraction. Proc Natl Acad Sci U S A 82:4142–4146

Berthold DR, Pond GR, Soban F, et al (2008) Docetaxel plus prednisone or mitoxantrone plus prednisone for advanced prostate cancer: updated survival in the TAX 327 study. J Clin Oncol 26:242–245

Brizel DM, Albers ME, Fisher SR, et al (1998) Hyperfractionated irradiation with or without concurrent chemotherapy for locally advanced head and neck cancer. N Engl J Med 338:1798–1804

Brunsvig PF, Andersen A, Aamdal S, et al (2007) Pharmacokinetic analysis of two different docetaxel dose levels in patients with non-small cell lung cancer treated with docetaxel as monotherapy or with concurrent radiotherapy. BMC Cancer 7:197

Buda A, Fossati R, Colombo N, et al (2005) Randomized trial of neoadjuvant chemotherapy comparing paclitaxel, ifosfamide, and cisplatin with ifosfamide and cisplatin followed by radical surgery in patients with locally advanced squamous cell cervical carcinoma: the SNAP01 Italian Collaborative Study. J Clin Oncol 23:4137–4145

Budach W, Gioioso D, Taghian A, et al (1997) Repopulation capacity during fractionated irradiation of squamous cell carcinomas and glioblastomas in vitro. Int J Radiat Oncol Biol Phys 39:743–750

Budach W, Paulsen F, Welz S, et al (2002) Mitomycin C in combination with radiotherapy as a potent inhibitor of tumour cell repopulation in a human squamous cell carcinoma. Br J Cancer 86:470–476

Budach V, Stuschke M, Budach W, et al (2005) Hyperfractionated accelerated chemoradiation with concurrent fluorouracil-mitomycin is more effective than dose-escalated hyperfractionated accelerated radiation therapy alone in locally advanced head and neck cancer: final results of the radiotherapy cooperative clinical trials group of the German Cancer Society 95-06 Prospective Randomized Trial. J Clin Oncol 23:1125–1135

Cao S, Durrani FA, Rustum YM (2005) Synergistic antitumor activity of capecitabine in combination with irinotecan. Clin Colorectal Cancer 4:336–343

Chang HJ, Jung KH, Kim DY, et al (2005) Bax, a predictive marker for therapeutic response to preoperative chemoradiotherapy in patients with rectal carcinoma. Hum Pathol 36:364–371

Clarke SJ, Rivory LP (1999) Clinical pharmacokinetics of docetaxel. Clin Pharmacokinet 36:99–114

Del Regato JA (1989) Magnus Strandqvist. Int J Radiat Oncol Biol Phys 17:631–642

Deo SV, Bhutani M, Shukla NK, et al (2003) Randomized trial comparing neo-adjuvant versus adjuvant chemotherapy in operable locally advanced breast cancer (T4b N0-2 M0). J Surg Oncol 84:192–197

Dische S, Saunders M, Barrett A, et al (1997) A randomised multicentre trial of CHART versus conventional radiotherapy in head and neck cancer. Radiother Oncol 44:123–136

Dreicer R, Magi-Galluzzi C, Zhou M, et al (2004) Phase II trial of neoadjuvant docetaxel before radical prostatectomy for locally advanced prostate cancer. Urology 63:1138–1142

Durand RE, LePard NE (1994) Modulation of tumor hypoxia by conventional chemotherapeutic agents. Int J Radiat Oncol Biol Phys 29:481–486

Durand RE, LePard NE (2000) Effects of mitomycin C on the oxygenation and radiosensitivity of murine and human tumours in mice. Radiother Oncol 56:245–252

Dy GK, Krook JE, Green EM, et al (2007) Impact of complete response to chemotherapy on overall survival in advanced colorectal cancer: results from intergroup N9741. J Clin Oncol 25:3469–3474

Earnshaw WC, Heck MM (1985) Localization of topoisomerase II in mitotic chromosomes. J Cell Biol 100:1716–1725

Efferth T, Volm M (2005) Pharmacogenetics for individualized cancer chemotherapy. Pharmacol Ther 107:155–176

Eliaz RE, Nir S, Marty C, Szoka FC Jr (2004) Determination and modeling of kinetics of cancer cell killing by doxorubicin and doxorubicin encapsulated in targeted liposomes. Cancer Res 64:711–718

Epstein RJ (1990) Drug-induced DNA damage and tumor chemosensitivity. J Clin Oncol 8:2062–2084

Evans TR, Yellowlees A, Foster E, et al (2005) Phase III randomized trial of doxorubicin and docetaxel versus doxorubicin and cyclophosphamide as primary medical therapy in women with breast cancer: an Anglo-Celtic cooperative oncology group study. J Clin Oncol 23:2988–2995

Farquhar C, Marjoribanks J, Basser R, et al (2005) High dose chemotherapy and autologous bone marrow or stem cell transplantation versus conventional chemotherapy for women with metastatic breast cancer. Cochrane Database Syst Rev:CD003142

Febbo PG, Richie JP, George DJ, et al (2005) Neoadjuvant docetaxel before radical prostatectomy in patients with high-risk localized prostate cancer. Clin Cancer Res 11:5233–5240

Ferriere JP, Assier I, Cure H, et al (1998) Primary chemotherapy in breast cancer: correlation between tumor response and patient outcome. Am J Clin Oncol 21:117–120

Forastiere AA, Goepfert H, Maor M, et al (2003) Concurrent chemotherapy and radiotherapy for organ preservation in advanced laryngeal cancer. N Engl J Med 349:2091–2098

Francini G, Paolelli L, Francini E (2008) Effect of neoadjuvant epirubicin and total androgen blockade on complete pathological response in patients with clinical stage T3/T4 prostate cancer. Eur J Surg Oncol 34:216–221

Geard CR, Jones JM (1994) Radiation and taxol effects on synchronized human cervical carcinoma cells. Int J Radiat Oncol Biol Phys 29:565–569

Geh JI, Bond SJ, Bentzen SM, et al (2006) Systemic overview of preoperative (neoadjuvant) chemoradiotherapy in patients with oesophageal cancer: evidence of a radiation and chemotherapy dose response. Radiother Oncol 78:236–244

Gerard J, Romestaing P, Bonnetain F, et al (2005) Preoperative chemoradiotherapy (CT-RT) improves local control in T3-4 rectal cancers: results of the FFCD 9203 randomized trial (abstract). Int J Radiat Oncol Biol Phys 63(suppl 1):S2–S3

Giocanti N, Hennequin C, Balosso J, et al (1993) DNA repair and cell cycle interactions in radiation sensitization by the topoisomerase II poison etoposide. Cancer Res 53:2105–2111

Gorodetsky R, Levdansky L, Ringel I, et al (1998) Paclitaxel-induced modification of the effects of radiation and alterations in the cell cycle in normal and tumor mammalian cells. Radiat Res 150:283–291

Graham CH, Kobayashi H, Stankiewicz KS, et al (1994) Rapid acquisition of multicellular drug resistance after a single exposure of mammary tumor cells to antitumor alkylating agents. J Natl Cancer Inst 86:975–982

Grau C, Overgaard J (1988) Effect of cancer chemotherapy on the hypoxic fraction of a solid tumor measured using a local tumor control assay. Radiother Oncol 13:301–309

Green JA, Kirwan JM, Tierney JF, et al (2001) Survival and recurrence after concomitant chemotherapy and radiotherapy for cancer of the uterine cervix: a systematic review and meta-analysis. Lancet 358:781–786

Grosu AL, Molls M, Zimmermann FB, et al (2006) High-precision radiation therapy with integrated biological imaging and tumor monitoring: evolution of the Munich concept and future research options. Strahlenther Onkol 182:361–368

Grothey A, Hedrick EE, Mass RD, et al. (2008) Response-independent survival benefit in metastatic colorectal cancer: a comparative analysis of N9741 and AVF2107. J Clin Oncol 26:183–189

Hartley A, Ho KF, McConkey C, Geh JI (2005) Pathological complete response following pre-operative chemoradiotherapy in rectal cancer: analysis of phase II/III trials. Br J Radiol 78:934–938

Helbekkmo N, Sundstrom S, Aasebo U, et al (2007) Vinorelbine/carboplatin versus gemcitabine/carboplatin in advanced NSCLC shows similar efficacy, but different impact of toxicity. Br J Cancer 97:283–289

Hennequin C, Giocanti N, Favaudon V (1996) Interaction of ionizing radiation with paclitaxel (Taxol) and docetaxel (Taxotere) in HeLa and SQ20B cells. Cancer Res 56:1842–1850

Hof H, Muenter M, Oetzel D, et al (2007) Stereotactic single-dose radiotherapy (radiosurgery) of early stage nonsmall-cell lung cancer. Cancer 110:148–155

Holden SA, Emi Y, Kakeji Y, et al (1997) Host distribution and response to antitumor alkylating agents of EMT-6 tumor cells from subcutaneous tumor implants. Cancer Chemother Pharmacol 40:87–93

Horiot JC, Lopez-Torrecilla J, Begg AC, et al (1997) Accelerated fractionation (AF) compared to conventional fractionation (CF) improves loco-regional control in the radiotherapy of advanced head and neck cancers: results of the EORTC 22851 randomized trial. Radiother Oncol 44:111–121

Hurley J, Doliny P, Reis I, et al (2006) Docetaxel, cisplatin, and trastuzumab as primary systemic therapy for human epidermal growth factor receptor 2-positive locally advanced breast cancer. J Clin Oncol 24:1831–1838

Jones B, Sanghera P (2007) Estimation of radiobiologic parameters and equivalent radiation dose of cytotoxic chemotherapy in malignant glioma. Int J Radiat Oncol Biol Phys 68:441–448

Joschko MA, Webster LK, Groves J, et al (1997) Enhancement of radiation-induced regrowth delay by gemcitabine in a human tumor xenograft model. Radiat Oncol Invest 5:62–71

Kallman RF, Bedarida G, Rapacchietta D (1992) Experimental studies on schedule dependence in the treatment of cancer with combinations of chemotherapy and radiotherapy. Front Radiat Ther Oncol 26:31–44

Karlsson YA, Malmstrom PO, Hatschek T, et al (1998) Multimodality treatment of 128 patients with locally advanced breast carcinoma in the era of mammography screening using standard polychemotherapy with 5-fluorouracil, epirubicin, and cyclophosphamide: prognostic and therapeutic implications. Cancer 83:936–947

Kasibhatla M, Kirkpatrick JP, Brizel DM (2007) How much radiation is the chemotherapy worth in advanced head and neck cancer? Int J Radiat Oncol Biol Phys 68:1491–1495

Khalil AA, Bentzen SM, Overgaard J (1997) Steepness of the dose-response curve as a function of volume in an experimental tumor irradiated under ambient or hypoxic conditions. Int J Radiat Oncol Biol Phys 39:797–802

Kim JJ, Tannock IF (2005) Repopulation of cancer cells during therapy: an important cause of treatment failure. Nat Rev Cancer 5:516–525

Kim JH, Kim SH, Kolozsvary A, Khil MS (1992) Potentiation of radiation response in human carcinoma cells in vitro and murine fibrosarcoma in vivo by topotecan, an inhibitor of DNA topoisomerase I. Int J Radiat Oncol Biol Phys 22:515–518

Korkaya H, Wicha MS (2007) Selective targeting of cancer stem cells: a new concept in cancer therapeutics. BioDrugs 21:299–310

Krause M, Prager J, Zhou X, et al (2007) EGFR-TK inhibition before radiotherapy reduces tumour volume but does not improve local control: differential response of cancer stem cells and nontumourigenic cells? Radiother Oncol 83:316–325

Lawrence JH, Tobiascarborn JL, Gottschalk A, Linfoot JA, Kling RP (1963) Alpha particle and proton beams in therapy. JAMA 186:236–245

Lawrence TS, Davis MA, Maybaum J (1994) Dependence of 5-fluorouracil-mediated radiosensitization on DNA-directed effects. Int J Radiat Oncol Biol Phys 29:519–523

Lawrence TS, Davis MA, Tang HY, Maybaum J (1996a) Fluorodeoxyuridine-mediated cytotoxicity and radiosensitization require S phase progression. Int J Radiat Biol 70:273–280

Lawrence TS, Davis MA, Loney TL (1996b) Fluoropyrimidine-mediated radiosensitization depends on cyclin E-dependent kinase activation. Cancer Res 56:3203–3206

Lawrence TS, Chang EY, Hahn TM (1996c) Radiosensitization of pancreatic cancer cells by 2′,2′-difluoro-2′-deoxycytidine. Int J Radiat Oncol Biol Phys 34:867–872

Lawrence TS, Chang EY, Hahn TM, Shewach DS (1997) Delayed radiosensitization of human colon carcinoma cells after a brief exposure to 2′,2′-difluoro-2′-deoxycytidine (gemcitabine). Clin Cancer Res 3:777–782

Lee JW, Park JK, Lee SH, et al (2006) Anti-tumor activity of heptaplatin in combination with 5-fluorouracil or paclitaxel against human head and neck cancer cells in vitro. Anticancer Drugs 17:377–384

Lee SS, Kim SB, Park SI, et al (2007) Capecitabine and cisplatin chemotherapy (XP) alone or sequentially combined chemoradiotherapy containing XP regimen in patients with three different settings of stage IV esophageal cancer. Jpn J Clin Oncol 37:829–835

Louis-Sylvestre C, Clough K, Asselain B, et al (2004) Axillary treatment in conservative management of operable breast cancer: dissection or radiotherapy? Results of a randomized study with 15 years of follow-up. J Clin Oncol 22:97–101

McGinn CJ, Miller EM, Lindstrom MJ, et al (1994) The role of cell cycle redistribution in radiosensitization: implications regarding the mechanism of fluorodeoxyuridine radiosensitization. Int J Radiat Oncol Biol Phys 30:851–859

McGinn CJ, Shewach DS, Lawrence TS (1996) Radiosensitizing nucleosides. J Natl Cancer Inst 88:1193–1203

Milas L, Hunter NR, Mason KA, et al (1994) Enhancement of tumor radioresponse of a murine mammary carcinoma by paclitaxel. Cancer Res 54:3506–3510

Milas L, Hunter NR, Mason KA, et al (1995) Role of reoxygenation in induction of enhancement of tumor radioresponse by paclitaxel. Cancer Res 55:3564–3568

Miller EM, Kinsella TJ (1992) Radiosensitization by fluorodeoxyuridine: effects of thymidylate synthase inhibition and cell synchronization. Cancer Res 52:1687–1694

Miller SJ, Lavker RM, Sun TT (2005) Interpreting epithelial cancer biology in the context of stem cells: tumor properties and therapeutic implications. Biochem Biophys Acta 1756:25–52

Minchinton AI, Tannock IF (2006) Drug penetration in solid tumours. Nat Rev Cancer 2006:583–592

Minna JD, Girard L, Xie Y (2007) Tumor mRNA expression profiles predict responses to chemotherapy. J Clin Oncol 25:4329–4334

Minsky BD, Pajak TF, Ginsberg RJ, et al (2002) INT 0123 (Radiation Therapy Oncology Group 94-05) phase III trial of combined-modality therapy for esophageal cancer: high-dose versus standard-dose radiation therapy. J Clin Oncol 20:1167–1174

Miyamoto T, Baba M, Sugane T, et al (2007) Carbon ion radiotherapy for stage I non-small cell lung cancer using a regimen of four fractions during 1 week. J Thorac Oncol 2:916–926

Modarress M, Maghami FQ, Golnavaz M, et al (2005) Comparative study of chemoradiation and neoadjuvant chemotherapy effects before radical hysterectomy in stage IB–IIB bulky cervical cancer and with tumor diameter greater than 4 cm. Int J Gynecol Cancer 15:483–488

Molls M, Vaupel P (1998) Blood perfusion and microenvironment of human tumors. Springer, Berlin Heidelberg New York

Moon Y, Todoroki T, Ohno T, et al (2000) Enhanced radiation killing by 5-fluorouracil of biliary tract cancer cell lines. Int J Oncol 16:987–994

Naida JD, Davis MA, Lawrence TS (1998) The effect of activation of wild-type p53 function on fluoropyrimidine-mediated radiosensitization. Int J Radiat Oncol Biol Phys 41:675–680

Nehls O, Okech T, Hsieh CJ, et al (2005) Low BAX protein expression correlates with disease recurrence in preoperatively irradiated rectal carcinoma. Int J Radiat Oncol Biol Phys 61:85–91

Nguyen PL, Zietman AL (2007) High-dose external beam radiation for localized prostate cancer: current status and future challenges. Cancer J 13:295–301

Nordsmark M, Bentzen SM, Rudat V, et al (2005) Prognostic value of tumor oxygenation in 397 head and neck tumors after primary radiotherapy. An international multicenter study. Radiother Oncol 77:18–24

Ota T, Takeshima N, Tabata T, et al (2007) Treatment of squamous cell carcinoma of the uterine cervix with radiation therapy alone: long-term survival, late complications, and incidence of second cancers. Br J Cancer 97:1058–1062

Paccagnella A, Oniga F, Bearz A, et al (2006) Adding gemcitabine to paclitaxel/carboplatin combination increases survival in advanced non-small cell lung cancer: results of a phase II–III study. J Clin Oncol 24:681–687

Pietras K, Hanahan D (2005) A multitargeted, metronomic, and maximum-tolerated dose "chemo-switch" regimen is antiangiogenic, producing objective responses and survival benefit in a mouse model of cancer. J Clin Oncol 23:939–952

Pinedo HM, Peters GF (1988) Fluorouracil: biochemistry and pharmacology. J Clin Oncol 6:1653–1664

Primeau AJ, Rendon A, Hedley D, et al (2005) The distribution of the anticancer drug doxorubicin in relation to blood vessels in solid tumors. Clin Cancer Res 11:8782–8788

Raitanen M, Rantanen V, Kulmala J, et al (2002) Supra-additive effect with concurrent paclitaxel and cisplatin in vulvar squamous cell carcinoma in vitro. Int J Cancer 100:238–243

Rau B, Sturm I, Lage H, et al (2003) Dynamic expression profile of p21WAF1/CIP1 and Ki-67 predicts survival in rectal carcinoma treated with preoperative radiochemotherapy. J Clin Oncol 21:3391–3401

Reitsamer R, Peintinger F, Prokop E, Hitzl W (2005) Pathological complete response rates comparing 3 versus 6 cycles of epidoxorubicin and docetaxel in the neoadjuvant setting of patients with stage II and III breast cancer. Anticancer Drugs 16:867–870

Richtig E, Ludwig R, Kerl H, et al (2005) Organ- and treatment-specific local response rates to systemic and local treatment modalities in stage IV melanoma. Br J Dermatol 153:925–931

Robert J, Morvan VL, Smith D, et al (2005) Predicting drug response and toxicity based on gene polymorphisms. Crit Rev Oncol Hematol 54:171–196

Robertson JM, Shewach DS, Lawrence TS (1996) Preclinical studies of chemotherapy and radiation therapy for pancreatic carcinoma. Cancer 78:674–679

Rockwell S (1982) Cytotoxicities of mitomycin C and X rays to aerobic and hypoxic cells in vitro. Int J Radiat Oncol Biol Phys 8:1035–1039

Rosier JF, Beauduin M, Bruniaux M, et al (1999) The effect of 2'-2' difluorodeoxycytidine (dFdC, gemcitabine) on radiation-induced cell lethality in two human head and neck squamous carcinoma cell lines differing in intrinsic radiosensitivity. Int J Radiat Biol 75:245–251

Rutqvist LE, Johansson H (2006) Long-term follow-up of the Stockholm randomized trials of postoperative radiation therapy versus adjuvant chemotherapy among 'high risk' pre- and postmenopausal breast cancer patients. Acta Oncol 45:517–527

Sauer R, Becker H, Hohenberger W, et al (2004) Preoperative versus postoperative chemoradiotherapy for rectal cancer. N Engl J Med 351:1731–1740

Schaake-Koning C, van den Bogaert W, Dalesio O, et al (1992) Effects of concomitant cisplatin and radiotherapy on inoperable non-small-cell lung cancer. N Engl J Med 326:524–530

Schulz-Ertner D, Nikoghosyan A, Hof H, et al. (2007) Carbon ion radiotherapy of skull base chondrosarcomas. Int J Radiat Oncol Biol Phys 67:171–177

Schütze C, Bergmann R, Yaromina A, et al (2007a) Effect of increase of radiation dose on local control relates to pretreatment FDG uptake in FaDu tumours in nude mice. Radiother Oncol 83:311–315

Schütze C, Dörfler A, Eicheler W, et al (2007b) Combination of EGFR/HER2 tyrosine kinase inhibition by BIBW2992 and BIBW2669 with irradiation in FaDu human squamous cell carcinoma. Strahlenther Onkol 182:256–264

Scott RB (1970) Cancer chemotherapy: the first 25 years. BMJ 4:259–265

Seifert P, Baker LH, Reed ML (1975) Comparison of continuously infused 5-FU with bolus injection in treatment of patients with colorectal carcinoma. Cancer 36:123–128

Shaked Y, Emmenegger U, Francia G, et al (2005) Low-dose metronomic combined with intermittent bolus-dose cyclophosphamide is an effective long-term chemotherapy treatment strategy. Cancer Res 65:7045–7051

Shewach DS, Hahn TM, Chang E, et al (1994) Metabolism of 2',2'-difluoro-2'-deoxycytidine and radiation sensitization of human colon carcinoma cells. Cancer Res 54:3218–3223

Shimizu D, Ishikawa T, Ichikawa Y, et al (2004) Current progress in the prediction of chemosensitivity for breast cancer. Breast Cancer 11:42–48

Shimoyama M (1975) The cytocidal action of alkylating agents and anticancer antibodies against in-vitro cultured Yoshida ascites sarcoma cells. J Jpn Soc Cancer Ther 10:63–72

Siewert JR, Molls M, Zimmermann F, Lordick F (2007) Esophageal cancer: clinical management. In: Kelsen DP, Daly JM, Kern SE, Levin B, Trepper JE, van Cutsem E (eds) Principles and practice of gastrointestinal oncology, 2nd edn. Lippincott Williams & Wilkins, Philadelphia, pp 203–230

Simoens C, Korst AE, De Pooter CM, et al (2003) In vitro interaction between ecteinascidin 743 (ET-743) and radiation, in relation to its cell cycle effects. Br J Cancer 89:2305–2311

Smith IE, A'Hern RP, Coombes GA, et al (2004) A novel continuous infusional 5-fluorouracil-based chemotherapy regimen compared with conventional chemotherapy in the neo-adjuvant treatment of early breast cancer: 5-year results of the TOPIC trial. Ann Oncol 15:751–758

Söderlund K, Stål O, Skoog L, et al (2007) Intact Mre11/Rad50/Nbs1 complex predicts good response to radiotherapy in early breast cancer. Int J Radiat Oncol Biol Phys 68:50–58

Stadler P, Becker A, Feldmann HJ, et al (1999) Influence of the hypoxic subvolume on the survival of patients with head and neck cancer. Int J Radiat Oncol Biol Phys 44:749–754

Staib P, Staltmeier E, Neurohr K (2005) Prediction of individual response to chemotherapy in patients with acute myeloid leukaemia using the chemosensitivity index Ci. Br J Haematol 128:783–791

Steel GG (1979) Terminology in the description of drug-radiation interactions. Int J Radiat Oncol Biol Phys 5:1145–1150

Steel GG, Peckham MJ (1979) Exploitable mechanisms in combined radiotherapy–chemotherapy: the concept of additivity. Int J Radiat Oncol Biol Phys 5:85–91

Stewart DJ, Chiritescu G, Dahrouge S, et al. (2007) Chemotherapy dose-response relationships in non-small cell lung cancer and implied resistance mechanisms. Cancer Treat Rev 33:101–137

Stupp R, Mason WP, van den Bent MJ, et al (2005) Radiotherapy plus concomitant and adjuvant temozolomide for glioblastoma. N Engl J Med 352:987–996

Sturm I, Petrowsky H, Volz R, et al (2001) Analysis of p53/BAX/p16(ink4a/CDKN2) in esophageal squamous cell carcinoma: high BAX and p16(ink4a/CDKN2) identifies patients with good prognosis. J Clin Oncol 19:2272–2281

Sui M, Dziadyk JM, Zhu X, Fan W (2004) Cell cycle-dependent antagonistic interactions between paclitaxel and gamma-radiation in combination therapy. Clin Cancer Res 10:4848–4857

Sundstrom S, Bremnes R, Aasebo U, et al (2004) Hypofractionated palliative radiotherapy (17 Gy per 2 fractions) in advanced non-small cell lung carcinoma is comparable to standard fractionation for symptom control and survival: a national phase III trial. J Clin Oncol 22:801–810

Taghian AG, Abi-Raad R, Assaad SI, et al (2005) Paclitaxel decreases the interstitial fluid pressure and improves oxygenation in breast cancers in patients treated with neoadjuvant chemotherapy: clinical implications. J Clin Oncol 23:1951–1961

Tannock IF (1989) Combined modality treatment with radiotherapy and chemotherapy. Radiother Oncol 16:83–101

Tannock IF (1992) Potential for therapeutic gain from combined-modality treatment. Front Radiat Ther Oncol 26:1–15

Tannock IF (1998) Conventional cancer therapy: promise broken or promise delayed? Lancet 351(suppl 2):SII9–SII16

Tannock IF, Lee CM, Tunggal JK, et al (2002) Limited penetration of anticancer drugs through tumor tissue: a potential cause of resistance of solid tumors to chemotherapy. Clin Cancer Res 8:878–884

Teicher BA, Lazo JS, Sartorelli AC (1981) Classification of antineoplastic agents by their selective toxicities toward oxygenated and hypoxic tumor cells. Cancer Res 41:73–81

Teicher BA, Herman TS, Holden SA, et al (1990) Tumor resistance to alkylating agents conferred by mechanisms operative only in vivo. Science 247:1457–1461

Thames HD, Suit HD (1986) Tumor radioresponsiveness versus fractionation sensitivity. Int J Radiat Oncol Biol Phys 12:687–691

Trott KR (1990) Cell repopulation and overall treatment time. Int J Radiat Oncol Biol Phys 19:1071–1075

Tsuji H, Ishikawa H, Yanagi T, et al (2007) Carbon-ion radiotherapy for locally advanced or unfavourably located choroidal melanoma: a phase I/II dose-escalation study. Int J Radiat Oncol Biol Phys 67:857–862

Ueno NT, Buzdar AU, Singletary SE, et al (1997) Combined-modality treatment of inflammatory breast carcinoma: twenty years of experience at M.D. Anderson Cancer Center. Cancer Chemother Pharmacol 40:321–329

Veyret C, Levy C, Chollet P, et al (2006) Inflammatory breast cancer outcome with epirubicin-based induction and maintenance chemotherapy: ten-year results from the French Adjuvant Study Group GETIS 02 trial. Cancer 107:2535–2544

Von Minckwitz G, Blohmer JU, Raab G, et al (2005) In vivo chemosensitivity-adapted preoperative chemotherapy in patients with early-stage breast cancer: the GEPARTRIO pilot study. Ann Oncol 16:56–63

Weber WA (2005) Use of PET for monitoring cancer therapy and for predicting outcome. J Nucl Med 46:983–995

Wouters BG, van den Beucken T, Magagnin MG, et al (2005) Control of the hypoxic response through regulation of mRNA translation. Semin Cell Dev Biol 16:487–501

Wu L, Tannock IF (2003) Repopulation in murine breast tumors during and after sequential treatments with cyclophosphamide and 5-fluorouracil. Cancer Res 63:2134–2138

Wurschmidt F, Bardenheuer MJ, Muller WU, Molls M (2000) Chromosomal aberrations induced in mice bone marrow by treating with cisplatin and irradiation. Strahlenther Onkol 176:319–323

Yang LX, Double EB, O'Hara JA, Wang HJ (1995) Production of DNA double-strand breaks by interactions between carboplatin and radiation: a potential mechanism for radiopotentiation. Radiat Res 143:309–315

Yaromina A, Krause M, Thames H, et al (2007) Pre-treatment number of clonogenic cells and their radiosensitivity are major determinants of local tumour control after fractionated irradiation. Radiother Oncol 83:304–310

Yasuda H, Yamaya M, Nakayama K, et al (2006) Randomized phase II trial comparing nitroglycerin plus vinorelbine and cisplatin plus vinorelbine and cisplatin alone in previously untreated stage IIIB/IV non-small cell lung cancer. J Clin Oncol 24:688–694

Yu YQ, Giocanti N, Averbeck D, et al (2000) Radiation-induced arrest of cells in G2 phase elicits hypersensitivity to DNA double-strand break inducers and an altered pattern of DNA cleavage upon re-irradiation. Int J Radiat Biol 76:901–912

Zelefsky MJ, Yamada Y, Kollmeier MA, et al (2008) Long-term outcome following three-dimensional conformal/intensity-modulated external-beam radiotherapy for clinical stage T3 prostate cancer. Eur Urol 53:1172–1179

Zhao L, West BT, Hayman JA, et al (2007) High radiation dose may reduce the negative effect of large gross tumor volume in patients with medically inoperable early-stage non-small cell lung cancer. Int J Radiat Oncol Biol Phys 68:103–110

Zimmermann FB, Geinitz H, Schill S, et al (2006) Stereotactic hypofractionated radiotherapy in stage I (T1-2 N0 M0) non-small-cell lung cancer (NSCLC). Acta Oncol 45:796–801

The Impact of Molecularly
Targeted Therapy in Multi-Modality Therapy

Shiyu Song, Paul Dent, and Steven Grant

CONTENTS

S. Song, MD
Department of Radiation Oncology, Massey Cancer Center,
Virginia Commonwealth University Health System, 401 College Street, Richmond, VA 23298, USA

P. Dent, PhD
Department of Biochemistry, Massey Cancer Center, Virginia
Commonwealth University Health System, 401 College Street,
Richmond, VA 23298, USA

S. Grant, MD
Departments of Medicine and Biochemistry, Massey Cancer
Center, Virginia Commonwealth University Health System,
401 College Street, Richmond, VA 23298, USA

- New classes of agents that target one or more of the processes that play important roles in the malignant phenotype are rapidly being introduced into clinical practice. These new drugs include specific antibodies against growth factors or their receptors and small molecules that interfere with signal transduction pathways regulating the cell cycle, gene transcription, and survival in cancer cells.
- Examples of targets are epidermal growth factor receptor family and platelet-derived growth factor receptors, as well as vascular endothelial cell growth factor and its respective receptors.
- Solid tumors usually have multiple abnormal pathways or genetic changes so that a single drug often is not sufficient for permanent tumor suppression.
- In metastatic colorectal cancer treatment, two agents were approved almost simultaneously, cetuximab and bevacizumab.
- Combined with radiotherapy, targeted drugs, such as cetuximab, have already demonstrated their clinical potential.
- Ongoing preclinical work has improved and will continue to improve our understanding of the underlying mechanisms and thus form the basis for further refinement.

11.1
Introduction

The development of a large number of targeted agents has introduced tremendous opportunities as well as challenges to the field of oncology. Although most agents show limited single drug potential for the cure of common solid neoplasms, they can prolong patient survival in selected tumor types and, most importantly, enhance the existing therapies for a variety of cancers. Improvements have been achieved in the treatment of hematological malignancies, colorectal cancer, renal cancer, lung cancer, head and neck cancer, breast cancer, and liver cancer. Because these agents do not cause side effects similar to those of cytotoxic drugs and radiation therapy, their combination with current conventional chemotherapy and radiotherapy is usually feasible. How to best combine these new agents with radiation and chemotherapy requires intensive and persistent efforts from both clinicians and research scientists.

The combination of radiation therapy and chemotherapy is shown to be superior to radiation alone in both tumor response and patient survival for a number of malignancies. New classes of agents are being developed and rapidly introduced into clinical use. These agents target one or more of the processes that play important roles in the malignant phenotype. These new drugs include specific antibodies against growth factors or their receptors and small molecules that interfere with signal transduction pathways regulating the cell cycle, gene transcription, and survival in cancer cells. Some of the drugs have a single specific target, whereas others may have multiple targets. A few have shown curative potential and others play a more adjuvant role. The rapid developments of such broad categories of drugs have created great challenges as well as the opportunity for basic, translational, and clinical researchers to evaluate and integrate them into clinical use. Importantly, because the targets of this therapy are processes that are dysregulated only in cancer cells, these agents do not share the same side effects in normal tissues of the conventional cytotoxic chemotherapy and radiation, their combination with radiation therapy has attracted significant interest among radiation oncologists.

11.2
Classes of Targeted Therapy Agents

A great number of molecularly targeted agents have been approved (Table 11.1) and more are being developed and are in various stage of clinical testing (Arora and Scholar 2005; Dancey and Chen 2006; Gerber 2008; Murdoch and Sager 2008). Because tyrosine kinase activity is involved in many key steps of signal transduction pathways, the majority of the agents are tyrosine kinase inhibitors (TKIs). Their targets are indicated in Fig. 11.1. Most signal transduction pathways initiate with receptor proteins with an extracellular domain for interaction with their ligands (usually growth factors) and an intracellular domain with tyrosine kinase activity. Once the receptors interact with ligands, the receptor kinase is activated, causing a cascade of reactions leading to gene transcription and protein production. Any elements in the signal transduction pathway can be potential targets. The first few approved agents were antibodies against surface antigens or growth receptors. Examples of these receptors are epidermal growth factor receptor (EGFR) family, such as her-2/neu and platelet-derived growth factor receptors (PDGFR). Some of the

Table 11.1. The targeted agents that are approved by the FDA for treatment of various malignancies. *EGFR* epidermal growth factor receptor, *Her-2* EGFR-2 (ERBB2), *VEGF* vascular endothelial growth factor, *VEGFR* VEGF receptor, *PDGFR* platelet-derived growth factor receptor, *c-KIT* a tyrosine kinase receptor encoded by c-kit oncogene, *FLT-3* Fms-like tyrosine kinase 3, *RET* a receptor tyrosine kinase encoded by proto-oncogene ret, *BCR-ABL* an oncogene protein and a tyrosine kinase encoded by a fusion oncogene by t(9:22) translocation, *SRC* a tyrosine kinase encoded by c-Src gene, a cellular version of viral oncogene v-Src, *m-TOR* mammalian target of rapamycin

Effects of agents	Target	Class of molecules	FDA-approved indications
Growth inhibition			
Trastuzumab (Herceptin)	Her-2/neu	Antibody	Her-2 overexpressing breast cancer
Cetuximab (Erbitux)	EGFR	Antibody	CRC, HNC
Panitumumab (Vectibix)	EGFR	Antibody	CRC
Gefitinib (Iressa)	EGFR	Small molecule	NSCLC
Erlotinib (Tarceva)	EGFR	Small molecule	NSCLC, pancreas cancer
Lapatinib (Tykerb)	EGFR, Her-2	Small molecule	Breast cancer
Bevacizumab (Avastin)	VEGF	Antibody	CRC and NSCLC
Sunitinib (Sutent)	VEGFR, PDGFR, c-KIT, FLT-3, RET	Small molecule	GIST, RCC
Sorafenib (Nexavar)	VEGFR, PDGFR, FLT3, Raf, RET	Small molecule	RCC, HCC
Protein turnover			
Bortezomib (Velcade)	Proteasome	Small molecule	Multiple myeloma
Oncoprotein			
Imatinib (Gleevec)	BCR-ABL, PDGFR, c-KIT	Small molecule	CML, ph(+) ALL, GIST
Dasatinib (Sprycel)	BCR-ABL, SRC, c-KIT	Small molecule	CML, ph(+) AML
Intracellular signal transduction			
Temsirolimus (Torisel)	m-TOR	Small molecule	RCC
Cell surface antigen			
Rituximab (Rituxan)	CD20	Antibody	Lymphoma

antibodies are against the growth factor itself, such as vascular endothelial cell growth factor (VEGF).

Among small-molecule TKIs, one of the more successful agents is imatinib mesylate. Imatinib mesylate is a TKI of the fusion oncoprotein Bcr-Abl, a gene product driving the development of chronic myelogenic leukemia (CML). A major reason for the effectiveness of Imatinib is CML transformation in many instances only requires Bcr-Abl. In these cases inhibition of Bcr-Abl activity is sufficient to provide long-term control of the disease. Solid tumors usually have multiple abnormal pathways or genetic changes so that a single drug usually is not sufficient for permanent tumor suppression.

Other classes of the targeted agents have demonstrated impressive activity in several tumor lines. In this chapter, we discuss the various classes of the targeted agents, provide examples of their use against common malignancies both alone and in combination with chemotherapy and radiation therapy, and discuss how these agents may be rationally combined in order to target multiple dysregulated pathways simultaneously. These agents can be divided into classes according to

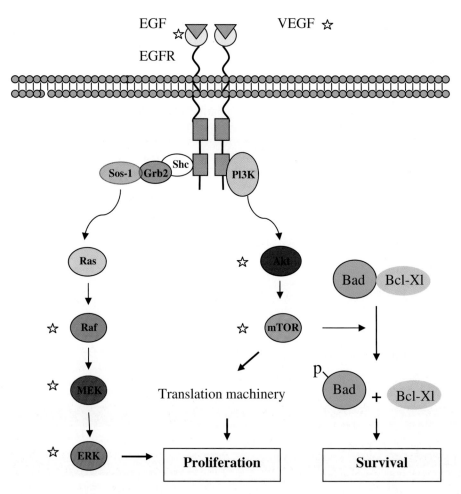

Fig. 11.1. Simplified representation of receptor tyrosine kinase pathways. Stars indicate the targets of currently approved agents. *EGF* epidermal growth factor, *EGFR* EGF receptor, *PI3K* phosphoinositide-3-kinase, *MEK* mitogen-activated protein kinase, *ERK* extracellular signal regulated kinase (also known as MAP kinase), *Shc src* homology collagen protein, *Akt* RAC-alpha serine/threonine-protein kinase or protein kinase B, *mTOR* mammalian target of rapamycin, *BAD* Bcl-Xl bcl family proteins, *SOS* son of sevenless (an activator of Ras protein), *Grb* Growth-factor receptor-bound protein

the type of molecules (antibodies vs small molecules) or their targeted cells (tumor cells vs angiogenesis). We discuss these agents according to their targeted biological processes.

11.2.1
Inhibitors of Kinase Signaling Pathways

As noted above, inhibitors of EGFR receptors and imatinib mesylate represent the prototypical forms of signaling inhibitors. Although imatinib mesylate is highly active in chronic phase CML, it is less active in acceler-

ated phase and blast phase disease (SAWYERS et al. 2002). It also has some, albeit limited, activity in Philadelphia+ acute lymphocytic leukemia (ALL; CHAMPAGNE et al. 2004). The Raf/MEK/ERK pathway is also frequently dysregulated in cancer. Such findings have prompted the development of multiple inhibitors of this pathway at the level of the MAP2K (MEK1/2), e.g., PD184352, and more recently, the multi-kinase Raf-1 inhibitor sorafenib. Mutations, particularly those associated with internal tandem repeats, in the Flt3 protein are found in as many as 20–30% of patients with acute myelogenic leukemia (AML), and are thought to contribute to the pathogenesis of the disease. Several FLT-3 inhibitors, including PKC412, are currently being evaluated in leukemia associated with FLT-3 mutations. Because dysregulation of these pathways in all likelihood contribute to—but are not primarily responsible for—the development of leukemia, the activity of the corresponding inhibitors as single agents is significantly less than that of imatinib mesylate in CML.

TKIs also include antibodies against growth factors and their receptors. Several antibody agents have been approved for clinical use for multiple cancers. Two examples of these agents are bevacizumab (Avastin) and cetuximab (Erbitux). Avastin is a recombinant humanized antibody that binds vascular endothelial growth factor (VEGF) and inhibits angiogenesis that is required for tumor growth. Erbitux is also a humanized monoclonal antibody and is against epidermal growth factor receptor (EGFR) and inhibits tumor growth by blocking EGF interaction with its receptors. Both agents were approved for the treatment of multiple solid tumors.

11.2.2
Cell Cycle Inhibitors

Dysregulation of the cell cycle traverse is a cardinal characteristic of neoplastic cells (KASTAN and BARTEK 2004). For this reason, the development of cell cycle inhibitors has become the focus of intense interest. Flavopiridol is a semisynthetic flavone that is a broad inhibitor of cyclin-dependent kinases (CDKs) and was the first CDK inhibitor to enter the clinic (SENDEROW-ICZ 1999). Flavopiridol kills human tumor cells at concentrations in the sub-micromolar range (ARGUELLO et al. 1998). Recently, the lethal effects of flavopiridol have been related to its ability to inhibit the cyclin T/cdk9 complex, which phosphorylates and activates RNA PolII, thereby down-regulating various short-lived pro-survival proteins, including MCL-1 and p21CIP1/WAF1 (CHAO and PRICE 2001). UCN-01 is also a CDK inhibitor that was originally developed as a PKC inhibitor, but which has subsequently been shown to inhibit various other signaling/cell cycle regulatory pathways, including PDK1/AKT and CHK1 (SATO et al. 2002; ZHAO et al. 2002). Most recently, the CDK inhibitor CYC202, the R-enantiomer of R-roscovitine, a purine analog CDK inhibitor, has entered the clinic.

11.2.3
Histone Deacetylase Inhibitors

Gene transcription is regulated by diverse factors, including those involved in the modification of chroma-

tin structure. The acetylation of core histones is reciprocally regulated by histone acetylases and deacetylases (HDACs; SENGUPTA and SETO 2004; PETERSON and LANIEL 2004). In general, acetylated histones assume a less compact structure rendering DNA more accessible to co-activator complexes thereby promoting gene transcription. HDACs also form complexes with co-repressors, and in so doing interfere with transcription of genes involved in leukemic cell maturation (MARKS et al. 2003). For these reasons, the development of HDAC inhibitors has been the focus of intense interest. Several classes of HDAC inhibitors have entered the clinical arena, including hydroxamates such as SAHA (vorinostat) and LAQ824, cyclic tetrapeptides such as depsipeptide, and short-chain fatty acids such as phenylbutyrate and valproic acid (MARKS and JIANG 2005; ROSATO and GRANT 2003). Initial single agent evidence of activity in patients has been noted (GAR-CIA-MANERO and ISSA 2005); however, while HDACIs have been shown to induce a differentiation response in tumor cells in vitro, their true anti-tumor activity may stem from their capacity to induce apoptosis. This phenomenon has been related to induction of oxidative damage, up-regulation of death receptors, and disruption of heat shock protein (HSP90) function, among other mechanisms (YU et al. 2002; RUEFLI et al. 2001; INSINGA et al. 2005).

11.2.4
Proteasome Inhibitors

The catalytic component of the 26S proteasome is responsible for the degradation of diverse cellular proteins, including those involved in regulation of signaling, cell cycle, and survival pathways, among others (ALMOND and COHEN 2002). Proteasome inhibitors have been shown to induce cell death in neoplastic cells while largely sparing their normal counterparts (AN et al. 1998). The mechanism by which proteasome inhibitors trigger the cell death process has not been clearly defined but may involve accumulation of pro-apoptotic proteins such as p53 and Bax (ALMOND and COHEN 2002; AN et al. 1998). In addition, proteasome inhibitors, by blocking proteasomal degradation of IκBα, disrupt the NF-κB pathway, which is critically involved in protection of cells from various noxious stimuli (PETERSON and LANIEL 2004). Recently, the boronic anhydride proteasome inhibitor Velcade has shown impressive activity in B-cell neoplasms, including multiple myeloma and certain forms of non-Hodgkin's lymphoma (ZANGARI et al. 2005).

11.2.5
HSP90 Antagonists

HSP90 is involved in the proper folding and maintenance of diverse proteins involved in cell cycle regulation and signaling (WORKMAN 2004). Disruption of HSP90 function results in protein misfolding, leading in turn to proteasomal degradation (NECKERS and IVY 2003). Geldanamycin analogs, such as 17AAG, have been shown to disrupt the function of a variety of signaling proteins, including Raf-1, AKT, EGFR2, and ERK1/2, among others, which can induce cell death and sensitize tumor cells to the actions of various cytotoxic drugs (HOSTEIN et al. 2001). As noted above, HDAC inhibitors, particularly those that interfere with the function of HDAC6, can induce acetylation of HSP90, and thus act as HSP90 antagonist mimetics (BALI et al. 2005).

11.2.6
Small-Molecule
BCL-2 Family Modulators

Cell death and survival decisions are reciprocally regulated by the balance between a large family of pro- (e.g., BAX, BAK, BAD, etc.) and anti-apoptotic (e.g., BCL-2, BCL-XL, MCL-1, A1, c-FLIP-s, XIAP etc) proteins (REED 1998). There has been extensive interest in attempts to shift the balance away from survival and toward apoptosis in tumor cells through the use of various molecules that regulate these apoptotic modulators. For example, antisense oligonucleotides directed against BCL-2 (G3139) have been employed clinically in an attempt to lower the apoptotic threshold for established cytotoxic drugs (MARCUCCI et al. 2003). An alternative approach involves the use of small molecules that interfere with the actions of various anti-apoptotic proteins, including BCL-2, BCL-XL and MCL-1 antagonists (HA14-1, ABT-737, Obatoclax; WANG et al. 2000; OLTERSDORF et al. 2005), and antagonists of XIAP (SCHIMMER et al. 2004). Lastly, efforts to activate the receptor-related, extrinsic apoptotic pathway have focused on the development of agents such as TRAIL (TNF-related apoptosis inducing ligand) and TRAIL agonist antibodies (PAN et al. 1997), which may selectively target neoplastic cells due to the presence of decoy receptors on normal host target tissues (SHERIDAN et al. 1997).

11.2.7
Translational Factor Inhibitors

Mammalian target of rapamycin (mTOR) is an intracellular serine/threonine kinase downstream of diverse signal transduction pathways such as those initiated by EGFR, VEGF, activated Ras, estrogen receptor, and nutrients. It is involved in regulation of cell proliferation, angiogenesis, and cell survival. Its main downstream targets are translational proteins (S6K1, 4E-BP1). Activation of mTOR leads to ribosome biogenesis, mRNA translation, and cell proliferation. It also is involved in mediating cell survival by regulating Bcl-2, Mcl-1, and cFlip. mTOR inhibitors are shown to cause cell growth arrest and cell death. Multiple mTOR inhibitors have been tested for the treatment of cancer. One example of these inhibitors is temsirolimus, which is shown to significantly improve the survival of patients with advanced renal cell carcinoma.

11.3
Targeted Therapy of Common Malignancies

11.3.1
Hematological Malignancies

11.3.1.1
Chronic Myelogenic Leukemia

Chronic myelogenic leukemia (CML) is caused by a chromosomal translocation that leads to the fusion of the ABL oncogene on chromosome 9q34 with the breakpoint cluster region (BCR) on chromosome 22q11.2, t(9;22)(q34;q11.2), cytogenetically termed the Philadelphia chromosome (Ph; NOWELL and HUNGERFORD 1961). Because Bcr-Abl protein is a constitutively active tyrosine kinase that activates many signal transduction pathways, including Ras/Raf/mitogen activated protein kinase (MAPK), phosphatidylinositol 3 kinase, STAT5/Janus kinase, and Myc, expression of Bcr-Abl alone is sufficient to trigger CML transformation. Imatinib mesylate is a highly active and specific tyrosine kinase inhibitor. In the pivotal phase-III trial, Imatinib demonstrated 98% response rate, 92% major cytogenetic responses, and 87% complete cytogenetic responses by 5 years (DRUKER et al. 2006). It now represents first-line standard therapy for CML. The majority of patients treated with imatinib mesylate are disease-free on maintenance doses; however, drug resistance occurs, either due to amplification of Bcr-Abl, or more frequently, mutations in the Bcr-Abl kinase domain. Recently, several new agents with high response rates and excellent tumor control have been approved for imatinib-resistant CML. FDA approved dasatinib after multiple phase-II clinical trials demonstrated 31–59% durable response in patients with CML refractory to imatinib (HOCHHAUS et al. 2007; CORTES et al. 2007; GUILHOT et al. 2007). One exception to this is resistance due to mutation of a specific gatekeeper region of the Bcr-Abl kinase (i.e., T315I), which confers resistance to both first- and second-generation Bcr-Abl kinase inhibitors (RAY et al. 2007). Interestingly, cells bearing such mutations appear sensitive to third-generation dual Bcr-Abl and aurora kinase inhibitors such as VX-680 (MK-0457), and good responses have been obtained with such agents in patients resistant to imatinib and dasatinib (DAI et al. 2008).

11.3.1.2
Acute Leukemia

Approximately 30% of patients with AML exhibit dysregulation of the FLT3 oncogene, due either to mutation or amplification of internal tandem repeats (ITD) (LEE et al. 2005). Such abnormalities carry a relatively poor prognosis. This has prompted the development of FLT3 inhibitors for such patients (e.g., PKC-412), either as monotherapy, or more commonly, in combination with standard anti-leukemic regimens (WEISBERG et al. 2002; STONE et al. 2005; FURUKAWA et al. 2007).

Epigenetic forms of therapy are also the subject of intense interest for the treatment of AML and related disorders such as the myelodysplastic syndrome (MDS). For example, inhibitors of DNA methyltransferase, such as 5-azacytidine or 5-deoxyazacytidine, have shown significant activity in patients with MDS (MOMPARLER 2005; WIJERMANS et al. 2005; MULLER et al. 2006). They are believed to act by inhibiting methylation of genes involved in cell differentiation, and allowing gene re-expression. In addition, combination regimens employing hypomethylating agents in combination with histone deacetylase inhibitors (e.g., vorinostat), which enhance gene expression by modifying chromatin acetylation, have also shown promising preliminary results in patients with MDS and AML.

11.3.1.3
Lymphoma

Rituximab is the first molecularly targeted agent approved for clinical use. It is an antibody against lymphocyte surface protein CD20. The function of CD20 and the mechanism of Rituximab cell killing are not clearly understood, but Rituximab rapidly reduces CD20 positive cells and therefore is effective against B-cell lymphomas, including aggressive large B-cell lymphoma, follicular lymphoma, and even the CD20-positive nodular lymphocyte-predominant Hodgkin's lymphoma. It has become standard treatment for non-Hodgkin's lymphomas, alone or in combination depending on the type of tumors. In addition, radiolabeled CD20 antibody (Zevalin and Bexxar) are also approved for chemorefractory lymphomas. Multiple new agents are in development and being tested in clinical trials.

11.3.1.4
Chronic Lymphocytic Leukemia

Chronic lymphocytic leukemia (CLL) is an accumulative disease of mature B lymphocytes. Rituximab, either alone or in combination with fludarabine, has proved to represent a highly effective form of therapy for this disease. In addition, Alemtuzumab (Campath; anti-CD52) has also been shown to be very active in CLL, although it has significant immunosuppressive activity. More recently, a novel infusional schedule of the CDK inhibitor flavopiridol has shown impressive activity in patients with refractory CLL.

11.3.1.5
Multiple Myeloma

Bortezomib (Velcade) is the first FDA-approved proteasome inhibitor for multiple myeloma. The ubiquitin–proteasome pathway is the major complex for degradation of intracellular proteins, including proteins that are involved in signal transduction pathway regulating cell growth and death. Inhibition of this system leads induction of apoptosis by mechanisms yet to be determined; however, it has been shown that myeloma cells are highly dependent upon activation of the NF-κB pathway for their survival, and that myeloma cells frequently display dysregulation of this pathway. It is thought that proteasome inhibitors, by blocking the degradation of IκBα, which binds to and sequesters NF-κB in the cytoplasm, thereby preventing nuclear translocation, inhibit NF-κB activation and thus induce myeloma cell death. Velcade has been approved for the treatment of myeloma refractory to other therapies, and more recently, relapsed mantle cell lymphoma.

In addition to proteasome inhibitors, immunomodulatory agents, such as thalidomide and lenalidomide, have also shown significant activity in multiple myeloma. The mechanism by which they act is not known with certainty but is felt to involve, at least in part, anti-angiogenic effects.

11.3.2
Breast Cancer

Twenty-five to 30% percent of breast cancers present with Her-2/neu (EGFR2) amplification and gene over-expression. The Her-2/neu oncoprotein is a receptor tyrosine kinase belonging to EGFR family. The antibody against Her-2/neu protein Trastuzumab (Herceptin) is a humanized monoclonal antibody that selectively binds with high affinity to the extracellular domain of the HER-2 receptor kinase. It was approved in 1998 for metastatic breast cancer with Her-2 amplification and was one of the first targeted therapy agents approved for breast cancer treatment. This approval was based on a large clinical trial of 469 patients with metastatic breast cancer and who were not previously treated for metastatic breast cancer. This study showed the combination of Herceptin with chemotherapy significantly increase tumor response rate, response time, and progression-free survival; there was a trend of overall survival benefits.

Herceptin was recently approved for early Her-2 positive breast cancer as adjuvant therapy following chemotherapy. In combined analysis of two multi-center trials (NSABP B31 and NCCTG N9831), adding 52 weeks of Herceptin to standard chemotherapy reduced recurrence (local, distant, or death) by 52%, and was associated with 33% reduction of deaths (Romond et al. 2005). This finding was also demonstrated in the European trial (Piccart-Gebhart et al. 2005). In these trials, Herceptin was found to be beneficial in all subgroups of early Her-2 positive breast cancers, regardless of tumor size, nodal status, and hormone receptor status. Herceptin is currently approved only for node-positive patients. One of the major toxicities of Herceptin is cardiomyopathy, which leads to left ventricular dysfunction and heart failure (2.9–4.1% in the combined analysis). This makes it problematic for combination treatment with paclitaxel, a standard chemotherapy agent for breast cancer with significant cardiac toxicity.

HER2 kinase is also a target for small-molecule inhibitors. One of the most exciting agents recently approved specifically for Her-2-positive breast cancer is lapatinib (Tykerb), an effective inhibitor against both EGFR and Her-2. This new agent was approved in March 2007 for use in combination with capecitabine for the treatment of patients with advanced or metastatic breast cancer whose tumors overexpress HER2 and who have received prior chemotherapy therapy including an anthracycline, a taxane, and Herceptin. The efficacy in combination with capecitabine in breast cancer were tested in a randomized trial (Geyer et al. 2006). Patients with locally advanced or metastatic HER2 over-expressing breast cancer who failed prior treatment, including taxanes, anthracyclines, and Herceptin, were randomized to receive either lapatinib plus capecitabine or capecitabine alone. The study was terminated early because interim analysis showed significant increase in time to progression (TTP; 27.1 vs 18.6 weeks) and in the response rates (23.7 vs 13.9%) favoring combination group. The most frequent adverse reactions during treatment with combination were diarrhea (65%), palmar-plantar erythrodysesthesia (PPE, 53%), nausea (44%), rash (28%), vomiting (26%), and fatigue (23%). In general, lapatinib is well tolerated.

Angiogenensis is a major target for cancer therapy, and it has been extensively studied in breast cancer. Avastin is recently approved for breast cancer. The effectiveness of Avastin in metastatic breast cancer is based on an improvement in progression free survival in two clinical trials (study 7 or E2100 and study 8 or AVF2119). In a randomized, multicenter study (study 7 or E2100) for first-line use, patients who had not received chemotherapy for locally recurrent or metastatic breast cancer were randomized to receive either paclitaxel alone or in combination with Avastin (Miller et al. 2007). The addition of Avastin to paclitaxel resulted in an improvement in PFS with no significant improvement in overall survival, but the median PFS was 11.3 vs 5.8 months for the Avastin plus paclitaxel arms vs the paclitaxel alone, respectively. Partial response rates in patients with measurable disease were higher with Avastin plus paclitaxel: 48.9 vs 22.2%, although no complete responses were observed. The use of Avastin for early breast cancer has been studied, showing promising results, but is not currently approved by FDA.

11.3.3
Colorectal Cancer

Two agents were approved almost simultaneously in early 2004 for metastatic colorectal cancer, Erbitux and Avastin. The efficacy of Erbitux alone or in combination with irinotecan were studied in a multicenter, randomized, controlled clinical trial (329 patients) and in combination with irinotecan in an open-label, single-arm trial (138 patients; Cunningham et al. 2004). All patients were diagnosed with EGFR-expressing, metastatic colorectal cancer, whose disease had progressed after receiving an irinotecan-containing regimen. The median duration of response in the overall population was 5.7 months in the combination arm and 4.2 months in the monotherapy arm. Compared with patients randomized to Erbitux alone, patients randomized to Erbitux and irinotecan experienced a significantly longer median time to disease progression. A single agent in a multicenter, open-label, single-arm clinical trial in patients with EGFR-expressing, metastatic colorectal cancer who progressed following an irinotecan-containing regimen showed a low response rate of 9%, with a median duration of response of 4.2 months (SALTZ et al. 2004). Interestingly, the response did not correlate with EGFR positivity. These studies led to its approval for the treatment of EGFR-expressing, metastatic colorectal carcinoma in patients who are refractory to irinotecan-based chemotherapy. Erbitux is also tested against best supportive care, showing a significant survival benefit (JONKER et al. 2007).

Avastin was approved nearly at the same time as Erbitux. Two randomized clinical trials evaluating Avastin in combination with intravenous 5-fluorouracil-based chemotherapy were conducted. The first study was a randomized, double-blind clinical trial of more than 800 patients testing Avastin as first-line treatment of metastatic colorectal cancer (HURWITZ et al. 2004). The primary end point was overall survival. The patients were treated with either bolus-IFL (irinotecan, 5-fluorouracil, and leucovorin) plus placebo (Arm 1), or bolus-IFL plus Avastin (Arm 2). This study showed a significant increase in overall survival (20.3 vs 15.6 months), progression-free survival (10.6 vs 6.2 months), and response rate (45 vs 35%) favoring Avastin group. The smaller second study was designed to evaluate Avastin in combination with 5-fluorouracil and leucovorin as the first-line treatment for metastatic colorectal cancers. This study also showed a significant increase in response rate as well as progression-free and overall survival (KABBINAVAR et al. 2005). In one of the largest studies, Avastin was also found to be effective as a second-line agent in combination with oxaliplatin, fluorouracil, and leucovorin (FOLFOX4) for previously treated metastatic colorectal cancer (GIANTONIO et al. 2007).

11.3.4
Lung Cancers

Lung cancer is a leading cause of cancer deaths worldwide, and the outcome of treatment has not significantly improved for decades. There is strong interest in molecularly targeted therapy for lung cancer in hope to improve survival. Again, there are two pathways that play an important role in lung cancer, EGFR and VEGF. EGFR is frequently overexpressed in non-small cell lung cancer (NSCLC) (>70%). The first agent for the treatment of NSCLC was gefitinib (Iressa), a small-molecule inhibitor of EGFR, which was approved by FDA under accelerated approval regulations for the treatment of patients with locally advanced or metastatic NSCLC after failure of both platinum-based and docetaxel chemotherapies. Multiple studies showed single-agent efficacy (KRIS et al. 2003; SIMON et al. 2003; SANTORO et al. 2004; FUKUOKA et al. 2003). Among the patients treated in the U.S., partial tumor responses occurred in 15 of 142 evaluable patients for a response rate of 10.6% overall. Responses occurred in 9 of 66 patients receiving 250 mg/day (13.6%) and 6 of 76 patients receiving 500 mg/day (7.9%). Median duration of response was 7.0 months (range 4.6–18.6+ months; COHEN et al. 2004). Iressa failed to improve treatment outcome or survival in combination with chemotherapy in multiple randomized clinical trials. Currently, Iressa is not actively used for NSCLC.

A second EGFR inhibitor approved in late 2004 is erlotinib (Tarceva). This approval was based on a large, randomized, double-blind, placebo-controlled phase-III trial (study BR.21) evaluated the use of single-agent Tarceva for the treatment of patients with locally advanced or metastatic NSCLC after failure of at least one prior chemotherapy regimen (SHEPHERD et al. 2005). There was statistically significant and clinically relevant prolongation in overall survival and progression-free survival for patients treated with Tarceva compared with patients receiving placebo. In this study, the hazard ratio (HR) for death in the Tarceva arm relative to the placebo arm estimated from the primary analysis was 0.73 indicating that Tarceva reduced the risk of death by 27% compared with placebo. Stable disease was observed in 35.1% of Tarceva-treated patients with measurable disease, compared with 26.5% of placebo-treated patients, for a CR+PR+SD rate of 44.0 and 27.5%, respectively. This difference was statistically significant ($p=0.004$). The responses obtained with Tarceva were durable: for patients with measurable disease, the median response duration was 34.3 weeks, ranging from 9.7 to 57.6+ weeks; however, as for Iressa, two randomized, double-blind, placebo-controlled phase-III trials (TALENT and TRIBUTE trials) investigated Tarceva in combination with standard chemotherapy as first-line treatment for patients with advanced NSCLC (GATZEMEIER et al. 2007; HERBST et al. 2005). Both trials failed to show survival benefit. The addition of Tarceva does not prolong survival over chemotherapy alone.

Mutational analysis of EGFR may help to identify patients who might respond to TKI. In a study of gefitinib for lung cancer, mutation was found in the tyrosine kinase domain of EGFR in 8 of 9 responders but in none of 7 patients who did not respond (LYNCH et al. 2004). Interestingly, adenocarcinoma histology, female gender, absence of smoking history, and Asian ethnicity appear to be predictive of gefitinib response; however, EGFR expression level may not be predictive.

Avastin was studied in NSCLC and approved in 2006 for NSCLC treatment in combination with carboplatin and paclitaxel for the initial systemic treatment of patients with unresectable, locally advanced, recurrent or metastatic, non-squamous, non-small cell lung cancer. An improvement in survival time was reported when Avastin was added to a standard chemotherapy regimen. A multi-center clinical trial supporting this approval enrolled 878 patients who had not received prior chemotherapy (SANDLER et al. 2006). The trial compared the effectiveness of Avastin plus carboplatin and paclitaxel with chemotherapy by carboplatin and paclitaxel alone. The median overall survival time for patients in the Avastin plus carboplatin and paclitaxel arm was 12.3 vs 10.3 months for patients receiving only carboplatin and paclitaxel.

11.3.5
Head and Neck Cancer

Despite the fact that many agents have been evaluated for head and neck cancer (HNC), the only FDA approved agent thus far is Erbitux, which is used in combination with radiation therapy (RT). The drug has shown a significant increase in locoregional tumor control and survival when combined with radiation as compared with radiation alone. In a phase-III randomized trial of 424 patients with stage-III/IV SCC of the oropharynx, hypopharynx, or larynx who had no prior therapy, patients were either treated with Erbitux plus RT (211 patients) or RT alone (213 patients; BONNER et al. 2006). Erbitux was administered as a 400 mg/m² initial dose, followed by 250 mg/m² weekly for the duration of RT (6–7 weeks), starting 1 week before RT. The RT was administered for 6–7 weeks as once daily, twice daily, or concomitant boost. The median survival time was 49 months on the Erbitux plus RT arm vs 29.3 months observed in patients receiving RT alone. The median duration of locoregional control was 24.4 months in patients receiving Erbitux plus RT vs 14.9 months for those receiving RT alone.

Erbitux has shown its efficacy in recurrent and metastatic HNC as well. A single-arm trial of Erbitux monotherapy in 103 patients with recurrent or metastatic SCCHN after failure of platinum-based therapy reported a response rate of 12.6%. Median response duration was 5.8 months (VERMORKEN et al. 2007). Combination of Erbitux with chemotherapy is much superior to chemotherapy alone in metastatic cancer patients. In a large European study of 442 patients with recurrent or metastatic SCCHN, the median survival was increased from 7.4 to 10.1 months with addition of Erbitux to chemotherapy (carboplatin or cisplatin plus 5-FU; presented at ASCO 2007). EGFR plays an important role in HNC, and a number of molecular agents are being tested in clinical trials, including Iressa and Tarceva. For the most part the clinical results appear to be disappointing.

11.3.6
Renal Cell Carcinoma

Newly available targeted therapy is particularly important for advanced renal cancer, because there is no existing effective chemotherapy for this disease. In the past two decades, immunotherapy has been the main treatment modality but with limited success. Recent development and approval of a few new agents provide a ray of hope for this patient population. The genetic or molecular changes in renal cancers provide ample targets for this new therapy. Besides the abnormal changes in signal transduction pathways seen in other cancers, a high proportion of renal cancers have abnormal von Hippel-Lindau (VHL), a tumor suppressor gene. Absence of the active VHL gene product causes dysfunction of the hypoxia-inducible system and accumulation of growth factors such as VEGF (KRIEG et al. 2000; NA et al. 2003). The search for molecular abnormalities proves to be fruitful. Thus far, there are four targeted agents approved for advanced or metastatic renal cancer, including sorafenib, sunitinib, temsirolimus, and Avastin.

The first agent approved by FDA for renal cancer is sorafenib (Nexavar), a multi-kinase inhibitor. Its targets include Raf-, VEGF-, and PDGF-signaling pathways. The Raf family kinase is part of a signal transduction cascade that transmits growth factor-mediated proliferative signals from the extracellular environment to the nucleus of the cell, it is also a part of pathway mediated by activated Ras. Nexavar is effective in tumors with raf gene mutations as well as with activated ras. In the larger phase-III, international, multicenter, randomized trial, the patients with advanced renal cell carcinoma who had received one prior systemic therapy were treated with Nexavar or placebo, the median time to tumor progression or death in the Nexavar treated arm was 167 days compared with 84 days in control group (Escudier et al. 2007a). However, only 2% of Nexavar patients had a confirmed partial response; therefore, the gain in PFS in Nexavar-treated patients was primarily due to stable disease. Overall survival was longer for Nexavar than placebo. In another randomized trial in patients with metastatic malignancies, including RCC, 202 patients with advanced RCC were enrolled into the study (Ratain et al. 2006). After the initial 12 weeks of Nexavar therapy, patients were monitored at week 24, for the 65 randomized patients, the progression-free rate was significantly higher in patients randomized to Nexavar (16 of 32, 50%) than in patients randomized to placebo (6 of 33, 18%). Progression-free survival was significantly longer in the Nexavar group (163 days) than in the placebo group (41 days).

Another Raf kinase inhibitor, sunitinib (Sutent), was approved in 2006 based on a multi-center, international randomized trial enrolling 750 patients with treatment-naïve metastatic renal cell carcinoma (Motzer et al. 2007). In that study, patients were randomized to receive either Sutent or interferon-α (IFN-α). Common metastatic sites included lung, lymph nodes, bone, and liver. There were 96 events (25.6%) of progression/death on Sutent compared with 154 events (41.1%) on IFN-α. Median progression-free survival was 47.3 weeks for Sutent-treated patients and 22.0 weeks for patients treated with IFN. Objective response rate on the Sutent arm was 27.5 vs 5.3% on IFN-α arm.

Temsirolimus is an mTOR (mammalian target of rapamycin) inhibitor. mTOR has multiple downstream targets, including cell translational machinery. Temsirolimus demonstrated clinical efficacy with significantly increased survival of renal cancer patients. In a clinical trial, 626 patients were randomized to one of three arms: interferon alfa (IFN) alone ($n = 207$); temsirolimus 25 mg alone ($n = 209$); or the combination of temsirolimus 15 mg and IFN ($n = 210$; Hudes et al. 2007). Temsirolimus was associated with a statistically significant improvement in overall survival when compared with IFN. The median OS was 10.9 months on the temsirolimus arm and 7.3 months on the IFN arm. Progression-free survival was 5.5 months on the temsirolimus arm and 3.1 months on the IFN arm. The combination of temsirolimus 15 mg and IFN did not increase survival over temsirolimus alone but was associated with increased toxicity.

Because VHL mutation leads to increase in angiogenesis, it plays a central role in renal cancer carcinogenesis (Na et al. 2003). Anti-angiogenesis has been proven to be a successful strategy. Avastin has been shown to improve progression-free survival of patients with metastatic RCC in phase-III trials both in the U.S. and Europe (Yang et al. 2003; Escudier et al. 2007b), and was approved for treatment of RCC.

11.3.7
Hepatocellular Carcinoma

In the past 30 years, no chemotherapy clinical trial for advanced hepatocellular carcinoma (HCC) has demonstrated any survival benefit for a long list of drugs. Recently, multiple new agents have been found to be effective against HCC, one of which is Nexavar, which has been approved for HCC. An international randomized placebo-controlled trial in patients with inoperable hepatocellular carcinoma showed a significant increase in survival (Llovet et al. 2008). The study was designed to compare the survival of a group of patients who received the drug against a group of similar patients who did not. A total of 602 patients were studied. Patients received either Nexavar or a placebo. The trial was stopped after a planned interim analysis showed a statistically significant advantage in overall survival for the patients who had received Nexavar. Patients who received Nexavar survived a median of 10.7 months, while patients who received placebo survived a median of 7.9 months. This study established Nexavar as first-line treatment for advanced HCC patients. Recently, this drug was tested in an Asian population and was found to be effective as well (presented at ASCO annual meeting 2008).

11.3.8
Others

Gastrointestinal stromal tumors (GIST) are the most common mesenchymal tumors of GI tract. GIST was found to have gain-of-function mutation of the kit gene. The Kit gene encodes KIT receptor tyrosine kinase, whose structure is similar to that of PDGFR. Imatinib mesylate, a potent inhibitor of Bcr-Abl oncoprotein, showed inhibitory effect on KIT. Imatinib was then successfully applied to the treatment of GISTs (Heinrich et al. 2003; van Oosterom et al. 2002; Blanke et al. 2008). Despite various mutations of Kit, and that PDFGR-alpha genes have been found in GISTs, most GISTs are imatinib sensitive. Imatinib is not only efficacious in advanced GIST, but also to reduce recurrence after resection for early GIST. After long-term administration of imatinib, however, new imatinib-resistant clones develop a secondary mutation of the Kit or PDGFR-alpha gene. New drugs and adjuvant regimens against such secondary progression are now being intensively explored. Sunitinib was later approved for the patients who develop resistance to, or who do not tolerate, imatinib.

11.4
Radiation and Targeted Therapy in Cancer Cell Killing

11.4.1
Ionizing Radiation and Activation of Common Signal Transduction Pathways

Ionizing radiation is used as a primary treatment for many types of cancer. Multiple laboratories have shown that EGFR is rapidly activated in response to the irradiation of multiple tumor cell types in vitro (WILLERS and HELD 2006; BENTZEN et al. 2005; ASTSATUROV et al. 2006; CHINNAIYAN et al. 2006; KIM et al. 2006; KAVANAGH et al. 1995; BALABAN et al. 1996). Low-dose, clinically relevant radiation exposure (~2 Gy) activates EGFR, and by heterodimerization, other members of the EGFR family (EGFR2, EGFR3, EGFR4); thus, although the irradiation of cells causes death, it also can enhance proliferation in the surviving fraction of cells and promote long-term resistance to multiple cytotoxic stresses. Exposure of carcinoma cells to clinically relevant low doses of ionizing radiation promotes the generation of reactive oxygen and reactive nitrogen species, with subsequent inactivation of protein tyrosine phosphatases, followed by the activation of the substrates of the tyrosine phosphatases, the growth factor receptor tyrosine kinases (TKs) in the plasma membrane (EGFR family of receptors). Receptor activation within several minutes of exposure enhances the activities of RAS family transducer molecules that mediate signaling from the membrane environment, causing the activation of multiple cytosolic signal transduction pathways. Intracellular pathways, such as the RAF-ERK1/2 and PI3K-AKT pathways, play a role in the long-term effects of cell survival from toxic stresses and the regulation of cell growth. Studies in the late 1990s argued that a ~2-Gy radiation exposure caused levels of EGFR1 and ERK1/2 pathway activation similar to those observed by growth-stimulatory EGF concentrations (0.1 nM) ~30 min after exposure (TODD et al. 1999; BOWERS et al. 2001); thus, ionizing radiation has the potential to promote the tyrosine phosphorylation and activation of intracellular pathways via PTPase inhibition at the level of the EGFR family receptor, and possibly, though not yet proved, also at the level of the tyrosine phosphorylated mitogen-activate protein kinase (MAPK) proteins.

11.4.2
EGFR Receptors and Paracrine Ligands as Survival Modules

After observations demonstrating the initial radiation-induced activation of the EGFR approximately 0–10 min after exposure, it became evident that the EGFR also were reactivated approximately 60–180+ min after irradiation. The primary mode of receptor activation at these later times occurred via a paracrine/autocrine mechanism (DENT et al. 1999; SHVARTSMAN et al. 2002). The initial activation of EGFR1 and the ERK1/2 pathway was directly responsible for the cleavage, release, and functional activation of pre-synthesized paracrine ligands, such as pro-transforming growth factor (TGF)-α, that fed back onto the irradiated tumor cell, and potentially in vivo onto unirradiated distant tumor cells, thereby re-energizing the signaling system (HAGAN et al. 2004). Increasing the radiation dose from 2 to 10 Gy enhances both the amplitude and duration of the secondary activation of EGFR1 and the secondary activation of the intracellular signaling pathways, suggesting that radiation can promote a dose-dependent increase in the cleavage of pro-TGF-α that reaches a plateau at approximately 10 Gy (DENT et al. 1999; SHVARTSMAN et al. 2002). In contrast to the secondary receptor and pathway activations, primary receptor and signaling pathway activations appear to come to a plateau at 3–5 Gy.

The expression of paracrine factors in tumor cells can change in the short-term (hours) and in the long-term (weeks) after irradiation, as potentially can the expression of the growth factor receptors that bind the factors. For example, in the instances of RAS–ERK1/2 signaling and p53 transcriptional function, the activities of which can be increased shortly following radiation exposure, in a variety of cells, these proteins act to enhance the expression of autocrine factors such as HB-EGF and epiregulin (FANG et al. 2001). However, loss of p53 function can also alter EGFR1 expression; for example, in comparing HCT116 wild-type and HCT116 p53 –/– cells, EGFR1 expression is reduced, and both wild-type and mutant p53 proteins have been shown to regulate the EGFR1 promoter (SHEIKH et al. 1997; NISHI et al. 2001). In MCF7 mammary carcinoma cells exposed to multiple low doses of radiation, the expression of EGFR1 and TGF-α was noted to rise, and the expression of the estrogen receptor to decline (SCHMIDT-ULLRICH et al. 1992). These findings argue that the activation by radiation of EGFR family receptors and downstream pathways has the potential to be influenced, in both the short- and long-term, by the amount of prior radiation exposure a cell has received and the mutational status of p53 and RAS proteins. Collectively, these observations argue that radiation generates signals within tumor cells that promote activation of growth factor receptors and signaling pathways that in turn promote the release of paracrine ligands from cells, leading to the reactivation of receptors and intracellular signaling pathways.

Signaling by EGFR family of receptors is, in general, believed to be pro-proliferative and cytoprotective, and inhibition of EGFR function has been explored in great detail by many drug companies and academic research laboratories as a mode of cancer therapy. Thus, when signaling from the EGFR family receptors is blocked, either by use of inhibitory antibodies (Cetuximab, Panitumumab, Matuzumab, Pertuzumab, Bevacizumab); or low molecular weight inhibitors of receptor TKs (Erlotinib, Gefitinib, Lapatinib, Canertinib), tumor cell growth can be reduced and in addition the sensitivity of these cells to being killed by a wide variety of noxious stresses increased (reviewed in SHELTON et al. 2005; BASELGA and ARTEAGA 2005; DASSONVILLE et al. 2007). In-vitro and xenograft tumor animal model studies have strongly argued that inhibition of EGFR function using single drug/antibody dosing has radiosensitizing effects (BIANCO et al. 2002; CHINNAIYAN et al. 2005; HARARI 2007). One example of the synergistic effects of the combination of radiation and anti-EGFR treatment was shown in animal studies; the combination of radiation and Erbitux produced lasting inhibition of tumor growth while radiation or Erbitux alone caused only temporal growth delay (HUANG and HARARI 2000). However, as a collective group, clinical trials in which the modulation of EGFR function was a primary goal for improved therapeutic outcomes have been considerably less successful in terms of tumor control than predicted based on in-vitro studies as well in animal studies (HARARI and HUANG 2006).

Several possible explanations could exist as to why a drug effect observed in vitro or in animals did not translate into as profound an anti-tumor effect in patients:

1. The required inhibitory concentration of the drug and the drug half-life are not achievable and are too short for a therapeutic effect, respectively, in patients.
2. The relative dependency (addiction) of cultured tumor cell isolates on EGFR signaling, including expression of hyperactive EGFR mutants (e.g., EGFR1 L858R), when compared with actual tumors in patients, may be biased based on in-vitro studies that use established cell lines. Additionally, the development of drug-resistant EGFR mutants in patients after long-term exposure to EGFR inhibitors (e.g., EGFR1 T790M) may preclude drug actions.
3. Exposure of tumor cells in vitro to kinase and other inhibitors, such as tamoxifen, has argued that compensatory activation of parallel growth factor receptors (such as the IGF-1 receptor and c-Kit) occurs to replace the loss of EGFR signaling caused by drug exposure, and acts to maintain tumor cell survival (KWAK et al. 2005; THOMAS et al. 2005; HUTCHESON et al. 2006).
4. The EGFR inhibitors that are often used in therapy only inhibit one EGFR family member, such as EGFR1, and, in a similar conceptual manner to the third point, other EGFR family members, such as EGFR2, may provide compensatory survival signaling to overcome loss of survival signaling from the inhibited receptor.
5. The development of other somatic mutations in survival signaling with the tumor cell, such as loss of PTEN (phosphatase and tensin homologue deleted in chromosome 10) function, which may be selected for in tumor cells undergoing EGFR inhibitor therapy, will lead to the development of tumor cells that are more resistant in general to the inhibitors of growth factor receptors.

11.4.3
Circumvention of EGFR Receptor Signaling Addiction: Activating Mutations in RAS and PI3K Signaling

The role of RAS signaling in terms of regulating radiosensitivity directly downstream of plasma membrane receptor TKs has also been investigated by many groups, with comparative data using cells from diverse genetic backgrounds arguing that mutated active H-, K-, and N-RAS proteins protect cells from the toxic effects of ionizing radiation by activating the PI3K pathway (YACOUB et al. 2006; IHLE et al. 2005; GUPTA et al. 2000, 2001). In HCT116 colon cancer cells expressing activated K-RAS D13, radiosensitivity was linked to signaling by the ERK1/2 pathway (CARON et al. 2005). Studies by others have also demonstrated that HCT116 cells expressing active K-RAS use the ERK1/2 pathway as a primary signal to protect themselves from the toxic effect of radiation and, in these experiments, isogenic HCT116 cells expressing active H-RAS V12 (with expression of active K-RAS D13 deleted) were noted to use the PI3K pathway as a primary signal to protect themselves from radiation toxicity (SHONAI et al. 2002). This suggests different RAS family members, H-RAS and K-RAS, have the potential to generate qualitatively different radioprotective signals via activating different downstream signal transduction pathways.

Data from several groups have demonstrated that the PI3K pathway is a key radio-protective pathway downstream of receptors and RAS proteins. Inhibition of PI3K pathway function by use of small-molecule inhibitors radiosensitizes tumor cells expressing mutant active RAS molecules or wild-type RAS molecules that are constitutively active due to upstream growth factor receptor signaling. It is possible that PI3K inhibitors may also exert a portion of their radiosensitizing properties by suppressing the function of proteins with PI3K-like kinase domains, such as ataxia–telangiectasia-mutated (ATM), ataxia–telangiectasia- and rad3-related (ATR), and DNA protein kinase (DNA-PK).

Growth factor-induced signaling from EGFR through the PI3K/AKT and RAF-1/ERK1/2 pathways can increase expression of multiple anti-apoptotic proteins, including BCL-XL, MCL-1, and c-FLIP isoforms, as well as the phosphorylation and inactivation of pro-apoptotic proteins including BAD, BIM, and pro-caspase 9 (Caro and Cederbaum 2006; Majumdar and Du 2006; Grethe and Porn-Ares 2006; Osaki et al. 2004). Radiation-induced ERK1/2 activation has also been linked to increased expression of the DNA repair proteins ERCC1, XRCC1, and XPC (Yacoub et al. 2003).

11.4.4
Novel Agents that Target Key Enzymes that Regulate the Transformed Phenotype and Play a Role in Maintaining Tumor Cell Survival

The initial portion of this chapter discussed how paracrine tumor cells which rely on EGFR for growth and survival can have their growth and radiosensitivity modulated by inhibitors of EGFR1–4. One prototypical example of treatment against cancer has been the development of the kinase inhibitor imatinib mesylate, the small-molecule inhibitor of the BCR-ABL kinase responsible for the development of CML (see above). In this disease, the Bcr/abl kinase is constitutively activated and signals downstream to diverse signaling/survival pathways (e.g., AKT, STAT5, BCL-XL) that collectively provide CML cells with a survival advantage over their normal counterparts. This success suggests that dysregulated kinases implicated in leukemogenesis may be associated with certain pro-apoptotic activities that can be unmasked by pharmacological inhibitors. The success of imatinib mesylate, and that of its successors (e.g., dasatinib), has prompted the development of numerous other agents targeting survival-signaling pathways for use in both hematological and non-hema-

tological malignancies. Similarly, in NSCLC expressing constitutively activated forms of EGFR1, treatment with EGFR1 inhibitors (Erlotinib, Gefitinib, Lapatinib, Canertinib) causes apoptosis of tumor cells and shrinkage of tumor in vivo.

11.5
Combination of Molecularly Targeted Agents with Conventional Therapies

Although a few of the agents are curative, many agents have low objective tumor response rate and short response duration. It is therefore logical to combine these new drugs with current standard therapies that have proven effectiveness, or combine two or more of these new drugs that may have synergistic effect against a specific cancer. Some of the combinations prove to be superior to the standard therapy. Examples of these combinations include: Avastin and chemotherapy for metastatic colorectal cancer; Erbitux and chemotherapy for colorectal cancer; Erbitux and radiation therapy for head and neck cancer (see specific disease section for details); and multiple agents against breast, renal, and various hematological malignancies.

Not all combinations produce better tumor response or survival, however. Combination of Iressa and Tarceva with cytotoxic chemotherapy failed to improved tumor response in NSCLC. In a phase-III trial testing the combination of Gefitinib and gemcitabine and cisplatin in advanced NSCLC (INTACT 1 trial), the addition of Gefitinib to chemotherapy did not improve tumor response and median survival over chemotherapy alone (Giaccone et al. 2004). A second phase-III trial comparing Gefitinib plus paclitaxel and carboplatin vs chemotherapy (INTACT 2 trial) again did not show improved tumor response rates, time to progression, and survival in newly diagnosed advanced lung cancers (Herbst et al. 2004). Similar failure was seen in combination of Erlotinib and chemotherapy in lung cancers (Gatzemeier et al. 2007).

11.5.1
Rationale for Combination Strategies Involving Molecularly Targeted Agents in Human Malignancies

While interest in the incorporation of molecularly targeted agents into the therapeutic armamentarium for human cancer expands, there is an emerging perception that with the exception of tumors with clearly defined molecular defects (e.g., dysregulated BCR/ABL), such agents may have relatively limited activity on their own. One logical approach to this problem is to combine such targeted agents with established chemotherapeutic drugs in order to lower the apoptotic threshold. Indeed, several preclinical studies have demonstrated enhanced tumor cell killing when various signal transduction inhibitors are combined with standard cytotoxic agents (Voigt et al. 2005; Choe et al. 2007; Shibuya et al. 2007; Baumann et al. 2007; Langer 2004); however, there is accumulating evidence that the combination of targeted agents may also be an extremely potent inhibitor of proliferation and inducer of death in malignant cells (Miller et al. 2007; Molhoek et al. 2005; Fleming et al. 2008; Sandler and Herbst 2006). One plausible explanation for increased cell killing is that neoplastic cells may mount a compensatory cytoprotective response when faced with an otherwise lethal insult, e.g., interruption of a key signaling or cell cycle regulatory pathway; thus, by interfering with activation of this secondary, compensatory pathway, one can theoretically render neoplastic cells helpless against the initial insult. An alternative possibility is just as neoplastic cells are primed to undergo apoptosis under certain circumstances, specific constellations of signaling and cell cycle events are recognized as harmful to the cell, and as a result, the apoptotic program is engaged. Whether either of these explanations can be validated, the fact remains that combining two of the targeted agents described above has been proven highly effective in triggering apoptosis in human tumor cells; thus, the possibility exists that anti-tumor strategies simultaneously targeting two or more cell cycle and signaling pathways may eventually have a role in the treatment of cancer. What follows below is a brief summary of some of the preclinical data supporting this approach, and examples of cases in which these strategies have entered the clinical arena. Because the number of targeted agents is growing logarithmically, the number of possible combination regimens is virtually limitless. Consequently, the following discussion is not meant to be an exhaustive summary of all possible therapeutic strategies; instead, its goal is to highlight some of the more promising avenues of investigation, with an emphasis on novel therapeutic approaches that might have clinical relevance.

11.5.2
Combination Strategies

To improve treatment outcome, the combination of agents should generate synergistic or additive effects on tumor cell killing. Synergistic effects could most likely be achieved by targeting multiple signal transduction pathways simultaneously that are potentially important for tumor cell growth and survival. Additive effect may be achieved by targeting the same target or same pathway by multiple agents as well as targeting multiple pathways.

11.5.2.1
Simultaneously Targeting Multiple Pathways

In many cancers, especially solid tumors, alternative pathway may confer the function of growth stimulation or survival signal when one pathway is inhibited. Similarly, tumors need multiple pathways to grow and progress. For example, a tumor needs both growth potential and environmental support, such as new vessel formation for blood supply. The combination of two agents to block growth signal and angiogenesis would significantly increase tumor inhibition and cell killing. The majority of the receptor kinases initiate multiple cascades downstream, leading to activation of proliferation as well as survival mechanisms. Simultaneously suppressing these cascades will enhance cell killing. Many clinical trials are investigating various combinations for improvement of treatment outcome. For example, Erbitux is combined with Avastin and chemotherapy for colorectal cancer (Tol et al. 2008; Tabernero 2007). A number of trials combine Erbitux or Avastin with small-molecule TKIs for the treatment of lung cancers, renal cancer, colorectal cancer, and various hematological malignancies (www.clinicaltrials.gov).

11.5.2.2
Combination of Targeted Agents Against Single Target

A treatment target may change due to mutation or it may exist in multiple variants. These mutations or variants render tumor resistance to single targeted agent therapy. Examples of this mutation are in Bcr-Abl and c-kit oncogenes that cause resistance to imatinib; however, cells with this mutation are sensitive to newer agents (such as dasatinib) that are approved for the treatment of imatinib-resistant leukemia. Clinical trials also demonstrated benefits of using multi-agents against a single target in solid tumors. For example, in breast cancer overexpressing Her-2, multiple agents against Her-2 protein is found to be more effective. The so-called total Her-2 blockage with lapatinib and Herceptin in a phase-III clinical trial in the patients who were heavily pretreated and progressed while on Herceptin showed significantly improved progression-free survival (reported at the ASCO Annual Meeting, 2008).

11.5.3
Future Candidate Combinations

11.5.3.1
Simultaneous CHK1 and MEK1/2 Inhibition

UCN-01 (7-hydroxystaurosporine) is currently being evaluated as an anti-neoplastic agent in clinical trials, both alone and in combination with chemotherapeutic agents and ionizing radiation (AKINAGA et al. 2000). UCN-01 exerts anti-proliferative activity both in vitro and in vivo, an action which initially was thought to be related to inhibition of protein kinase C (PKC) isoforms (TAKAHASHI et al. 1989). Based on the fact that many PKC isoforms have been linked to cytoprotective signaling within cells, the ability of UCN-01 to block signaling by this family of kinases and to cause cell death appears, on the surface, to be a reasonable hypothetical mode of action for this drug. More recently, UCN-01 has also been shown to inhibit the downstream effector of PI3 kinase, PDK-1, in the same concentration range as PKC isoforms (SATO et al. 2002); however, as a single agent, UCN-01 toxicity, evident in tumor cells over the range 150–500 nM, is an order of magnitude above the in-vitro IC50 of the drug for PKC isoforms and PDK-1. At lower clinically relevant concentrations (<100 nM), UCN-01 as a single agent is marginally toxic but enhances the lethality of established chemotherapeutic agents by several postulated mechanisms, in particular by inhibition of CHK1 (GRAVES et al. 2000). Inhibition of CHK1 may directly promote activation of the protein phosphatase CDC25C and can also interfere with CDC25C elimination by blocking its binding to 14-3-3 proteins and subsequent degradation. Down-regulation of CDC25C function results in enhanced phosphorylation and inactivation of cyclin-dependent kinases (CDKs), such as p34CDC2, which are critically involved in G2/M cell cycle arrest following DNA damage (KASTAN 2001); thus, UCN-01 can function as a checkpoint abrogator capable of enhancing the lethal actions of DNA-damaging agents, including ionizing radiation (CARTEE et al. 2002), cisplatin (BUNCH and EASTMAN 1996), Ara-C (TANG et al. 2000), and campothecins (SHAO et al. 1997). It has been argued that UCN-01, administered at pharmacologically achievable concentrations, promotes sensitization to cell killing via CHK1 inhibition and CDK dephosphorylation rather than by inhibition of PKC family enzymes and the PI3 kinase effector PDK-1.

Multiple intracellular signal transduction pathways, e.g., RAS/RAF-1/ERK1/2, RAS/IKK/NFκB, and RAS/PI3K/PDK-1/AKT/p70S6 kinase, are often highly activated in tumor cells, frequently due to alterations in proto-oncogene function, and have been proposed by many laboratories as therapeutic targets in preventing cancer cell growth in a wide variety of malignancies. Furthermore, inhibition of chemotherapeutic drug and radiation-induced growth factor receptor or signaling pathway activation by novel inhibitors of kinase domains has been shown by many groups to enhance the toxicity of established chemotherapy/radiation modalities, e.g., use of EGFR1 and EGFR2 inhibitors. An alternative approach, however, to killing tumor cells without using established cytotoxic therapies is to exploit tumor cell reliance (i.e., addiction) to high levels of signaling pathway activity within multiple pathways to maintain their growth and viability.

Several years ago, it was shown under in-vitro conditions, that UCN-01 at clinically relevant concentrations causes activation of the ERK1/2 pathway in multiple transformed cell types (DAI et al. 2001, 2002; MCKINSTRY et al. 2002). Prevention of ERK1/2 pathway activation, by blockade of MEK1/2 signaling by use of small-molecule kinase inhibitors or of RAS function by use of farnesyltransferase inhibitors (FTIs), rapidly promoted UCN-01-induced tumor cell death in a synergistic fashion (DAI et al. 2004b, 2005a). Non-transformed cells from multiple tissue types were noted in several studies to be insensitive to apoptosis-induction by this strategy. More recent work has translated these in-vitro findings into a xenograft animal model system using estrogen-dependent (MCF7) and independent human mammary carcinoma (MDA-MB-231) cell lines. In both MDA-MB-231 and MCF7 cells a transient 2-day in-vivo exposure of established tumors to a MEK1/2 inhibitor and UCN-01 resulted in profound induction of tumor cell death in animals receiving combined drug exposure, and tumor control ratios for both cell lines of 0.36, 30 days after drug administration. Irradiation of mammary tumors after MEK1/2 inhibitor and UCN-01 exposure caused a profound increase in tumor radiosensitivity.

The primary mechanism of lethality for MEK1/2 inhibitor/FTI and UCN-01 treatment was similar in both hematological and solid tumor cell types: MEK1/2 inhibitor/FTI and UCN-01 treatment caused activation of JNK1/2 signaling and an activating conformational change in the pro-apoptotic protein BAX, resulting in mitochondrial dysfunction leading, collectively, to activation of the intrinsic apoptosis pathway. In carcinoma cells, caspase 8 appeared to play a facilitating role in the amplification of mitochondrial dysfunction (McKinstry et al. 2002). Constitutive overexpression of mitochondrial protective proteins, such as BCL-2 and BCL-XL, suppressed cell death after MEK1/2 inhibitor/FTI and UCN-01 treatment, a protective effect which could be overcome when cells were simultaneously exposed to the novel clinically relevant death receptor agonist/extrinsic apoptosis pathway activator TRAIL (Dai et al. 2003c). In multiple myeloma cells MEK1/2 inhibitor/FTI and UCN-01-mediated lethality was not attenuated by conventional resistance mechanisms to cytotoxic drugs (e.g., melphalan or dexamethasone), addition of exogenous interleukin-6 or insulin-like growth factor I, or the presence of stromal cells. Furthermore, in multiple myeloma cells under conditions of MEK1/2 inhibitor and UCN-01-induced lethality IL-6 was still capable of promoting AKT activation, arguing that growth factor-induced PDK-1 activation was not compromised by concentrations of UCN-01 that can promote MEK1/2 lethality (Dai et al. 2002).

Other downstream cytoprotective components of RAS have also been investigated for a cytotoxic interaction with UCN-01. In multiple myeloma cells, the output from MEK1/2 is believed to be one upstream activating signal for the protective transcription factor NFκB. In agreement with this concept, inhibitors of NFκB function also interact with UCN-01 to promote myeloma cell death via activation of the intrinsic apoptosis pathway, which is not further enhanced by co-administration of MEK1/2 inhibitors in agreement with ERK1/2 being an upstream activation of NFκB in MM cells. The semi-synthetic antibiotic based on geldanamycin, 17AAG, also has been observed to interact with UCN-01 to promote leukemia cell death (Jia et al. 2003). As 17AAG inhibits HSP90 function, it is probable that 17AAG-induced down-regulation of Raf-1 and AKT expression and phosphorylation plays a major role in the death-inducing process when combined with UCN-01. It is also noteworthy, based on studies showing ectopic expression of BCL-2 protecting cells from MEK1/2 inhibitor and UCN-01-induced lethality, that 17AAG and UCN-01 also act to suppress expression of mitochondrial protective proteins such as BCL-2 and MCL-1. As noted previously, UCN-01 was initially characterized from a therapeutic standpoint as a PKC inhibitor; however, in leukemia cells it was discovered that co-exposure of human leukemia cells to 17AAG and the "specific" PKC inhibitor bisindolylmaleimide (GFX) did not result in enhanced lethality, arguing against the possibility that the PKC inhibitory actions of UCN-01 are responsible for synergistic cell-killing interactions.

Downstream of RAS, the PI3 kinase and MEK1/2 signaling pathways converge to promote activation of p70 S6 kinase. The activity of p70 S6 kinase is important for the regulation of translation, and this kinase is coordinately regulated by PI3 kinase signaling via PDK-1, AKT, and mTOR. ERK1/2 phosphorylation of p70 S6 kinase releases auto-inhibitory domain repression permitting full activation of the kinase. The mTOR inhibitor rapamycin has been frequently used to block p70 S6 kinase activation and rapamycin has been shown to interact with UCN-01 to promote cell death in leukemia cells (Hahn et al. 2005). In a manner similar to that of 17AAG and UCN-01, combined rapamycin and UCN-01 treatment suppressed expression of anti-apoptotic mitochondrial proteins such as BCL-2. Furthermore, in contrast to MEK1/2 inhibitor and UCN-01 treatment, rapamycin and UCN-01-induced mitochondrial dysfunction was a secondary, caspase-dependent event. Collectively, these findings suggest that 17AAG and rapamycin may represent small-molecule signaling inhibitors with greatest utility in promoting UCN-01 lethality, due to the fact that, regardless of whether tumor cells display low or elevated expression levels of mitochondrial protective proteins, significant killing will occur secondary to suppression of protective protein expression and activation of pro-apoptotic BH3 protein function.

Finally, it is noted that the overall concept that blocking compensatory survival pathway activation responses leads to leukemic cell killing has been extended by several groups using a variety of small-molecule inhibitors of kinases and other enzymes, including, for example, flavopiridol and PI3 kinase inhibitors, flavopiridol and histone deacetylase inhibitors, histone deacetylase inhibitors and perifosine, MEK1/2 inhibitors, and imatinib mesylate.

11.5.3.2
Histone Deacetylase Inhibitor Combinations

As noted previously, HDAC inhibitors exert multiple actions, and potentially kill cells through disparate mechanisms. It is therefore hardly surprising that HDACIs interact synergistically with a variety of other signal transduction and cell cycle modulators. For example, flavopiridol is a cell cycle inhibitor, and can arrest cells in the G1 phase of the cell cycle (Han et al. 2000). Because differentiation induction in any cell type, including that triggered by HDAC inhibitors (Dai et al. 2003a), requires G1 arrest, it seems reasonable to speculate that flavopiridol might enhance the differentiation-inducing ability of HDAC inhibitors; however, contrary to expectations, flavopiridol did not enhance differentiation induction by the HDACI vorinostat; instead, it blocked differentiation and dramatically enhanced apoptosis (ALMENARA et al. 2002). This phenomenon stems from several flavopiridol-mediated actions, including inhibition of DNA polymerase-II phosphorylation and resulting down-regulation of p21$^{CIP1/WAF1}$ (ROSATO et al. 2001) as well as inhibition of NF-κB (GAO et al. 2004). Clinical trials evaluating the in-vivo activity of this regimen in patients with leukemia and solid malignancies will begin shortly. Recent studies have focused on the capacity of HDAC inhibitors to disrupt, through inhibition of HDAC6, the function of HSP90 (RUEFLI et al. 2001; INSINGA et al. 2005). Perhaps not surprisingly, several groups have reported that HDAC inhibitors, such as vorinostat and LAQ824, interact synergistically with HSP90 antagonists such as 17AAG in human tumor cells (GEORGE et al. 2005; RAHMANI et al. 2003b). In the case of BCR/ABL+ leukemias, this phenomenon was associated with diminished association of BCR/ABL with HSP90 and enhanced proteasomal degradation (RAHMANI et al. 2003b). In view of evidence that mutant activated kinase proteins are claimed to be particularly susceptible to interference / down-regulation by use of agents that interfere with protein folding (GORRE et al. 2002), this strategy may also be effective in tumor cell types associated with specific mutant proteins, e.g., FLT3 (GEORGE et al. 2005), B-Raf, and activated EGFR1 proteins.

The lethal effects of HDACIs can also be influenced by inhibitors of various signal transduction pathways. For example, the PI3K/AKT pathway protects cells from apoptosis through multiple mechanisms, including phosphorylation/inactivation of BAD and inhibition of caspase-9, among other actions (DATTA et al. 1999). Inhibition of PI3K, and by extension, AKT, by the kinase inhibitor LY294002 has been shown to enhance the lethal effects of HDACIs in malignant cells (RAHMANI et al. 2003a). More recently, the alkylysophospholipid perifosine, which is currently undergoing clinical evaluation, has been reported to disrupt this pathway by interfering with the membrane association of AKT (KONDAPAKA et al. 2003). In human leukemia cells, including those of lymphoid origin, perifosine interacts synergistically with HDACIs such as vorinostat and sodium butyrate in association with generation of the pro-apoptotic lipid second messenger ceramide (RAHMANI et al. 2003b). Together, these findings suggest that a regimen combining perifosine and HDACIs, such as vorinostat, warrants investigation as an antitumor strategy.

Among their other lethal actions, HDACIs trigger cell death, at least in part, through induction of oxidative damage (e.g., generation of ROS). This capacity may also account for, or contribute to, their therapeutic selectivity. For example, it has recently been shown that HDACIs selectively induce the antioxidant enzyme thioredoxin in normal compared with transformed cells, resulting in preferential oxidative injury in the latter (UNGERSTEDT et al. 2005). Such findings raise the possibility that HDACIs might selectively enhance the lethality of other agents acting via production of ROS. A logical candidate agent for such a therapeutic strategy is the estrogen derivative 2-methoxyestradiol (2-ME). In human leukemia cells, 2-ME selectively induces oxidative injury by inhibiting the activity of the important antioxidant enzyme superoxide dismutase (SOD; HUANG et al. 2000). Notably, this process appears to occur preferentially in neoplastic cells (HUANG et al. 2000) and involves down-regulation of the AKT pathway (GAO et al. 2006). Given the putatively selective induction of oxidative injury by both HDACIs and 2-ME, the possibility arises that combining these agents might result in further potentiation of anti-tumor cell activity and selectivity. In fact, results of a recent study indicate that simultaneous exposure of human tumor cells to sub-toxic concentrations of 2-ME and HDACIs (e.g., vorinostat and sodium butyrate) resulted in a dramatic increase in lethality in association with a pronounced increase in ROS levels (GAO et al. 2006). As observed in the case of 2-ME alone, combined exposure of cells to 2-ME and HDACIs resulted in the marked inactivation of AKT accompanied by activation of the stress-related JNK pathway. Together, these findings support the concept that combining HDACIs with agents that induce oxidative injury may be an effective and potentially selective therapeutic strategy in cancer.

11.5.3.3
Proteasome and Other Inhibitors of the NFκB Pathway

The 26S proteasome represents the major non-lysosomal mechanism by which unwanted proteins are degraded (CIECHANOVER 2005). Following ubiquination by various ubiquitin ligases, such proteins are channeled into the 20S catalytic core of the proteasome, where they are degraded via multiple activities, e.g., chymotryptic. Proteasome function plays a critical role in regulation of diverse proteins involved in signal transduction, cell cycle, and survival regulation (ADAMS 2004). Because proteasomes are so ubiquitous, it seemed unlikely that proteasome inhibition represented a viable therapeutic strategy. Nevertheless, multiple preclinical studies have demonstrated that proteasome inhibitors effectively kill transformed cells, and that such actions may selectively spare normal tissues. This work has culminated in the development of Velcade, a highly potent proteasome inhibitor which has shown impressive activity in patients with multiple myeloma, including those who are resistant to standard therapy (O'Connor et al. 2005). The mechanism by which Velcade and other proteasome inhibitors kill neoplastic cells is not known with certainty, but attention has largely been focused on the NFκB pathway. Interference with proteasome function leads to accumulation of members of the IκB family, particularly IκBα, which bind to NFκB, thereby opposing nuclear translocation and transcriptional activity. This, in turn, results in down-regulation of diverse anti-apoptotic genes, including BCL-XL and XIAP, among others. Interference with proteasome function can also promote apoptosis via up-regulation of pro-apoptotic proteins, including p53 and BAX (Insinga et al. 2005; Almond and Cohen 2002).

There is evidence to suggest that interference with proteasome function can potently enhance HDACI lethality in various neoplastic cell types. For example, combined proteasome and HDAC inhibition was initially shown to promote apoptosis in retinoblastoma cells (Giuliano et al. 1999), and subsequent studies demonstrated similar interactions in human leukemia and myeloma cells (Yu et al. 2003a; Pei et al. 2004a). In this context, it is unlikely to be coincidental that both proteasome (Yu et al. 2004) and HDAC inhibitors have been shown to kill cells through induction of reactive oxygen species. In fact, co-treatment of leukemic cells with Velcade and HDAC inhibitors (e.g., vorinostat) was associated with a marked increase in oxidative damage, and conversely, attenuated by addition of free radical scavengers (Pei et al. 2004a).

Aside from this possibility, other possible mechanisms exist which might account for synergistic interactions between HDAC and proteasome inhibitors, particularly those related to perturbations in NFκB. For example, HDACIs are known to induce acetylation of diverse proteins in addition to histones, including p53, HSP90, and NFκB, among others. It has also been shown that acetylation of NFκB, or more specifically p65, leads to activation of NFκB via multiple mechanisms, including increased nuclear transport and diminished binding to IκBα, among others (Chen and Greene 2003). Activation of NFκB by HDACIs may lead to induction of certain antioxidant enzymes, particularly Mn-SOD, which could attenuate HDACI-mediated oxidative injury; thus, interruption of the NFκB pathway may prevent certain HDACI-mediated actions which limit the lethality of this class of compounds, thereby lowering the threshold for apoptosis. Based on these concepts,

regimens combining clinically relevant HDACIs and proteasome inhibitors, such as Velcade, warrant consideration in anti-cancer therapy.

These findings may theoretically be extended to include other classes of agents that interrupt the NF-κB pathway. For example, degradation of IκBα generally involves phosphorylation by members of the IKK family, particularly IKKβ (Chen and Greene 2004), which promotes ubiquitination and subsequent proteasomal degradation. Recently, a series of IKK inhibitors have been developed which have the net effect of blocking IκBα phosphorylation, thereby sparing it from proteasomal destruction, and allowing it to sequester NF-κB in the cytosol (Tergaonkar et al. 2003). This has the net effect of antagonizing activation of NFκB-responsive genes, including those exerting anti-apoptotic functions. Although IKK inhibitors are currently the focus of interest in view of their potential anti-inflammatory actions, the possibility exists that these agents may display anti-neoplastic activities as well, and may also promote the lethality of other targeted agents. For example, as noted above, blockade of proteasomal degradation of IκBα may contribute to synergistic interactions between HDAC inhibitors and proteasome inhibitors such as Velcade. Analogously, interference with IKK phosphorylation (e.g., by IKK inhibitors), rather than proteasomal degradation of IκBα, may exert the same net effect on HDACI-induced apoptosis. In fact, results of a recent study demonstrated that inhibition of IKK by the IKK inhibitor Bay 11-7082 markedly enhanced the lethal effects of the second-generation HDACIs MS275 and vorinostat in tumor cells in association with diminished acetylation of RelA, reduced DNA binding, and interference with RelA/IκBα association (Dai et al. 2005b). These events were also associated with enhanced oxidative damage (e.g., ROS generation) and diminished expression of the antioxidant enzyme Mn-SOD, an NFκB target, as well as down-regulation of XIAP and activation of JNK (Dai et al. 2005b). Based on these considerations, it is tempting to speculate that HDACIs exert certain intrinsic pro-apoptotic actions e.g., induction of mitochondrial injury and generation of ROS (Insinga et al. 2005; Almond and Cohen 2002); however, their capacity to acetylate NFκB, and in so doing, to activate anti-apoptotic genes (e.g., Mn-SOD, XIAP), may oppose these events. By blocking the latter actions, either by inhibiting proteasomal degradation of IκBα (e.g., by proteasome inhibitors), or by preventing its phosphorylation (e.g., by IKK inhibitors), the pro-apoptotic actions of HDACIs may be left unopposed; thus, a therapeutic strategy combining proteasome or IKK inhibitors with HDACIs warrants consideration in the treatment of cancer.

11.5.3.4
Proteasome
and CDK Inhibition

There is now evidence to suggest that combined pro-teasome and CDK inhibition may represent a rational strategy in the treatment of cancer. As noted previously, CDK inhibitors, such as flavopiridol and R-roscovitine (CYC202), have recently entered the clinical arena. Although it is logical to postulate that the lethal effects of these agents stem from inhibition of CDKs and result-ing disruption of the cell cycle traverse, it has become apparent that these agents exert pleiotropic actions which may be responsible for, or contribute to, their anti-tumor activities. For example, as discussed pre-viously, both flavopiridol and roscovitine inhibit the cyclin T/CDK9 transcriptional regulatory apparatus, and thus down-regulate a number of short-lived anti-apoptotic proteins including XIAP and MCL-1 (WHIT-TAKER et al. 2004). More recently, it has been shown that flavopiridol is also a potent inhibitor of IKK, and as a consequence, may function as an NFκB antagonist. For example, TAKADA and colleagues (2005) demon-strated that flavopiridol potently inhibited NFκB DNA binding in cells exposed to TNFα. Based on these find-ings, it seems reasonable to postulate that further dis-ruption of the NFκB pathway might lower the thresh-old for flavopiridol-mediated lethality. In fact, results of a recent study have shown that co-administration of flavopiridol with proteasome inhibitors in tumor cells resulted in a dramatic increase in mitochondrial dam-age and apoptosis in association with activation of the stress-related JNK pathway, and down-regulation of the anti-apoptotic proteins XIAP and MCL-1 (DAI et al. 2003b). Significantly, co-administration of flavopiridol and proteasome inhibitors resulted in a pronounced reduction in NFκB DNA binding, consistent with the notion that these agents cooperate to block IKK phos-phorylation (flavopiridol) as well as proteasomal degra-dation (proteasome inhibitors). These findings were not restricted to flavopiridol in that synergistic anti-tumor interactions between proteasome inhibitors and rosco-vitine were also observed. Subsequently, a strategy com-bining flavopiridol with Velcade was shown to be highly effective in inducing apoptosis in BCR/ABL+ leukemia cells, including several lines highly resistant to imatinib mesylate (DAI et al. 2004a). Based in part upon these findings, a phase-I trial of Velcade and flavopiridol has recently been launched in patients with refractory/progressive B-cell malignancies including multiple my-eloma, indolent non-Hodgkin's lymphoma, and mantle cell lymphoma.

11.5.3.5
MAP2K (MEK1/2) Inhibitor Combinations

As noted previously, it has been established that the net output of stress (e.g., JNK) vs survival (e.g., MEK1/2-ERK1/2)-related pathways can determine whether a cell lives or dies (XIA et al. 1995). Although the mechanism(s) by which the MEK1/2-ERK1/2 path-way promotes survival is not known with certainty, it is known that JNK may be directly involved in the induc-tion of mitochondrial injury (TOURNIER et al. 2000), and that induction of ERK1/2 can oppose the action of certain pro-apoptotic proteins (e.g., capase-9, BIM, BAD) (ALLAN et al. 2003; GISE et al. 2001). These con-siderations served as the basis for the development of pharmacological MEK1/2 inhibitors, such as PD184352 (CI-1040), which have shown activity in preclinical animal models and have also been shown to be biologi-cally active in humans (RINEHART et al. 2004). In pre-clinical systems, MEK1/2 inhibitors have been shown to potentiate the lethality of a variety of cytotoxic agents, including taxanes, ara-C, and novel agents such as UCN-01; however, a growing body of evidence sug-gests that MEK1/2 inhibition can lower the threshold for cell death for a variety of other targeted agents, and that such synergistic interactions are, if anything, more impressive than those seen with established cytotoxic agents.

Several lines of evidence suggest that the lethal ac-tions of proteasome inhibitors are critically dependent upon the status of the MEK/ERK pathway. For example, proteasome inhibitor (i.e., Velcade) lethality has been associated with the reciprocal induction of JNK and the inactivation of MEK/ERK (PEI et al. 2004b). Further-more, in another study, both pharmacological and ge-netic approaches revealed that interruption of MEK1/2-ERK1/2 lowered the threshold of transformed cells to proteasome inhibitor-mediated cell death (ORLOWSKI et al. 2002). In this context, it may be relevant that Vel-cade lethality has been related to ROS generation (PEI et al. 2004b), and that the MEK1/2-ERK1/2 pathway rep-resents an important cellular defense to oxidative stress (CHU et al. 2004). Whatever the mechanism underlying proteasome/MEK1/2 inhibitor synergism, such find-ings raise the possibility that regimens combining Vel-cade with clinically relevant MEK1/2 inhibitors warrant scrutiny as a cancer therapeutic.

MEK1/2 inhibition also has the potential to lower the threshold for other targeted agents, including those directed against leukemia. For example, the MEK1/2-ERK1/2 pathway is known to be activated by the BCR/ABL kinase, and may be perturbed by BCR/ABL kinase inhibitors such as imatinib mesylate (ORLOWSKI et al. 2002). Interestingly, some BCR/ABL+ cells can respond to imatinib mesylate with an increase in ERK1/2 activation (CHU et al. 2004) which may represent a compensatory response to the initial insult. Consequently, it is not surprising that MEK1/2 inhibitors, such as PD184352, have been shown to interact synergistically with imatinib mesylate in BCR/ABL+ leukemia cells (YU et al. 2003b). This phenomenon was associated with down-regulation of phospho-ERK1/2, CREB, MCL-1, and BCL-XL, and activation of JNK and p38MAPK. Notably, synergism was observed in some leukemia cells resistant to imatinib mesylate. Such findings raise the possibility that co-administration of imatinib mesylate (or other BCR/ABL kinase inhibitors) with pharmacologically relevant MEK1/2 inhibitors might play a useful role in BCR/ABL+ hematological malignancies, including Ph+ ALL.

Lastly, it has been observed that the lethal effects of HDAC inhibitors toward human tumor cells are reciprocally related to the induction of stress-related kinases (e.g., JNK) and the down-regulation of survival-signaling pathways (e.g., MEK1/2-ERK1/2). Consequently, the concept of combining HDAC with MEK1/2 inhibitors has a logical basis. In fact, it has recently been shown that co-administration of the HDAC inhibitor vorinostat with MEK1/2 inhibitors, such as PD184352 and U0126, leads to a dramatic increase in mitochondrial injury and apoptosis in BCR/ABL+ human leukemia cells, including those resistant to imatinib mesylate (YU et al. 2005). Notably, these events were related to enhanced oxidative damage (i.e., ROS generation) and increased levels of the pro-apoptotic lipid second-messenger ceramide. Given evidence that HDAC inhibitors kill cells through a free radical-dependent mechanism, and that the MEK1/2-ERK1/2 pathway represents a major cellular defense of cells to oxidative stress, it is tempting to speculate that HDAC and MEK1/2 inhibitors cooperate to promote apoptosis in BCR/ABL+ leukemia cells through an oxidative damage-related mechanism.

11.5.3.6
Combination Regimens Involving Modulators of the Apoptotic Pathway

There has been considerable interest in the development of agents capable of modulating the apoptotic pathway. Such agents generally fall into two major categories: (a) those that antagonize the actions of anti-apoptotic proteins; and (b) those that mimic the action of pro-apoptotic proteins. The former group includes small-molecule inhibitors of BCL-2, BCL-XL, and XIAP, such as HA14-1, ABT-737, Obatoclax, and XIAP-antagonist peptides. The latter group includes mimetics of Smac (SUN et al. 2004) and death receptor agonists such as TRAIL (WANG and EL-DEIRY 2003).

Several preclinical studies have documented synergistic interactions between small-molecule BCL-2 antagonists and signal transduction modulators in various cell types, including those of leukemic origin. For example, synergistic interactions between the BCL-2 antagonist HA14-1, which disrupts the ability of BCL-2 to block mitochondrial injury (e.g., cytochrome c release), and the CDK inhibitor flavopiridol, have been reported in myeloma cells (PEI et al. 2004b). This phenomenon was associated with MCL-1 down-regulation and activation of the stress-related JNK kinase. Analogously, synergistic induction of mitochondrial injury and apoptosis were reported in myeloma cells exposed to HA14-1 and the proteasome inhibitor Velcade, although in contrast to results with flavopiridol, enhanced lethality was only observed when the proteasome inhibitor preceded HA14-1 (PEI et al. 2003). Under these circumstances, a marked increase in oxidative damage (ROS generation) was noted, and the lethal effects of this combination were antagonized by the antioxidant N-acetylcysteine. Collectively, these findings suggest that combined exposure to these agents kills cells by promoting oxidative injury, a concept consistent with the documented ability of BCL-2 and related proteins to act as an antioxidant (GOTTLIEB et al. 2000), and proteasome inhibitors to kill cells in association with free radical generation (LING et al. 2003).

Small-molecule BCL-2 inhibitors can also promote the lethal effects of survival signal transduction inhibitors. For example, in tumor cells, combined exposure to HA14-1 and the MEK1/2 inhibitor PD184352 resulted in a dramatic increase in lethality (MILELLA et al. 2001). Such findings are consistent with evidence that interruption of the MEK1/2 pathway acts, at least in part, by modifying caspase activity as well as the activity of certain pro-apoptotic proteins (e.g., BIM and BAD). They also raise the possibility that as small-molecule BCL-2 inhibitors are developed, combination strategies involving, in addition to standard chemotherapeutic compounds, novel signaling agents warrant attention as cancer therapeutics.

Synergistic anti-tumor interactions between signaling/cell cycle inhibitors and TRAIL have also been reported. Upon binding to its cognate receptor, TRAIL activates, through the FADD (Fas-associated death domain)-related component of death receptors, procaspase-8, which in turn cleaves and activates Bid, a potent inducer of mitochondrial injury and cytochrome C release (Li et al. 1998; THORBURN 2004). A theoretical basis for the selectivity of TRAIL and related molecules is the fact that its actions are opposed by inactive decoy receptors, which are generally not expressed or expressed at very low levels in tumor cells; therefore, to the extent that signaling or cell cycle inhibitory agents selectively target transformed cells, combination regimens involving TRAIL offer the possibility of amplifying the extent of anti-tumor selectivity.

A strong rationale exists for combining HDACIs with TRAIL. For example, simultaneous activation of the intrinsic, mitochondrial pathway (i.e., by HDACIs) and the extrinsic, receptor-related pathway (i.e., by TRAIL) would logically be expected to result in amplification of activation of the apoptotic cascade. In fact, simultaneous administration of clinically relevant HDACIs (e.g., vorinostat) with TRAIL has been shown by several investigators to potently induce apoptosis in human leukemia cells (ROSATO et al. 2003; GUO et al. 2004). Furthermore, very recent studies have demonstrated that tumor cells can selectively respond to HDACIs with up-regulation of death receptors (e.g., DR4 and DR5), as well as CD95 and Fas-L (INSINGA et al. 2005); therefore, the up-regulation of death receptors by HDACIs would logically be expected to enhance the lethal effects of agents such as TRAIL, the lethality of which is dependent upon activation of such receptors.

Similar interactions have been observed with the CDK inhibitor flavopiridol. Initial studies demonstrated that flavopiridol interacted synergistically with TNF to induce apoptosis in lung cancer cells. Subsequently, it was shown that co-administration of TRAIL with flavopiridol resulted in a marked increase in mitochondrial damage and apoptosis in other tumor cell types (SENDEROWICZ 1999; ROSATO et al. 2004). Given evidence that flavopiridol acts at least in part to induce apoptosis in tumor cells via induction of mitochondrial injury, it seems plausible to propose that the potent tumoricidal effects of a regimen combining TRAIL with flavopiridol, as in the case of HDACIs, stems from simultaneous activation of the intrinsic and extrinsic apoptotic pathways.

11.6

Conclusion

The development of the novel targeted agents has introduced tremendous opportunities as well as challenges to clinicians. Although most agents for solid tumors show limited single-drug cure potential, they can prolong patient survival in selected tumor types, and most importantly enhance the existing therapies for a variety of cancers. The most notable success includes treatment of hematological malignancies, particularly CML, colorectal cancers, GIST, renal cancer, lung cancer, head and neck cancer, breast cancer, and liver cancer. Because these agents do not cause side effects similar to those of cytotoxic drugs and radiation therapy, their combination with current conventional chemotherapy and radiotherapy is usually feasible. They do cause a spectrum of toxicities, some of which can be life threatening, such as thromboembolic events, bleeding, perforation, and cardiotoxicities in the case of Avastin. How to best combine these new agents with radiation and chemotherapy requires intensive and persistent efforts from both clinicians and research scientists.

References

Adams J (2004) The proteasome: a suitable antineoplastic target. Nat Rev Cancer 4:349–360

Akinaga S, Sugiyama K, Akiyama T (2000) UCN-01 (7-hydroxystaurosporine) and other indolocarbazole compounds: A new generation of anti-cancer agents for the new century? Anticancer Drug Des 15:43–52

Allan LA, Morrice N, Brady S et al. (2003) Inhibition of caspase-9 through phosphorylation at Thr 125 by ERK MAPK. Nat Cell Biol 5:647–654

Almenara J, Rosato R, Grant S (2002) Synergistic induction of mitochondrial damage and apoptosis in human leukemia cells by flavopiridol and the histone deacetylase inhibitor suberoylanilide hydroxamic acid (SAHA). Leukemia 16:1331–1343

Almond JB, Cohen GM (2002) The proteasome: a novel target for cancer chemotherapy. Leukemia 16:433–443

An B, Goldfarb RH, Siman R et al. (1998) Novel dipeptidyl proteasome inhibitors overcome Bcl-2 protective function and selectively accumulate the cyclin-dependent kinase inhibitor p27 and induce apoptosis in transformed, but not normal, human fibroblasts. Cell Death Differ 5:1062–1075

Arguello F, Alexander M, Sterry JA et al. (1998) Flavopiridol induces apoptosis of normal lymphoid cells, causes immunosuppression, and has potent antitumor activity in vivo against human leukemia and lymphoma xenografts. Blood 91:2482–2490

Arora A, Scholar EM (2005) Role of tyrosine kinase inhibitors in cancer therapy. J Pharmacol Exp Ther 315:971–979

Astsaturov I, Cohen RB, Harari P (2006) Targeting epidermal growth factor receptor signaling in the treatment of head and neck cancer. Expert Rev Anticancer Ther 6:1179–1193

Balaban N, Moni J, Shannon M et al. (1996) The effect of ionizing radiation on signal transduction: antibodies to EGF receptor sensitize A431 cells to radiation. Biochim Biophys Acta 1314:147–156

Bali P, Pranpat M, Bradner J et al. (2005) Inhibition of histone deacetylase 6 acetylates and disrupts the chaperone function of heat shock protein 90: a novel basis for antileukemia activity of histone deacetylase inhibitors. J Biol Chem 280:26729–26734

Baselga J, Arteaga CL (2005) Critical update and emerging trends in epidermal growth factor receptor targeting in cancer. J Clin Oncol 23:2445–2459

Baumann M, Krause M, Dikomey E et al. (2007) EGFR-targeted anti-cancer drugs in radiotherapy: preclinical evaluation of mechanisms. Radiother Oncol 83:238–248

Bentzen SM, Atasoy BM, Daley FM et al. (2005) Epidermal growth factor receptor expression in pretreatment biopsies from head and neck squamous cell carcinoma as a predictive factor for a benefit from accelerated radiation therapy in a randomized controlled trial. J Clin Oncol 23:5560–5567

Bianco C, Tortora G, Bianco R et al. (2002) Enhancement of antitumor activity of ionizing radiation by combined treatment with the selective epidermal growth factor receptor-tyrosine kinase inhibitor ZD1839 (Iressa). Clin Cancer Res 8:3250–3258

Blanke CD, Rankin C, Demetri GD et al. (2008) Phase III randomized, intergroup trial assessing imatinib mesylate at two dose levels in patients with unresectable or metastatic gastrointestinal stromal tumors expressing the kit receptor tyrosine kinase: S0033. J Clin Oncol 26:626–632

Bonner JA, Harari PM, Giralt J et al. (2006) Radiotherapy plus cetuximab for squamous-cell carcinoma of the head and neck. N Engl J Med 354:567–578

Bowers G, Reardon D, Hewitt T et al. (2001) The relative role of ErbB1-4 receptor tyrosine kinases in radiation signal transduction responses of human carcinoma cells. Oncogene 20:1388–1397

Bunch RT, Eastman A (1996) Enhancement of cisplatin-induced cytotoxicity by 7-hydroxystaurosporine (UCN-01), a new G2-checkpoint inhibitor. Clin Cancer Res 2:791–797

Caro AA, Cederbaum AI (2006) Role of phosphatidylinositol 3-kinase/AKT as a survival pathway against CYP2E1-dependent toxicity. J Pharmacol Exp Ther 318:360–372

Caron RW, Yacoub A, Li M et al. (2005) Activated forms of H-RAS and K-RAS differentially regulate membrane association of PI3K, PDK-1, and AKT and the effect of therapeutic kinase inhibitors on cell survival. Mol Cancer Ther 4:257–270

Cartee L, Sankala H, Davis C et al. (2002) 7-hydroxystaurosporine (UCN-01) and ionizing radiation combine to inhibit the growth of Bcl-2-overexpressing U937 leukemia cells through a non-apoptotic mechanism. Int J Oncol 21:351–359

Champagne MA, Capdeville R, Krailo M et al. (2004) Imatinib mesylate (STI571) for treatment of children with Philadelphia chromosome-positive leukemia: results from a Children's Oncology Group phase 1 study. Blood 104:2655–2660

Chao SH, Price DH (2001) Flavopiridol inactivates P-TEFb and blocks most RNA polymerase II transcription in vivo. J Biol Chem 276:31793–31799

Chen LF, Greene WC (2003) Regulation of distinct biological activities of the NF-kappaB transcription factor complex by acetylation. J Mol Med 81:549–557

Chen LF, Greene WC (2004) Shaping the nuclear action of NF-kappaB. Nat Rev Mol Cell Biol 5:392–401

Chinnaiyan P, Huang S, Vallabhaneni G et al. (2005) Mechanisms of enhanced radiation response following epidermal growth factor receptor signaling inhibition by erlotinib (Tarceva). Cancer Res 65:3328–3335

Chinnaiyan P, Allen GW, Harari PM (2006) Radiation and new molecular agents, part II: targeting HDAC, HSP90, IGF-1R, PI3K, and Ras. Semin Radiat Oncol 16:59–64

Choe MS, Chen Z, Klass CM et al. (2007) Enhancement of docetaxel-induced cytotoxicity by blocking epidermal growth factor receptor and cyclooxygenase-2 pathways in squamous cell carcinoma of the head and neck. Clin Cancer Res 13:3015–3023

Chu S, Holtz M, Gupta M et al. (2004) BCR/ABL kinase inhibition by imatinib mesylate enhances MAP kinase activity in chronic myelogenous leukemia CD34+ cells. Blood 103:3167–3174

Ciechanover A (2005) Intracellular protein degradation: from a vague idea, through the lysosome and the ubiquitin-proteasome system, and onto human diseases and drug targeting (Nobel lecture). Angew Chem Int Ed Engl 44:5944–5967

Cohen MH, Williams GA, Sridhara R et al. (2004) United States Food and Drug Administration Drug Approval summary:Gefitinib (ZD1839; Iressa) tablets. Clin Cancer Res 10:1212–1218

Cortes J, Rousselot P, Kim DW et al. (2007) Dasatinib induces complete hematologic and cytogenetic responses in patients with imatinib-resistant or -intolerant chronic myeloid leukemia in blast crisis. Blood 109:3207–3213

Cunningham D, Humblet Y, Siena S et al. (2004) Cetuximab monotherapy and cetuximab plus irinotecan in irinotecan-refractory metastatic colorectal cancer. N Engl J Med 351:337–345

Dai Y, Yu C, Singh V et al. (2001) Pharmacological inhibitors of the mitogen-activated protein kinase (MAPK) kinase/MAPK cascade interact synergistically with UCN-01 to induce mitochondrial dysfunction and apoptosis in human leukemia cells. Cancer Res 61:5106–5115

Dai Y, Landowski TH, Rosen ST et al. (2002) Combined treatment with the checkpoint abrogator UCN-01 and MEK1/2 inhibitors potently induces apoptosis in drug-sensitive and -resistant myeloma cells through an IL-6-independent mechanism. Blood 100:3333–3343

Dai Y, Rahmani M, Grant S (2003a) An intact NF-kappaB pathway is required for histone deacetylase inhibitor-induced G1 arrest and maturation in U937 human myeloid leukemia cells. Cell Cycle 2:467–472

Dai Y, Rahmani M, Grant S (2003b) Proteasome inhibitors potentiate leukemic cell apoptosis induced by the cyclin-dependent kinase inhibitor flavopiridol through a SAPK/JNK- and NF-kappaB-dependent process. Oncogene 22:7108–7122

Dai Y, Dent P, Grant S (2003c) Tumor necrosis factor-related apoptosis-inducing ligand (TRAIL) promotes mitochondrial dysfunction and apoptosis induced by 7-hydroxystaurosporine and mitogen-activated protein kinase kinase inhibitors in human leukemia cells that ectopically express Bcl-2 and Bcl-xL. Mol Pharmacol 64:1402–1409

Dai Y, Rahmani M, Pei XY et al. (2004a) Bortezomib and flavopiridol interact synergistically to induce apoptosis in chronic myeloid leukemia cells resistant to imatinib mesylate through both Bcr/Abl-dependent and -independent mechanisms. Blood 104:509–518

Dai Y, Pei XY, Rahmani M et al. (2004b) Interruption of the NF-kappaB pathway by Bay 11-7082 promotes UCN-01-mediated mitochondrial dysfunction and apoptosis in human multiple myeloma cells. Blood 103:2761–2770

Dai Y, Rahmani M, Pei XY et al. (2005a) Farnesyltransferase inhibitors interact synergistically with the Chk1 inhibitor UCN-01 to induce apoptosis in human leukemia cells through interruption of both Akt and MEK/ERK pathways and activation of SEK1/JNK. Blood 105:1706–1716

Dai Y, Rahmani M, Dent P et al. (2005b) Blockade of histone deacetylase inhibitor-induced RelA/p65 acetylation and NF-kappaB activation potentiates apoptosis in leukemia cells through a process mediated by oxidative damage, XIAP downregulation, and c-Jun N-terminal kinase 1 activation. Mol Cell Biol 25:5429–5444

Dai Y, Chen S, Venditti CA et al. (2008) Vorinostat synergistically potentiates MK-0457 lethality in chronic myelogenous leukemia cells sensitive and resistant to imatinib mesylate. Blood 112:793–804

Dancey JE, Chen HX (2006) Strategies for optimizing combinations of molecularly targeted anticancer agents. Nat Rev Drug Discov 5:649–659

Dassonville O, Bozec A, Fischel JL et al. (2007) EGFR targeting therapies: monoclonal antibodies versus tyrosine kinase inhibitors. Similarities and differences. Crit Rev Oncol Hematol 62:53–61

Datta SR, Brunet A, Greenberg ME (1999) Cellular survival: a play in three Akts. Genes Dev 13:2905–2927

Dent P, Reardon DB, Park JS et al. (1999) Radiation-induced release of transforming growth factor alpha activates the epidermal growth factor receptor and mitogen-activated protein kinase pathway in carcinoma cells, leading to increased proliferation and protection from radiation-induced cell death. Mol Biol Cell 10:2493–2506

Druker BJ, Guilhot F, O'Brien SG et al. (2006) Five-year follow-up of patients receiving imatinib for chronic myeloid leukemia. N Engl J Med 355:2408–2417

Escudier B, Eisen T, Stadler WM et al. (2007a) Sorafenib in advanced clear-cell renal-cell carcinoma. N Engl J Med 356:125–134

Escudier B, Pluzanska A, Koralewski P et al. (2007b) Bevacizumab plus interferon alfa-2a for treatment of metastatic renal cell carcinoma: a randomised, double-blind phase III trial. Lancet 370:2103–2111

Fang L, Li G, Liu G et al. (2001) p53 induction of heparin-binding EGF-like growth factor counteracts p53 growth suppression through activation of MAPK and PI3K/Akt signaling cascades. Embo J 20:1931–1939

Fleming IN, Hogben M, Frame S et al. (2008) Synergistic inhibition of ErbB signaling by combined treatment with seliciclib and ErbB-targeting agents. Clin Cancer Res 14:4326–4335

Fukuoka M, Yano S, Giaccone G et al. (2003) Multi-institutional randomized phase II trial of gefitinib for previously treated patients with advanced non-small-cell lung cancer (The IDEAL 1 Trial) [corrected]. J Clin Oncol 21:2237–2246

Furukawa Y, Vu HA, Akutsu M et al. (2007) Divergent cytotoxic effects of PKC412 in combination with conventional antileukemic agents in FLT3 mutation-positive versus -negative leukemia cell lines. Leukemia 21:1005–1014

Gao N, Dai Y, Rahmani M et al. (2004) Contribution of disruption of the nuclear factor-kappaB pathway to induction of apoptosis in human leukemia cells by histone deacetylase inhibitors and flavopiridol. Mol Pharmacol 66:956–963

Gao N, Rahmani M, Shi X et al. (2006) Synergistic antileukemic interactions between 2-medroxyestradiol (2-ME) and histone deacetylase inhibitors involve Akt down-regulation and oxidative stress. Blood 107:241–249

Garcia-Manero G, Issa JP (2005) Histone deacetylase inhibitors: a review of their clinical status as antineoplastic agents. Cancer Invest 23:635–642

Gatzemeier U, Pluzanska A, Szczesna A et al. (2007) Phase III study of erlotinib in combination with cisplatin and gemcitabine in advanced non-small-cell lung cancer: the Tarceva Lung Cancer Investigation Trial. J Clin Oncol 25:1545–1552

George P, Bali P, Annavarapu S et al. (2005) Combination of the histone deacetylase inhibitor LBH589 and the hsp90 inhibitor 17-AAG is highly active against human CML-BC cells and AML cells with activating mutation of FLT-3. Blood 105:1768–1776

Gerber DE (2008) Targeted therapies: a new generation of cancer treatments. Am Fam Physician 77:311–319

Geyer CE, Forster J, Lindquist D et al. (2006) Lapatinib plus capecitabine for HER2-positive advanced breast cancer. N Engl J Med 355:2733–2743

Giaccone G, Herbst RS, Manegold C et al. (2004) Gefitinib in combination with gemcitabine and cisplatin in advanced non-small-cell lung cancer: a phase III trial – INTACT 1. J Clin Oncol 22:777–784

Giantonio BJ, Catalano PJ, Meropol NJ et al. (2007) Bevacizumab in combination with oxaliplatin, fluorouracil, and leucovorin (FOLFOX4) for previously treated metastatic colorectal cancer: results from the Eastern Cooperative Oncology Group Study E3200. J Clin Oncol 25:1539–1544

Gise A von, Lorenz P, Wellbrock C et al. (2001) Apoptosis suppression by Raf-1 and MEK1 requires MEK- and phosphatidylinositol 3-kinase-dependent signals. Mol Cell Biol 21:2324–2336

Giuliano M, Lauricella M, Calvaruso G et al. (1999) The apoptotic effects and synergistic interaction of sodium butyrate and MG132 in human retinoblastoma Y79 cells. Cancer Res 59:5586–5595

Gorre ME, Ellwood-Yen K, Chiosis G et al. (2002) BCR-ABL point mutants isolated from patients with imatinib mesylate-resistant chronic myeloid leukemia remain sensitive to inhibitors of the BCR-ABL chaperone heat shock protein 90. Blood 100:3041–3044

Gottlieb E, Vander Heiden MG, Thompson CB (2000) Bcl-x(L) prevents the initial decrease in mitochondrial membrane potential and subsequent reactive oxygen species production during tumor necrosis factor alpha-induced apoptosis. Mol Cell Biol 20:5680–5689

Graves PR, Yu L, Schwarz JK et al. (2000) The Chk1 protein kinase and the Cdc25C regulatory pathways are targets of the anticancer agent UCN-01. J Biol Chem 275:5600–5605

Grethe S, Porn-Ares MI (2006) p38 MAPK regulates phosphorylation of Bad via PP2A-dependent suppression of the MEK1/2-ERK1/2 survival pathway in TNF-alpha induced endothelial apoptosis. Cell Signal 18:531–540

Guilhot F, Apperley J, Kim DW et al. (2007) Dasatinib induces significant hematologic and cytogenetic responses in patients with imatinib-resistant or -intolerant chronic myeloid leukemia in accelerated phase. Blood 109:4143–4150

Guo F, Sigua C, Tao J et al. (2004) Cotreatment with histone deacetylase inhibitor LAQ824 enhances Apo-2L/tumor necrosis factor-related apoptosis inducing ligand-induced death inducing signaling complex activity and apoptosis of human acute leukemia cells. Cancer Res 64:2580–2589

Gupta AK, Bernhard EJ, Bakanauskas VJ et al. (2000) RAS-Mediated radiation resistance is not linked to MAP kinase activation in two bladder carcinoma cell lines. Radiat Res 154:64–72

Gupta AK, Bakanauskas VJ, Cerniglia GJ et al. (2001) The Ras radiation resistance pathway. Cancer Res 61:4278–4282

Hagan M, Yacoub A, Dent P (2004) Ionizing radiation causes a dose-dependent release of transforming growth factor alpha in vitro from irradiated xenografts and during palliative treatment of hormone-refractory prostate carcinoma. Clin Cancer Res 10:5724–5731

Hahn M, Li W, Yu C et al. (2005) Rapamycin and UCN-01 synergistically induce apoptosis in human leukemia cells through a process that is regulated by the Raf-1/MEK/ERK, Akt, and JNK signal transduction pathways. Mol Cancer Ther 4:457–470

Han JW, Ahn SH, Park SH et al. (2000) Apicidin, a histone deacetylase inhibitor, inhibits proliferation of tumor cells via induction of p21WAF1/Cip1 and gelsolin. Cancer Res 60:6068–6074

Harari PM (2007) Stepwise progress in epidermal growth factor receptor/radiation studies for head and neck cancer. Int J Radiat Oncol Biol Phys 69:S25–S27

Harari PM, Huang S (2006) Radiation combined with EGFR signal inhibitors: head and neck cancer focus. Semin Radiat Oncol 16:38–44

Heinrich MC, Corless CL, Demetri GD et al. (2003) Kinase mutations and imatinib response in patients with metastatic gastrointestinal stromal tumor. J Clin Oncol 21:4342–4349

Herbst RS, Giaccone G, Schiller JH et al. (2004) Gefitinib in combination with paclitaxel and carboplatin in advanced non-small-cell lung cancer: a phase III trial: INTACT 2. J Clin Oncol 22:785–794

Herbst RS, Prager D, Hermann R et al. (2005) TRIBUTE: a phase III trial of erlotinib hydrochloride (OSI-774) combined with carboplatin and paclitaxel chemotherapy in advanced non-small-cell lung cancer. J Clin Oncol 23:5892–5899

Hochhaus A, Kantarjian HM, Baccarani M et al. (2007) Dasatinib induces notable hematologic and cytogenetic responses in chronic-phase chronic myeloid leukemia after failure of imatinib therapy. Blood 109:2303–2309

Hostein I, Robertson D, DiStefano F et al. (2001) Inhibition of signal transduction by the Hsp90 inhibitor 17-allylamino-17-demethoxygeldanamycin results in cytostasis and apoptosis. Cancer Res 61:4003–4009

Huang SM, Harari PM (2000) Modulation of radiation response after epidermal growth factor receptor blockade in squamous cell carcinomas: inhibition of damage repair, cell cycle kinetics, and tumor angiogenesis. Clin Cancer Res 6:2166–2174

Huang P, Feng L, Oldham EA et al. (2000) Superoxide dismutase as a target for the selective killing of cancer cells. Nature 407:390–395

Hudes G, Carducci M, Tomczak P et al. (2007) Temsirolimus, interferon alfa, or both for advanced renal-cell carcinoma. N Engl J Med 356:2271–2281

Hurwitz H, Fehrenbacher L, Novotny W et al. (2004) Bevacizumab plus irinotecan, fluorouracil, and leucovorin for metastatic colorectal cancer. N Engl J Med 350:2335–2342

Hutcheson IR, Knowlden JM, Jones HE et al. (2006) Inductive mechanisms limiting response to anti-epidermal growth factor receptor therapy. Endocr Relat Cancer 13 (Suppl 1):S89–S97

Ihle NT, Paine-Murrieta G, Berggren MI et al. (2005) The phosphatidylinositol-3-kinase inhibitor PX-866 overcomes resistance to the epidermal growth factor receptor inhibitor gefitinib in A-549 human non-small cell lung cancer xenografts. Mol Cancer Ther 4:1349–1357

Insinga A, Monestiroli S, Ronzoni S et al. (2005) Inhibitors of histone deacetylases induce tumor-selective apoptosis through activation of the death receptor pathway. Nat Med 11:71–76

Jia W, Yu C, Rahmani M et al. (2003) Synergistic antileukemic interactions between 17-AAG and UCN-01 involve interruption of RAF/MEK- and AKT-related pathways. Blood 102:1824–1832

Jonker DJ, O'Callaghan CJ, Karapetis CS et al. (2007) Cetuximab for the treatment of colorectal cancer. N Engl J Med 357:2040–2048

Kabbinavar FF, Schulz J, McCleod M et al. (2005) Addition of bevacizumab to bolus fluorouracil and leucovorin in first-line metastatic colorectal cancer: results of a randomized phase II trial. J Clin Oncol 23:3697–3705

Kastan MB (2001) Cell cycle. Checking two steps. Nature 410:766–767

Kastan MB, Bartek J (2004) Cell-cycle checkpoints and cancer. Nature 432:316–323

Kavanagh BD, Lin PS, Chen P et al. (1995) Radiation-induced enhanced proliferation of human squamous cancer cells in vitro: a release from inhibition by epidermal growth factor. Clin Cancer Res 1:1557–1562

Kim DW, Huamani J, Fu A et al. (2006) Molecular strategies targeting the host component of cancer to enhance tumor response to radiation therapy. Int J Radiat Oncol Biol Phys 64:38–46

Kondapaka SB, Singh SS, Dasmahapatra GP et al. (2003) Perifosine, a novel alkylphospholipid, inhibits protein kinase B activation. Mol Cancer Ther 2:1093–1103

Krieg M, Haas R, Brauch H et al. (2000) Up-regulation of hypoxia-inducible factors HIF-1alpha and HIF-2alpha under normoxic conditions in renal carcinoma cells by von Hippel-Lindau tumor suppressor gene loss of function. Oncogene 19:5435–5443

Kris MG, Natale RB, Herbst RS et al. (2003) Efficacy of gefitinib, an inhibitor of the epidermal growth factor receptor tyrosine kinase, in symptomatic patients with non-small cell lung cancer: a randomized trial. J Am Med Assoc 290:2149–2158

Kwak EL, Sordella R, Bell DW et al. (2005) Irreversible inhibitors of the EGF receptor may circumvent acquired resistance to gefitinib. Proc Natl Acad Sci U S A 102:7665–7670

Langer CJ (2004) Emerging role of epidermal growth factor receptor inhibition in therapy for advanced malignancy: focus on NSCLC. Int J Radiat Oncol Biol Phys 58:991–1002

Lee BH, Williams IR, Anastasiadou E et al. (2005) FLT3 internal tandem duplication mutations induce myeloproliferative or lymphoid disease in a transgenic mouse model. Oncogene 24:7882–7892

Li H, Zhu H, Xu CJ et al. (1998) Cleavage of BID by caspase 8 mediates the mitochondrial damage in the Fas pathway of apoptosis. Cell 94:491–501

Ling YH, Liebes L, Zou Y et al. (2003) Reactive oxygen species generation and mitochondrial dysfunction in the apoptotic response to Bortezomib, a novel proteasome inhibitor, in human H460 non-small cell lung cancer cells. J Biol Chem 278:33714–33723

Llovet JM, Ricci S, Mazzaferro V et al. (2008) Sorafenib in advanced hepatocellular carcinoma. N Engl J Med 359:378–390

Lynch TJ, Bell DW, Sordella R et al. (2004) Activating mutations in the epidermal growth factor receptor underlying responsiveness of non-small-cell lung cancer to gefitinib. N Engl J Med 350:2129–2139

Majumdar AP, Du J (2006) Phosphatidylinositol 3-kinase/Akt signaling stimulates colonic mucosal cell survival during aging. Am J Physiol Gastrointest Liver Physiol 290:G49–G55

Marcucci G, Byrd JC, Dai G et al. (2003) Phase 1 and pharmacodynamic studies of G3139, a Bcl-2 antisense oligonucleotide, in combination with chemotherapy in refractory or relapsed acute leukemia. Blood 101:425–432

Marks PA, Jiang X (2005) Histone deacetylase inhibitors in programmed cell death and cancer therapy. Cell Cycle 4:549–551

Marks PA, Miller T, Richon VM (2003) Histone deacetylases. Curr Opin Pharmacol 3:344–351

McKinstry R, Qiao L, Yacoub A et al. (2002) Inhibitors of MEK1/2 interact with UCN-01 to induce apoptosis and reduce colony formation in mammary and prostate carcinoma cells. Cancer Biol Ther 1:243–253

Milella M, Kornblau SM, Estrov Z et al. (2001) Therapeutic targeting of the MEK/MAPK signal transduction module in acute myeloid leukemia. J Clin Invest 108:851–859

Miller K, Wang M, Gralow J et al. (2007) Paclitaxel plus bevacizumab versus paclitaxel alone for metastatic breast cancer. N Engl J Med 357:2666–2676

Molhoek KR, Brautigan DL, Slingluff CL Jr (2005) Synergistic inhibition of human melanoma proliferation by combination treatment with B-Raf inhibitor BAY43-9006 and mTOR inhibitor Rapamycin. J Transl Med 3:39

Momparler RL (2005) Epigenetic therapy of cancer with 5-aza-2'-deoxycytidine (decitabine). Semin Oncol 32:443–451

Motzer RJ, Hutson TE, Tomczak P et al. (2007) Sunitinib versus interferon alfa in metastatic renal-cell carcinoma. N Engl J Med 356:115–124

Muller CI, Ruter B, Koeffler HP et al. (2006) DNA hypermethylation of myeloid cells, a novel therapeutic target in MDS and AML. Curr Pharm Biotechnol 7:315–321

Murdoch D, Sager J (2008) Will targeted therapy hold its promise? An evidence-based review. Curr Opin Oncol 20:104–111

Na X, Wu G, Ryan CK et al. (2003) Overproduction of vascular endothelial growth factor related to von Hippel-Lindau tumor suppressor gene mutations and hypoxia-inducible factor-1 alpha expression in renal cell carcinomas. J Urol 170:588–592

Neckers L, Ivy SP (2003) Heat shock protein 90. Curr Opin Oncol 15:419–424

Nishi H, Senoo M, Nishi KH et al. (2001) p53 Homologue p63 represses epidermal growth factor receptor expression. J Biol Chem 276:41717–41724

Nowell PC, Hungerford DA (1961) Chromosome studies in human leukemia. II. Chronic granulocytic leukemia. J Natl Cancer Inst 27:1013–1035

O'Connor OA, Wright J, Moskowitz C et al. (2005) Phase II clinical experience with the novel proteasome inhibitor bortezomib in patients with indolent non-Hodgkin's lymphoma and mantle cell lymphoma. J Clin Oncol 23:676–684

Oltersdorf T, Elmore SW, Shoemaker AR et al. (2005) An inhibitor of Bcl-2 family proteins induces regression of solid tumours. Nature 435:677–681

Orlowski RZ, Small GW, Shi YY (2002) Evidence that inhibition of p44/42 mitogen-activated protein kinase signaling is a factor in proteasome inhibitor-mediated apoptosis. J Biol Chem 277:27864–27871

Osaki M, Kase S, Adachi K et al. (2004) Inhibition of the PI3K-Akt signaling pathway enhances the sensitivity of Fas-mediated apoptosis in human gastric carcinoma cell line, MKN-45. J Cancer Res Clin Oncol 130:8–14

Pan G, Ni J, Wei YF et al. (1997) An antagonist decoy receptor and a death domain-containing receptor for TRAIL. Science 277:815–818

Pei XY, Dai Y, Grant S (2003) The proteasome inhibitor bortezomib promotes mitochondrial injury and apoptosis induced by the small molecule Bcl-2 inhibitor HA14-1 in multiple myeloma cells. Leukemia 17:2036–2045

Pei XY, Dai Y, Grant S (2004a) Synergistic induction of oxidative injury and apoptosis in human multiple myeloma cells by the proteasome inhibitor bortezomib and histone deacetylase inhibitors. Clin Cancer Res 10:3839–3852

Pei XY, Dai Y, Grant S (2004b) The small-molecule Bcl-2 inhibitor HA14-1 interacts synergistically with flavopiridol to induce mitochondrial injury and apoptosis in human myeloma cells through a free radical-dependent and Jun NH2-terminal kinase-dependent mechanism. Mol Cancer Ther 3:1513–1524

Peterson CL, Laniel MA (2004) Histones and histone modifications. Curr Biol 14:R546–R551

Piccart-Gebhart MJ, Procter M, Leyland-Jones B et al. (2005) Trastuzumab after adjuvant chemotherapy in HER2-positive breast cancer. N Engl J Med 353:1659–1672

Rahmani M, Yu C, Reese E et al. (2003a) Inhibition of PI-3 kinase sensitizes human leukemic cells to histone deacetylase inhibitor-mediated apoptosis through p44/42 MAP kinase inactivation and abrogation of p21(CIP1/WAF1) induction rather than AKT inhibition. Oncogene 22:6231–6242

Rahmani M, Yu C, Dai Y et al. (2003b) Coadministration of the heat shock protein 90 antagonist 17-allylamino-17-demethoxygeldanamycin with suberoylanilide hydroxamic acid or sodium butyrate synergistically induces apoptosis in human leukemia cells. Cancer Res 63:8420–8427

Ratain MJ, Eisen T, Stadler WM et al. (2006) Phase II placebo-controlled randomized discontinuation trial of sorafenib in patients with metastatic renal cell carcinoma. J Clin Oncol 24:2505–2512

Ray A, Cowan-Jacob SW, Manley PW et al. (2007) Identification of BCR-ABL point mutations conferring resistance to the Abl kinase inhibitor AMN107 (nilotinib) by a random mutagenesis study. Blood 109:5011–5015

Reed JC (1998) Bcl-2 family proteins. Oncogene 17:3225–3236

Rinehart J, Adjei AA, Lorusso PM et al. (2004) Multicenter phase II study of the oral MEK inhibitor, CI-1040, in patients with advanced non-small-cell lung, breast, colon, and pancreatic cancer. J Clin Oncol 22:4456–4462

Romond EH, Perez EA, Bryant J et al. (2005) Trastuzumab plus adjuvant chemotherapy for operable HER2-positive breast cancer. N Engl J Med 353:1673–1684

Rosato RR, Grant S (2003) Histone deacetylase inhibitors in cancer therapy. Cancer Biol Ther 2:30–37

Rosato RR, Wang Z, Gopalkrishnan RV et al. (2001) Evidence of a functional role for the cyclin-dependent kinase-inhibitor p21WAF1/CIP1/MDA6 in promoting differentiation and preventing mitochondrial dysfunction and apoptosis induced by sodium butyrate in human myelomonocytic leukemia cells (U937). Int J Oncol 19:181–191

Rosato RR, Almenara JA, Dai Y et al. (2003) Simultaneous activation of the intrinsic and extrinsic pathways by histone deacetylase (HDAC) inhibitors and tumor necrosis factor-related apoptosis-inducing ligand (TRAIL) synergistically induces mitochondrial damage and apoptosis in human leukemia cells. Mol Cancer Ther 2:1273–1284

Rosato RR, Dai Y, Almenara JA et al. (2004) Potent antileukemic interactions between flavopiridol and TRAIL/Apo2L involve flavopiridol-mediated XIAP downregulation. Leukemia 18:1780–1788

Ruefli AA, Ausserlechner MJ, Bernhard D et al. (2001) The histone deacetylase inhibitor and chemotherapeutic agent suberoylanilide hydroxamic acid (SAHA) induces a cell-death pathway characterized by cleavage of Bid and production of reactive oxygen species. Proc Natl Acad Sci U S A 98:10833–10838

Saltz LB, Meropol NJ, Loehrer PJ Sr et al. (2004) Phase II trial of cetuximab in patients with refractory colorectal cancer that expresses the epidermal growth factor receptor. J Clin Oncol 22:1201–1208

Sandler A, Herbst R (2006) Combining targeted agents: blocking the epidermal growth factor and vascular endothelial growth factor pathways. Clin Cancer Res 12:4421s–4425s

Sandler A, Gray R, Perry MC et al. (2006) Paclitaxel-carboplatin alone or with bevacizumab for non-small-cell lung cancer. N Engl J Med 355:2542–2550

Santoro A, Cavina R, Latteri F et al. (2004) Activity of a specific inhibitor, gefitinib (Iressa, ZD1839), of epidermal growth factor receptor in refractory non-small-cell lung cancer. Ann Oncol 15:33–37

Sato S, Fujita N,Tsuruo T (2002) Interference with PDK1-Akt survival signaling pathway by UCN-01 (7-hydroxystaurosporine). Oncogene 21:1727–1738

Sawyers CL, Hochhaus A, Feldman E et al. (2002) Imatinib induces hematologic and cytogenetic responses in patients with chronic myelogenous leukemia in myeloid blast crisis: results of a phase II study. Blood 99:3530–3539

Schimmer AD, Welsh K, Pinilla C et al. (2004) Small-molecule antagonists of apoptosis suppressor XIAP exhibit broad antitumor activity. Cancer Cell 5:25–35

Schmidt-Ullrich RK, Valerie K, Chan W et al. (1992) Expression of oestrogen receptor and transforming growth factor-alpha in MCF-7 cells after exposure to fractionated irradiation. Int J Radiat Biol 61:405–415

Senderowicz AM (1999) Flavopiridol: the first cyclin-dependent kinase inhibitor in human clinical trials. Invest New Drugs 17:313–320

Sengupta N, Seto E (2004) Regulation of histone deacetylase activities. J Cell Biochem 93:57–67

Shao RG, Cao CX, Shimizu T et al. (1997) Abrogation of an S-phase checkpoint and potentiation of camptothecin cytotoxicity by 7-hydroxystaurosporine (UCN-01) in human cancer cell lines, possibly influenced by p53 function. Cancer Res 57:4029–4035

Sheikh MS, Carrier F, Johnson AC et al. (1997) Identification of an additional p53-responsive site in the human epidermal growth factor receptor gene promotor. Oncogene 15:1095–1101

Shelton JG, Steelman LS, Abrams SL et al. (2005) The epidermal growth factor receptor gene family as a target for therapeutic intervention in numerous cancers: What's genetics got to do with it? Expert Opin Ther Targets 9:1009–1030

Shepherd FA, Rodrigues Pereira J, Ciuleanu T et al. (2005) Erlotinib in previously treated non-small-cell lung cancer. N Engl J Med 353:123–132

Sheridan JP, Marsters SA, Pitti RM et al. (1997) Control of TRAIL-induced apoptosis by a family of signaling and decoy receptors. Science 277:818–821

Shibuya K, Komaki R, Shintani T et al. (2007) Targeted therapy against VEGFR and EGFR with ZD6474 enhances the therapeutic efficacy of irradiation in an orthotopic model of human non-small-cell lung cancer. Int J Radiat Oncol Biol Phys 69:1534–1543

Shonai T, Adachi M, Sakata K et al. (2002) MEK/ERK pathway protects ionizing radiation-induced loss of mitochondrial membrane potential and cell death in lymphocytic leukemia cells. Cell Death Differ 9:963–971

Shvartsman SY, Hagan MP, Yacoub A et al. (2002) Autocrine loops with positive feedback enable context-dependent cell signaling. Am J Physiol Cell Physiol 282:C545–C559

Simon GR, Ruckdeschel JC, Williams C et al. (2003) Gefitinib (ZD1839) in previously treated advanced non-small-cell lung cancer: experience from a single institution. Cancer Control 10:388–395

Stone RM, DeAngelo DJ, Klimek V et al. (2005) Patients with acute myeloid leukemia and an activating mutation in FLT3 respond to a small-molecule FLT3 tyrosine kinase inhibitor, PKC412. Blood 105:54–60

Sun H, Nikolovska-Coleska Z, Yang CY et al. (2004) Structure-based design, synthesis, and evaluation of conformationally constrained mimetics of the second mitochondria-derived activator of caspase that target the X-linked inhibitor of apoptosis protein/caspase-9 interaction site. J Med Chem 47:4147–4150

Tabernero J (2007) The role of VEGF and EGFR inhibition: implications for combining anti-VEGF and anti-EGFR agents. Mol Cancer Res 5:203–220

Takada Y, Kobayashi Y, Aggarwal BB (2005) Evodiamine abolishes constitutive and inducible NF-kappaB activation by inhibiting IkappaBalpha kinase activation, thereby suppressing NF-kappaB-regulated antiapoptotic and metastatic gene expression, up-regulating apoptosis, and inhibiting invasion. J Biol Chem 280:17203–17212

Takahashi I, Saitoh Y, Yoshida M et al. (1989) UCN-01 and UCN-02, new selective inhibitors of protein kinase C. II. Purification, physico-chemical properties, structural determination and biological activities. J Antibiot (Tokyo) 42:571–576

Tang L, Boise LH, Dent P et al. (2000) Potentiation of 1-beta-D-arabinofuranosylcytosine-mediated mitochondrial damage and apoptosis in human leukemia cells (U937) overexpressing bcl-2 by the kinase inhibitor 7-hydroxystaurosporine (UCN-01). Biochem Pharmacol 60:1445–1456

Tergaonkar V, Bottero V, Ikawa M et al. (2003) IkappaB kinase-independent IkappaBalpha degradation pathway:functional NF-kappaB activity and implications for cancer therapy. Mol Cell Biol 23:8070–8083

Thomas RK, Greulich H, Yuza Y et al. (2005) Detection of oncogenic mutations in the EGFR gene in lung adenocarcinoma with differential sensitivity to EGFR tyrosine kinase inhibitors. Cold Spring Harb Symp Quant Biol 70:73–81

Thorburn A (2004) Death receptor-induced cell killing. Cell Signal 16:139–144

Todd DG, Mikkelsen RB, Rorrer WK et al. (1999) Ionizing radiation stimulates existing signal transduction pathways involving the activation of epidermal growth factor receptor and ERBB-3, and changes of intracellular calcium in A431 human squamous carcinoma cells. J Recept Signal Transduct Res 19:885–908

Tol J, Koopman M, Rodenburg CJ et al. (2008) A randomised phase III study on capecitabine, oxaliplatin and bevacizumab with or without cetuximab in first-line advanced colorectal cancer, the CAIRO2 study of the Dutch Colorectal Cancer Group (DCCG). An interim analysis of toxicity. Ann Oncol 19:734–738

Tournier C, Hess P, Yang DD et al. (2000) Requirement of JNK for stress-induced activation of the cytochrome c-mediated death pathway. Science 288:870–874

Ungerstedt JS, Sowa Y, Xu WS et al. (2005) Role of thioredoxin in the response of normal and transformed cells to histone deacetylase inhibitors. Proc Natl Acad Sci U S A 102:673–678

Van Oosterom AT, Judson IR, Verweij J et al. (2002) Update of phase I study of imatinib (STI571) in advanced soft tissue sarcomas and gastrointestinal stromal tumors: a report of the EORTC Soft Tissue and Bone Sarcoma Group. Eur J Cancer 38 (Suppl 5):S83–S87

Vermorken JB, Trigo J, Hitt R et al. (2007) Open-label, uncontrolled, multicenter phase II study to evaluate the efficacy and toxicity of cetuximab as a single agent in patients with recurrent and/or metastatic squamous cell carcinoma of the head and neck who failed to respond to platinum-based therapy. J Clin Oncol 25:2171–2177

Voigt W, Pickan V, Pfeiffer C et al. (2005) Preclinical evaluation of ZD1839 alone or in combination with oxaliplatin in a panel of human tumor cell lines: implications for clinical use. Onkologie 28:482–488

Wang S, El-Deiry WS (2003) TRAIL and apoptosis induction by TNF-family death receptors. Oncogene 22:8628–8633

Wang JL, Liu D, Zhang ZJ et al. (2000) Structure-based discovery of an organic compound that binds Bcl-2 protein and induces apoptosis of tumor cells. Proc Natl Acad Sci U S A 97:7124–7129

Weisberg E, Boulton C, Kelly LM et al. (2002) Inhibition of mutant FLT3 receptors in leukemia cells by the small molecule tyrosine kinase inhibitor PKC412. Cancer Cell 1:433–443

Whittaker SR, Walton MI, Garrett MD et al. (2004) The cyclin-dependent kinase inhibitor CYC202 (R-roscovitine) inhibits retinoblastoma protein phosphorylation, causes loss of Cyclin D1, and activates the mitogen-activated protein kinase pathway. Cancer Res 64:262–272

Wijermans PW, Lubbert M, Verhoef G et al. (2005) An epigenetic approach to the treatment of advanced MDS; the experience with the DNA demethylating agent 5-aza-2'-deoxycytidine (decitabine) in 177 patients. Ann Hematol 84 (Suppl 1):9–17

Willers H, Held KD (2006) Introduction to clinical radiation biology. Hematol Oncol Clin North Am 20:1–24

Workman P (2004) Altered states: selectively drugging the Hsp90 cancer chaperone. Trends Mol Med 10:47–51

Xia Z, Dickens M, Raingeaud J et al. (1995) Opposing effects of ERK and JNK-p38 MAP kinases on apoptosis. Science 270:1326–1331

Yacoub A, McKinstry R, Hinman D et al. (2003) Epidermal growth factor and ionizing radiation up-regulate the DNA repair genes XRCC1 and ERCC1 in DU145 and LNCaP prostate carcinoma through MAPK signaling. Radiat Res 159:439–452

Yacoub A, Park MA, Hanna D et al. (2006) OSU-03012 promotes caspase-independent but PERK-, cathepsin B-, BID-, and AIF-dependent killing of transformed cells. Mol Pharmacol 70:589–603

Yang JC, Haworth L, Sherry RM et al. (2003) A randomized trial of bevacizumab, an anti-vascular endothelial growth factor antibody, for metastatic renal cancer. N Engl J Med 349:427–434

Yu X, Guo ZS, Marcu MG et al. (2002) Modulation of p53, ErbB1, ErbB2, and Raf-1 expression in lung cancer cells by depsipeptide FR901228. J Natl Cancer Inst 94:504–513

Yu C, Rahmani M, Conrad D et al. (2003a) The proteasome inhibitor bortezomib interacts synergistically with histone deacetylase inhibitors to induce apoptosis in Bcr/Abl+ cells sensitive and resistant to STI571. Blood 102:3765–3774

Yu C, Rahmani M, Almenara J et al. (2003b) Histone deacetylase inhibitors promote STI571-mediated apoptosis in STI571-sensitive and -resistant Bcr/Abl+ human myeloid leukemia cells. Cancer Res 63:2118–2126

Yu C, Rahmani M, Dent P et al. (2004) The hierarchical relationship between MAPK signaling and ROS generation in human leukemia cells undergoing apoptosis in response to the proteasome inhibitor Bortezomib. Exp Cell Res 295:555–566

Yu C, Dasmahapatra G, Dent P et al. (2005) Synergistic interactions between MEK1/2 and histone deacetylase inhibitors in BCR/ABL+ human leukemia cells. Leukemia 19:1579–1589

Zangari M, Esseltine D, Lee CK et al. (2005) Response to bortezomib is associated to osteoblastic activation in patients with multiple myeloma. Br J Haematol 131:71–73

Zhao B, Bower MJ, McDevitt PJ et al. (2002) Structural basis for Chk1 inhibition by UCN-01. J Biol Chem 277:46609–46615

Target-Based Interventions to Treat Radiation-Induced Lung Injury

Isabel L. Jackson, Mitchell S. Anscher, and Zeljko Vujaskovic

CONTENTS

KEY POINTS

- Delivery of the therapeutically optimum dose of radiation to achieve local tumor control and improved survival is limited by the risk of unacceptable normal tissue toxicity.
- Improved understanding of the molecular mechanisms underlying radiation-induced normal tissue injury has identified a number of molecular pathways, pro-fibrogenic growth factors, inflammatory cytokines, and chronic oxidative stress that can be targeted to ameliorate normal tissue injury.
- Approaches to prevent, mitigate, and/or treat radiation-induced normal tissue injury have been investigated in pre-clinical and clinical studies with varying degrees of success.
- Better understanding of normal tissue radiobiology will lead to improved therapeutic targeting to prevent, mitigate, and/or treat radiation-induced normal tissue toxicity.
- Therapeutic modalities to prevent, mitigate, and/or treat radiation-induced normal tissue toxicity will allow a higher clinically achievable therapeutic dose, improve local tumor control, diminish the negative consequences of radiation toxicity on quality of life, and potentially improve overall patient survival.

I. L. Jackson, B.S.
Department of Radiation Oncology, Box 3455 MSRB, Duke University Medical Center, Durham, NC 27705, USA

M. S. Anscher, MD, FACR, FACRO
Florence and Hyman Meyers Professor and Chair
Department of Radiation Oncology, Virginia Commonwealth University School of Medicine, 401 College Street, P.O. Box 980058, Richmond, VA 23298, USA

Z. Vujaskovic, MD, PhD
Department of Radiation Oncology, Box 3455 MSRB, Duke University Medical Center, Durham, NC 27705, USA

Abstract

The ability to achieve local tumor control and improved overall survival with radiation therapy is limited by the risk of unacceptable normal tissue toxicity. A number of therapeutic interventions targeting the molecular pathways responsible for the development of acute and long-term injury have been investigated in pre-clinical and clinical studies. These interventions have primarily targeted apoptosis, growth factors, and pro-inflammatory and pro-fibrogenic pathways in an attempt to prevent, mitigate, or treat radiation-induced injury. As the mechanisms underlying radiation-induced normal tissue injury are better elucidated, the identification of new potential targets and improved therapeutic interventions will allow patient-stratified dose escalation and improve long-term response rates. The following chapter outlines current target-based interventions being investigated and discusses the recent discovery of novel pathways that may be targeted in the future.

12.1
Introduction

The number of cancer survivors in the US alone now exceeds 10 million people. As the number of cancer survivors increases, the percentage of survivors with chronic health conditions related to treatment toxicity has grown. For the majority of patients diagnosed with cancer, radiation therapy with curative or palliative intent will be an important component of treatment. The likelihood for developing radiation-induced normal tissue toxicity has broad implications not only for the cancer survivor population, but also for patients in which more aggressive cytotoxic treatment strategies might be beneficial both for achieving tumor control and improvement in survival. Thus, the probability for normal tissue complications during or after radiotherapy limits the maximum effective dose that can be delivered to the tumor (Stone et al. 2003). The maximum tolerated dose is unknown for most tissues, and the ability to predict individual patient risk for the development of delayed injury is challenging. Formal dose escalation studies in radiation oncology have rarely been done. Thus, the clinically accepted tolerated doses have been mostly empirically derived through clinical observation and experience (Emami et al. 1991; Milano et al. 2007), and these doses are well below those required to achieve local control for most solid tumors. While these tolerance doses may be reasonable estimates for large populations of patients, the radiosensitivity of an individual cannot be determined accurately at this time.

The clinical significance of this problem can best be illustrated using the example of non-small cell lung cancer (NSCLC). Non-small cell carcinoma of the lung (NSCLC) is one of the most common cancers in the United States, with more than 172,000 cases diagnosed in 2005 (Jemal et al. 2005). It remains the most common cause of cancer deaths in this country. About one-

third of these patients will present with non-metastatic, but locally advanced or medically inoperable disease. For these patients, radiation therapy has been the mainstay of treatment.

Despite the high frequency of distant metastases in patients with unresectable NSCLC, local failure remains a significant clinical problem. The Radiation Therapy Oncology Group (RTOG) trials have reported radiographically assessed local failure rates of 35–58% in this patient population (Perez et al. 1986). Arriagada et al. (1991) reported on a series of 353 patients more rigorously assessed for local control following either radiotherapy alone (65 Gy in 2.5-Gy fractions) or the same radiotherapy plus chemotherapy (vindesine, cyclophosphamide, cisplatin, and lomustine) for unresectable NSCLC. In this randomized trial, patients underwent routine bronchoscopy and biopsy 3 months after radiotherapy and at 6-month intervals thereafter. The actuarial local control rate at 1 year was only 15–17% with radiotherapy + chemotherapy; chemotherapy did not improve local control.

Several investigators have noted the importance of local control in the treatment of NSCLC. In patients with unresectable NSCLC, Perez et al. (1986) demonstrated that intrathoracic tumor control at 6 months following radiotherapy predicted improved survival. These authors reported a 20% 3-year survival in complete responders compared to 4% in partial responders. Saunders et al. (1984) noted a similar finding, with 65% of complete responders alive at 2 years, compared to none of the partial responders. The uncertainties in defining local control in unresectable lung cancer make it difficult to be certain that improvements in local control are achievable with higher radiation doses and that this reduction in local relapse will translate into an increase in survival. Nevertheless, the available data suggest that the total tumor dose appears to significantly influence both local control and survival in NSCLC. The RTOG reported local failure rates of 53%, 49%, and 35% for patients irradiated to total doses of 40 Gy, 50 Gy, and 60 Gy, respectively (Perez et al. 1986). Median survivals in these three groups were 7 months, 9 months, and 10 months, respectively. Other investigators have confirmed the findings of Perez. For example, when controlling for tumor size, Dosoretz et al. (1993) noted a better disease-free survival for doses above 65 Gy versus doses of 60–65 Gy. As a result of findings, investigators at several institutions have instituted pilot, phase I, and phase II radiation dose escalation studies in patients with NSCLC (Cox et al. 1990; Anscher et al. 2001; Roseman et al. 2002; Zhao et al. 2007; Socinski et al. 2008). Much higher doses have been achieved using the modern radiotherapy techniques of three-dimensional conformal (3DCRT), intensity-modulated radiotherapy (IMRT) and image-guided adaptive radiation therapy (IGRT) (ROBERTSON et al. 1997; KEALL et al. 2006; SCHILD et al. 2006). Despite the highly sophisticated approaches to radiation dose delivery utilized in these studies, normal tissue injury remains a significant problem.

Certain factors affecting normal tissue tolerability include the anatomic location of the tumor, the cellular kinetics and organization of surrounding tissue, pre-existing pathologic conditions, genetic variability, and physical factors (fractionation scheme, total dose, and volume irradiated). The effect of normal tissue complications on the physical and emotional quality of life for cancer survivors depends on the tissue affected and severity of injury. For a minority of these patients, the long-term effect of treatment is worse than the disease itself. As the number of long-term cancer survivors increases, late complications of cancer therapy are becoming an increasingly important concern to both physicians and patients. For the radiation oncologist, a better understanding of the molecular events underlying normal tissue injury will permit a more rational approach to its prevention and treatment (ANSCHER et al. 1994). Currently, the physician must try to prevent complications primarily through restricting the dose and volume to be irradiated (VUJASKOVIC et al. 2000). The relationship between dose, volume, complications, and tumor control is complex and not precisely defined for most cancers and normal tissues (EMAMI et al. 1991; VUJASKOVIC et al. 2000; MILANO et al. 2007). Only recently have investigators attempted to better delineate these relationships by taking advantage of innovations in radiation dose delivery and imaging technology.

The relationship between the probability of local tumor control and probability for normal tissue toxicity is defined by the therapeutic ratio (Fig. 12.1). Both have sigmoid dose response curves, and a number of therapeutic interventions have been investigated to either improve tumor sensitivity to radiation or reduce the deleterious effects of radiation on normal tissue without negatively affecting tumor response (BRIZEL 2007). Treatment options for radiation-induced injury are defined as (1) prophylactic agents, typically given prior to irradiation, (2) mitigators, agents given after irradiation, but prior to symptomatic injury, or (3) treatment given at the time of symptomatic injury to reverse tissue damage (MOULDER 2003).

Over the past several years, major advances in the tools of molecular biology have enabled scientists to move rapidly toward a better understanding of underly-

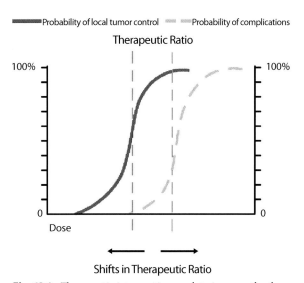

Fig. 12.1. Therapeutic interventions seek to improve the therapeutic ratio by increasing normal tissue tolerance to radiation or through radiosensitization of the tumor. Reproduced from BRIZEL (2005)

ing mechanisms responsible for radiation-induced normal tissue injury. It has been known for decades that the biologic response to ionizing radiation begins with the generation of reactive oxygen species (ROS) (RILEY 1994). More recently, researchers have described how these immediate biochemical events rapidly trigger a series of genetic and molecular phenomena leading to clinically and histologically recognizable injury (BRACH et al. 1991; BARCELLOS-HOFF 1993; HONG et al. 1995; JOHNSTON et al. 1995; RUBIN et al. 1995; HAUER-JENSEN et al. 1999; VUJASKOVIC et al. 2001; HALLAHAN et al. 2002; HONG et al. 2003). This response to radiation is dynamic and involves a number of mediators of inflammation and fibrosis produced by macrophages, epithelial cells, and fibroblasts. These events appear to be sustained for months to years beyond the completion of therapy; however, the mechanisms responsible for maintaining the injured phenotype, until recently, have remained unknown (VUJASKOVIC et al. 2001) .

As in tumor biology, the improvement in knowledge of ongoing molecular processes in radiation-induced injury has provided new mechanisms and insights for modulating the cellular and tissue response using target-based strategies to ameliorate normal tissue injury. This chapter will review potential molecular and physiological targets and respective therapeutic interventions, focusing on protection of normal tissues as a model for translational studies for target-based therapies.

12.2
Molecular and Physiological Basis of Normal Tissue Injury

It was originally assumed normal tissue injury was an unavoidable, untreatable, and irreversible consequence of radiation therapy. The classical radiobiology concept supported the target cell hypothesis, which suggested the effects of radiation were mostly the result of clonogenic cell death (MICHALOWSKI 1984). The acute versus late tissue effects therefore corresponded to the rate of cell turnover in the irradiated tissue (MICHALOWSKI 1984). However, since the early to mid-1990s, the target cell hypothesis has come under increasing scrutiny. Although cell kinetics play a role in radiation-induced injury, it has now been acknowledged that radiation-induced normal tissue injury is a consequence of dynamic interactions among various cells of the tissue, inflammatory mediators, and the vascular endothelium beginning at the time of irradiation and continuing throughout the time to disease progression (RUBIN et al. 1995; VUJASKOVIC et al. 2001; FLECKENSTEIN et al. 2007b). This is particularly relevant for late-responding tissue (lung, liver, and spinal cord) in which there is a latent period lasting months to years before which symptoms may appear.

The acute phase of radiation injury develops during the course of radiation therapy or immediately after and is primarily characterized by injury to tissues with rapidly proliferating stem cell compartments such as the salivary glands (xerostomia), gastrointestinal mucosa (mucositis, diarrhea), or skin (erythema). Likewise, late injury develops in tissues with slow proliferation indexes (lung, liver, and CNS). The new molecular-based paradigm has renewed interest to develop therapeutic interventions for radiation-induced normal tissue toxicity to target the series of ongoing events leading to the development of symptomatic injury.

The biological effects of ionizing radiation begin with the transient increase in reactive oxygen species (ROS), such as superoxide ($O2^-$), hydrogen peroxide (H_2O_2), and hydroxyl radical ($HO^.$) at the time of irradiation (RILEY 1994). The direct effect is injury to cellular components, chromosomal damage, and cell-mediated death (RUBIN et al. 1995). Within days post-radiation, there are noticeable effects on vascular endothelial function, including increased leukocyte-endothelial interac-

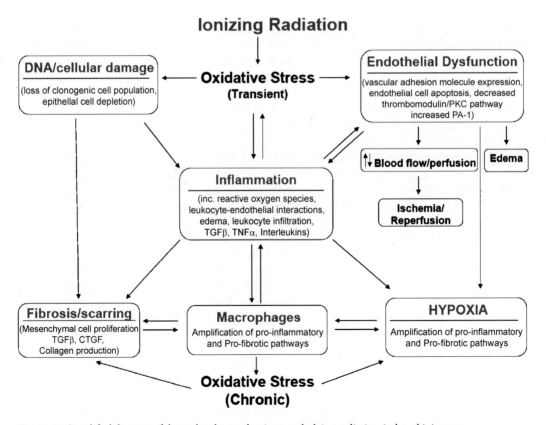

Fig. 12.2. Simplified diagram of the molecular mechanisms underlying radiation-induced injury

tions, detachment of endothelial cells from the basal lamina, endothelial cell apoptosis, and loss of microvessel density, resulting in reduced blood flow and tissue hypoxia (DEWHIRST et al. 1987; WANG et al. 2007a). The immediate cellular injury and vascular dysfunction are followed by an acute and progressive inflammatory cell infiltration and activation of an ongoing cytokine cascade, leading to chronic oxidative stress. These cellular events are ongoing throughout the "latent" period prior to the development of symptomatic injury. The end result is an environment characterized by endothelial dysfunction, extravasation of plasma proteins and edema, inflammatory cell infiltration and activation, lipid peroxidation, fibrin accumulation in the extracellular matrix, and functional tissue damage (Fig. 12.2) (STONE et al. 2003; BRUSH et al. 2007; DELANIAN et al. 2007; RODEMANN et al. 2007b; ZHAO et al. 2007).

A number of cytokines, growth factors, and oxidant-generating enzymes have been implicated in the aforementioned processes and have been used as potential targets in an attempt to ameliorate and/or treat radiation-induced normal tissue injury. A growing body of evidence points toward a complex web of protein interactions as being important in the pathogenesis of abnormal fibrogenesis (see Table 12.1). For example, HUANG et al. (2002) have found that IL-7, a cytokine that enhances T cell function and IFN-γ production, inhibits both TGFß production and signaling, and protects against the development of bleomycin-induced pulmonary fibrosis. FEDOROCKO et al. (2002) showed that radiation exposure could increase cytokine production both directly (IL-6, TNF-α) and indirectly (GM-CSF), either by locally acting paracrine or endocrine effects or as a result of systemic effects of early proinflammatory mediators such as IL-1 or TNF-α. There is no doubt that protein production is a dynamic process, which will change as a result of cancer treatment. HONG et al. (2003) have documented temporal and spatial changes in the expression of proinflammatory cytokines (TNF-α, IL-1α, and IL-1ß) following thoracic irradiation in mice.

Table 12.1 lists proteins that might be potential targets for intervention, since they are components in all of the major pathways thought to be involved in the response of cells to radiation (SCHMIDT-ULLRICH et al. 2000; TSOUTSOU et al. 2006).

Table 12.1. Summary of the function of candidate proteins

Protein	Function
IL-1ß	Inflammation, growth factor expression
IL-5	Proinflammatory
IL-6	Proinflammatory, decrease apoptosis of activated lung fibroblasts
IL-7	Proinflammatory
IL-8	Angiogenesis, leukocyte chemotaxis, collagen synthesis
IL-10	Anti-inflammatory (decrease TNFα production, decrease upregulation of endothelial cell adhesion molecules)
IL-13	Proinflammatory
MCP-1	Inflammation, chemoattraction of monocytes
MIP-1alpha	Antiproliferative
PDGF BB	Angiogenesis, recruit smooth muscle cells
VEGF	Angiogenesis and increased vascular permeability
EGF	Epithelial cell motility, mitogenicity, and differentiation
EGFR	Receptor for EGF, initial component of EGF signaling pathway
NFkappaB	Pleotropic gene transcription responses
HIF-1	Transcription factor for genes regulating angiogenesis

Table 12.1. (*continued*) Summary of the function of candidate proteins

Protein	Function
TGF-alpha	Cell motility and proliferation
FGF 2	Angiogenesis and fibroblast proliferation
MMP-1	Degradation of collagen and extracellular matrix proteins
MMP-2	Matrix remodeling, growth factor release
MMP-3	Matrix remodeling, growth factor release
MMP-13	Matrix remodeling, growth factor release
SMAD 2/3	Signal transduction in the TGFß pathway
IGF-1R	Binding of IGF-1 (reepithialization and granulation tissue formation)
TNF-alpha	Growth factor expression, inflammation, matrix production, and remodeling
TGFß	Profibrotic, immunosuppression, angiogenesis, metastasis
Beta-catenin	Epithelial-mesenchymal transition
Nitric-oxide synthases	Inflammation
Superoxide dismutases	Endogenous anti-inflammatory regulator

12.3
Target-Based Therapeutic Strategies

12.3.1
Transforming Growth Factor Beta (TGFβ)

Over the past 20 years, the role of TGFβ in post-radiation injury has been extensively studied in experimental models of radiation-induced cellular and tissue injury. Since MARTIN et al. (2000) described TGFβ signaling to be the *master switch* in radiation-induced fibroproliferative disease, investigators have sought to mitigate the severity of injury through TGFβ targeting. TGFβ, a pleuripotent cytokine, is a critical mediator of cell growth and proliferation, extracellular matrix remodeling, inhibition of matrix degradation, chronic inflammatory disease, and angiogenesis (ROBERTS 1999; FLANDERS 2004). Latent TGFβ is sequestered in the extracellular environment until it is activated by proteases, free radicals, or radiation (BARCELLOS-HOFF et al. 1996). The latency-associated peptide (LAP) bound to TGFβ acts as a molecular chaperone and sensor of oxidative stress (BAECELLOS-HOFF 1993; 1996; BARCELLOS-HOFF et al. 1994, 1996; VODOVOTZ et al. 1999; JOBLING et al. 2006). Recently, JOBLING et al. (2006) used free radical scav-

engers to determine that hydroxyl radical bioavailability, which can be produced by radiolytic hydrolysis, is the primary oxidizing agent responsible for activation of latent TGFβ. It is therefore plausible to assume that oxidation of LAP explains the rapid increase in active TGFβ observed within hours post radiation (FLECKENSTEIN et al. 2007a). The biologically active form of TGFβ readily binds the ubiquitously expressed TGFβ type I and II receptors (ROBERTS 1999; FLANDERS 2004; ANDRAWEWA et al. 2007a, 2007b). Stabilization of the type II/type I receptor complex by their cytoplasmic domains leads to downstsream phosphorylation of Smad 2/3 proteins, which then form an active heterooligomeric complex with Smad 4 that can bind DNA and initiate transcription (Fig. 12.3) (ROBERTS 1999).

In a recent paper by FLECKENSTEIN et al. (2007b), 28-Gy single-dose irradiation to the right hemithorax resulted in increased TGFβ production within 24 h post-radiation followed by a bi-phasic decrease in perfusion, development of tissue hypoxia, and infiltration and accumulation of macrophages with a concomitant increase in oxidative stress.

Other studies aimed at identifying TGFβ as a key mediator in the pathological response to radiation have used antagonists to TGFβ or components of its signal transduction pathway (RABBINI et al. 2003; NISHIOKA

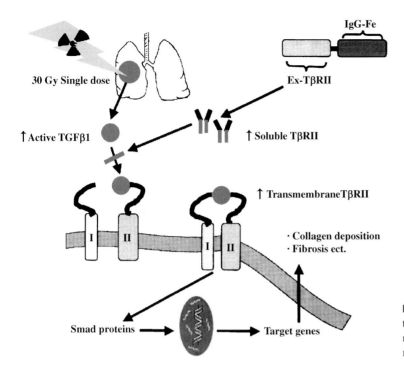

Fig. 12.3. TGFβ signaling pathway and therapeutic targeting with soluble TGFβ receptor (TβRII). Reproduced from Rabbani et al. (2003)

et al. 2004; Anscher et al. 2006, 2008). Anscher and Vujaskovic (2008) found a small molecule kinase inhibitor targeting the TGFβ pathway preserved the structural integrity of the lung and prevented organ dysfunction using both biological and functional parameters to assess the severity of lung injury after 28-Gy single-dose right hemithoracic irradiation. Their 2007 study was consistent with studies conducted between 1995 and 2006 (Ehrhart et al. 1997; Nishioka et al. 2004; Anscher et al. 2006) in which several authors found blockade of the TGFβ signaling pathway using an anti-TGFβ antibody or adenoviral vector expressing a soluble TGFβ receptor to neutralize the protein in vivo significantly protected lung tissue from radiation injury. In Anscher and Vujaskovic's studies (2006), histological and morphologic comparison among animals at the end of the follow-up period (6 months) showed a decrease in macrophage infiltration and inflammation, reduced alveolar wall thickness and collage deposition, and an improvement in overall lung function (Rabbini et al. 2003). These results are supported by Nishioka and colleagues (2004), who reported similar findings using an adenoviral vector expressing soluble TGFβ receptor in their experimental model of hemithoracic lung injury using 30-Gy single-dose irradiation.

12.3.2
Keratinocyte Growth Factor

Keratinocyte growth factor (KGF) is a member of the fibroblast growth factor family. KGF is produced by mesenchymal cells (i.e., fibroblasts, γδT-cells) and is specific for epithelial cells expressing a splice variant of FGFR2. KGF stimulates proliferation and differentiation to facilitate re-epithelialization of injured tissue. A number of studies have sought to mitigate radiation-induced injury through modulation of cellular proliferation, particular for acute responding tissues, such as the oral mucosa. The best data for the utility of KGF in mitigation or treatment of radiation-induced injury come from animal models of oral mucositis, a common complication from treatment of the head and neck cancer. Dorr and colleagues (2001, 2002, 2005c) in Dresden have provided much of the evidence regarding the protective effect of rHuKGF in pre-clinical settings using both single-dose and fractionated radiation. In a 2005 study, Dorr found a dose-response effect of rHuKGF (palifermin) in a mouse model of oral mucositis following fractionated irradiation. The highest ED50 values for mucosal tolerance were achieved with 15 mg/kg or 22.5 mg/kg; however, the authors found doses as low as 1 mg/kg offered significant protection against mouse tongue ulceration (DORR et al. 2005b). rHuKGF given during the course of radiotherapy appears to be more effective in models of oral mucositis rather than when given prior to the start of radiation treatment. Studies by Dorr suggest doses above 30 mg/kg offer no improvement over those seen at 15 and 22.5 mg/kg (DORR et al. 2005b). In those studies, the optimum therapeutic strategy involved three applications of rHuKGF during the course of radiation therapy; however, greater than three did not offer any significant improvement (DORR et al. 2005c). Thus, it appears there is a cumulative dose threshold for which no greater protection is achieved with higher doses or further treatment. The radioprotective effect was preserved when chemotherapy (5-FU and cisplatin) was combined with radiation (DORR et al. 2005a).

KGF has been shown to be a direct stimulator of type II pneumocytes both in vitro and in vivo (ULICH et al. 1994; TERRY et al. 2004). CHEN et al. (2004) found high doses of recombinant human KGF (15 mg/kg) given i.v. 15 min prior to the last fraction of radiation offered significant protection against radiation-induced pulmonary injury. The protective effect was assessed using functional injury (breathing frequency) and histological, morphological, and immunohistochemical staining for architectural/structural distortion, collagen deposition, and activation of the TGFβ/Smad signaling pathway. The protective effect of rHuKGF on the lung is described to be a result of type II pneumocyte differentiation to type I pneumocytes, which normally comprise 95% of the alveolar surface area, concurrent with apoptosis of hyperplastic alveolar type II cells (FEHRENBACH et al. 1999, 2000, 2002). TERRY et al. (2004) described an actively proliferating pulmonary environment after stimulation with rHuKGF. Terry found whole thorax irradiation to mice at the time of increased alveolar epithelial cellularity (after KGF delivery) resulted in a right shift in the dose response curve for radiation-induced pneumonitis. Jaal and Dorr recently completed a new study to investigate the effect of rHuKGF on mouse urinary bladder. A single dose of 15 mg/kg given subcutaneously prior to irradiation reduced both the early and late effects of bladder toxicity. The same effect was not observed when given after irradiation (JAAL et al. 2007); however, longer administration of the drug post-irradiation may provide better results.

12.3.3
Angiotensin-Converting Enzyme (ACE)

The success of angiotensin-converting enzyme inhibitors and AngII receptor antagonists for reducing the development of late injury has been shown in a number of published studies during the past 2 decades (MOULDER et al. 1993, 1996, 197a, 1997b, 1998a, 1998b, 1998c, 2003, 2007b; COHEN et al. 1997; MOLTENI et al. 2000; 2007). Indirect evidence for the role of a renin-angiotensin system in radiation-induced delayed injury stems from studies using ACE inhibitors to successfully reduce the severity of delayed radiation nephropathy; however, no evidence of alterations in either the enzyme renin or its substrate, angiotensin II, have been found.

The utility of ACE inhibitors has been investigated primarily in animal models of radiation nephropathy. Radiation nephropathy is characterized by tubulointerstitial fibrosis and glomerulosclerosis, leading to renal failure (ROBBINS et al. 2006). Within 5 weeks after bilateral or total body irradiation followed by bone marrow transplant, there is an increase in the number of cells staining positive for proliferating cell nuclear antigen, suggesting irradiation induces an increase in renal tubular cell proliferation. It was thought cellular proliferation or chronic oxidative stress may be a target for ACE inhibitors and AII blockers (MOULDER et al. 2002). However, non-thiol-containing ACE inhibitors, such as enalapril, were also effective at reducing the severity of radiation-induced renal injury diminishing the enthusiasm for chronic oxidative stress as the underlying target. The thiol-containing captopril was one of the first ACE inhibitors proven to both prevent and treat radiation nephropathy. MOULDER and colleagues (1998a) found the actuarial risk of renal failure after bilateral irradiation in a rat model was significantly reduced with continuous treatment of Captopril (62.5 mg/l and 500 mg/l) or AII blocker (L 158,809) when treatment started 24 weeks post exposure during the time of established injury. MOULDER and colleagues (1998b) demonstrated the protective effect of Captopril was independent of the pharmacologic dose and found low doses achieved equally effective mitigation of nephropathy assessed by a decrease in azotemia, proteinurea, and histopathologic damage. The same group determined the better efficacy of AII blocker as a prophylactic agent compared to Captopril was suggestive of dual mechanisms underlying the acute and delayed renal responses to radiation. At doses below the human MTD, Captopril increased survival from 49 weeks (irradiated alone) to 74 weeks (P < 0.0001). In these studies, Captopril or AII blocker was only effective when given continuously after the development of injury. In subsequent studies, the authors found ACE inhibitors delivered for short time intervals (3-6 weeks) could be effective when delivered between 3 to 10 weeks post-irradiation, before or after which the effectiveness diminished (COHEN et al. 1997; MOULDER et al. 1998b), coinciding with the time of renal tubular cell and glomerular proliferation. However, in those same studies, Moulder and colleagues found that AII blockers inhibited renal tubular cell proliferation, but had no effect on glomerular cell proliferation. Consequentially, in experimental models of radiation-induced pneumonitis and fibrosis, cessation of treatment with ACEI has been followed by a rapid deterioration in lung injury (ROBBINS et al. 2006).

Based on promising animal work, COHEN et al. (2008) launched a phase III trial of Captopril vs. placebo after hematopoeitic stem cell transplant to mitigate chronic renal failure. The study included both adults and children with various types of leukemia or myelodysplastic syndrome. Patients received total body irradiation to 14 Gy in nine fractions, with the dose to the kidney limited to 9.8 Gy. Captopril was started after engraftment was confirmed, beginning at a dose of 6.25 mg b.i.d. and escalating to a dose of 25 mg t.i.d. (12.5 mg t.i.d. in children). Unfortunately, the study was unable to meet its accrual goals. Despite this problem, however, there was a trend toward better preservation of renal function in the Captopril-treated group, as measured by glomerular filtration rate at 1 year ($P = 0.07$). Thus, this study supports the conclusion that an ACE inhibitor may mitigate chronic renal failure after radiation-based hematopoeitc stem cell transplant. This study awaits confirmation.

12.3.4
Statins

The molecular and cellular events leading to late toxicity after RT begin virtually immediately after the first exposure to ionizing radiation. Endothelial cell damage plays an important role in this process, and recent evidence suggests that the capillary endothelial cell may be the first cellular element to be damaged by RT (PARIS et al. 2001). Late vascular effects include, in addition to telangiectasia development, capillary collapse, thickening of the basement membrane, and loss of clonogenic capacity (PENA et al. 2000). Capillaries also may be the most sensitive component of the vascular system (RODEMANN et al. 2007a). Vascular damage is important in the phenotype of RT-induced rectal injury, where telangiectatic vessels are often responsible for the bleeding characteristic of this condition (GARG et al. 2006).

The molecular pathways involved in endothelial cell death probably involve both DNA damage-dependent and -independent mechanisms (Fig. 12.4). At higher doses (10–20 Gy), radiation-induced apoptosis, mediated through the generation of ceramide via the sphinomyelin pathway (LI et al. 2003), appears to be the dominant mechanism. Ceramide mediates the activation of three major pathways of endothelial cell apoptosis: the MAPK 8 pathway, the mitochondrial pathway, and the death receptor (TNF) pathway (RODEMANN et al. 2007a). The MAPK 8 pathway seems dominant, and this pathway results in apoptosis through the action of effector caspases (RODEMANN et al. 2007a). Similar processes are thought to mediate a number of other chronic conditions, including coronary artery disease (FORRESTER et al. 2007).

The cholesterol-lowering agents 3-hydroxy-methylglutaryl Co-A reductase (HMG Co-A reductase) inhibitors (statins) have been demonstrated to reduce the risk

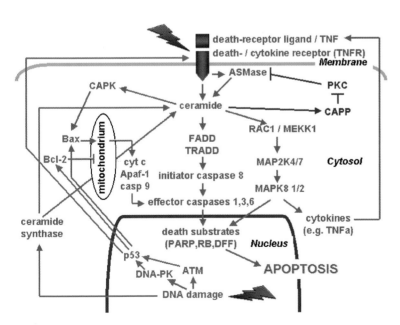

Fig. 12.4. Pathways of endothelial cell apoptosis following exposure to ionizing radiation. Reproduced from RODEMANN (2007a)

of myocardial infarction, in part, through their vascular protective effects, which are not dependent on changes in serum cholesterol levels (ROSENSON 2001). In vitro, statins have been shown to inhibit the expression and/or activity of mediators of inflammation, including reactive oxygen species, TNFα, cyclooxygenase-2, matrix metalloproteinases, and thromboxane A2, while increasing the expression of anti-inflammatory effectors, such as nitric oxide synthase (FORRESTER et al. 2007).

Emerging evidence suggests that statins may afford protection against the deleterious effects of ionizing radiation. In vitro, statins have been shown to protect human endothelial cells from ionizing radiation (GAUGLER et al. 2005; BOERMA et al. 2006; NUBEL et al. 2006). Multiple mechanisms appear to be involved, including attenuation of extracellular stress responses (RIKITAKE et al. 2001; MORIKAWA et al. 2002), down-regulation of chemokines and chemokine receptors (WAEHRE et al. 2003), and by exerting anti-inflammatory and antithrombotic effects (UNDAS et al. 2002; PEREZ-GUERRERO et al. 2003; SHI et al. 2003; BOERMA et al. 2006) on these cells. After irradiation, there is an early increase in pro-inflammatory cytokines (IL-6, TNF-α) and transcription factors (NFκB) leading to the development of lymphedema and tissue fibrosis. Statins have been shown to reduce vascular endothelial cell activation and inflammatory cytokine and transcription factor production, specifically IL-6, TNFα, and NFκB (HAYDONT et al. 2007a; PARK et al. 2008a, 2008b).

The biological rationale for statins as an interventional approach to mitigate radiation-induced injury has recently been postulated to result from inhibition of the Rho/Rock pathway, which exerts influence over vascular function and pro-inflammatory and pro-fibrotic cytokines (HAYDONT et al. 2007b). Gene arrays of irradiated tissue have shown divergent expression of genes coding for the Rho/Rock pathway from normal tissue (BOURGIER et al. 2005). Furthermore, BOURGIER and colleagues (2005) treated isolated primary intestinal smooth muscle cells from ileal biopsies taken from patients with late radiation enteritis with Rho inhibitor to determine whether it could alter the cells pro-fibrogenic phenotype. Inhibition of the Rho pathway decreased expression of both connective tissue growth factor and collagen type I. The decrease in fibrogenic activity was in contrast to isolated untreated cells, which showed cytoskeletal rearrangement, alteration in Rho pathway gene expression, and increased connective tissue growth factor (CTGF) and collagen secretion. Thus, the ability of statins to reduce inflammation and fibrotic activity (including downregulation of CTGF) when given post-radiation suggests potential mediation through the Rho/ROCK pathway. In a subsequent study by HAYDONT et al. (2005), Pravastatin, a hydrophilic statin, reduced CTGF, TGFβ, and collagen production from intestinal smooth muscle cells isolated from patients with radiation enteritis and improved radiation enteropathy in an animal model (HAYDONT et al. 2007a).

Two independent investigators found statins had a limited effect on the early, acute effects of radiation on normal intestine; however, they significantly ameliorated delayed injury, resulting in less collagen deposition and reduced mucosal injury (HAYDONT et al. 2007c; WANG et al. 2007b). HAYDONT et al. further evaluated the effect of Pravastatin on three tumor cell lines in vivo and demonstrated no protective effect on tumor response to radiation. Thus, statins may have the potential to protect against RT-induced late effects, and, in fact, atorvastatin is currently being evaluated as a treatment to prevent progression of carotid artery intima-media damage after RT to the head and neck in the Netherlands (F. Stewart, personal communication).

12.3.5
Pentoxifylline and α-Tocopherol

A number of successful clinical trials carried out over the last decade have demonstrated treatment with Pentoxifylline (PTX) and alpha-tocopherol (vitamin E) during the course of radiation therapy and up to 2 years thereafter reverses superficial fibrosis and mitigates lung injury. DELANIAN and colleagues (1999) enrolled 52 patients with symptomatic radiation-induced superficial fibrosis between 1995 and 1997. Patients were treated with a combination of 400 mg PTX and 500 IU vitamin E twice per day for 1 year after the development of fibrosis. Significant regression (mean RIF surface area) and functional improvement (SOMA) were observed 3 months to 1 year after the start of treatment with PTX-vitamin E. No unacceptable toxicity with PTX and vitamin E was observed in any of the enrolled patients. The precise mechanism of action of PTX and vitamin E is unknown; however, multiple pre-clinical and clinical studies have shown combined treatment is more effective than either given alone, suggesting a synergistic mechanism of action (LEFAIX et al. 1999). In a follow-up study published in 2005 in the *Journal of Clinical Oncology*, DELANIAN and colleagues (2005) compared short-term (6 to 12 months) versus long-term (24 to 48 months) treatment of symptomatic radiation-induced fibrosis with PTX-vitamin E. Patients receiving PTX-vitamin E had a 68% reduction in fibrosis at 24 months. However, the authors found recurrence of radiation-induced fibrosis when PTX-vitamin E treatment was discontinued (6 to 12 month treatment arm). The most significant and long-term regression of fibrosis occurred in patients treated for 3 or more years. The same year, HADDAD et al. (2005) published the results of a phase II clinical trial with 34 patients treated for 3 months with 800 mg PTX and 1,000 U vitamin E daily for superficial radiation-induced fibrosis. Patients were followed for fibrotic surface area regression and grade of fibrosis (SOMA scale). Out of the 29 patients who completed the study, the mean surface area regression at 3 months had decreased by 43% (±19%; P < 0.001). Eighteen patients who continued on PTX-vitamin E for 6 months had a 72% (±15%) reduction in surface area. MISIRLIOGLU et al. (2007) evaluated the radioprotective benefit of PTX-vitamin E in lung cancer patients receiving thoracic irradiation. Forty-four patients received 400 mg PTX three times per day and vitamin E 300 mg twice per day during the course of radiation therapy and thereafter for 3 months. Patients treated with PTX-vitamin E had significantly less acute, subacute, and long-term radiation-induced injury (RTOG/EORTC scale). These studies, taken together, suggest PTX-vitamin E is most effective when given continuously for months to years after radiation. Furthermore, the recurrence of fibrosis after cessation of treatment suggests PTX-vitamin E disrupts the ongoing processes responsible for facilitating radiation-induced fibrosis; however, it does not permanently irradicate the underlying cause. More work is needed to better define the underlying mechanisms behind the success of this therapy.

12.4
Targeting Chronic Oxidative Stress

Redox changes in tissue can have profound effects on cellular signaling and tissue interactions. In the last decade, superoxide (O_2^-) and other ROS have been shown to play important roles in intracellular signaling and cytokine induction and activation (BAI et al. 1993; RILEY 1994; MCBRIDE 1995; SCHMIDT-ULLRICH et al. 2000; DELANIAN et al. 2001; DHAR et al. 2002; MIKKELSEN et al. 2003; CUZZOCREA et al. 2004; MOELLER et al. 2004). It is becoming increasingly well known that ROS/RNS affect DNA binding and activation of several key redox-sensitive transcription factors, such as SP-1, AP-1, NF-κB, HIF-1α, and NRF1, and growth factors (TGFβ) thought to be involved in radiation-induced normal tissue injury. Experimental studies demonstrate the collapse of antioxidant status, characterized by decreased levels of Cu/Zn-SOD and gluthione peroxides, occurs within hours following radiation (ERKAL et al. 2006; BENDERITTER et al. 2007; PARK et al. 2007). The prolonged imbalance between oxygen-derived free radicals and antioxidant capacity following the initial exposure to radiation leads to amplification of signal transduction pathways involved in inflammation and fibrogenesis (FLECKENSTEIN et al. 2007b). Thus, the result is an uncontrolled and progressive increase in oxidative/nitroxidative stress leading to post-translational modification of proteins, changes in transcriptional patterns of genes regulating DNA repair, cell cycle arrest and proliferation, altered cell signaling, release of cytokines and growth factors, and inflammation.

A number of biochemical compounds, such as cysteine, cysteamine, and pentoxifylline/tocopherol, Mn salens, Mn porphyrins, Mn cyclic polyamines, and fullerenes, have been used to target oxygen-derived free radicals in an attempt to reduce radiation-induced damage. Most notably, thiol compounds (amifostine in particular) have been shown in preclinical and clinical settings to reduce normal tissue toxicity from radiation (BRIZEL et al. 2000; KOUKOURAKIS and YANNAKAKIS 2001; VUJASKOVIC et al. 2002, 2007). Thus far, amifostine has been the only FDA-approved drug for protection against radiation-induced injury in the clinical setting. In the pre-clinical setting, superoxide dismutase-based strategies have been shown to offer the most effective and efficient antioxidant capability. It has been extensively shown that overexpression of SOD or therapeutic delivery of exogenous SOD inhibits radiation-induced changes in a number of biological endpoints, including enzyme activity, membrane integrity, DNA damage, cell transformation, and cell and animal survival (SANCHIZ et al. 1996; EPPERLY et al. 1999; VOZENIN-BROTONS et al. 2001; VUJASKOVIC et al. 2002a; EPPERLY et al. 2003; KHAN et al. 2003; RABBANI et al. 2007a; STINIVASAN et al. 2007).

The mitigating effect of superoxide dismutases (Cu, Zn-SOD; MnSOD) is the result of its catalytic dismutation of superoxide anion (O_2^-) in a two-step process to oxygen and water. Vujaskovic and colleagues have shown manganese porphyrin mimetics of superoxide dismutase act as pulmonary radioprotectors in vivo as a result of their potent ROS scavenging abilities (VUJASKOVIC et al. 2002b; RABBANI et al. 2007a, 2007c; GAUTER-FLECKENSTEIN et al. 2007). In those studies, long-term administration of MnSOD mimetic improved pulmonary function and reduced morphological and histological damage after radiation (RABBANI et al. 2007a). Most importantly, activation of redox-sensitive transcription factors and signaling molecules involved in inflammation, angiogenesis, and fibrosis, such as TGF-β, HIF-1α, and NFκB, were greatly reduced. In other studies, MnSOD mimetics attenuated levels of macrophage inflammatory protein and interleukin-6 following ischemia/reperfusion injury. In a study by JACKSON et al. (2007), TGF-β production by hypoxic macrophages in vitro could be alleviated by incubation with an SOD mimetic, MnTE-2-PyP^{5+}.

In studies by EPPERLY et al. (1999), a time-dependent progression in pathologic fibrosis after irradiation

Table 12.2. Summary of pre-clinical and clinical studies using target based interventions

	Injury type	Reference
Transforming growth factor-beta (TGFβ) targets	Radiation pneumonitis/fibrosis	Preclinical: NISHIOKA et al. 2004; RABBANI et al. 2003; SCHULTZE-MOSGAU et al. 2003; ANSCHER et al. 2006, 2008
Recombinant human keratinocyte growth factor (rHuKGF/Palifermin)	Radiation pneumonitis/fibrosis	Preclinical: CHEN et al. 2004; YI et al. 1996
	Esophagitis/nucositis/xerostomia	Preclinical: DORR et al. 2001, 2005c, 2005b, clinical: RADTKE et al. 2005; BRIZEL et al. 2008
	Gastrointestinal	Preclinical: FARRELL et al. 1998
	Bladder	Preclinical: JAAL et al. 2007
Angiotensin-converting enzyme (ACE) inhibitors (butylaminiperindopril, captopril)	Radiation pneumonitis/fibrosis	Preclinical: WARD et al. 1988, 1989; MOLTENI et al. 2000; MATEJ et al. 2007
		Preclinical: MOULDER et al. 1997a
	Gastrointestinal	Preclinical: MOULDER et al. 1993, 1998a, 2007a; COHEN et al. 1997 Clinical: COHEN et al. 2008
	Radiation nephropathy	KIM et al. 2004; RYU et al. 2007
	Optical neuropathy	
Statins	Radiation induced enteropathy	Preclinical: HAYDONT et al. 2007c; WANG et al. 2007b Preclinical: WILLIAMS et al. 2004).
	Pulmonary fibrosis	
Pentoxifylline ± alpha-tocopherol (vitamin E)	Radiation pneumonitis/fibrosis	Preclinical: RUBE et al. 2002; KOH et al. 1995 Clinical: MISIRLIOGLU et al. 2007; OZTURK et al. 2004
	Subcutaneous fibrosis	Clinical: HADDAD et al. 2005; OKUNIEFF et al. 2004; DELANIAN et al. 2003; LEFAIX et al. 1999; DELANIAN 1998
	Uterine	Clinical: LETUR-KONIRSCH et al. 2002
Amifostine	Multiple	Preclinical: VUJASKOVIC et al. 2002c;
		Clinical: VEERASARN et al. 2006; ANTONADOU et al. 2003, 2001; KOMAKI et al. 2004; KOUKOURAKIS et al. 2001; PHAN et al. 2001; MOVSAS et al. 2005; BRIZEL et al. 2000; TROG et al. 1999
		Preclinical: VUJASKOVIC et al. 2007
Superoxide dismutase-based strategies	Radiation pneumonitis/fibrosis	Preclinical: GAUTER-FLECKENSTEIN et al. 2007; RABBANI et al. 2007c, 2007b, 2005; EPPERLY et al. 2004, 2002a; GUO et al. 2003

indicated increased IL-1 mRNA levels correlated with early radiation pneumonitis, followed by an increase in TGF-β during the development of fibrotic disease and mortality. Moreover, EPPERLY et al. (2000b) found manganese-SOD plasmid/liposome complex could prevent DNA double-strand breaks, inhibit mitochondrial-dependent apoptosis, reduce vascular adhesion molecule expression (EPPERLY et al. 2002c), and decrease early onset of TGFβ, IL-1, and TNF-α mRNA levels (EPPERLY et al. 2000a), as well as improve median survival time (EPPERLY et al. 2000b). A series of SOD gene therapy studies in animals have also suggested the protective effect of SOD from radiation toxicity in the esophagus and lung (EPPERLY et al. 2000a). Furthermore, it has been shown that the administration of liposomal Cu/Zn-SOD and MnSOD up to 6 months after irradiation in an experimental animal model was shown to reverse radiation-induced fibrosis (LEFAIX et al. 1996). Studies using a combined treatment of Cu/Zn-SOD and L-NAME was effective against indirect damage caused by reactive species generated in rat lung tissue after radiation (KHAN et al. 2003). Currently, Cu/Zn-SOD has been used in the clinical application of radiation therapy in Europe to reduce the severity of mucositis, cystitis, and fibrosis (SANCHIZ et al. 1996; VALENCIA et al. 2002; ESCO et al. 2004). Cu/Zn-SOD has been shown to reduce DNA damage and chromosomal aberrations, decrease activation of pro-inflammatory transcription factors and signaling molecules, and ameliorate radiation-induced injury (BREUER et al. 1992; LEFAIX et al. 1996; DELANIAN et al. 2001; PETER et al. 2001; VOZENIN-BROTONS et al. 2001). Multiple studies have shown superoxide dismutase-based strategies reduce expression of pro-inflammatory and profibrogenic cytokines and growth factors, as well as cellular adhesion molecules diminishing leukocyte recruitment into the injured tissue. Furthermore, the elimination of free-radical bioavailability to activate TGF-β results in decreased extracellular matrix formation and increased matrix degradation. The consequence is decreased inflammation and fibro-proliferation and mitigation of architectural/structural damage and overall reduction in lung injury. Table 12.2 outlines a summary of relevant findings.

12.5

Stem Cell Therapy

Recent insight into the role of stem cells in radiation-induced injury has opened the door to new therapeutic interventions focused on mobilization of bone marrow-derived stem cells to replenish the depleted cell population and restore tissue function after radiation. It has been hypothesized that radiation-induced depletion of stem cells in the gastrointestinal villi and salivary glands contribute to the development of acute and long-term injury in these tissues. Several investigators have hypothesized the dose effect of radiation injury was characteristic of the number of stem cells killed after radiation. For example, it has been suggested hyposalivation following radiation for head and neck cancer results from the depletion of the progenitor cell population and inability to regenerate acinar and ductal cells for normal salivary gland function. LOMBAERT et al. (2006) delivered 15-Gy single-dose irradiation to the salivary glands of female mice transplanted with eGFP+ bone marrow from male mice. The dose was sufficient to induce morphological, histological, and functional injury to the submandibular salivary glands. Salivary glands from irradiated control mice had complete reduction in saliva production at 90 days and substantial atrophy of the glands, decrease in perfusion, and acinar and ductal cell apoptosis at 130 days after irradiation. Bone marrow stem cells from irradiated chimeric mice were stimulated at 10, 30, or 60 days with granulocyte-colony stimulating factor (GCSF). GCSF-stimulated mice showed significantly improved tissue function measured by increased saliva production, reduced salivary gland atrophy, improved gland color and increased gland weight, and restoration of the number of acinar and ductal gland cells. Unexpectedly, neither the acinar nor ductal cells of the irradiated eGFP+ chimeric mice expressed eGFP/Y chromosome upon histological examination, suggesting the increased number of acinar and ductal cells was not bone marrow derived. Based on the proximity of eGFP signal to myoepithelial cells, the authors could not rule out bone marrow origin of myoepithelial cells. However, the presence of co-localized CD31 and eGFP in mesenchymal cells led the authors to conclude that the majority of the bone marrow-derived stem cells in the irradiated tissue were endothelial/mesenchymal and that these cells played a major role in the restoration of gland function and amelioration of histological and morphological injury. Studies by MOUISEDDINE et al. (2007) support the conclusions by Lombaert's study that stem cells of mesenchymal origin may play a role in amelioration of radiation-induced injury. MOUISSEDINE et al. (2007) found human bone marrow-derived cells migrated to irradiated tissue and tissue outside the irradiated field after local or total body irradiation (FRANCOIS et al. 2006). These promising studies encourage further exploration of the potentially beneficial role of stem cell therapy for amelioration of radiation-induced normal tissue injury.

12.6
Additional Targets

The aforementioned therapeutic interventions have been the most well studied; however, as our understanding of the molecular mechanisms of radiation-induced normal tissue injury has grown, novel pathways have emerged that might be targeted to prevent, mitigate, or treat radiation-induced normal tissue. In a recent issue of *Science*, BURDELYA and colleagues (2008) used a novel agent, CBLB502, to target Toll-like receptor 5, a ligand for NFκB expressed on enterocytes, dendritic and endothelial cells. Burdelya hypothesized CBLB502, a potent NFκB activator, would prevent NFκB-mediated p53-dependent apoptosis and improve overall survival. In those studies, CBLB502 rescued 87% of mice from lethal total body irradiation in the range of 10–13 Gy. Similarly, Burdelya found compounds that did not activate NFκB in vitro also did not protect mice from lethal total body irradiation. These results, along with studies using TLR5 knockout mice in which CBLB502 was ineffective as a radiation protector, led the authors to conclude that NFκB-mediated activation of TLR5 signaling is necessary for protection against radiation-induced lethality. Molecular analysis of tissue from CBLB502-treated animals demonstrated reduced small intestine toxicity with CBLB502 as compared to irradiated controls, including significantly less apoptosis of cells in the lamina propria and endothelial cells. However, CBLB502 was only effective when given prophylactically, thus limiting its use to therapeutic radiation rather than use for accidental or deliberate exposures, such as in the case of a nuclear accident or attack. At lower radiation doses (<9 Gy), CBLB502 improved overall animal survival (7% controls vs. 40% treated) when given within an hour post-exposure. CBLB502 underwent further evaluation in non-human primate studies. In these studies, CBLB502 did not exhibit any signs of toxicity. Non-human primates received 6.5 Gy total body irradiation ($LD_{50/70}$) 45 min after a single injection of 0.04 mg/kg CBLB502. CBLB502 increased the 40-day survival from 25 to 64%. Likewise, CBLB502 has been shown to have no radioprotective effect on tumors, making this compound an ideal agent for clinical trial.

Other novel pathways for therapeutic intervention have focused on neuroimmune interactions and the use of neuropeptides. The enteric nervous system has in gastrointestinal homeostasis, for example, regulation of secretion, motility, immune function, microcirculation, as well as orchestrates interactions between the immune system and fibroproliferation (WANG et al. 2007c). Thus, Wang, Hauer-Jensen, and colleagues have performed several studies to further explore the role of the neuroimmune system in radiation-induced gastrointestinal injury. In earlier studies, the group found mast cells to be an integral component of the gastrointestinal response to radiation. Mast cell-mediated regulation of epithelial barrier function and vascular permeability, two key components dysregulated in the gastrointestinal syndrome, is under the control of sensory enteric nerves. Thus, the neuroimmune interactions between these cells provide a potential target for therapeutic intervention (WANG et al. 2007a). In a 2006 study, sensory nerve ablation using a neuropeptide increased acute gastrointestinal toxicity (inflammation, mucosal surface area), yet proved effective in reducing fibrosis by a mast-cell dependent mechanism (WANG et al. 2006b). In further studies, WANG and colleagues (2006a) found two neuropeptides, substance P and calcitonin gene-related peptide (CGRP) were increased after localized irradiation of the intestine. Using substance P and CGRP antagonists, the authors found these neuropeptides have opposing effects on the intestinal mucosa during the development of radiation-induced intestinal injury. The authors concluded CGRP antagonists may be beneficial as radioprotectors, and further evaluation is warranted to evaluate their ability to mitigate radiation-induced intestinal injury.

12.7
Conclusions

The identification of molecular pathways involved in radiation-induced normal tissue injury has resulted in the identification of potential candidates for targeted therapies. To date, few of these compounds have been tested in the clinic. The most thoroughly investigated agents for use as mitigators and/or treatment for radiation-induced normal tissue injury have been antioxidant compounds, ACE inhibitors, and growth factors. Interest in this area of research, however, is growing, and newer agents will be developed that may prevent the development of radiation-induced injury in the future. Agents already in the clinic for other purposes, such as the statins, are being tested because of mechanisms of action that are relevant to radiation protection. Thus, in the near future we should have more to offer patients currently suffering from normal tissue injury from cancer therapy.

References

Andarawewa KL, Erickson AC, Chou WS et al. (2007a) Ionizing radiation predisposes nonmalignant human mammary epithelial cells to undergo transforming growth factor beta induced epithelial to mesenchymal transition. Cancer Res 67: 8662–8670

Andarawewa KL, Paupert J, Pal A et al. (2007b) New rationales for using TGFbeta inhibitors in radiotherapy. Int J Radiat Biol 83: 803–811

Anscher MS, Murase T, Prescott DM et al. (1994) Changes in plasma TGF beta levels during pulmonary radiotherapy as a predictor of the risk of developing radiation pneumonitis. Int J Radiat Oncol Biol Phys 30: 671–676

Anscher MS, Marks LB, Shafman TD et al. (2001) Using plasma transforming growth factor beta-1 during radiotherapy to select patients for dose escalation. J Clin Oncol 19: 3758–3765

Anscher MS, Thrasher B, Rabbani Z et al. (2006) Antitransforming growth factor-beta antibody 1D11 ameliorates normal tissue damage caused by high-dose radiation. Int J Radiat Oncol Biol Phys 65: 876–881

Anscher MS, Thrasher B, Zgonjanin L et al. (2008) Small molecular inhibitor of transforming growth factor-beta protects against development of radiation-induced lung injury. Int J Radiat Oncol Biol Phys 71: 829–837

Antonadou D, Coliarakis N, Synodinou M et al. (2001) Randomized phase III trial of radiation treatment +/− amifostine in patients with advanced-stage lung cancer. Int J Radiat Oncol Biol Phys 51: 915–922

Antonadou D, Throuvalas N, Petridis A et al. (2003) Effect of amifostine on toxicities associated with radiochemotherapy in patients with locally advanced non-small-cell lung cancer. Int J Radiat Oncol Biol Phys 57: 402–408

Arriagada R, Le Chevalier T, Quoix E et al. (1991) ASTRO (American Society for Therapeutic Radiology and Oncology) plenary: Effect of chemotherapy on locally advanced non-small cell lung carcinoma: a randomized study of 353 patients. GETCB (Groupe d'Etude et Traitement des Cancers Bronchiques), FNCLCC (Federation Nationale des Centres de Lutte contre le Cancer) and the CEBI trialists. Int J Radiat Oncol Biol Phys 20: 1183–1190

Bai Y, Wang D, Wang L et al. (1993) The role of free radicals in the development of radiation interstitial pneumonitis. J Env Pathol Toxicol Oncol 12: 199–204

Barcellos-Hoff MH (1993) Radiation-induced transforming growth factor beta and subsequent extracellular matrix reorganization in murine mammary gland. Cancer Res 53: 3880–3386

Barcellos-Hoff MH, Derynck R, Tsang ML et al. (1994) Transforming growth factor-beta activation in irradiated murine mammary gland. J Clin Invest 93: 892–899

Barcellos-Hoff MH (1996) Latency and activation in the control of TGF-beta. J Mammary Gland Biol Neoplasia 1: 353–363

Barcellos-Hoff MH, Dix TA (1996) Redox-mediated activation of latent transforming growth factor-beta 1. Mol Endocrinol 10: 1077–1083

Benderitter M, Isoir M, Buard V et al. (2007) Collapse of skin antioxidant status during the subacute period of cutaneous radiation syndrome: a case report. Radiat Res 167: 43–50

Boerma M, Burton GR, Wang J et al. (2006) Comparative expression profiling in primary and immortalized endothelial cells: changes in gene expression in response to hydroxy methylglutaryl-coenzyme A reductase inhibition. Blood Coagul Fibrinolysis 17: 173–180

Bourgier C, Haydont V, Milliat F et al. (2005) Inhibition of Rho kinase modulates radiation induced fibrogenic phenotype in intestinal smooth muscle cells through alteration of the cytoskeleton and connective tissue growth factor expression. Gut 54: 336–343

Brach MA, Hass R, Sherman ML et al. (1991) Ionizing radiation induces expression and binding activity of the nuclear factor kappa B. J Clin Invest 88: 691–695

Breuer R, Tochner Z, Conner MW et al. (1992) Superoxide dismutase inhibits radiation-induced lung injury in hamsters. Lung 170: 19–29

Brizel DM, Wasserman TH, Henke M et al. (2000) Phase III randomized trial of amifostine as a radioprotector in head and neck cancer. J Clin Oncol 18: 3339–3345

Brizel DM (ed):(2005) Strategies for protecting normal tissue in the treatment of head and neck cancer. In: Adelstein DJ, ed: Squamous Cell Head and Neck Cancer Recent Clinical Progress and Prospects for the Future. Totowa, NJ, Humana Press, pp 228

Brizel DM (2007) Pharmacologic approaches to radiation protection. J Clin Oncol 25: 4084–4089

Brizel DM, Murphy BA, Rosenthal DI et al. (2008) Phase II study of palifermin and concurrent chemoradiation in head and neck squamous cell carcinoma. J Clin Oncol 26: 2489–2496

Brush J, Lipnick SL, Phillips T et al. (2007) Molecular mechanisms of late normal tissue injury. Semin Radiat Oncol 17: 121–130

Burdelya LG, Krivokrysenko VI, Tallant TC et al. (2008) An agonist of toll-like receptor 5 has radioprotective activity in mouse and primate models. Science 320: 226–230

Chen L, Brizel DM, Rabbani ZN et al. (2004) The protective effect of recombinant human keratinocyte growth factor on radiation-induced pulmonary toxicity in rats. Int J Radiat Oncol Biol Phys 60: 1520–1529

Cohen EP, Fish BL, and Moulder JE (1997) Successful brief captopril treatment in experimental radiation nephropathy. J Lab Clin Med 129: 536–547

Cohen EP, Irving AA, Drobyski WR et al. (2008) Captopril to mitigate chronic renal failure after hematopoietic stem cell transplantation: a randomized controlled trial. Int J Radiat Oncol Biol Phys 70: 1546–1551

Cox JD, Azarnia N, Byhardt RW et al. (1990) A randomized phase I/II trial of hyperfractionated radiation therapy with total doses of 60.0 Gy to 79.2 Gy: possible survival benefit with greater than or equal to 69.6 Gy in favorable patients with Radiation Therapy Oncology Group stage III non-small-cell lung carcinoma: report of Radiation Therapy Oncology Group 83–11. J Clin Oncol 8: 1543–1555

Cuzzocrea S, Pisano B, Dugo L et al. (2004) Superoxide-related signaling cascade mediates nuclear factor-kB activation in acute inflammation. Antioxidants and Redox Signaling 6: 699–704

Delanian S (1998) Striking regression of radiation-induced fibrosis by a combination of pentoxifylline and tocopherol. Br J Radiol 71: 892–894

Delanian S, Balla-Mekias S, Lefaix JL (1999) Striking regression of chronic radiotherapy damage in a clinical trial of combined pentoxifylline and tocopherol. J Clin Oncol 17: 3283–3290

Delanian S, Martin M, Bravard A et al. (2001) Cu/Zn superoxide dismutase modulates phenotypic changes in cultured fibroblasts from human skin with chronic radiotherapy damage. Radiother Oncol 58: 325–331

Delanian S, Porcher R, Balla-Mekias S et al. (2003) Randomized, placebo-controlled trial of combined pentoxifylline and tocopherol for regression of superficial radiation-induced fibrosis. J Clin Oncol 21: 2545–2550

Delanian S, Porcher R, Rudant J et al. (2005) Kinetics of response to long-term treatment combining pentoxifylline and tocopherol in patients with superficial radiation-induced fibrosis. J Clin Oncol 23: 8570–8579

Delanian S, Lefaix JL (2007) Current management for late normal tissue injury: radiation-induced fibrosis and necrosis. Semin Radiat Oncol 17: 99–107

Dewhirst MW, Gustafson C, Gross JF et al. (1987) Temporal effects of 5.0 Gy radiation in healing subcutaneous microvasculature of a dorsal flap window chamber. Radiat Res 112: 581–591

Dhar A, Young MR, Colburn NH (2002) The role of AP-1, NF-kB and ROS/NOS in skin carcinogenesis: The JB-6 model is predictive. Mol Cell Biochem 234/235: 185–193

Dorr W, Noack R, Spekl K et al. (2001) Modification of oral mucositis by keratinocyte growth factor: single radiation exposure. Int J Radiat Biol 77: 341–347

Dorr W, Spekl K, Farrell CL (2002) The effect of keratinocyte growth factor on healing of manifest radiation ulcers in mouse tongue epithelium. Cell Prolif 35 Suppl 1: 86–92

Dorr W, Bassler S, Reichel S et al. (2005a) Reduction of radiochemotherapy-induced early oral mucositis by recombinant human keratinocyte growth factor (palifermin): experimental studies in mice. Int J Radiat Oncol Biol Phys 62: 881–887

Dorr W, Heider K, Spekl K (2005b) Reduction of oral mucositis by palifermin (rHuKGF): dose-effect of rHuKGF. Int J Radiat Biol 81: 557–565

Dorr W, Reichel S, Spekl K (2005c) Effects of keratinocyte growth factor (palifermin) administration protocols on oral mucositis (mouse) induced by fractionated irradiation. Radiother Oncol 75: 99–105

Dosoretz DE, Galmarini D, Rubenstein JH et al. (1993) Local control in medically inoperable lung cancer: an analysis of its importance in outcome and factors determining the probability of tumor eradication. Int J Radiat Oncol Biol Phys 27: 507–516

Ehrhart EJ, Segarini P, Tsang ML et al. (1997) Latent transforming growth factor beta1 activation in situ: quantitative and functional evidence after low-dose gamma-irradiation. Faseb J 11: 991–1002

Emami B, Lyman J, Brown A et al. (1991) Tolerance of normal tissue to therapeutic irradiation. Int J Radiat Oncol Biol Phys 21: 109–122

Epperly MW, Travis EL, Sikora C et al. (1999) Manganese [correction of Magnesium] superoxide dismutase (MnSOD) plasmid/liposome pulmonary radioprotective gene therapy: modulation of irradiation-induced mRNA for IL-I, TNF-alpha, and TGF-beta correlates with delay of organizing alveolitis/fibrosis. Biol Blood Marrow Transplant 5: 204–214

Epperly MW, Defilippi S, Sikora C et al. (2000a) Intratracheal injection of manganese superoxide dismutase (MnSOD) plasmid/liposomes protects normal lung but not orthotopic tumors from irradiation. Gene Ther 7: 1011–1018

Epperly MW, Epstein CJ, Travis EL et al. (2000b) Decreased pulmonary radiation resistance of manganese superoxide dismutase (MnSOD)-deficient mice is corrected by human manganese superoxide dismutase-Plasmid/Liposome (SOD2-PL) intratracheal gene therapy. Radiat Res 154: 365–374

Epperly MW, Defilippi S, Sikora C et al. (2002a) Radioprotection of lung and esophagus by overexpression of the human manganese superoxide dismutase transgene. Mil Med 167: 71–73

Epperly MW, Sikora CA, DeFilippi SJ et al. (2002b) Manganese superoxide dismutase (SOD2) inhibits radiation-induced apoptosis by stabilization of the mitochondrial membrane. Radiat Res 157: 568–577

Epperly MW, Sikora CA, DeFilippi SJ et al. (2002c) Pulmonary irradiation-induced expression of VCAM-I and ICAM-I is decreased by manganese superoxide dismutase-plasmid/liposome (MnSOD-PL) gene therapy. Biol Blood Marrow Transplant 8: 175–187

Epperly MW, Gretton JE, Sikora CA et al. (2003) Mitochondrial localization of superoxide dismutase is required for decreasing radiation-induced cellular damage. Radiat Res 160: 568–578

Epperly MW, Carpenter M, Agarwal A et al. (2004) Intraoral manganese superoxide dismutase-plasmid/liposome (MnSOD-PL) radioprotective gene therapy decreases ionizing irradiation-induced murine mucosal cell cycling and apoptosis. In Vivo 18: 401–410

Erkal HS, Batcioglu K, Serin M et al. (2006) The evaluation of the oxidant injury as a function of time following brain irradiation in a rat model. Neurochem Res 31: 1271–1277

Esco R, Valencia J, Coronel P et al. (2004) Efficacy of orgotein in prevention of late side effects of pelvic irradiation: a randomized study. Int J Radiat Oncol Biol Phys 60: 1211–1219

Farrell CL, Bready JV, Rex KL et al. (1998) Keratinocyte growth factor protects mice from chemotherapy and radiation-induced gastrointestinal injury and mortality. Cancer Res 58: 933–939

Fedorocko P, Egyed A, Vacek A (2002) Irradiation induces increased production of haemopoietic and proinflammatory cytokines in the mouse lung. Int J Radiat Biol 78: 305–313

Fehrenbach H, Kasper M, Tschernig T et al. (1999) Keratinocyte growth factor-induced hyperplasia of rat alveolar type II cells in vivo is resolved by differentiation into type I cells and by apoptosis. Eur Respir J 14: 534–544

Fehrenbach H, Kasper M, Koslowski R et al. (2000) Alveolar epithelial type II cell apoptosis in vivo during resolution of keratinocyte growth factor-induced hyperplasia in the rat. Histochem Cell Biol 114: 49–61

Fehrenbach H, Fehrenbach A, Pan T et al. (2002) Keratinocyte growth factor-induced proliferation of rat airway epithelium is restricted to Clara cells in vivo. Eur Respir J 20: 1185–1197

Flanders KC (2004) Smad3 as a mediator of the fibrotic response. Int J Exp Pathol 85: 47–64

Fleckenstein K, Zgonjanin L, Chen L et al. (2007a) Temporal onset of hypoxia and oxidative stress after pulmonary irradiation. Int J Radiat Oncol Biol Physics 68: 196–204

Fleckenstein K, Zgonjanin L, Chen L et al. (2007b) Temporal onset of hypoxia and oxidative stress after pulmonary irradiation. Int J Radiat Oncol Biol Phys 68: 196–204

Forrester JS, Libby P (2007) The inflammation hypothesis and its potential relevance to statin therapy. Am J Cardiol 99: 732–738

Francois S, Bensidhoum M, Mouiseddine M et al. (2006) Local irradiation not only induces homing of human mesenchymal stem cells at exposed sites but promotes their widespread engraftment to multiple organs: a study of their quantitative distribution after irradiation damage. Stem Cells 24: 1020–1029

Garg AK, Mai WY, McGary JE et al. (2006) Radiation proctopathy in the treatment of prostate cancer. Int J Radiat Oncol Biol Phys 66: 1294–1305

Gaugler MH, Vereycken-Holler V, Squiban C et al. (2005) Pravastatin limits endothelial activation after irradiation and decreases the resulting inflammatory and thrombotic responses. Radiat Res 163: 479–487

Gauter-Fleckenstein B, Fleckenstein K, Owzar K et al. (2007) Comparison of two Mn porphyrin-based mimics of superoxide dismutase in pulmonary radioprotection. Free Radic Biol Med 44: 982–989

Guo HL, Wolfe D, Epperly MW et al. (2003) Gene transfer of human manganese superoxide dismutase protects small intestinal villi from radiation injury. J Gastrointest Surg 7: 229–235; discussion 235–236

Haddad P, Kalaghchi B, Amouzegar-Hashemi F (2005) Pentoxifylline and vitamin E combination for superficial radiation-induced fibrosis: a phase II clinical trial. Radiother Oncol 77: 324–326

Hallahan DE, Geng L, Shyr Y (2002) Effects of intercellular adhesion molecule 1 (ICAM-1) null mutation on radiation-induced pulmonary fibrosis and respiratory insufficiency in mice. J Natl Cancer Inst 94: 733–741

Hauer-Jensen M, Kong FM, Fink LM et al. (1999) Circulating thrombomodulin during radiation therapy of lung cancer. Radiat Oncol Invest 7: 238–242

Haydont V, Mathe D, Bourgier C et al. (2005) Induction of CTGF by TGF-beta1 in normal and radiation enteritis human smooth muscle cells: Smad/Rho balance and therapeutic perspectives. Radiother Oncol 76: 219–225

Haydont V, Bourgier C, Pocard M et al. (2007a) Pravastatin Inhibits the Rho/CCN2/extracellular matrix cascade in human fibrosis explants and improves radiation-induced intestinal fibrosis in rats. Clin Cancer Res 13: 5331–5340

Haydont V, Bourgier C, Vozenin-Brotons MC (2007b) Rho/ROCK pathway as a molecular target for modulation of intestinal radiation-induced toxicity. Br J Radiol 80 Spec No 1: S32–40

Haydont V, Gilliot O, Rivera S et al. (2007c) Successful mitigation of delayed intestinal radiation injury using pravastatin is not associated with acute injury improvement or tumor protection. Int J Radiat Oncol Biol Phys 68: 1471–1482

Hong JH, Chiang CS, Campbell IL et al. (1995) Induction of acute phase gene expression by brain irradiation. Int J Radiat Oncol Biol Phys 33: 619–626

Hong JH, Jung SM, Tsao TC et al. (2003) Bronchoalveolar lavage and interstitial cells have different roles in radiation-induced lung injury. Int J Radiat Biol 79: 159–167

Huang M, Sharma S, Zhu LX et al. (2002) IL-7 inhibits fibroblast TGF-beta production and signaling in pulmonary fibrosis. J Clin Invest 109: 931–937

Jaal J, Dorr W (2007) Effect of recombinant human keratinocyte growth factor (rHuKGF, Palifermin) on radiation-induced mouse urinary bladder dysfunction. Int J Radiat Oncol Biol Phys 69: 528–533

Jackson IL, Chen L, Batinic-Haberle I et al. (2007) Superoxide dismutase mimetic reduces hypoxia-induced O2*-, TGF-beta, and VEGF production by macrophages. Free Radic Res 41: 8–14

Jemal A, Murray T, Ward E et al. (2005) Cancer statistics, 2005. CA Cancer J Clin 55: 10–30

Jobling MF, Mott JD, Finnegan MT et al. (2006) Isoform-specific activation of latent transforming growth factor beta (LTGF-beta) by reactive oxygen species. Radiat Res 166: 839–848

Johnston CJ, Piedboeuf B, Baggs R et al. (1995) Differences in correlation of mRNA gene expression in mice sensitive and resistant to radiation-induced pulmonary fibrosis. Radiat Res 142: 197–203

Keall P, Vedam S, George R et al. (2006) The clinical implementation of respiratory-gated intensity-modulated radiotherapy. Med Dosim 31: 152–162

Khan MA, Van Dyk J, Yeung IW et al. (2003) Partial volume rat lung irradiation; assessment of early DNA damage in different lung regions and effect of radical scavengers. Radiother Oncol 66: 95–102

Kim JH, Brown SL, Kolozsvary A et al. (2004) Modification of radiation injury by ramipril, inhibitor of angiotensin-converting enzyme, on optic neuropathy in the rat. Radiat Res 161: 137–142

Koh WJ, Stelzer KJ, Peterson LM et al. (1995) Effect of pentoxifylline on radiation-induced lung and skin toxicity in rats. Int J Radiat Oncol Biol Phys 31: 71–77

Komaki R, Lee JS, Milas L et al. (2004) Effects of amifostine on acute toxicity from concurrent chemotherapy and radiotherapy for inoperable non-small-cell lung cancer: report of a randomized comparative trial. Int J Radiat Oncol Biol Phys 58: 1369–1377

Koukourakis MI, Yannakakis D (2001) High dose daily amifostine and hypofractionated intensively accelerated radiotherapy for locally advanced breast cancer. A phase I/II study and report on early and late sequellae. Anticancer Res 21: 2973–2978

Lefaix JL, Delanian S, Leplat JJ et al. (1996) Successful treatment of radiation-induced fibrosis using Cu/Zn-SOD and Mn-SOD: an experimental study. Int J Radiat Oncol Biol Phys 35: 305–312

Lefaix JL, Delanian S, Vozenin MC et al. (1999) Striking regression of subcutaneous fibrosis induced by high doses of gamma rays using a combination of pentoxifylline and alpha-tocopherol: an experimental study. Int J Radiat Oncol Biol Phys 43: 839–847

Letur-Konirsch H, Guis F, Delanian S (2002) Uterine restoration by radiation sequelae regression with combined pentoxifylline-tocopherol: a phase II study. Fertil Steril 77: 1219–1226

Li YQ, Chen P, Haimovitz-Friedman A et al. (2003) Endothelial apoptosis initiates acute blood-brain barrier disruption after ionizing radiation. Cancer Res 63: 5950–5956

Lombaert IM, Wierenga PK, Kok T et al. (2006) Mobilization of bone marrow stem cells by granulocyte colony-stimulating factor ameliorates radiation-induced damage to salivary glands. Clin Cancer Res 12: 1804–1812

Martin M, Lefaix J, Delanian S (2000) TGF-beta1 and radiation fibrosis: a master switch and a specific therapeutic target? Int J Radiat Oncol Biol Phys 47: 277–290

Matej R, Housa D, Pouckova P et al. (2007) Radiation-induced production of PAR-1 and TGF-beta 1 mRNA in lung of C57Bl6 and C3H murine strains and influence of pharmacoprophylaxis by ACE inhibitors. Pathol Res Pract 203: 107–114

McBride WH (1995) Cytokine cascades in late normal tissue radiation responses. Int J Radiat Oncol Biol Phys 33: 233–234

Michalowski A (1984) A critical appraisal of clonogenic survival assays in the evaluation of radiation damage to normal tissues. Radiother Oncol 1: 241–246

Mikkelsen RB, Wardman P (2003) Biological chemistry of reactive oxygen and nitrogen and radiation-induced signal transduction mechanisms. Oncogene 22: 5734–5754

Milano MT, Constine LS, Okunieff P (2007) Normal tissue tolerance dose metrics for radiation therapy of major organs. Semin Radiat Oncol 17: 131–140

Misirlioglu CH, Demirkasimoglu T, Kucukplakci B et al. (2007) Pentoxifylline and alpha-tocopherol in prevention of radiation-induced lung toxicity in patients with lung cancer. Med Oncol 24: 308–311

Moeller BJ, Cao Y, Li CY et al. (2004) Radiation activates HIF-1 to regulate vascular radiosensitivity in tumors: Role of reoxygenation, free radicals, and stress granules. Cancer Cell 5: 429–441

Molteni A, Moulder JE, Cohen EF et al. (2000) Control of radiation-induced pneumopathy and lung fibrosis by angiotensin-converting enzyme inhibitors and an angiotensin II type 1 receptor blocker. Int J Radiat Biol 76: 523–532

Molteni A, Wolfe LF, Ward WF et al. (2007) Effect of an angiotensin II receptor blocker and two angiotensin converting enzyme inhibitors on transforming growth factor-beta (TGF-beta) and alpha-actomyosin (alpha SMA), important mediators of radiation-induced pneumopathy and lung fibrosis. Curr Pharm Des 13: 1307–1316

Morikawa S, Takabe W, Mataki C et al. (2002) The effect of statins on mRNA levels of genes related to inflammation, coagulation, and vascular constriction in HUVEC. Human umbilical vein endothelial cells. J Atheroscler Thromb 9: 178–183

Mouiseddine M, Francois S, Semont A et al. (2007) Human mesenchymal stem cells home specifically to radiation-injured tissues in a non-obese diabetes/severe combined immunodeficiency mouse model. Br J Radiol 80 Spec No 1: S49–55

Moulder JE, Fish BL, Cohen EP (1993) Treatment of radiation nephropathy with ACE inhibitors. Int J Radiat Oncol Biol Phys 27: 93–99

Moulder JE, Fish BL, Cohen EP et al. (1996) Angiotensin II receptor antagonists in the prevention of radiation nephropathy. Radiat Res 146: 106–110

Moulder JE, Fish BL (1997a) Angiotensin converting enzyme inhibitor captopril does not prevent acute gastrointestinal radiation damage in the rat. Radiat Oncol Investig 5: 50–53

Moulder JE, Fish BL, Cohen EP (1997b) Noncontinuous use of angiotensin converting enzyme inhibitors in the treatment of experimental bone marrow transplant nephropathy. Bone Marrow Transplant 19: 729–735

Moulder JE, Fish BL, Cohen EP (1998a) Radiation nephropathy is treatable with an angiotensin converting enzyme inhibitor or an angiotensin II type-1 (AT1) receptor antagonist. Radiother Oncol 46: 307–315

Moulder JE, Fish BL, Cohen EP (1998b) Angiotensin II receptor antagonists in the treatment and prevention of radiation nephropathy. Int J Radiat Biol 73: 415–421

Moulder JE, Fish BL, Cohen EP (1998c) Brief pharmacological intervention in experimental radiation nephropathy. Radiat Res 150: 535–541

Moulder JE, Fish BL, Cohen EP (2002) Dietary sodium modification and experimental radiation nephropathy. Int J Radiat Biol 78: 903–911

Moulder JE (2003) Pharmacological intervention to prevent or ameliorate chronic radiation injuries. Semin Radiat Oncol 13: 73–84

Moulder JE, Fish BL, Cohen EP (2003) ACE inhibitors and AII receptor antagonists in the treatment and prevention of bone marrow transplant nephropathy. Curr Pharm Des 9: 737–749

Moulder JE, Cohen EP (2007a) Future strategies for mitigation and treatment of chronic radiation-induced normal tissue injury. Semin Radiat Oncol 17: 141–148

Moulder JE, Fish BL, Cohen EP (2007b) Treatment of radiation nephropathy with ACE inhibitors and AII type-1 and type-2 receptor antagonists. Curr Pharm Des 13: 1317–1325

Movsas B, Scott C, Langer C et al. (2005) Randomized trial of amifostine in locally advanced non-small-cell lung cancer patients receiving chemotherapy and hyperfractionated radiation: radiation therapy oncology group trial 98-01. J Clin Oncol 23: 2145–2154

Nishioka A, Ogawa Y, Mima T et al. (2004) Histopathologic amelioration of fibroproliferative change in rat irradiated lung using soluble transforming growth factor-beta (TGF-beta) receptor mediated by adenoviral vector. Int J Radiat Oncol Biol Phys 58: 1235–1241

Nubel T, Damrot J, Roos WP et al. (2006) Lovastatin protects human endothelial cells from killing by ionizing radiation without impairing induction and repair of DNA double-strand breaks. Clin Cancer Res 12: 933–939

Okunieff P, Augustine E, Hicks JE et al. (2004) Pentoxifylline in the treatment of radiation-induced fibrosis. J Clin Oncol 22: 2207–2213

Ozturk B, Egehan I, Atavci S et al. (2004) Pentoxifylline in prevention of radiation-induced lung toxicity in patients with breast and lung cancer: a double-blind randomized trial. Int J Radiat Oncol Biol Phys 58: 213–219

Paris F, Fuks Z, Kang A et al. (2001) Endothelial apoptosis as the primary lesion initiating intestinal radiation damage in mice. Science 293: 293–297

Park EM, Ramnath N, Yang GY et al. (2007) High superoxide dismutase and low glutathione peroxidase activities in red blood cells predict susceptibility of lung cancer patients to radiation pneumonitis. Free Radic Biol Med 42: 280–287

Park KW, Hwang KK, Cho HJ et al. (2008a) Simvastatin enhances endothelial differentiation of peripheral blood mononuclear cells in hypercholesterolemic patients and induces pro-angiogenic cytokine IL-8 secretion from monocytes. Clin Chim Acta 388: 156–166

Park SY, Lee JS, Ko YJ et al. (2008b) Inhibitory effect of simvastatin on the TNF-alpha- and angiotensin II-induced monocyte adhesion to endothelial cells is mediated through the suppression of geranylgeranyl isoprenoid-dependent ROS generation. Arch Pharm Res 31: 195–204

Pena LA, Fuks Z, Kolesnick RN (2000) Radiation-induced apoptosis of endothelial cells in the murine central nervous system: protection by fibroblast growth factor and sphingomyelinase deficiency. Cancer Res 60: 321–327

Perez-Guerrero C, Alvarez de Sotomayor M, Jimenez L et al. (2003) Effects of simvastatin on endothelial function after chronic inhibition of nitric oxide synthase by L-NAME. J Cardiovasc Pharmacol 42: 204–210

Perez CA, Bauer M, Edelstein S et al. (1986) Impact of tumor control on survival in carcinoma of the lung treated with irradiation. Int J Radiat Oncol Biol Phys 12: 539–547

Peter Y, Rotman G, Lotem J et al. (2001) Elevated Cu/Zn-SOD exacerbates radiation sensitivity and hematopoietic abnormalities of Atm-deficient mice. Embo J 20: 1538–1546

Phan TP, Crane CH, Janjan NA et al. (2001) WR-2721 reduces intestinal toxicity from concurrent gemcitabine and radiation treatment. Int J Pancreatol 29: 19–23

Rabbani ZN, Anscher MS, Zhang X et al. (2003) Soluble TGF beta type II receptor gene therapy ameliorates acute radiation-induced pulmonary injury in rats. Int J Radiat Oncol Biol Phys 57: 563–572

Rabbani ZN, Anscher MS, Folz RJ et al. (2005) Overexpression of extracellular superoxide dismutase reduces acute radiation induced lung toxicity. BMC Cancer 5: 59

Rabbani ZN, Batinic-Haberle I, Anscher MS et al. (2007a) Long-term administration of a small molecular weight catalytic metalloporphyrin antioxidant, AEOL 10150, protects lungs from radiation-induced injury. Int J Radiat Oncol Biol Phys 67: 573–580

Rabbani ZN, Batinic-Haberle I, Anscher MS et al. (2007b) Long-term administration of a small molecular weight catalytic metalloporphyrin antioxidant, AEOL 10150, protects lungs from radiation-induced injury. Int J Radiat Oncol Biol Physics 67: 573–580

Rabbani ZN, Salahuddin FK, Yarmolenko P et al. (2007c) Low molecular weight catalytic metalloporphyrin antioxidant AEOL 10150 protects lungs from fractionated radiation. Free Radic Res 41: 1273–1282

Radtke ML, Kolesar JM (2005) Palifermin (Kepivance) for the treatment of oral mucositis in patients with hematologic malignancies requiring hematopoietic stem cell support. J Oncol Pharm Pract 11: 121–125

Rikitake Y, Kawashima S, Takeshita S et al. (2001) Anti-oxidative properties of fluvastatin, an HMG-CoA reductase inhibitor, contribute to prevention of atherosclerosis in cholesterol-fed rabbits. Atherosclerosis 154: 87–96

Riley PA (1994) Free radicals in biology: oxidative stress and the effects of ionizing radiation. Int J Radiat Biol 65: 27–33

Robbins ME, Diz DI (2006) Pathogenic role of the renin-angiotensin system in modulating radiation-induced late effects. Int J Radiat Oncol Biol Phys 64: 6–12

Roberts AB (1999) TGF-beta signaling from receptors to the nucleus. Microbes Infect 1: 1265–1273

Robertson JM, Ten Haken RK, Hazuka MB et al. (1997) Dose escalation for non-small cell lung cancer using conformal radiation therapy. Int J Radiat Oncol Biol Phys 37: 1079–1085

Rodemann H, Blaese M (2007a) Responses of normal cells to ionizing radiation. Semin Radiat Oncol (in press)

Rodemann HP, Blaese MA (2007b) Responses of normal cells to ionizing radiation. Semin Radiat Oncol 17: 81–88

Rosenman JG, Halle JS, Socinski MA et al. (2002) High-dose conformal radiotherapy for treatment of stage IIIA/IIIB non-small-cell lung cancer: technical issues and results of a phase I/II trial. Int J Radiat Oncol Biol Phys 54: 348–356

Rosenson RS (2001) Pluripotential mechanisms of cardioprotection with HMG-CoA reductase inhibitor therapy. Am J Cardiovasc Drugs 1: 411–420

Rube CE, Wilfert F, Uthe D et al. (2002) Modulation of radiation-induced tumour necrosis factor alpha (TNF-alpha) expression in the lung tissue by pentoxifylline. Radiother Oncol 64: 177–187

Rubin P, Johnston CJ, Williams JP et al. (1995) A perpetual cascade of cytokines postirradiation leads to pulmonary fibrosis. Int J Radiat Oncol Biol Phys 33: 99–109

Ryu S, Kolozsvary A, Jenrow KA et al. (2007) Mitigation of radiation-induced optic neuropathy in rats by ACE inhibitor ramipril: importance of ramipril dose and treatment time. J Neurooncol 82: 119–124

Sanchiz F, Milla A, Artola N et al. (1996) Prevention of radio-induced cystitis by orgotein: a randomized study. Anticancer Res 16: 2025–2028

Saunders MI, Barltrop MA, Rassa PM et al. (1984) The relationship between tumor response and survival following radiotherapy for carcinoma of the bronchus. Int J Radiat Oncol Biol Phys 10: 503–508

Schild SE, McGinnis WL, Graham D et al. (2006) Results of a phase I trial of concurrent chemotherapy and escalating doses of radiation for unresectable non-small-cell lung cancer. Int J Radiat Oncol Biol Phys 65: 1106–1111

Schmidt-Ullrich RK, Dent P, Grant S et al. (2000) Signal transduction and cellular radiation responses. Radiat Res 153: 245–257

Schultze-Mosgau S, Wehrhan F, Amann K et al. (2003) In vivo TGF-beta 3 expression during wound healing in irradiated tissue. An experimental study. Strahlenther Onkol 179: 410–416

Shi J, Wang J, Zheng H et al. (2003) Statins increase thrombomodulin expression and function in human endothelial cells by a nitric oxide-dependent mechanism and counteract tumor necrosis factor alpha-induced thrombomodulin downregulation. Blood Coagul Fibrinolysis 14: 575–585

Socinski MA, Blackstock AW, Bogart JA et al. (2008) Randomized phase II trial of induction chemotherapy followed by concurrent chemotherapy and dose-escalated thoracic conformal radiotherapy (74 Gy) in stage III non-small-cell lung cancer: CALGB 30105. J Clin Oncol 26: 2457–2463

Stinivasan V, Doctrow S, Singh V et al. (2007) Radiation counterneasure efficacy of superoxide dismutase (SOD)/catalase (CAT) mimetic EUK-189 in mice exposed to cobalt-60 gamma radiation. In: 13th International Congress of Radiation Research, San Francisco

Stone HB, Coleman CN, Anscher MS et al. (2003) Effects of radiation on normal tissue: consequences and mechanisms. Lancet Oncol 4: 529–536

Terry NH, Brinkley J, Doig AJ et al. (2004) Cellular kinetics of murine lung: model system to determine basis for radioprotection with keratinocyte growth factor. Int J Radiat Oncol Biol Phys 58: 435–444

Trog D, Bank P, Wendt TG et al. (1999) Daily amifostine given concomitantly to chemoradiation in head and neck cancer. A pilot study. Strahlenther Onkol 175: 444–449

Tsoutsou PG, Koukourakis MI (2006) Radiation pneumonitis and fibrosis: mechanisms underlying its pathogenesis and implications for future research. Int J Radiat Oncol Biol Phys 66: 1281–1293

Ulich TR, Yi ES, Longmuir K et al. (1994) Keratinocyte growth factor is a growth factor for type II pneumocytes in vivo. J Clin Invest 93: 1298–1306

Undas A, Brozek J, Musial J (2002) Anti-inflammatory and antithrombotic effects of statins in the management of coronary artery disease. Clin Lab 48: 287–296

Valencia J, Velilla C, Urpegui A et al. (2002) The efficacy of orgotein in the treatment of acute toxicity due to radiotherapy on head and neck tumors. Tumori 88: 385–389

Veerasarn V, Phromratanapongse P, Suntornpong N et al. (2006) Effect of Amifostine to prevent radiotherapy-induced acute and late toxicity in head and neck cancer patients who had normal or mild impaired salivary gland function. J Med Assoc Thai 89: 2056–2067

Vodovotz Y, Chesler L, Chong H et al. (1999) Regulation of transforming growth factor beta1 by nitric oxide. Cancer Res 59: 2142–2149

Vozenin-Brotons MC, Sivan V, Gault N et al. (2001) Antifibrotic action of Cu/Zn SOD is mediated by TGF-b1 repression and phenotypic reversion of myofibroblasts. Free Radical Biol Med 30: 30–42

Vujaskovic Z, Marks LB, Anscher MS (2000) The physical parameters and molecular events associated with radiation-induced lung toxicity. Semin Radiat Oncol 10: 296–307

Vujaskovic Z, Anscher MS, Feng QF et al. (2001) Radiation-induced hypoxia may perpetuate late normal tissue injury. Int J Radiat Oncol Biol Phys 50: 851–855

Vujaskovic Z, Batinic-Haberle I, Rabbani ZN et al. (2002a) A small molecular weight catalytic metalloporphyrin antioxidant with superoxide dismutase (SOD) mimetic properties protects lungs from radiation-induced injury. Free Radical Biol Med 33: 857–863

Vujaskovic Z, Batinic-Haberle I, Rabbani ZN et al. (2002b) A small molecular weight catalytic metalloporphyrin antioxidant with superoxide dismutase (SOD) mimetic properties protects lungs from radiation-induced injury. Free Radic Biol Med 33: 857–863

Vujaskovic Z, Feng QF, Rabbani ZN et al. (2002c) Radioprotection of lungs by amifostine is associated with reduction in profibrogenic cytokine activity. Radiat Res 157: 656–660

Vujaskovic Z, Thrasher BA, Jackson IL et al. (2007) Radioprotective effects of amifostine on acute and chronic esophageal injury in rodents. Int J Radiat Oncol Biol Phys 69: 534–540

Waehre T, Damas JK, Gullestad L et al. (2003) Hydroxymethylglutaryl coenzyme a reductase inhibitors down-regulate chemokines and chemokine receptors in patients with coronary artery disease. J Am Coll Cardiol 41: 1460–1467

Wang J, Qiu X, Kulkarni A et al. (2006a) Calcitonin gene-related peptide and substance P regulate the intestinal radiation response. Clin Cancer Res 12: 4112–4118

Wang J, Zheng H, Kulkarni A et al. (2006b) Regulation of early and delayed radiation responses in rat small intestine by capsaicin-sensitive nerves. Int J Radiat Oncol Biol Phys 64: 1528–1536

Wang J, Boerma M, Fu Q et al. (2007a) Significance of endothelial dysfunction in the pathogenesis of early and delayed radiation enteropathy. World J Gastroenterol 13: 3047–3055

Wang J, Boerma M, Fu Q et al. (2007b) Simvastatin ameliorates radiation enteropathy development after localized, fractionated irradiation by a protein C-independent mechanism. Int J Radiat Oncol Biol Phys 68: 1483–1490

Wang J, Hauer-Jensen M (2007c) Neuroimmune interactions: potential target for mitigating or treating intestinal radiation injury. Br J Radiol 80 Spec No 1: S41–48

Ward WF, Kim YT, Molteni A et al. (1988) Radiation-induced pulmonary endothelial dysfunction in rats: modification by an inhibitor of angiotensin converting enzyme. Int J Radiat Oncol Biol Phys 15: 135–140

Ward WF, Molteni A, Ts'ao CH (1989) Radiation-induced endothelial dysfunction and fibrosis in rat lung: modification by the angiotensin converting enzyme inhibitor CL242817. Radiat Res 117: 342–350

Williams JP, Hernady E, Johnston CJ et al. (2004) Effect of administration of lovastatin on the development of late pulmonary effects after whole-lung irradiation in a murine model. Radiat Res 161: 560–567

Yi ES, Williams ST, Lee H et al. (1996) Keratinocyte growth factor ameliorates radiation- and bleomycin-induced lung injury and mortality. Am J Pathol 149: 1963–1970

Zhao W, Diz DI, Robbins ME (2007) Oxidative damage pathways in relation to normal tissue injury. Br J Radiol 80 Spec No 1: S23–31

Mechanisms of Treatment Resistance: Molecular and Clinical Examples for Radio- and Chemotherapy

Carsten Nieder

CONTENTS

C. Nieder, MD
Professor, University of Tromsø
Department of Internal Medicine – Oncology, Nordlandssyke-
huset HF Hospital, Prinsensgate 164, 8092 Bodø, Norway

KEY POINTS

- DNA damage response mechanisms encompass pathways of DNA repair, cell cycle checkpoint arrest, and apoptosis. Together, these mechanisms function to maintain genomic stability in the face of exogenous and endogenous DNA damage, including damage induced by cancer therapy.
- The induction of DNA damage is probably one of the most crucial events after irradiation of cells. In this regard, ionizing radiation triggers a wide array of lesions including base damage, single-strand breaks, and double-strand breaks. Persisting damage results in micronuclei formation, chromosome aberrations, and cell death.
- Two major repair pathways, homologous recombination and non-homologous end-joining, have evolved to deal with double-strand breaks.
- More recently a novel link between epidermal growth factor receptor (EGFR) signaling pathways and DNA repair mechanisms, especially non-homologous end-joining, could be demonstrated.
- Cell death and survival decisions are reciprocally regulated by the balance between a large family of pro- and antiapoptotic proteins.
- Drug resistance in experimental tumors might be caused by upregulation of drug transporters or by interference with apoptosis/senescence.
- Membrane proteins, notably MDR, MRP, and BCRP of the ATP binding cassette transporter family encoding efflux pumps, play important roles in the development of multidrug resistance.
- Overexpression of these transporters has been observed frequently in many types of human malignancies and correlated with poor responses to chemotherapeutic agents.

Abstract

The clinical experience from numerous well-controlled large-scale studies trying to improve the results of radio- and pharmacotherapy of advanced malignant tumors by, e.g., dose escalation and/or addition of new drugs or other treatment modifiers suggests that great expectations based on sound rationales often result in small improvements of outcome. This has led to experimental and translational studies of the mechanisms that allow cancer cells to escape cytotoxic treatment or develop resistance. The present chapter summarizes our current knowledge on selected mechanisms and pathways, e.g., related to DNA damage repair.

13.1
Introduction

The human body is continuously exposed to a large number of damaging agents, and among these are various types of ionizing radiation. Defense or detoxification and repair mechanisms are thus necessary to ensure survival of individual cells and the whole organism in a challenging environment. Misrepair of DNA damage might lead to permanent mutations and eventually carcinogenesis. While in principle useful and beneficial strategies, the different components of repair create serious obstacles to effective killing of unwanted cells, such as those having acquired a malignant phenotype and thereby threatening the organism by their ability to undergo uncontrolled divisions and metastasis to distant sites. It has recently been suggested that cancer stem cells are relatively quiescent cells, which are especially difficult to eradicate (EYLER and RICH 2008; VISVADER and LINDEMANN 2008). Contributing factors include lower levels of apoptosis, more rapid damage repair, basal activation of DNA damage checkpoints, expression of drug pumps, and production of higher amounts of growth factors such as vascular endothelial growth factor. However, this subject has already been discussed in more detail in other chapters of this book and will not be repeated here. This chapter provides a condensed overview of the most important mechanisms and pathways that allow malignant cells to escape the damaging effects of commonly used treatments, particularly radio- and chemotherapy (Table 13.1). DNA damage response mechanisms encompass pathways of DNA repair, cell cycle checkpoint arrest, and apoptosis. Together, these mechanisms function to maintain genomic stability in the face of exogenous and endogenous DNA damage.

Table 13.1. Factors that contribute to treatment resistance and failure

Low inherent radiosensitivity
Large number of malignant cells
Proliferation status and cell cycle phase
Ability to repair damage and/or respond to stress
Deficient cell death mechanisms
Use of agents that modify the response, e.g., radical scavengers
Use of antagonistic combinations of drugs
Intrinsic and acquired resistance to cytotoxic drugs, hormonal treatment, angiogenesis inhibition, etc.
Physiological mechanisms as summarized in Chap. 15

13.2
Radiotherapy

The induction of DNA damage is probably one of the most crucial events after irradiation of cells. In this regard, ionizing radiation triggers a wide array of lesions including base damage, single-strand breaks, and, notably, double-strand breaks (DSB). Persisting damage results in micronuclei formation, chromosome aberrations, and cell death. After irradiation, different molecular systems are involved in recognition and repair of the damage (KAO et al. 2005). Ataxia telangiectasia mutated (ATM) is activated in response to DSBs and initiates cell cycle checkpoint arrest (JEGGO and LÖBRICH 2006). The response to DNA breaks requires the coordinated effort of the ATM-CHK2-p53 and ATR-CHK1 DNA damage-sensing pathways and DNA repair (e.g., DNA-PK and RAD51 complexes). The turnover of many of these DNA damage-associated proteins is controlled by the 26S proteasome (CHOUDHURY et al. 2006). Accumulating evidence also indicates that the transcription factor nuclear factor-kappaB (NF-kappaB) plays a critical role in cellular protection against a variety of genotoxic agents including ionizing radiation, and inhibition of NF-kappaB leads to radiosensitization in radioresistant cancer cells. NF-kappaB was found to be defective in cells from patients with A-T (ataxia-telangiectasia) who are highly sensitive to DNA damage induced by ionizing radiation and UV lights. Both ATM and NF-kappaB deficiencies result in increased sensitivity to

DNA DSBs. p53, the guardian of the genome, has long been considered a major player in determining the outcome of cancer treatment because of its role as a mediator of growth arrest and apoptosis after exposure to chemo- and radiotherapy (Nieder et al. 2000; Thames et al. 2002; Bassett et al. 2008; Williams et al. 2008). However, not all cancer cell lines that contain mutant p53 are resistant to treatment (Hiro et al. 2008). Clinical data also confirm that other factors outweigh the influence of p53, among these the results from the large trial by the Danish Breast Cancer Group where tissue microarray sections of 1,000 breast cancer patients were stained by immunohistochemical methods for p53 and BCL-2 (Kyndi et al. 2008).

Whereas most of the induced damage is quickly repaired, DSB repair is slow and unrepaired DSBs are important for the final induction of cell death. In higher eukaryotic cells, DSBs in chromatin promptly initiate the phosphorylation of the histone H2A variant, H2AX, at serine 139 to generate gamma-H2AX. This phosphorylation event requires the activation of the phosphatidylinositol-3-OH-kinase-like family of protein kinases, DNA-protein kinase (PK)$_{CS}$, ATM, and ATR, and serves as a landing pad for the accumulation and retention of the central components of the signaling cascade initiated by DNA damage. Regions in chromatin with gamma-H2AX are conveniently detected by immunofluorescence microscopy and serve as beacons of DSBs. This has allowed the development of an assay that has proved particularly useful in the molecular analysis of the processing of DSBs.

Many chemotherapeutic agents, especially those known to be of value in combination with radiation, also induce considerable DNA damage or interfere with effective DNA repair. Cisplatin, for example, acts by complex formation with guanosine residues and subsequent adduct formation ultimately resulting in intra- and interstrand crosslinks. This type of damage is mostly removed by base excision repair and mismatch repair. Several sets of data suggest that single-strand damage induced by radiation in close vicinity to DNA damage triggered by cisplatin results in a mutual inhibition of the damage-specific repair system; thus, the amount of resulting damage leads to an increased net cell kill (Begg 1990; Yang et al. 1995). ERCC1, a structure-specific endonuclease involved in nucleotide excision repair and homologous recombination (HR), confers resistance to cisplatin. Patients with ERCC1-negative non-small cell lung cancer were shown to benefit from adjuvant cisplatin-based chemotherapy.

The biochemical pathways implicated in DNA repair and DNA synthesis overlap in several regards; thus, drugs acting on the synthesis of DNA putatively also interfere with the repair of DNA damage induced by ionizing radiation. Several prototypical radiation sensitizers may act via these mechanisms. Besides cisplatin, 5-fluorouracil (5-FU) is probably the most commonly employed drug in clinical combined modality settings. Basically, 5-FU inhibits thymidylate synthase thereby reducing the intracellular pool of nucleoside triphosphates (Pinedo and Peters 1988; Miller and Kinsella 1992). In addition, the drug is integrated into DNA via fluorodeoxyuridine, also contributing to its antineoplastic effects. Several lines of evidence suggest that the amount of 5-FU integrated into DNA directly correlates with the radiosensitizing effect.

Two major pathways, HR and non-homologous end-joining (NHEJ), have evolved to deal with DSBs, and are conserved from yeast to vertebrates. Despite the conservation of these pathways, their relative contribution to DSB repair varies greatly between these two species. HR plays a dominant role in any DSB repair in yeast, whereas NHEJ significantly contributes to DSB repair in vertebrates. Much more details on this issue are provided in chapter 14. NHEJ is a pathway that rejoins DNA ends, usually after removal of a limited number of base pairs. It is initiated by the Ku70/Ku80 heterodimer, which binds to DNA ends and recruits the DNA-PK$_{CS}$. The latter can phosphorylate a variety of repair proteins.

More recently a novel link between epidermal growth factor receptor (EGFR) signaling pathways and DNA repair mechanisms, especially NHEJ repair, could be demonstrated (Rodemann et al. 2007). After observations demonstrating the initial radiation-induced activation of the EGFR approximately 0–10 min after exposure, it became evident that the EGFR also is re-activated approximately 60–180+ min after irradiation. The primary mode of receptor activation at these later times occurred via a paracrine/autocrine mechanism (Dent et al. 1999; Shvartsman et al. 2002). The initial activation of EGFR1 and the ERK1/2 pathway was directly responsible for the cleavage, release, and functional activation of presynthesized paracrine ligands, such as pro-transforming growth factor (TGF)-alpha, that fed back onto the irradiated tumor cell, thereby re-energizing the signaling system (Hagan et al. 2004). Signaling by the EGFR family of receptors is, in general, believed to be pro-proliferative and cytoprotective. In vitro and xenograft tumor animal model studies have strongly argued that inhibition of EGFR function using single drug/antibody dosing has radiosensitizing effects (Bianco et al. 2002; Chinnaiyan et al. 2005; Harari 2007). Data from several groups have demonstrated that the PI3K pathway is a key radioprotective pathway downstream of receptors and RAS proteins. Inhibition of PI3K pathway function by use of small molecule inhibitors radiosensitizes tumor cells expressing mutant active RAS molecules or wild-type RAS molecules that are constitutively active due to upstream growth factor receptor signaling. It is possible that PI3K inhibitors may also exert a portion of their radiosensitizing properties by suppressing the function of proteins with PI3K-like kinase domains, such as ATM, ataxia-telangiectasia- and rad3-related (ATR), and DNA-PK.

Growth factor-induced signaling from EGFR through the PI3K/AKT and RAF-1/ERK1/2 pathways can increase expression of multiple antiapoptotic proteins, including BCL-XL, MCL-1, and c-FLIP isoforms, as well as the phosphorylation and inactivation of pro-apoptotic proteins including BAD, BIM, and pro-caspase 9 (Osaki et al. 2004; Caro and Cederbaum 2006; Grethe and Porn-Ares 2006; Majumdar and Du 2006). Radiation-induced ERK1/2 activation has also been linked to increased expression of the DNA repair proteins ERCC1, XRCC1, and XPC (Yacoub et al. 2003).

Single-strand breaks (SSBs) can occur in cells either directly, or indirectly following initiation of base excision repair. SSBs generally have blocked termini lacking the conventional 5'-phosphate and 3'-hydroxyl groups and require further processing prior to DNA synthesis and ligation. XRCC1 is devoid of any known enzymatic activity, but it can physically interact with other proteins involved in all stages of the overlapping SSB repair and base excision repair pathways, including those that conduct the rate-limiting end-tailoring, and in many cases can stimulate their enzymatic activities. XRCC1(−/−) cells are also sensitized by PARP inhibition demonstrating that PARP-mediated poly(ADP-ribosyl)ation plays a role in modulation of cytotoxicity beyond recruitment of XRCC1 to sites of DNA damage (Horton et al. 2008).

13.3
Chemotherapy

Solid tumors usually have multiple abnormal pathways or genetic changes so that a single drug usually is not sufficient for permanent tumor suppression. Many anticancer drugs are cell-cycle specific and therefore most active against cells that are proliferating. Thus, the non-proliferating fraction is difficult to eradicate. Tumor regrowth in between cycles of therapy also contributes to limited efficacy. Pharmacotherapy is limited by the fact that the dose of the active, cell killing form of the compound is variable within the tumor and its cells. This results from problems in the delivery of drugs (perfusion,

interstitial fluid pressure, tissue pH, protein binding, etc.), cellular uptake, efflux, metabolization, inactivation, and resistance. In fact, the pharmacokinetic profile of anticancer drugs is characterized by substantial interpatient variability where two- to threefold variation is not uncommon. These issues even gain complexity with simultaneous administration of two or more drugs. Depending on variations in actual drug concentration, a fixed combination of two drugs might either show additivity or antagonism in the same tumor cells. Borst et al. (2007) have studied mouse mammary tumors induced by conditional deletion of Brca1 and p53. These tumors responded to monotherapy with the maximal tolerable dose of doxorubicin, or docetaxel, but eventually always became resistant to the drugs. Resistance in most tumors was caused by upregulation of drug transporters and not by interference with apoptosis/senescence.

As the importance of drug transporters in the clinical pharmacokinetics of drugs is recognized, genetic polymorphisms of drug transporters have emerged as one of the determinant factors to produce the interindividual variability of pharmacokinetics. Many clinical studies have shown the influence of genetic polymorphisms of drug transporters on the pharmacokinetics and subsequent pharmacological and toxicological effects of drugs. The functional change in a transporter in clearance organs such as liver and kidney affects the drug concentration in the blood circulation, while that in the pharmacological or toxicological target can alter the local concentration at the target sites without changing its plasma concentration. As for the transporters for organic anions, some single nucleotide polymorphisms (SNPs) or haplotypes occurring with high frequency in organic anion transporting polypeptide (OATP) 1B1, multidrug resistance 1 (MDR1), and breast cancer resistance protein (BCRP) have been extensively investigated in both human clinical studies and in vitro functional assays (Maeda and Sugiyama 2008). Membrane proteins, notably MDR, multidrug resistance protein (MRP), and BCRP of the ATP binding cassette (ABC) transporter family encoding efflux pumps, play important roles in the development of multidrug resistance. Overexpression of these transporters has been observed frequently in many types of human malignancies and correlated with poor responses to chemotherapeutic agents. Evidence has accumulated showing that redox signals are activated in response to drug treatments that affect the expression and activity of these transporters by multiple mechanisms, including (a) conformational changes in the transporters, (b) regulation of the biosynthesis cofactors required for the transporter's function, (c) regulation of the expression of transporters at transcriptional, posttranscriptional, and epigenetic levels, and (d) amplification of the copy number of genes encoding these transporters (Kuo 2009).

Cells surviving initial chemotherapy may upregulate active resistance mechanisms, which allows for growth despite therapy (Stewart et al. 2007). Furthermore, cells may survive until therapy cessation by downregulating metabolism/cycling, becoming temporarily quiescent. Expression levels of intact tumor suppressor proteins and molecular targets of antineoplastic agents are critical in defining cancer cell drug sensitivity; however, the intracellular location of a specific protein may be as important. Many tumor suppressor proteins must be present in the cell nucleus to perform their policing activities or for the cell to respond to chemotherapeutic agents. Nuclear proteins needed to prevent cancer initiation or progression or to optimize chemotherapeutic response include the tumor suppressor proteins p53, APC/beta-catenin, and FOXO family genes; negative regulators of cell cycle progression and survival such as p21(CIP1) and p27(KIP1); and chemotherapeutic targets such as DNA topoisomerases I and IIalpha. Mislocalization of a nuclear protein into the cytoplasm can render it ineffective as a tumor suppressor or as a target for chemotherapy. During disease progression or in response to the tumor environment, cancer cells appear to acquire intracellular mechanisms to export anticancer nuclear proteins. These mechanisms generally involve modification of nuclear proteins, causing the proteins to reveal leucine-rich nuclear export signal protein sequences. Subsequent export is mediated by CRM1 (Turner and Sullivan 2008).

13.3.1
The Glioblastoma Example

The main prerequisites of successful chemotherapy are sensitivity of the tumor cells to the mechanisms of the drug and sufficient drug exposure. The key issues of tumor heterogeneity with primary and acquired resistance as well as pharmacokinetics, pharmacodynamics, and tumor microenvironment deserve particular attention because of several facts that are specific for brain tumors. First of all, the intact blood-brain barrier (BBB) prevents access to the brain for several compounds. Even in areas of BBB disturbance, as present for example in high-grade glioma, the effects of contemporary drug treatment are not satisfactory. Thus, achieving therapeutic concentrations in distal, seemingly intact areas that also are known to contain infiltrating tumor cells remains an enormous challenge. Various strate-

gies of modified application or increased dose have been explored, including intra-arterial, intrathecal, and intratumoral delivery as well as disruption of the BBB. Furthermore, many patients with brain tumors are able to metabolize chemotherapy drugs more rapidly than other tumor patients because of concomitant enzyme-inducing medications that are necessary to treat or prevent seizures (Nieder et al. 2006). Phenytoin, carbamazepine, and phenobarbital induce hepatic cytochrome P450 enzymes, resulting for example in higher maximum tolerated drug doses. It is also important to notice the possibility of decreased drug effectiveness from corticosteroid treatment. Possible drug resistance mechanisms include the cell membrane protein P-glycoprotein (PGP), an energy-dependent drug efflux pump removing a wide range of lipophilic chemotherapy agents. PGP expression has been described in tumor blood vessels as well as neoplastic cells of high-grade glioma (Von Bossanyi et al. 1997). Another mechanism is intracellular drug inactivation or transformation as a result of increased concentrations of detoxifying enzymes such as glutathione S-transferases (GST), O^6-methylguanine methyltransferase (MGMT), or PARP. GST catalyzes the conjugation of glutathione with a large number of compounds with an electrophilic center, including chemotherapeutic agents. Nitrosoureas may be deactivated by denitrosylation via GST or methylation by MGMT. Belanich et al. (1996) showed that BCNU-treated patients with high levels of MGMT had a significantly shorter time to progression and overall survival than those with lower levels. Friedman et al. (1998) reported that MGMT level might be a valuable predictive factor for response to temozolomide. It has recently been investigated whether *MGMT* promoter methylation in glioblastoma tissue from 206, i.e., 36% of all, patients in the randomized EORTC/NCIC trial is associated with a benefit from temozolomide (Hegi et al. 2005). Of these samples, 45% had detectable methylation, which leads to a loss of MGMT expression and reduced DNA repair capacity. Unrepaired lesions might trigger cell-death cascades. Consistent with these facts, overall survival was better in patients with methylated promoter in both groups (radiotherapy and radiotherapy plus temozolomide). Furthermore, patients with methylated promoter and reduced MGMT expression treated with radiotherapy had a median survival of 15 months, and those treated with radiation plus temozolomide of 22 months ($p=0.007$). In the unmethylated group, the difference in median survival was only 1 month ($p=0.06$). Especially for these patients, alternative treatments need to be studied. Pretreatment with O^6-methylguanine, which inactivates the enzyme, may overcome resistance.

13.3.2
Epidermal Growth Factor Receptor Inhibition

The observation that only a minority of patients respond to EGFR-targeted therapies, in combination with their toxicity and high costs, has driven the search for molecular markers predictive of response. It has recently been discovered that mutations in the KRAS oncogene constitute a negative predictive marker in the setting of colorectal cancer, namely that their presence can be used to predict which patients are unlikely to benefit from treatment with EGFR-directed therapy (GARCIA et al. 2008).

Growth and proliferation responses mediated by the ErbB family of receptor tyrosine kinases are often dysregulated in breast cancer, resulting in an aggressive course of disease and, historically, a poorer prognosis. The inhibition of ErbB-mediated signaling using recently developed monoclonal antibodies and small molecule tyrosine kinase inhibitors has resulted in significant clinical benefit for patients with this tumor phenotype in the metastatic and adjuvant settings. However, many ErbB2-positive cancers exhibit intrinsic resistance, and the widespread development of acquired resistance to ErbB-targeted agents remains a substantial clinical problem. There are many potential mechanisms for resistance to this type of therapy, including the formation of alternative ErbB signaling complexes and crosstalk with other pathways. Lapatinib is a selective small molecule inhibitor of ErbB2 and EGFR tyrosine kinases that was recently approved for ErbB2+ breast cancers that progressed on trastuzumab-based therapy. The efficacy of lapatinib as a monotherapy or in combination with chemotherapy, however, is limited by the development of therapeutic resistance that typically occurs within 12 months of starting therapy. In contrast to small molecule inhibitors targeting other receptor tyrosine kinases where resistance has been attributed to mutations within the targeted receptor, ErbB2 mutations have not been commonly found in breast tumors. Instead, acquired resistance to lapatinib seems to be mediated by redundant survival pathways that are activated as a consequence of marked inhibition of ErbB2 kinase activity. For example, inhibition of phosphatidylinositol 3 kinase-Akt in lapatinib-treated cells leads to derepression of FOXO3A, a transcription factor that upregulates estrogen receptor (ER) signaling, resulting in a switch in the regulation of survival factors (e.g., survivin) and cell survival from ErbB2 alone to ER and ErbB2 in resistant cells (CHEN et al. 2008).

Several possible explanations exist as to why a drug effect observed in vitro or in animals does not translate into a profound antitumor effect in patients:

1. The required inhibitory concentration of the drug and the drug half-life are not achievable and are too short for a therapeutic effect, respectively, in patients.

2. The relative dependency (addiction) of cultured tumor cell isolates on EGFR signaling, including expression of hyperactive EGFR mutants (e.g., EGFR1 L858R), when compared to actual tumors in patients, may be biased based on in vitro studies that use established cell lines. Also, the development of drug-resistant EGFR mutants in patients after long-term exposure to EGFR inhibitors (e.g., EGFR1 T790M) may preclude drug actions.

3. Exposure of tumor cells in vitro to kinase and other inhibitors, such as tamoxifen, has argued that compensatory activation of parallel growth factor receptors (such as the IGF-1 receptor and c-Kit) occurs to replace the loss of EGFR receptor signaling caused by drug exposure and acts to maintain tumor cell survival (KWAK et al. 2005; THOMAS et al. 2005; HUTCHESON et al. 2006).

4. The EGFR inhibitors that are often used in therapy only inhibit one EGFR family member, such as EGFR1, and, in a similar conceptual manner to the third point just listed, other EGFR family members, such as EGFR2, may provide compensatory survival signaling to overcome loss of survival signaling from the inhibited receptor.

5. The development of other somatic mutations in survival signaling with the tumor cell, such as loss of PTEN (phosphatase and tensin homologue deleted in chromosome 10) function, which may be selected for in tumor cells undergoing EGFR inhibitor therapy, will lead to the development of tumor cells that are more resistant in general to the inhibitors of growth factor receptors.

13.3.3
Small Molecule BCL-2 Family Modulators

Cell death and survival decisions are reciprocally regulated by the balance between a large family of pro- (e.g., BAX, BAK, BAD, etc.) and antiapoptotic (e.g., BCL-2, BCL-XL, MCL-1, A1, c-FLIP-s, XIAP, etc.) proteins (REED 1998). There has been extensive interest in attempts to shift the balance away from survival and toward apoptosis in tumor cells through the use of various molecules that regulate these apoptotic modulators. For example, antisense oligonucleotides directed against BCL-2 have been employed clinically in an attempt to lower the apoptotic threshold for established cytotoxic drugs (MARCUCCI et al. 2003). An alternative approach involves the use of small molecules that interfere with the actions of various antiapoptotic proteins (WANG et al. 2000; OLTERSDORF et al. 2005) and antagonists of XIAP (SCHIMMER et al. 2004).

As noted previously, it has been established that the net output of stress-related versus survival-related pathways can determine whether a cell lives or dies (XIA et al. 1995). Although the mechanism(s) by which the MEK1/2-ERK1/2 pathway promotes survival is not known with certainty, it is known that JNK may be directly involved in the induction of mitochondrial injury (TOURNIER et al. 2000), and that induction of ERK1/2 can oppose the action of certain pro-apoptotic proteins (e.g., caspase-9, BIM, BAD) (ALLAN et al. 2003; VON GISE et al. 2001). However, a growing body of evidence suggests that MEK1/2 inhibition can lower the threshold for cell death for a variety of other targeted agents, and that such synergistic interactions might improve combined drug treatment.

References

Allan LA, Morrice N, Brady S, et al (2003) Inhibition of caspase-9 through phosphorylation at Thr 125 by ERK MAPK. Nat Cell Biol 5:647–654

Bassett EA, Wang W, Rastinejad F, El-Deiry WS (2008) Structural and functional basis for therapeutic modulation of p53 signaling. Clin Cancer Res 14:6376–6386

Begg AC (1990) Cisplatin and radiation: interaction probabilities and therapeutic possibilities. Int J Radiat Oncol Biol Phys 19:1183–1189

Belanich M, Pastor M, Randall T, et al (1996) Retrospective study of the correlation between DNA repair protein alkyltransferase and survival of brain tumor patients treated with carmustine. Cancer Res 56:783–788

Bianco C, Tortora G, Bianco R, et al (2002) Enhancement of antitumor activity of ionizing radiation by combined treatment with the selective epidermal growth factor receptor-tyrosine kinase inhibitor ZD1839 (Iressa). Clin Cancer Res 8:3250–3258

Borst P, Jonkers J, Rottenberg S (2007) What makes tumors multidrug resistant? Cell Cycle 6:2782–2787

Caro AA, Cederbaum AI (2006) Role of phosphatidylinositol 3-kinase/AKT as a survival pathway against CYP2E1-dependent toxicity. J Pharmacol Exp Ther 318:360–372

Chen FL, Xia W, Spector NL (2008) Acquired resistance to small molecule ErbB2 tyrosine kinase inhibitors. Clin Cancer Res 14:6730–6734

Chinnaiyan P, Huang S, Vallabhaneni G, et al (2005) Mechanisms of enhanced radiation response following epidermal growth factor receptor signaling inhibition by erlotinib (Tarceva). Cancer Res 65:3328–3335

Choudhury A, Cuddihy A, Bristow RG (2006) Radiation and new molecular agents part I: targeting ATM-ATR checkpoints, DNA repair, and the proteasome. Semin Radiat Oncol 16:51–58

Dent P, Reardon DB, Park JS, et al (1999) Radiation-induced release of transforming growth factor alpha activates the epidermal growth factor receptor and mitogen-activated protein kinase pathway in carcinoma cells, leading to increased proliferation and protection from radiation-induced cell death. Mol Biol Cell 10:2493–2506

Eyler CE, Rich JN (2008) Survival of the fittest: cancer stem cells in therapeutic resistance and angiogenesis. J Clin Oncol 26:2839–2845

Friedman HS, McLendon RE, Kerby T, et al (1998) DNA mismatch repair and O6-alkylguanine-DNA alkyltransferase analysis and response to Temodal in newly diagnosed malignant glioma. J Clin Oncol 16:3851–3857

Garcia J, Riely GJ, Nafa K, Ladanyi M (2008) KRAS mutational testing in the selection of patients for EGFR-targeted therapies. Semin Diagn Pathol 25:288–294

Grethe S, Porn-Ares MI (2006) p38 MAPK regulates phosphorylation of Bad via PP2A-dependent suppression of the MEK1/2-ERK1/2 survival pathway in TNF-alpha induced endothelial apoptosis. Cell Signal 18:531–540

Hagan M, Yacoub A, Dent P (2004) Ionizing radiation causes a dose-dependent release of transforming growth factor alpha in vitro from irradiated xenografts and during palliative treatment of hormone-refractory prostate carcinoma. Clin Cancer Res 10:5724–5731

Harari PM (2007) Stepwise progress in epidermal growth factor receptor/radiation studies for head and neck cancer. Int J Radiat Oncol Biol Phys 69:S25–27

Hegi ME, Diserens AC, Gorlia T, et al (2005) *MGMT* gene silencing and benefit from temozolomide in glioblastoma. N Engl J Med 352:997–1003

Hiro J, Inoue Y, Toiyama Y, et al (2008) Mechanism of resistance to chemoradiation in p53 mutant human colon cancer. Int J Oncol 32:1305–1310

Horton JK, Watson M, Stefanick DF, et al (2008) XRCC1 and DNA polymerase beta in cellular protection against cytotoxic DNA single-strand breaks. Cell Res 18:48–63

Hutcheson IR, Knowlden JM, Jones HE, et al (2006) Inductive mechanisms limiting response to anti-epidermal growth factor receptor therapy. Endocr Relat Cancer 13(suppl 1):S89–S97

Jeggo PA, Löbrich M (2006) Contribution of DNA repair and cell cycle checkpoint arrest to the maintenance of genomic stability. DNA Repair (Amst) 5:1192–1198

Kao J, Rosenstein BS, Peters S, Milano MT, Kron SJ (2005) Cellular response to DNA damage. Ann N Y Acad Sci 1066:243–258

Kuo MT (2009) Redox regulation of multidrug resistance in cancer chemotherapy: molecular mechanisms and therapeutic opportunities. Antioxid Redox Signal 11:99–133

Kwak EL, Sordella R, Bell DW, et al (2005) Irreversible inhibitors of the EGF receptor may circumvent acquired resistance to gefitinib. Proc Natl Acad Sci U S A 102:7665–7670

Kyndi M, Sørensen FB, Knudsen H, et al (2008) Impact of BCL2 and p53 on postmastectomy radiotherapy response in high-risk breast cancer. A subgroup analysis of DBCG82 b&c. Acta Oncol 47:608–617

Maeda K, Sugiyama Y (2008) Impact of genetic polymorphisms of transporters on the pharmacokinetic, pharmacodynamic and toxicological properties of anionic drugs. Drug Metab Pharmacokinet 23:223–235

Majumdar AP, Du J (2006) Phosphatidylinositol 3-kinase/Akt signaling stimulates colonic mucosal cell survival during aging. Am J Physiol Gastrointest Liver Physiol 290:G49–G55

Marcucci G, Byrd JC, Dai G, et al (2003) Phase 1 and pharmacodynamic studies of G3139, a Bcl-2 antisense oligonucleotide, in combination with chemotherapy in refractory or relapsed acute leukemia. Blood 101:425–432

Miller EM, Kinsella TJ (1992) Radiosensitization by fluorodeoxyuridine: effects of thymidylate synthase inhibition and cell synchronization. Cancer Res 52:1687–1694

Nieder C, Petersen S, Petersen C, Thames HD (2000) The challenge of p53 as prognostic and predictive factor in gliomas. Cancer Treat Rev 26:67–73

Nieder C, Adam M, Grosu AL (2006) Combined modality treatment of glioblastoma multiforme: the role of temozolomide. Rev Recent Clin Trials 1:43–51

Oltersdorf T, Elmore SW, Shoemaker AR, et al (2005) An inhibitor of Bcl-2 family proteins induces regression of solid tumours. Nature 435:677–681

Osaki M, Kase S, Adachi K, et al (2004) Inhibition of the PI3K-Akt signaling pathway enhances the sensitivity of Fas-mediated apoptosis in human gastric carcinoma cell line, MKN-45. J Cancer Res Clin Oncol 130:8–14

Pinedo HM, Peters GF (1988) Fluorouracil: biochemistry and pharmacology. J Clin Oncol 6:1653–1664

Reed JC (1998) Bcl-2 family proteins. Oncogene 17:3225–3236

Rodemann HP, Dittmann K, Toulany M (2007) Radiation-induced EGFR-signaling and control of DNA-damage repair. Int J Radiat Biol 83:781–791

Schimmer AD, Welsh K, Pinilla C, et al (2004) Small-molecule antagonists of apoptosis suppressor XIAP exhibit broad antitumor activity. Cancer Cell 5:25–35

Shvartsman SY, Hagan MP, Yacoub A, et al (2002) Autocrine loops with positive feedback enable context-dependent cell signaling. Am J Physiol Cell Physiol 282:C545–C559

Stewart DJ, Chiritescu G, Dahrouge S, et al (2007) Chemotherapy dose-response relationships in non-small cell lung cancer and implied resistance mechanisms. Cancer Treat Rev 33:101–137

Thames HD, Petersen C, Petersen S, Nieder C, Baumann M (2002) Immunohistochemically detected p53 mutations in epithelial tumors and results of treatment with chemotherapy and radiotherapy. A treatment-specific overview of the clinical data. Strahlenther Onkol 178:411–421

Thomas RK, Greulich H, Yuza Y, et al (2005) Detection of oncogenic mutations in the EGFR gene in lung adenocarcinoma with differential sensitivity to EGFR tyrosine kinase inhibitors. Cold Spring Harb Symp Quant Biol 70:73–81

Tournier C, Hess P, Yang DD, et al (2000) Requirement of JNK for stress-induced activation of the cytochrome c-mediated death pathway. Science 288:870–874

Turner JG, Sullivan DM (2008) CRM1-mediated nuclear export of proteins and drug resistance in cancer. Curr Med Chem 15:2648–2655

Visvader JE, Lindeman GJ (2008) Cancer stem cells in solid tumours: accumulating evidence and unresolved questions. Nat Rev Cancer 8:755–768

Von Bossanyi P, Diete S, Dietzmann K, et al (1997) Immunohistochemical expression of P-glycoprotein and glutathione S-transferases in cerebral gliomas and response to chemotherapy. Acta Neuropathol 94:605–611

von Gise A, Lorenz P, Wellbrock C, et al (2001) Apoptosis suppression by Raf-1 and MEK1 requires MEK- and phosphatidylinositol 3-kinase-dependent signals. Mol Cell Biol 21:2324–2336

Wang JL, Liu D, Zhang ZJ, et al (2000) Structure-based discovery of an organic compound that binds Bcl-2 protein and induces apoptosis of tumor cells. Proc Natl Acad Sci U S A 97:7124–7129

Williams JR, Zhang Y, Zhou H, et al (2008) A quantitative overview of radiosensitivity of human tumor cells across histological type and TP53 status. Int J Radiat Biol 84:253–264

Xia Z, Dickens M, Raingeaud J, et al (1995) Opposing effects of ERK and JNK-p38 MAP kinases on apoptosis. Science 270:1326–1331

Yacoub A, McKinstry R, Hinman D, et al (2003) Epidermal growth factor and ionizing radiation up-regulate the DNA repair genes XRCC1 and ERCC1 in DU145 and LNCaP prostate carcinoma through MAPK signaling. Radiat Res 159:439–452

Yang LX, Double EB, O'Hara JA, Wang HJ (1995) Production of DNA double-strand breaks by interactions between carboplatin and radiation: a potential mechanism for radiopotentiation. Radiat Res 143:309–315

DNA Repair and Cell Cycle Regulation
After Ionizing Irradiation

George Iliakis, Jochen Dahm-Daphi, and Ekkehard Dikomey

CONTENTS

G. Iliakis, PhD
Institute of Medical Radiation Biology, University of Duisburg–Essen Medical School, Hufelandstraße 55, 45122 Essen, Germany

J. Dahm-Daphi, MD
Laboratory of Radiobiology and Experimental Radio-Oncology, University Medical Center Hamburg-Eppendorf, Martinistraße 52, 20246 Hamburg, Germany

E. Dikomey, PhD
Laboratory of Radiobiology and Experimental Radio-Oncology, University Medical Center Hamburg-Eppendorf, Martinistraße 52, 20246 Hamburg, Germany

KEY POINTS

- DNA damage is now known to affect every aspect of the cellular metabolism and to include extensive modifications in transcriptional regulation, as well as life-or-death decisions.
- Simple DNA lesions can be repaired by excision of damaged nucleotides and resynthesis of the missing segments of the molecule by using the intact strand as template.
- Complex lesions affecting both DNA strands cause a failure of the fundamental requirement for repair, i.e., the presence of an intact complementary strand.
- The generation of localized, multiple ionization events by single-particle traversals is a unique property of ionizing radiation (IR) and the main cause for the high efficiency of induction of double-stranded breaks (DSBs) and other complex DNA lesions.
- Critical for damage responses are kinases of the phosphatidylinositol 3–like kinase family, mainly DNA-PK, ATM, and ATR.
- The repair kinetics of X-ray–induced DSBs are described by a biphasic curve eventually reaching a plateau. For most cell lines, the fast component includes about 30%, and the slow component about 60%, of all DSBs induced. The plateau reflects the number of nonrejoined DSBs but may also include misjoining events.
- Repair of DSBs in mammalian cells is dominated by the efficient repair pathway of nonhomologous endjoining (NHEJ). Homology-dependent pathways can also be employed, but they appear restricted to the S–G2 phase of the cell cycle.
- The NHEJ pathway operates with very fast kinetics and has been shown to require a set of "core" proteins performing well-described

functions. Lack of core proteins renders cells remarkably repair deficient and highly sensitive to IR and other DSB-inducing agents.

- Endjoining components like Ku or XRCC4 exert a dominant role in this repair pathway in the sense that their presence prevents the utilization of other pathways such as B-NHEJ, HRR, or SSA.
- Homologous recombination repair uses a perfect homologous sequence to restore exactly the DNA sequence disrupted by the DSB. This homology is usually provided postreplication by the sister chromatid.
- Repair of DSBs will benefit from a regulatory linkage with the cell cycle engine suppressing DNA replication and cell division when DSBs are detected.
- Epidermal growth factor receptor up-regulation is suggested to stimulate the respective DNA repair pathways leading thus to radioresistance.

Abstract

Ionizing radiation (IR) induces a diverse spectrum of DNA lesions, among which the DNA double-stranded break (DSB) is the most critical; both with respect to cell lethality, as well as with respect to the induction of mutations leading to genomic instability and cancer. Mammalian cells have developed multifaceted machinery to detect and restore this type of damage. As a result, most IR-induced DSBs are repaired efficiently. However, despite efficient repair, the probability for error-prone processing remains considerably higher for DNA DSBs than for other IR-induced DNA lesions. Therefore, after exposure to IR, unrepaired or misrepaired DSBs are the main cause of cell lethality and mutation induction. Here, we review the molecular processes elicited in mammalian cells on induction of DSBs. In addition to the pathways recruited for their repair, we describe signaling processes that detect this lesion and interphase with the cell cycle engine in an effort to delay cell cycle transitions that could interfere with repair. Molecular characterization of these pathways and processes offers unique opportunities for defining useful predictors of cellular response to IR and appropriate targets for optimizing the application of radiation in the clinical setting for the treatment of human cancer.

14.1
Introduction

Ionization events in the nucleus damage constituents of the DNA – the primary target of most adverse radiation effects in higher eukaryotes. Single ionizations break the sugar–phosphate backbone of the DNA to generate single-strand breaks (SSB), which need to be resealed, or damage bases in the interior of the helix that require replacement. Such simple DNA lesions can be repaired by excision of damaged nucleotides and resynthesis of the missing segments of the molecule, using the intact strand as template (CALDECOTT 2008; DAVID et al. 2007). It is thought that the double-stranded nature of DNA evolved mainly to ensure its preservation through repair mechanisms developed on the principle of strand complementarity. As a result, isolated, single DNA lesions are repaired efficiently in a predominantly error-free manner and carry only a low probability for lethality or mutagenicity. Similar isolated DNA lesions can also be produced by ongoing cellular metabolic processes. Indeed, it is estimated that as a result of the intracellular oxidative metabolism as well as of spontaneous base hydrolysis and deamination, thousands of DNA lesions are produced per cell every day. Then what is the discriminating feature of ionizing radiation (IR) that underlies its highly cytotoxic and mutagenic potential?

Ionization events generated by charged particles are not evenly distributed but are instead localized along their trajectories, particularly at the end of tracks, generating blobs and spurs of energy deposition (GOODHEAD 2006; NIKJOO et al. 1998). This leads to accumulation of chemically distinct damages in a small segment of the DNA, referred to as a locally multiply damage site (LMDS), or simply as a complex lesion. Complex lesions affecting both DNA strands cause a failure of the above-discussed fundamental requirement for repair, i.e., the presence of an intact complementary strand. Among complex radiation-induced DNA lesions, the simplest is the DNA double-strand break (DSB), formed by two SSBs generated in close proximity in the complementary DNA strands. In principle, one DSB can be originated either from one or from two different particles. However, the linear yield of DSBs with dose implicates coordinated ionizations within a single track in their induction. The generation of localized, multiple ionization events by single-particle traversals is a unique property of IR and the main cause for the high efficiency of induction of DSBs and other complex DNA lesions.

Because the number of ionizations induced in the DNA by spurs and blobs is not limited to two and can actually reach considerable numbers, particularly after exposure to high linear-energy-transfer (LET) radiation, highly complex lesions can be envisioned, comprising SSBs, as well as non-strand-disrupting sugar and base damages. As a result, sections of DNA many base pairs long can be shuttered, ultimately leading, directly or indirectly, to the formation of a DSB. Under these conditions, the extensive form of damage present in both DNA strands jeopardizes complementarity-based repair. Lesions of further complexity can be envisioned when considering the organization of DNA in chromatin loops. Blobs localized at the loop attachment site can induce several DSBs simultaneously, which together may destabilize the intervening chromatin and may cause the loss of entire DNA segments. It is evident from this outline that the term *DSB* is broad, comprising a spectrum of lesions, from simple breaks that could be repaired by replacing a couple of damaged terminal nucleotides to extensive accumulations of damage that will require the replacement of substantial portions of the DNA molecule. Repair systems operating on such lesions should therefore have such processing flexibility built in.

Because metabolic activities taking place in the DNA during the cell cycle such as replication and mitosis-associated chromatin condensation can interfere with DNA repair, DSB processing is directly coupled to cell cycle progression. Salient features of this coupling are delays in cell cycle progression observed in irradiated cells, which have been studied extensively by radiation biologists during the last 40 years. Although these delays were initially considered passive cellular responses, it is now a well-established fact that they represent active responses mediated by activation through DNA damage of signaling pathways, which slow down cell cycle progression by downregulating the cell cycle engine. The term *checkpoints* is now widely used to describe this active coupling of cell cycle progression with DNA damage and is thought essential for optimal repair. The molecular processes associated with checkpoint activation are described in the following sections. Importantly, DNA damage is now known to affect every aspect of cellular metabolism and to include extensive modifications in transcriptional regulation, as well as life-or-death decisions. All these cellular responses are commonly integrated under the phrase *biological responses to DNA damage*.

The molecular description of DSB processing and checkpoint activation would have been a role of specialists, if it did not have direct relevance to cancer research and radiation therapy. Indeed, recent advances in the field clearly demonstrate the importance of these processes in genomic stability and implicate their partial abrogation in the development of cancer. Furthermore, DSB repair and checkpoint response are major determinants of cellular radiosensitivity to killing and therefore of direct relevance to radiation therapy. Evidence accumulates that participating proteins display activity differences among individuals, which may underlie well-known variations in individual radiosensitivity. Furthermore, tumor-associated modifications in the constitution of these proteins may alter the radiosensitivity of tumor cells and may underlie the development of tumor radioresistance. In addition, molecular understanding of the pathways involved is expected to uncover molecular targets for the development of specific inhibitors, with the aim of improving treatment with IR of human tumors.

14.2
DSB Repair

The above outline considers intrinsic properties of IR and points to DSBs and other complex lesions ultimately disrupting DNA continuity as major candidates for the observed effects resulting from complications and problems in their processing. However, it is important to stress that the evolutionary pressure for the development of mechanisms dealing with DSBs may not originate from IR but from the fact that DSBs also are either the unwanted side effect of certain DNA metabolic activities or the required initiators of important DNA-modifying cellular activities. As a result, selective pressure must have existed for organisms to evolve systems for processing DSBs. Programmed DSBs at predetermined genomic locations are integral to meiosis, and are induced during VDJ and class switch recombination required for the development of the adaptive immune system in higher eukaryotes. On the other hand, DSBs can be induced at random genomic locations when replication forks collapse on encountering SSBs or base damages. Mechanisms to repair DSBs will therefore benefit cells not only in their response to IR, but also in their ability to perform essential biological functions and to protect themselves from replication errors.

The nature of DSBs directly implies that processing mechanisms need to solve the problem of DNA destabilization caused by the disruption in the continuity of the molecule, the problem of sequence restoration near the DSB, and possibly also the problem generated by the presence of other forms of DNA damage near the break. The information summarized in the following sections indicates that despite these extra requirements, cells are successful in developing powerful mechanisms for DSB processing. However, despite success, the probability for error-prone processing for DSBs remains considerably higher than for any other IR-induced DNA lesion. As a result, unrepaired or misrepaired DSBs are the main cause of cell lethality and mutation induction after exposure to IR.

14.2.1
Methods to Assay for DSBs

Before proceeding to the molecular descriptions of DSB repair and checkpoint activation, methodologies commonly employed to assay DSBs are briefly outlined. These methods can be separated between those that are based on changes in the physical characteristics of the DNA and those that are based on biochemical modifications associated with DSB repair.

14.2.1.1
Physical Methods of DSB Detection

Physical methods of DSB detection are based on changes in the size-sensitive properties of the DNA molecule. Although these methods allow very straightforward and precise DNA size determinations for relatively small molecules (up to 100 kbp), they frequently fail when applied to DNA molecules the size of human chromosomes (average of 150 Mbp).

Neutral sucrose-gradient centrifugation is the method of choice for DSB determination in bacteria and yeast, due to its quantitative nature and the well-understood theoretical background. In this method, cells are lysed to free up DNA, which is then allowed to sediment under the influence of high-speed centrifugation in a neutral sucrose gradient. Small molecules will sediment slower than will large molecules, which allows evaluation of fragmentation by IR. Despite its theoreti-

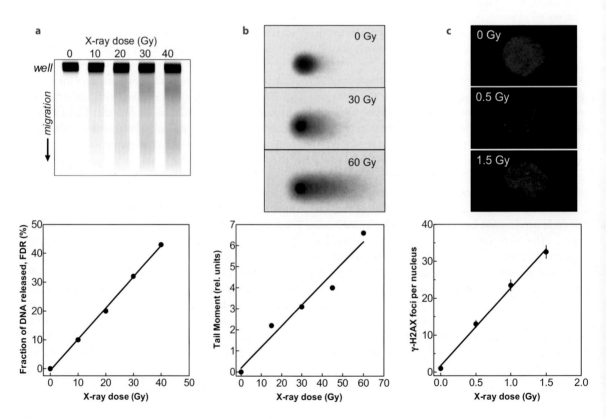

Fig. 14.1a–c. Detection of radiation-induced DSBs by **a** pulsed-field gel electrophoresis, **b** neutral comet assay, or **c** γ-H2AX foci formation. Measurements were performed either immediately (**a, b**) or 60 min after (**c**) irradiation on ice. (Fig. 14.1a was kindly provided by Dr. Minli Wang, Institute of Medical Radiobiology, Essen, Germany; Fig. 14.1b by Dr. Holger Klammer, Institute of Medical Radiobiology, Essen, Germany; and Fig. 14.1c by Drs. Andrea Kinner and Christian Staudt, Institute of Medical Radiobiology, Essen, Germany)

cal advantages, neutral sucrose-gradient centrifugation is tedious, and for human DNA, it requires special care to avoid sedimentation artifacts.

Gel electrophoresis performed at constant field strength is extensively used to size DNA molecules but fails to separate them at sizes above 30 kbp, due to reptation problems. This limitation can be overcome by periodic changes in strength and orientation of the electric field, to allow DNA relaxation between pulses. An array of pulsed-field gel electrophoresis (PFGE) methods have been derived from this concept and used to measure induction and repair of DSBs. Although sizing is not always quantitative when using these methods, they are widely used in the field and have helped to generate a substantial amount of valuable data. Typical gel obtained with cells exposed to IR and analyzed immediately after irradiation is shown in Fig. 14.1a. PFGE methods require relatively large radiation doses for a reliable determination of the DSB load.

It has been demonstrated that useful data can also be obtained when gel electrophoresis of irradiated DNA in higher eukaryotes is performed in a constant field (constant-field gel electrophoresis [CFGE]), and the fraction of DNA released is taken as a measure of the DSB load (DAHM-DAPHI and DIKOMEY 1995). Although DNA sizing is under these conditions not possible, the method is useful, particularly due to its low demands in specialized equipment.

Single-cell gel electrophoresis can be regarded as a special variation of CFGE and allows determination of DNA DSB in individual cells. This offers certain distinct advantages including low requirements for biological material and direct possibilities for analyses of repair throughout the cell cycle. This assay, which is also known as the "comet" assay is illustrated in Fig. 14.1b.

The above-described techniques only measure DNA size and ascribe reductions to the induction of DSBs. Conversely, repair is assayed by evaluating increases in DNA size as a function of time after exposure to IR. As outlined above, after exposure of cells to IR, a spectrum of DNA-disrupting lesions with potentially different repair requirements is induced, all of which are seen by all these assays as DSBs. This is an important limitation of these assays that should be kept in mind. Furthermore, "repair" in these assays will imply restoration of molecular size but will not imply in any way that the DNA molecule was restored to its original state. Additions or deletions of a few or of thousands of bases around the DSB will not be detected, and in a similar fashion, misrejoining events will also remain undetected. This is also important to keep in mind, particularly since, as we will see later, mammalian cells employ quite differ-

ent systems to repair DSBs, which have very different abilities in restoring the DNA molecule.

14.2.1.2
Biochemical Approaches: γ-H2AX Foci Detection

Each DSB will activate signaling pathways that modify a large array of cellular responses to optimize repair and life-or-death decisions. Critical for these responses are kinases of the phosphatidylinositol 3–like kinase family, mainly DNA-PK, ATM, and ATR. Ten years ago it was demonstrated that activation of these kinases in the vicinity (about 10 Mbp) of the DSB leads to phosphorylation of the histone variant H2AX at serine 139, to generate γ-H2AX, which can be visualized as a focus, using specific antibodies and fluorescence microscopy (JEGGO and LOBRICH 2005; LOBRICH and JEGGO 2007). γ-H2AX foci formation has been shown a reliable surrogate for DSBs and is used extensively to measure induction and repair of DSBs. Typical results obtained with this method are shown in Fig. 14.1c. This technique is extremely sensitive and can be used to detect DSB even after X-ray doses as low as few milligrays (JEGGO and LOBRICH 2005; LOBRICH and JEGGO 2007). Since γ-H2AX foci formation requires the above-mentioned kinases and is orchestrated by a complex biochemical pathway involving a large array of proteins, not all of which contribute to DSB repair, care must be taken when interpreting the results (KINNER et al. 2008).

14.2.2
Induction and Repair Kinetics of DNA DSBs

In mammalian cells, DSBs are induced linearly with dose (Fig. 14.1). For X-rays, on average 20–30 DSBs are induced per Gray and per normal mammalian cell with a diploid genome (DAHM-DAPHI and DIKOMEY 1995; ROTHKAMM and LOBRICH 2003). While there is no pronounced variation in the induction of DSBs for normal cells, neither between different tissues nor between different individuals (DIKOMEY et al. 1998, 2000; RÜBE et al. 2008; WURM et al. 1994), significant differences were found for tumor cells, even after normalizing to the respective DNA content (see Fig. 14.2a) (EL-AWADY et al. 2003; MCMILLAN et al. 1990; RUIZ DE ALMODO-VAR et al. 1994). This variation in DSB induction, which might result from changes in chromatin structure frequently occurring in tumor cells, was often reported correlated with the respective differences in cellular

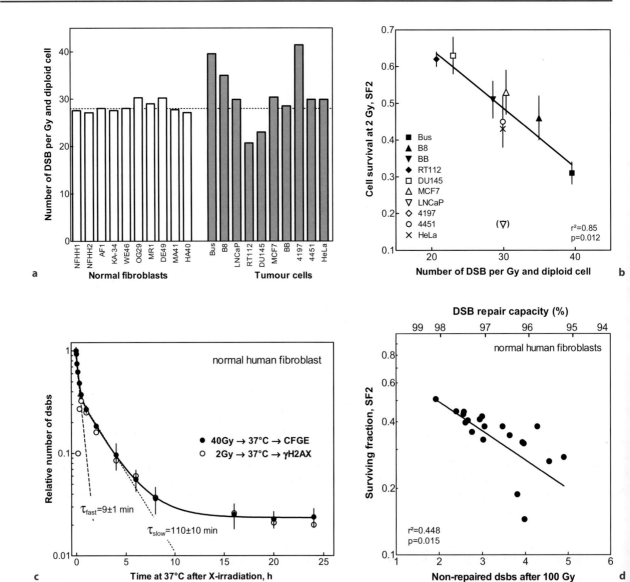

Fig. 14.2a–d. Induction and repair of DSBs after X-irradiation. **a** Variation of the initial number of DSBs in normal human fibroblasts and tumor cells as detected by CFGE; **b** correlation between the initial number of DSBs and cellular sensitivity (*SF2*) in human tumor cells (data are from El-Awady et al. 2003); **c** repair kinetics of DSBs in normal human fibroblasts detected either by CFGE or by γ-H2AX foci scoring (data for CFGE are from Kasten-Pisula et al. 2005, or were kindly provided by Dr. Ulla Kasten-Pisula, Laboratory of Radiobiology & Experimental Radiation Oncology, University Medical Center Hamburg-Eppendorf, Hamburg, Germany); **d** correlation between residual DSBs measured with CFGE 24 h after irradiation and SF2, as found for normal human fibroblasts (data are taken from Kasten-Pisula et al. 2005)

radiosensitivity (see Fig. 14.2b) (El-Awady et al. 2003; McMillan et al. 1990; Ruiz de Almodovar et al. 1994). Likely this variation in DSB induction is one of the main reasons for the large differences of the cellular radiosensitivity observed for many tumor entities.

The repair kinetics of X-ray-induced DSBs as measured by PFGE or CFGE are described by a biphasic curve eventually reaching a plateau (as illustrated in Fig. 14.2c) for a human fibroblast strain exposed to a X-ray dose of 40 Gy (Kasten-Pisula et al. 2005). Generally, there is a fast exponential component with a half-time ranging between 5 and 30 min, and a slow component with a half-time ranging between 2 and 5 h (Dahm-Daphi and Dikomey 1996). For most cell lines, the fast component includes about 30%, and the slow component about 60%, of all DSBs induced. The plateau reflects the number of nonrejoined DSBs but may also include misjoining events. An almost identical curve is obtained when DSBs are assessed by γ-H2AX foci, scoring after a much lower X-ray dose of only 2 Gy (see Fig. 14.2c, open symbols) (ROTHKAMM and LOBRICH 2003). However, since these foci are formed with time after irradiation, their number first increases with increasing time after irradiation, generally reaching a maximum at about 30 min, which is followed by a decline similar to that seen when DSBs are measured by CFGE. Due to these differences in the kinetics, the fast DSB repair component is generally not detected when using the γ-H2AX technique (STIFF et al. 2004).

The kinetics of DSB repair depend on the type of radiation used, with an increase in both the slow component of rejoining as well as in the final plateau reached with increasing LET (ESPOSITO et al. 2005; TAUCHER-SCHOLZ et al. 1996). Since there is an increase by a factor of about 3 in the total number of DSBs remaining for radiations of LET between 50 and 100 KeV/μ, it is thought that the increase in unrepaired DSBs can explain the respective rise in cellular radiosensitivity to killing (ESPOSITO et al. 2005, 2006; TAUCHER-SCHOLZ et al. 1996).

DSB repair also depends not only on several parameters such as cell cycle position, proliferation, cell matrix proximity, etc., but also (especially) on oxygen concentration. Reduction in oxygen results in a reduced formation of DSBs (which is nevertheless only seen after low- and not high-LET radiation), but also reduces the overall repair capacity (FRANKENBERG-SCHWAGER et al. 1991; HIRAYAMA et al. 2005; PRISE et al. 1987; WHITAKER and McMILLAN 1992). Consequently, hypoxic cells are much more radioresistant but show less recovery.

The interindividual variation of the DSB repair kinetics, as measured for normal human fibroblasts, is very small, with little change in the final plateau, indicating that these cells differ only in the total DSB repair capacity (DIKOMEY et al. 2000). This capacity was found to vary only between 95 and 99%, but to have a strong correlation with the respective cellular radiosensitivity (see Fig. 14.2d) (KASTEN-PISULA et al. 2005). This observation illustrates that for normal cells – in contrast to tumor cells – variation in cellular radiosensitivity appears to result primarily from differences in DSB repair capacity.

Overall, the DSB repair kinetics measured for human tumor cells are similar to those observed for normal human fibroblasts, but with slightly greater variation in both the slow component of rejoining as well as in the final plateau (EL-AWADY et al. 2003). However, it should be noted that these kinetics are also affected by many other parameters, as outlined above, so that a clear-cut comparison with normal cells is not possible. In addition, these kinetics might be affected by the occurrence of apoptotic cells, often observed in tumor cells.

For some cell lines, a clear deviation from these kinetics is observed, with either an increase in the slow component or in the respective half-time, and/or a higher final plateau. These deviations can be taken as an indication of either a defect in one of the DSB repair pathways involved or in the regulation of these pathways. This is outlined in more detail in Sect. 14.2.3, which also includes some prominent examples.

14.2.3
Pathways of DSB Repair

14.2.3.1
Nonhomologous Endjoining

The observation made about 15 years ago that mammalian cells do not prefer homologous recombination for the repair of DSB but instead use a simple system based on clearance of DNA ends and ligation was a considerable surprise in the field. This repair system does not require a homologous sequence. It can operate on any type of DNA end and was hence named nonhomologous endjoining (NHEJ). Specific proteins assemble at the DNA, hold broken ends in close proximity, and prepare them at the same time for ligation. This end processing is particularly important after IR exposure, since only a small minority of radiation-induced lesions is directly ligatable. The broken DNA termini generated after IR typically carry 3'phosphates and phosphoglycolates, which cannot be processed by ligases and, thus, need to be removed. The subsequent ligation restores the continuity of the DNA molecule but not the exact DNA sequence around the DSB. NHEJ is hence considered in most cases error prone. This pathway operates with very fast kinetics and has been shown to require a set of "core" proteins performing well-described functions that are summarized in Fig. 14.3a.

Within seconds after induction, the DSB is bound by a heterodimer of Ku70 and Ku80, which keeps the ends in proximity and immediately recruits a third large protein, the catalytic subunit (DNA-PKcs), into a holocomplex called DNA-dependent protein kinase (DNA-PK). DNA-PK executes several key functions and orchestrates the entire process, which is, hence, also called DNA-PK–dependent nonhomologous endjoin-

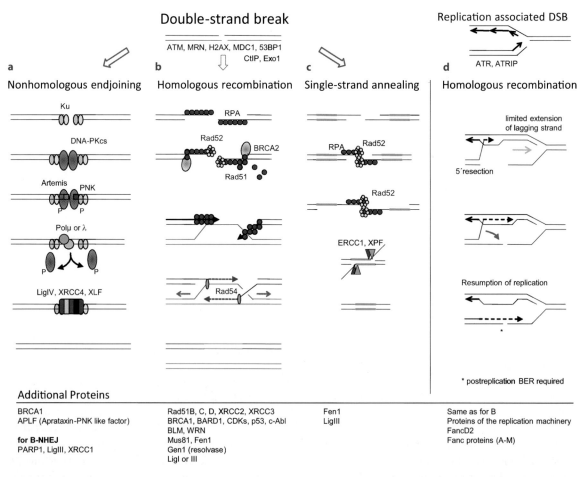

Fig. 14.3a–d. DSB repair pathways in mammalian cells. **a** Nonhomologous endjoining (*NHEJ*), **b** homologous recombination repair (HRR), **c** single-strand annealing (SSA), **d** repair of replication associated DSBs by homologous recombination

ing (D-NHEJ). In addition to providing an important shelter for the vulnerable free termini, the DNA-PK complex phosphorylates a number of downstream targets including itself (autophosphorylation). DNA-PK also binds to and regulates the activity of Artemis, an endo-/exonuclease involved in the tailoring of "dirty" ends for ligation. The Ku components of the DNA-PK complex are required for recruitment of the ligation complex, and DNA-PKcs modulates its activity. The complex of DNA–ligase IV and its cofactors XRCC4 and XLF build the second functional bridge, stabilizing the chromatin structure until both ends have been definitively rejoined. This bridge provides support for groups of enzymes involved in NHEJ. DNA polymerases of the Pol X family (Pol μ, Pol λ), and polynucleotide kinase (PNK) or terminal deoxynucleotidyl transferase (TdT) can modify ends and/or replenish small sequence gaps by fill-in synthesis.

The kinase function of DNA-PK not only modulates components of the NHEJ, but appears to also timely coordinate this pathway with cell cycle progression and with other repair pathways (see below).

Most of the core D-NHEJ proteins are essential for this pathway, as they have unique functions and cannot be replaced by other enzymes. Lack of core proteins renders cells remarkably repair deficient and highly sensitive to IR and other DSB-inducing agents (DIKOMEY et al. 1998; LIEBER et al. 2003; RIBALLO et al. 2004). Knockout mice have, in addition a deficient immune response because D-NHEJ also executes VDJ and class switch recombination, essential processes for the generation of an antibody and T-cell receptor arsenal. In addition, these mice have growth defects, neurological abnormalities, and experience premature aging. Ligase IV and XRCC4 deficiency even confers embryonic lethality. Ku-, DNA-PKcs- and Artemis-deficient mice are viable but severely radiosensitive and immune compromised. Interestingly, very few examples of human NHEJ defects exist, presumably underscoring the essential nature of this pathway. The rare Artemis syndrome is a prominent exception, with severe immunodefects, radiosensitivity, and a short life span. It has been identified as a recent founder mutation in Native American tribes.

14.2.3.2
Backup Pathways of NHEJ

For many years, scientists appreciated that a considerable amount of DSBs could be repaired even in the complete absence of core D-NHEJ proteins such as Ku, DNA-PK, XRCC4, or ligase IV. In addition, the frequency of chromosomal aberrations was significantly enhanced, including not only frank chromosome breaks, but also translocations. In particular, the latter was enigmatic. It was thought that without the DNA-PK or DNA ligation complexes, DSB ends could not be held in close proximity. Thus, free DNA ends might diffuse and come into contact with distal chromosomal breaks. But how could they be rejoined without the specific tools described above? Molecular analysis of break sites in mice and humans revealed in most cases no extended homology, excluding the involvement of homologous recombination repair in this process.

Two parallel lines of discoveries during the last few years have shed light on this repair phenotype. It was observed that indeed DSB ends could be rejoined by an alternative repair pathway, which operates independently of a functional DNA-PK complex. To be active, this pathway requires the absence of the classic core components and can hence be considered a backup pathway (therefore named B-NHEJ). Although important details regarding the function of this pathway are lacking, current evidence suggests that it uses the DNA ligase III–PARP-1–XRCC1 module, normally involved in the repair of SSBs and base damage (Audebert et al. 2004; Windhofer et al. 2007). This pathway is more error prone, leads to longer deletions, and typically makes use of longer microhomologies to generate sufficient stability for annealing and rejoining of the ends (Schulte-Uentrop et al. 2008). It was further shown that the use of this alternative endjoining is associated with frequent chromosomal translocations, possibly representing a significant source for oncogenic mutations (Nussenzweig and Nussenzweig 2007). Notably, this alternative pathway is intimately involved in class switch and under certain conditions in VDJ recombination in cases when D-NHEJ is compromised

(Corneo et al. 2007; Yan et al. 2007). Together, current data suggest that B-NHEJ functions predominantly when factors such as Ku-DNA-PKcs or LigIV-XRCC4, which keep DNA ends in close proximity and protect them from degradation, are lacking. Indeed, how stable DNA ends remain may be decisive for the usage of classic D-NHEJ or one of the alternative repair pathways including B-NHEJ and homologous recombination (for more details about the regulation of repair pathways, see Sect. 14.2.3.5).

14.2.3.3
Homologous Recombination Repair

In mammalian cells, the second important DSB repair pathway is known as homologous recombination repair (HRR). It was described about 40 years ago and is best characterized for prokaryotes and yeast cells, in which it plays a dominant role. If one defines *repair* the restoration of the DNA molecule in its original state, then only the HRR pathway will deserve this characterization. HRR uses a perfect homologous sequence to restore exactly the DNA sequence disrupted by the DSB. This homology is usually provided postreplication by the sister chromatid. Between the S phase and mitosis, both sisters lay in close proximity and are kept together by numerous protein bridges known as cohesins. This connection enables efficient search for homology and strand exchange. Accordingly, these structural proteins are also termed the structural maintenance of chromosomes (SMC) family and play a critical role in HRR (Lehmann 2005). Interestingly, another well-established HRR protein, Rad50 (see below), shares extensive homologies with the SMC group and likely has the identical function to physically hold recombination partners together (Hopfner et al. 2002).

Other homologous sequences present in a cell are much less convenient recombination partners than the sister chromatid is. The diploid mammalian genome includes a second allele with extended sequence homology. Both homologous chromosomes, however, frequently occupy remote loci in the cell nucleus, making synapsis and information exchange unlikely. Pseudogenes and repetitive elements are widespread in the mammalian genome, but usually do not share sufficiently long homologies as required for conservative recombination. Together, these constraints underscore the preferred use of the sister chromatid and likely restrict HRR to the postreplicative S–G2 phase. Further support to this notion comes from the cyclic expression of key HRR proteins, such as Rad51, Rad52, Rad54, BRCA1, BRCA2, and CtIP, all of which peak during the S–G2 phase (CHEN et al. 2008; ESSERS et al. 2002; NAROD and FOULKES 2004). The low level of these proteins in G1 might indirectly help to suppress HRR in a phase of the cell cycle wherein strand exchange with inappropriate partners may cause fatal chromosomal aberrations, gene amplification, or loss of heterozygosity (LOH).

The current knowledge on the mechanism of homologous recombination is summarized in Fig. 14.3b. The ultimate purpose of all participating steps is for the damaged strand to copy the sequence from the undamaged strand. It is believed that the initiating step of HRR is the resection of the 5'strands at the DSB, leaving long 3' single-stranded overhangs that are able to invade the undamaged homologous double DNA strand and to serve as primer for subsequent repair synthesis. The resection step requires as a minimum the presence of MRN (a complex comprising Mre11, Rad50 and nibrin, the protein defective in Nijmegen breakage syndrome [NBS]) and CtIP. It is, however, not clear whether the nuclease function of Mre11 is directly involved. The long, single DNA strands generated by this function are immediately covered and stabilized by replication protein A (RPA). RPA is subsequently replaced by polymers of Rad51, which are wrapped around the single strands, thus forming a so-called nucleoprotein filament. Rad51 loading is governed by BRCA2, the tumor suppressor of breast and ovarian malignancies. Rad51 is the principal recombinase catalyzing the key steps of HRR, the homology search, strand invasion to generate the so-called D-loop, and finally, strand exchange. The branched, triplex DNA structure formed during this exchange is named the Holiday junction. A double Holliday junction consists of both free DSB ends invading the intact duplex in opposite directions. The copying process, driven by polymerase η, moves the branched structure along the DNA strands (branch migration). This translocation is promoted by Rad54 and presumably supported by a complex of the Rad51 homologues XRCC3 and Rad51C. On ATP cleavage, Rad51 dissociates from the DNA to allow completion of the recombination process. After a sufficient number of bases have been copied (gene conversion usually replicates 30–100 bp), the Holliday junction has to be resolved, and the strands need to separate and reanneal to close the DSB. Apparently, the XRCC3–Rad51C complex is engaged in this resolution, perhaps together or alternatively to helicases of the RecQ family (BLM, WRN, RecQ) and topoisomerase III. Depending on how the heteroduplex is cleaved and religated, gene conversion yields noncrossover or crossover recombinants (sister chromatid exchange).

The central process of HRR, the engagement of Rad51 recombinase with DNA damage, is also extensively studied by visualization of repair foci. A fraction of nuclear γ-H2AX foci (see above) are also stained for Rad51, and it is believed that this reflects the assembly of hundreds of Rad51 molecules at those DSBs that are processed by HRR. The proper foci formation is not only dependent on the loading factor BRCA2, but also on the various Rad51 paralogues. The heterodimer XRCC3–Rad51C is already described; less well understood is the second complex composed of Rad51B,C,D and XRCC2. This BCDX2 complex preferably binds Y-shaped DNA structures resembling those at stalled replication forks, which also require HRR for resumption of DNA synthesis, although they do not necessarily involve a frank DSB. From these and other more recent observations in the bacterium *Caenorhabditis elegans* (WARD et al. 2007), it is speculated that the Rad51 paralogues are tools that discriminate between the various DNA lesions and guide the appropriate assembly of Rad51.

During the last decade, it became evident that the classic double Holliday junction is not the only valid HRR model. For repairing the break, it is sufficient that repair synthesis extends only one DNA end beyond the DSB. This single new strand can then separate from the intact double helix, flip back to its original partner strand, and anneal. Fill-in synthesis would replenish the remaining gap. This synthesis-dependent strand annealing (SDSA) may be employed even more frequently than the classic gene conversion model. This is particularly true during the S phase, when numerous DSBs are formed through SSBs colliding with the replication fork (Fig. 14.3d). The collision leaves a single double-stranded end (also termed one-ended DSB), which has no second end as a natural partner to connect to and carry out NHEJ. Figure 14.3d shows a gap located on the "leading" strand of DNA replication. This structure is unstable and leads to a collapse of the replication fork. HRR-guided invasion of the interrupted 3' end into the second newly replicated double helix would prevent the local dissociation of the replication machinery. Limited DNA synthesis across the gap, resolution of the triple helix, and reannealing to the damaged strand would allow resumption of replication. The remaining SSB could be subsequently closed by an excision-type of repair. The model depicted is the simplest one; others ("template switch," "replication fork reversal," "replication fork regression") have been suggested, mainly based on data from *Escherichia coli*. However, it is not known which one best applies for higher eukaryotes.

All proteins involved in HRR are confirmed important for the survival of cells after IR, particularly in the S–G2 phase. Indeed, cells with defects in proteins involved, if at all viable, are known to be more or less radiosensitive. It was therefore a great surprise to see no real defect in DSB rejoining as measured by PFGE (Wang et al. 2001; Rothkamm et al. 2003). In contrast to those methods of physical DSB detection of DSBs, γ-H2AX foci scoring revealed a small, cell cycle–specific repair defect at low radiation doses (Rothkamm and Lobrich 2003). The reasons for those differences are not understood at present. The results clearly demonstrate, however, that in mammals, HRR is not a repair option for the entirety of IR-induced DSBs – in contrast to yeast and bacteria – but to be specific for a subset of DSBs. It is important to elucidate whether some of the chemical characteristics of DSBs play a defining role in the selection of this repair pathway. Alternatively, the possibility should be considered that location in chromatin and the levels of condensation of the surrounding chromatin play a defining role in the recruitment of HRR for the repair of DSBs. Further genetic factors that direct the pathway choice are discussed in Sect. 14.2.3.5.

14.2.3.4
Single-Strand Annealing

Single-strand annealing (SSA), which is seen as another variant of HRR, was originally characterized in yeast, but evidence has accumulated that it may also be a relevant repair pathway in higher eukaryotes. This pathway can be active when a DSB is located between two identical repeat sequences whose homology is utilized in repair. SSA is therefore considered a form of HRR. It shares the initial steps of the above-described HRR pathway, which requires the generation of free 3' single-stranded ends (Fig. 14.3c). The homologous sequences are identified on both ends by a yet-unknown mechanism and subsequently, the complementary single strands anneal. These steps are governed by the heptamer-ring formed by the Rad52 protein. Nonmatching ends are removed by the ERCC1-XPF endonuclease. In contrast to other variants of HRR, SSA is obligatorily mutagenic. One of the repeat copies and the intervening sequence are always lost. In mammalian cells sequence repeats, such as long interspersed nucleotide element (LINE) and short interspersed nucleotide element (SINE) sequences, are particularly abundant in heterochromatic regions, where the loss of sequence may be of no consequence. On the other hand, it was recently shown that SSA-like recombination could also involve distant loci on different chromosomes, resulting in oncogenic translocations (Elliott et al. 2005; Weinstock et al. 2006). To what degree SSA contributes to overall repair of DSBs remains to be determined. Importantly, in mammalian cells, loss of Rad52 does not result in a radiosensitive phenotype, either because critical steps of the SSA pathway are redundantly controlled by other proteins, or because other forms of HRR such as gene conversion with crossover substitute when SSA is not functional.

14.2.3.5
Regulation of DSB Repair

Four levels of regulation of DSB repair are described here, which are considered examples for a complex network that is only now beginning to be elucidated:
1. Regulation at the level of executer proteins
2. Regulation via upstream signaling, protein recruitment, and protein activation
3. Regulation via modification of the DNA end structure
4. Regulation via modification of a single repair protein, DNA-PK

Another increasingly important parameter, the structural modulation of chromatin to accommodate DNA repair, is not considered further here.

14.2.3.5.1
Regulation at the Level of Executer Proteins

The principal goal of DSB repair is to reestablish the chromosomal continuity and thus to prevent loss of genetic information. To this end, DNA ends must be held together and reconnected by simple means. This is best achieved by the classic NHEJ system. It was indeed shown that endjoining components like Ku or XRCC4 exert a dominant role in this repair pathway in the sense that their presence prevents the utilization of other pathways such as B-NHEJ, HRR, or SSA (Mansour et al. 2008; Stark et al. 2004). In particular, the abundant nuclear protein Ku with its high affinity for DNA ends can regulate the choice of pathways by outcompeting other proteins (i.e., PARP1 or Rad52), which would otherwise shuttle repair into alternative directions (Ristic et al. 2003; Windhofer et al. 2007). The second aim of DSB repair, to accurately maintain the genetic code, would be best served by conservative HRR in the S–G2 phase, using the sister chromatid as template. Homology search beyond this spatiotemporal framework would be associated with illegitimate recombination events (translocations) or with failure of the repair process all together. To avoid this from happening, cells have developed additional mechanisms to tightly control the utilization of the different repair pathways and thus to minimize deleterious consequences associated with inappropriate use.

14.2.3.5.2
Regulation via Upstream Signaling, Protein Recruitment, and Protein Activation

The cellular response to DSBs is initiated by a not-fully-elucidated damage recognition process, leading to the binding of MRN, which in turn is required for activation and recruitment of ATM (PAULL and LEE 2005), the major regulator of DDR with respect to repair and checkpoint response. The role of ATM in the phosphorylation of H2AX has been described above. This chromatin modification near a DSB provides the stage for the recruitment of two further mediator proteins, MDC1 and 53BP1. MDC1 appears to preferably support HRR, while 53BP1 exerts a control function in NHEJ and the related VDJ and class switch recombination (DIFILIPPANTONIO et al. 2008; WARD et al. 2004; XIE et al. 2007). MDC1 is one of the numerous phosphorylation targets of ATM besides nibrin, DNA-PKcs, CHK2, SMC1, BRCA1, and CtIP.

14.2.3.5.3
Regulation via Modification of the DNA End Structure

MRN, BRCA1, and CtIP form an inactive complex that can be activated by phosphorylation by both ATM and CDK1. Thus, BRCA1 is derepressed as it dissociates from the complex and functions as regulator of cell cycle checkpoints and repair fidelity. MRN, together with CtIP, initiates the resection of 5' ends to generate 3' single-stranded overhangs, presumably via Mre11 nuclease activity (Fig. 14.3b). As a result, this end modification critically determines repair pathway choice. As long as the DNA ends remain stable, repair proceeds by NHEJ. However, as soon as ATM–mediated resection starts, repair is shuttled toward HRR, or less likely SSA (HUERTAS et al. 2008; SARTORI et al. 2007). Recent results also suggest that CtIP–MRN-mediated resection might also promote alternative endjoining, which is also accompanied by extensive end degradation (BENNARDO et al. 2008).

14.2.3.5.4
Regulation via Modification of a Single Repair Protein, DNA-PK

During DSB processing, DNA-PKcs becomes phosphorylated at distinct clusters of amino acid residues, either by itself or by ATM. Depending on which cluster is phosphorylated, DNA-PK becomes activated or inhib-ited. Inhibition of DNA-PK not only reduces D-NHEJ, but also actively guides repair toward HRR (SHRIVASTAV et al. 2008). A second, more passive possibility to shuttle repair into a recombination path arises when DNA-PK dissociates from the DNA ends. This dissociation, a result of autophosphorylation (Fig. 14.3a), is an integral part NHEJ to allow further steps in the end-joining process. However, it might also open the door for HRR proteins to bind to the damage site and thus terminate NHEJ.

In conclusion, repair of DSBs in mammalian cells is dominated by the efficient repair pathway of NHEJ. Homology-dependent pathways such as HRR, and to lesser degree SSA, can also be employed, but they appear restricted to the S–G2 phase of the cell cycle. Pathway utilization is tightly regulated at various levels to minimize the deleterious consequences of erroneous repair. It is of eminent importance to elucidate whether the genetic control of repair is relaxed in tumor cells, as this may explain their increased genomic instability. Enhanced utilization of "backup" pathways, on the other hand, may increase survival chances when pathways used as first line of defense fail, which may enhance the genomic instability of the tumor and thus its radioresistance. For additional reading, several reviews on DSB repair and its regulation are available (HELLEDAY et al. 2007; KINNER et al. 2008; LIEBER et al. 2003; SHRIVASTAV et al. 2008; WYMAN and KANAAR 2006).

14.3
Radiation Induced Cell Cycle Checkpoints

The above description of DSB repair pathways assumes an idle, double-stranded DNA molecule that is randomly broken by IR. In a multicellular organism, this condition may be approximated by the majority of cells that are not actively dividing, but are instead terminally differentiated and arrested in the G0 phase. However, the development of a multicellular organism from a fertilized egg requires a great number of cell divisions. Also, adult multicellular organisms require cell division for maintenance and self-renewal. It is therefore likely that DSBs will occur in the DNA of dividing cells that are in different stages of the cell cycle.

During the cell cycle, cells replicate their DNA and subsequently distribute it evenly in the daughter cells. The replication of DNA during the S phase, as well as its distribution to the daughter cells at mitosis, are complex processes associated with radical changes in the organization of DNA in chromatin. One can therefore deduce that during such chromatin reorganization, re-

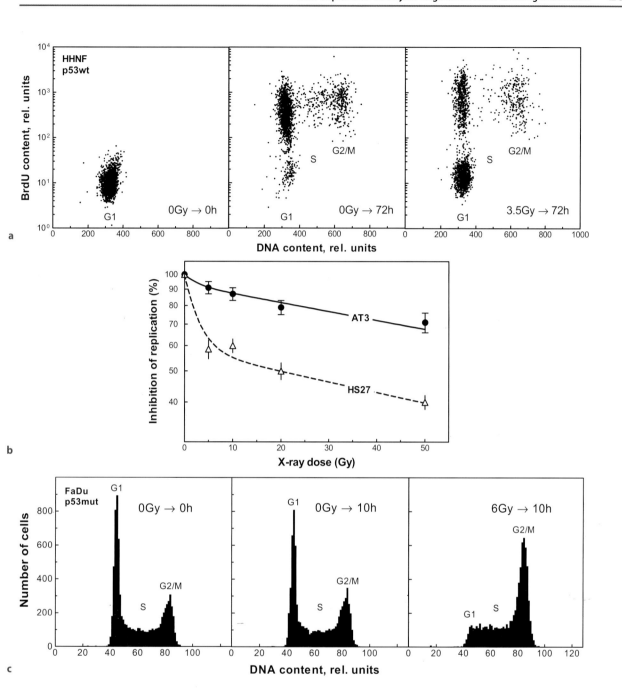

Fig. 14.4a–c. Radiation-induced cell cycle delays in irradiated mammalian cells. **a** Delay in G1, as detected in the normal human fibroblast strain HHNF irradiated with 3.5 Gy. Confluent cells were stimulated into the cell cycle, and proliferating cells were identified by BrdU incorporation, which was followed by antibody staining and analysis by flow cytometry (kindly provided by Dr. Ingo Brammer, Laboratory of Radiobiology & Experimental Radiation Oncology, University Medical Center Hamburg-Eppendorf, Hamburg, Germany). **b** Inhibition of DNA replication after exposure to IR. Replication activity was measured via incorporation of radioactively labeled thymidine (data are from PAINTER 1986). **c** Delay in G2, as detected in the mutant p53 human squamous cell carcinoma strain FaDu after irradiation with 6 Gy. Exponentially growing cells were irradiated with 6 Gy, and the cell cycle distribution was measured by flow cytometry

pair of DSBs is compromised. The following examples illustrate possible scenarios as to how this might happen. The unstopped progression of a replication fork to a DSB will not only cause the collapse of the replication fork, but it will also generate such a destabilizing condition in the DNA that may abrogate subsequent repair. Even an SSB, normally a harmless DNA lesion, can cause the collapse of an advancing replication fork and lead to the formation of a one-sided DSB (see above). During mitosis, the decondensed chromatin of the interphase nucleus condenses to chromosomes, a process associated with extensive chromatin remodeling. The presence of DSBs in the genome during such remodeling activity is likely to pull the ends of the DSB apart, thus interfering with or compromising subsequent repair.

From the potential complications outlined above, it becomes obvious that repair of DSBs will benefit from a regulatory linkage with the cell cycle engine, suppressing DNA replication and cell division when DSBs are detected. Indeed, early studies on the effect of radiation on cell proliferation have uncovered delays that could be attributed to specific inhibition in the progression of cells from G1 into the S phase, and from the G2 into the M phase, as well as a less pronounced inhibition of DNA replication during the S phase. Typical experiments demonstrating these cell cycle–specific delays in the progression of cells through the cell cycle are summarized in Fig. 14.4.

Delay or arrest in the G1 phase (Fig. 14.4a) is especially known for normal human fibroblasts expressing wild-type p53 (Di Leonardo et al. 1994; Li et al. 1995; Nagasawa et al. 1995), but it also occurs in other cell types. In fibroblast cultures grown to confluence, most cells are in G1 (Fig. 14.4a, left panel). When these cells are stimulated into the cell cycle by reseeding at a lower density, proliferating cells can easily be separated via incorporation of BrdU. After 72 h, most cells are triggered into the cell cycle, and there are only few cells remaining in G1 (Fig. 14.4a, middle panel). However, this fraction clearly increases when prior to stimulation cells are irradiated with 3.5 Gy. This demonstrates a radiation-induced delay in G1 (Fig. 14.4a, left panel).

Radiation also reduces the rate of DNA synthesis during the S phase (Fig. 14.4b). There is a dose-dependent biphasic reduction, suggesting inhibition of at least two different steps in replication. It is now known that the radiosensitive component reflects inhibition of replicon cluster initiation, whereas the radioresistant component reflects inhibition of DNA chain elongation (Painter and Young 1980). This inhibition is reduced in cells from ataxia telangiectasia (AT) patients, suggesting that it reflects an active cellular response to the radiation insult, rather than a passive consequence of DNA damage.

Delay in the G2 phase (Fig. 14.4c) is generally observed when exponentially growing cells are exposed to IR and is especially pronounced in cells with p53MUT, because these cells are not arrested in G1. This dose-dependent accumulation in the G2 phase is observed few hours later, suggesting a delay in traversing this phase of the cell cycle.

While it was initially thought that DNA damage passively causes these delays, it is now well documented that the observed delays derive from active cellular responses, termed checkpoints, linking DNA repair with the cell cycle engine in an effort to optimize repair and to maximize genomic stability. The molecular characterization of DNA damage checkpoints is a hot topic of modern biology, with direct connections not only to radiation biology, but also to the field of cancer. A brief summary on the current state of knowledge on this topic is given below.

14.3.1
DNA Damage Checkpoints

The molecular machinery of the DNA damage checkpoint must be capable of detecting damage in the DNA and of interphasing with the cell cycle machinery in a regulatory way. To achieve this, the participating proteins must be able to sense DNA damage and to transduce the information to the cell cycle engine. Therefore, proteins participating in the DNA damage checkpoint are grouped into sensors of the DNA damage signal (see Sect. 14.3.2.1), transducers of the signal and effectors that modify the cell cycle (see Sect. 14.3.2.2).

14.3.1.1
DNA Damage Sensors

Damage in the DNA is associated with direct or indirect alterations in its structure or its organization in chromatin. Sensors of damage must therefore be able to detect these changes. Indeed, sensors of DNA damage are known able to detect single- and double-stranded interruptions, the presence of single-stranded regions in the DNA, as well as changes in chromatin structure. Typically, sensors are proteins whose activity, often kinase activity, is regulated by DNA damage or its consequences.

Sensor capacity is associated with DNA-PK, which through its double-stranded DNA end-binding component Ku is activated by DSBs. Activation of this kinase leads to the phosphorylation of several substrates involved in the repair of DSBs by NHEJ (see Sect. 14.2.2.1) and may also contribute through yet-incompletely characterized mechanisms to the maintenance of checkpoints in the cell cycle (Guan et al. 2000). DSB sensing ability is also attributed to ATM kinase (Shiloh 2006). Activation of this kinase is thought mediated either by the DSB directly, by the resulting changes in chromatin conformation, or through interactions with the MRN protein complex described in the HRR discussion above. The ATM kinase features prominently in DNA damage–induced checkpoints in every phase of the cell cycle. A related kinase, ATR, is activated by single-stranded DNA through its accessory protein ATRIP, which in turn recognizes the single-stranded DNA-binding protein RPA. Single-stranded DNA is transiently generated during the repair of several DNA lesions. During DSB repair, single-stranded DNA is generated in the DNA end-processing stages of HRR (see above). ATR, like ATM, is a key component of the DNA damage checkpoint mechanism.

DSBs are lesions induced in relatively low numbers after exposure to IR. For every 1,000–2,000 SSBs and base damages induced per Gray, only 20–40 DSBs are generated. How is then possible for few lesions to initiate the global responses shown in Fig. 14.4? An important recognition in the field of checkpoints is that DSB sensing and processing is associated with a characteristic local modification and/or specific relocalization of proteins to DSB sites, generating distinct subnuclear structures observable by immunofluorescence microscopy, which are commonly referred to as foci. When such foci are induced by IR, they are referred to as IR-induced nuclear foci (IRIF) (Fernandez-Capetillo et al. 2003, 2004). The H2AX phosphorylation and γ-H2AX foci formation described above is one of the most widely studied such modifications. Many more have now been described. An accumulation of proteins near DSBs provides resources for repair and opportunities for signal amplification, which may facilitate the mounting of global responses.

The signal required for IRIF formation can be initiated by the direct or indirect activation by DSBs of ATM, ATR, or DNA-PK. One important phosphorylation target of these kinases is serine 139 of H2AX to generate γ-H2AX (see above). γ-H2AX has been shown to attract a number of chromatin-remodeling and checkpoint-associated proteins. The most specific of these interactions is probably that with MDC1. Indeed, the BRCT repeats of MDC1 are considered the predominant recognition module of γ-H2AX (Lukas et al. 2004; Stewart et al. 2003; Stucki et al. 2005). The interaction between MDC1 and γ-H2AX sets the

stage for further protein interactions around the DSB because there is evidence that MDC1 interacts directly with NBS1 (Goldberg et al. 2003), which in the form of the MRN complex is required for the activation of ATM (Falck et al. 2005; You et al. 2005) and is also involved in HRR (see above). The latter interaction, by bringing the MRN complex to the DSB and thus providing further ATM activation, generates a positive feedback loop that extends H2AX phosphorylation.

In addition to MDC1, 53BP1 also has the ability to detect changes in chromatin on the induction of DSBs. This protein also forms foci in cells exposed to IR, with kinetics similar to those of γ-H2AX (Schultz et al. 2000) and appears to detect DNA damage–induced changes in chromatin conformation. Recruitment of 53BP1 to sites of DSBs depends on a region of the protein that contains two consecutive Tudor domains that can bind directly to methylated histone H3 (Huyen et al. 2004; Iwabuchi et al. 2003; Ward et al. 2003). Because this methylation is constitutive under physiological conditions, only structural modifications are required to reveal it for a 53BP1 molecule to anchor to it.

In addition to phosphorylation, ubiquitinylation (Bennett and Harper 2008) also contributes to damage sensing and checkpoint signal generation. Thus, ATM-mediated phosphorylation of MDC1 leads to the recruitment of RNF8 E3 ubiquitin ligase to the sites of DSBs, which mediates the ubiquitination of H2A and H2AX (Huen et al. 2007; Mailand et al. 2007). This modification is thought to reinforce, through yet-uncharacterized mechanisms, the recruitment to chromatin of 53BP1, as well as the association of BRCA1-BARD1 complex on IRIF.

14.3.1.2
Signal Transducers and Effectors

The above-described choreography that involves sensors and mediator proteins sets the stage for a modulation of the cell cycle progression. Thus, activation of ATM and ATR, together with the associated signal amplification described above, leads to activation through direct phosphorylation of the downstream checkpoint kinases CHK1 and CHK2. Once activated, these kinases directly interphase with the cell cycle through regulation of the CDC25 family of phosphatases.

The CDC25 family of phosphatases is required for the activation of cyclin-dependent kinases (CDKs), which catalyze the transition of cells from one phase of the cell cycle to the next. Thus, CDC25C removes inhibitory phosphate residues from CDK1 and initiates in this way the transition of a nonirradiated cell from the

G2 phase into mitosis. CDC25A has a similar effect on DNA replication associated processes.

Depending on the cell cycle phase in which the cell is irradiated, CHK1 and/or CHK2 phosphorylate the Cdc25 member regulating the corresponding cell cycle activities. This phosphorylation targets the phosphatase for ubiquitinylation, translocation from the nucleus into the cytoplasm, and ultimate degradation. In the absence of active CDC25, the corresponding CDK remains inactive, and the cell fails to carry out processes required for the normal progression through the cycle – it remains arrested or delayed in the cell cycle phase where it received the radiation insult. This elegant mechanism imposes delays in the progression through all phases of the cell cycle except mitosis as soon as damage is detected by sensor proteins.

An additional component of the checkpoint machinery involves the actions of the p53 protein. This protein has received considerable attention by virtue of its tumor suppressor properties and its mutated status in over 50% of human tumors. In a nonirradiated cell, wild-type p53 is quickly degraded through direct interaction with MDM2, which targets the protein for ubiquitinylation. As a result, the protein is unable to function, and the cell remains unaffected in its progression through the cell cycle. DNA damage and the associated activation of ATM and ATR stabilize p53 through direct phosphorylation, as well through phosphorylation and inactivation of its inhibitor MDM2. Accumulated p53 initiates through its transcriptional activity the expression of the CDK inhibitor, p21, which suppresses the activation of CDK2 and thus the progression of cells through G1 and into the S phase. In this way, an additional hurdle is generated in the progression of irradiated cells from G1 into the S phase.

A direct prediction of the mechanism described above is that the loss of p53 function seen in many tumor cell lines will be associated with an attenuation of the IR-induced delay in G1. While such association is generally observed in nontransformed cells, it is erratic in tumor cells with the p53 status unable to predict the presence of a G1 checkpoint (Li et al. 1995; Little et al. 1995).

While the ATM–ATR-initiated activation of CHK1 and CHK2 regulates the checkpoint in every phase of the cell cycle, the p53 response is firmly associated mainly with the IR-induced delay in G1. Is p53 then a protein acting specifically in the G1 phase of the cell cycle? There is evidence for a role of p53 in radiation-induced delays in other phases of the cell cycle as well, but the evidence is less solid than it is the delay in the G1 phase (Powell et al. 1995). Thus, more work is required to evaluate the possible involvement of the p53

component of the checkpoint response in other phases of the cell cycle.

14.4
Clinical Implications

In radiotherapy, information gained about the molecular and cellular aspects of DSB repair has stimulated a broad spectrum of research in several different directions. This information is utilized especially to establish prognostic and predictive assays for tumor response after radiotherapy and to define new, tumor-specific targets.

14.4.1
Prediction and Prognosis

Predictive assays are required for the radiosensitivity of both normal and tumor tissue. For normal tissue, radiosensitivity is considered a critical factor for the risk of development of both acute and late effects after radiotherapy (Borgmann et al. 2002, 2008; De Ruyck et al. 2005; Hoeller et al. 2003; West et al. 2001). It was found that radiosensitivity is mostly determined by genetic factors (Borgmann et al. 2007), and that is best assessed by measuring chromosome aberrations in human lymphocytes irradiated in vitro (Borgmann et al. 2007). No clear correlation with side effects was seen when the individual radiosensitivity was determined by using human fibroblasts, irrespective of whether radiosensitivity was assessed via repair proteins, residual DSBs, or chromosomal damage (Borgmann et al. 2002; Dickson et al. 2002; El-Awady et al. 2005). The reason for this difference is unknown, but it is thought that the correlation between radiosensitivity in situ and radiosensitivity in vitro is not as good for fibroblasts, due to changes occurring during in vitro maintenance (Borgmann et al. 2008), possibly as a result of a change in their differentiation status (Herskind et al. 2000).

Overall variation of normal tissue radiosensitivity is best described by a Gaussian distribution with a coefficient of variation (CV) of 10–20% (Dikomey et al. 2003b). The genetic factors leading to this variation remain unknown, but do not derive from gross changes in major DNA repair enzymes (Dikomey et al. 2003a). It is thought that this variation is the result of slight fluctuations in the abundance or activity of many different proteins contributing to DDR mediated by single-nucleotide polymorphisms (SNPs).

After exposure to IR, tumor cells are mainly inactivated via lethal chromosome aberrations resulting from non- or misrejoined DSBs. Radiation-induced primary apoptosis and terminal differentiation are thought of minor importance (Borgmann et al. 2004; Gudkov and Komarova 2003; Kasten-Pisula et al. 2008). Nevertheless, when comparing different tumor cell lines, there is only a weak correlation between cellular radiosensitivity and the number of either residual DSBs or lethal chromosome aberrations scored. This is probably because these parameters are affected by primary or secondary apoptosis, changes in cell cycle (Akudugu et al. 2004; Eastham et al. 2001; El-Awady et al. 2003; Nunez et al. 1995; Olive et al. 1994), or DNA ploidy (Coco Martin et al. 1999). As a result, neither parameter is useful for the estimation of tumor cell radiosensitivity in the clinical routine.

Recent data suggest that the level of DSB repair proteins, as detected by immunohistochemistry, is a good candidate for a predictor of tumor radiosensitivity. Overall tumor cells appear to have a higher level of DSB repair proteins than has the normal surrounding tissue, and this seems true for both NHEJ as well as HRR proteins. It was shown that the level of the heterodimer Ku70–Ku80 might be associated with tumor radiosensitivity and with that, tumor outcome (Harima et al. 2003; Komuro et al. 2002; Lee et al. 2005; Wilson et al. 2000). Tumors with low Ku levels showed significantly less recurrences when compared with tumors with high Ku levels. No such clear association, however, was seen for DNA PKcs, ATM, or the MRN complex (Lee et al. 2005; Soderlund et al. 2007).

Also, the levels of Rad51, the key protein of HRR (see above), appear of relevance for the prognosis of tumor response after radiotherapy. For this protein, expression was found enhanced, especially in grade 3 tumors, and there is an association between this expression and tumor prognosis (Maacke et al. 2000a,b; Qiao et al. 2005). It was suggested that a high level of Rad51 might either lead to increased genomic instability (Paffett et al. 2005; Richardson et al. 2004) and with that, to poor prognosis, or that it might enhance the survival potential of tumor cells by rendering them more resistant to treatment or to apoptosis (Maacke et al. 2000a).

14.4.2
Tumor Targets

In radiotherapy, there is great need to identify new molecular targets that will allow the specific inactivation of tumor cells. In this context, certain receptors such as epidermal growth factor receptor (EGFR) are considered of great relevance (Baumann et al. 2007; Harrington et al. 2007; Magne et al. 2008). This receptor is involved in several important endpoints such as proliferation and differentiation, angiogenesis, metastasis, and in the DNA damage response after both radio- as well as chemotherapy (Nyati et al. 2006; Rodemann et al. 2007; Song et al. 2005). In many tumors, this receptor is overexpressed and – most importantly – upregulated after irradiation (Contessa et al. 1999; Dittmann et al. 2005; Valerie et al. 2007; Yacoub et al. 2006). Activation of EGFR by both natural ligands and X-irradiation was also found to result in an increased expression of specific repair proteins such as ERCC2, XRCC1, as well as DNA PKcs (Dittmann et al. 2005; Yacoub et al. 2003). This upregulation is suggested to stimulate the respective DNA repair pathways, leading thus to radioresistance. Therefore, inhibition of EGFR either by antibodies or by specific tyrosine-kinase inhibitors was found to inhibit repair and to enhance cell killing (Toulany et al. 2006). Notably, the same treatment is without effect in normal cells, but it is also unlikely to achieve radiosensitization in all cells composing a tumor (Toulany et al. 2006). The reason for the latter variation in response is unknown, but may be the result of genetic differences among tumors or among cells in the same tumor. Thus, it could be shown that radiosensitization by EGFR inhibition may be restricted to those tumor cells in which K-Ras is mutated, and therefore the EGFR pathway permanently upregulated (Toulany et al. 2005). More work is needed to conclusively characterize the parameters determining the response of tumor cells to radiation and to develop strategies that optimally exploit their genetic background.

References

Akudugu JM, Theron T, Serafin AM et al (2004) Influence of DNA double-strand break rejoining on clonogenic survival and micronucleus yield in human cell lines. Int J Radiat Biol 80:93–104

Audebert M, Salles B, Calsou P (2004) Involvement of poly(ADP-ribose) polymerase-1 and XRCC1/DNA ligase III in an alternative route for DNA double-strand breaks rejoining. J Biol Chem 279:55117–55126

Baumann M, Krause M, Dikomey E et al (2007) EGFR-targeted anti-cancer drugs in radiotherapy: preclinical evaluation of mechanisms. Radiother Oncol 83:238–248

Bennardo N, Cheng A, Huang N et al (2008) Alternative NHEJ is a mechanistically distinct pathway of mammalian chromosome break repair. PLoS Genet 4:e1000110

Bennett EJ, Harper JW (2008) DNA damage: ubiquitin marks the spot. Nat Struct Mol Biol 15:20–22

Borgmann K, Roper B, El-Awady R et al (2002) Indicators of late normal tissue response after radiotherapy for head and neck cancer: fibroblasts, lymphocytes, genetics, DNA repair, and chromosome aberrations. Radiother Oncol 64:141–152

Borgmann K, Dede M, Wrona A et al (2004) For X-irradiated normal human fibroblasts, only half of cell inactivation results from chromosomal damage. Int J Radiat Oncol Biol Phys 58:445–452

Borgmann K, Haeberle D, Doerk T et al (2007) Genetic determination of chromosomal radiosensitivities in G0- and G2-phase human lymphocytes. Radiother Oncol 83:196–202

Borgmann K, Hoeller U, Nowack S et al (2008) Individual radiosensitivity measured with lymphocytes may predict the risk of acute reaction after radiotherapy. Int J Radiat Oncol Biol Phys 71:256–264

Caldecott KW (2008) Single-strand break repair and genetic disease. Nat Rev Genet 9:619–631

Chen L, Nievera CJ, Lee AY et al (2008) Cell cycle-dependent complex formation of BRCA1.CtIP.MRN is important for DNA double-strand break repair. J Biol Chem 283:7713–7720

Coco Martin JM, Mooren E, Ottenheim C et al (1999) Potential of radiation-induced chromosome aberrations to predict radiosensitivity in human tumour cells. Int J Radiat Biol 75:1161–1168

Contessa JN, Reardon DB, Todd D et al (1999) The inducible expression of dominant-negative epidermal growth factor receptor CD533 results in radiosensitization of human mammary carcinoma cells. Clin Cancer Res 5:405–411

Corneo B, Wendland RL, Deriano L et al (2007) Rag mutations reveal robust alternative end joining. Nature 449:483–486

Dahm-Daphi J, Dikomey E (1995) Separation of DNA fragments induced by ionizing irradiation using a graded-field gel electrophoresis. Int J Radiat Biol 67:161–168

Dahm-Daphi J, Dikomey E (1996) Rejoining of DNA double-strand breaks in X-irradiated CHO cells studied by constant- and graded-field gel electrophoresis. Int J Radiat Biol 69:615–621

David SS, O'Shea VL, Kundu S (2007) Base-excision repair of oxidative DNA damage. Nature 447:941–950

De Ruyck K, Van Eijkeren M, Claes K et al (2005) Radiation-induced damage to normal tissues after radiotherapy in patients treated for gynecologic tumors: association with single nucleotide polymorphisms in *XRCC1*, *XRCC3*, and *OGG1* genes and in vitro chromosomal radiosensitivity in lymphocytes. Int J Radiat Oncol Biol Phys 62:1140–1149

Di Leonardo A, Linke SP, Clarkin K et al (1994) DNA damage triggers a prolonged p53-dependent G1 arrest and long-term induction of Cip1 in normal human fibroblasts. Genes Dev 8:2540–2551

Dickson J, Magee B, Stewart A et al (2002) Relationship between residual radiation-induced DNA double-strand breaks in cultured fibroblasts and late radiation reactions: a comparison of training and validation cohorts of breast cancer patients. Radiother Oncol 62:321–326

Difilippantonio S, Gapud E, Wong N et al (2008) 53BP1 facilitates long-range DNA end-joining during V(D)J recombination. Nature 456:529–533

Dikomey E, Dahm-Daphi J, Brammer I et al (1998) Correlation between cellular radiosensitivity and non-repaired double-strand breaks studied in nine mammalian cell lines. Int J Radiat Biol 73:269–278

Dikomey E, Brammer I, Johansen J et al (2000) Relationship between DNA double-strand breaks, cell killing, and fibrosis studied in confluent skin fibroblasts derived from breast cancer patients. Int J Radiat Oncol Biol Phys 46:481–490

Dikomey E, Borgmann K, Brammer I et al (2003a) Molecular mechanisms of individual radiosensitivity studied in normal diploid human fibroblasts. Toxicology 193:125–135

Dikomey E, Borgmann K, Peacock J et al (2003b) Why recent studies relating normal tissue response to individual radiosensitivity might have failed and how new studies should be performed. Int J Radiat Oncol Biol Phys 56:1194–1200

Dittmann K, Mayer C, Fehrenbacher B et al (2005) Radiation-induced epidermal growth factor receptor nuclear import is linked to activation of DNA-dependent protein kinase. J Biol Chem 280:31182–31189

Eastham AM, Atkinson J, West CM (2001) Relationships between clonogenic cell survival, DNA damage and chromosomal radiosensitivity in nine human cervix carcinoma cell lines. Int J Radiat Biol 77:295–302

El-Awady RA, Dikomey E, Dahm-Daphi J (2003) Radiosensitivity of human tumour cells is correlated with the induction but not with the repair of DNA double-strand breaks. Br J Cancer 89:593–601

El-Awady RA, Mahmoud M, Saleh EM et al (2005) No correlation between radiosensitivity or double-strand break repair capacity of normal fibroblasts and acute normal tissue reaction after radiotherapy of breast cancer patients. Int J Radiat Biol 81:501–508

Elliott B, Richardson C, Jasin M (2005) Chromosomal translocation mechanisms at intronic Alu elements in mammalian cells. Mol Cell 17:885–894

Esposito G, Antonelli F, Belli M et al (2005) DNA DSB induced by iron ions in human fibroblasts: LET dependence and shielding efficiency. Adv Space Res 35:243–248

Esposito G, Belli M, Campa A et al (2006) DNA fragments induction in human fibroblasts by radiations of different qualities. Radiat Prot Dosimetry 122:166–168

Essers J, Hendriks RW, Wesoly J et al (2002) Analysis of mouse Rad54 expression and its implications for homologous recombination. DNA Repair (Amst) 1:779–793

Falck J, Coates J, Jackson SP (2005) Conserved modes of recruitment of ATM, ATR and DNA-PKcs to sites of DNA damage. Nature 434:605–611

Fernandez-Capetillo O, Celeste A, Nussenzweig A (2003) Focusing on foci: H2AX and the recruitment of DNA-damage response factors. Cell Cycle 2:426–427

Fernandez-Capetillo O, Lee A, Nussenzweig M et al (2004) H2AX: the histone guardian of the genome. DNA Repair (Amst) 3:959–967

Frankenberg-Schwager M, Frankenberg D, Harbich R (1991) Different oxygen enhancement ratios for induced and un-rejoined DNA double-strand breaks in eukaryotic cells. Radiat Res 128:243–250

Goldberg M, Stucki M, Falck J et al (2003) MDC1 is required for the intra-S phase DNA damage checkpoint. Nature 421:952–956

Goodhead DT (2006) Energy deposition stochastics and track structure: what about the target? Radiat Prot Dosimetry 122:3–15

Guan J, DiBiase S, Iliakis G (2000) The catalytic subunit DNA-dependent protein kinase (DNA-PKcs) facilitates recovery from radiation-induced inhibition of DNA replication. Nucleic Acids Res 28:1183–1192

Gudkov AV, Komarova EA (2003) The role of p53 in determining sensitivity to radiotherapy. Nat Rev Cancer 3:117–129

Harima Y, Sawada S, Miyazaki Y et al (2003) Expression of Ku80 in cervical cancer correlates with response to radiotherapy and survival. Am J Clin Oncol 26:e80–e85

Harrington K, Jankowska P, Hingorani M (2007) Molecular biology for the radiation oncologist: the 5Rs of radiobiology meet the hallmarks of cancer. Clin Oncol (R Coll Radiol) 19:561–571

Helleday T, Lo J, van Gent DC et al (2007) DNA double-strand break repair: from mechanistic understanding to cancer treatment. DNA Repair (Amst) 6:923–935

Herskind C, Johansen J, Bentzen SM et al (2000) Fibroblast differentiation in subcutaneous fibrosis after postmastectomy radiotherapy. Acta Oncol 39:383–388

Hirayama R, Furusawa Y, Fukawa T et al (2005) Repair kinetics of DNA-DSB induced by X-rays or carbon ions under oxic and hypoxic conditions. J Radiat Res (Tokyo) 46:325–332

Hoeller U, Borgmann K, Bonacker M et al (2003) Individual radiosensitivity measured with lymphocytes may be used to predict the risk of fibrosis after radiotherapy for breast cancer. Radiother Oncol 69:137–144

Hopfner KP, Craig L, Moncalian G et al (2002) The Rad50 zinc-hook is a structure joining Mre11 complexes in DNA recombination and repair. Nature 418:562–566

Huen MS, Grant R, Manke I et al (2007) RNF8 transduces the DNA-damage signal via histone ubiquitylation and checkpoint protein assembly. Cell 131:901–914

Huertas P, Cortes-Ledesma F, Sartori AA et al (2008) CDK targets Sae2 to control DNA-end resection and homologous recombination. Nature 455:689–692

Huyen Y, Zgheib O, Ditullio RA, Jr. et al (2004) Methylated lysine 79 of histone H3 targets 53BP1 to DNA double-strand breaks. Nature 432:406–411

Iwabuchi K, Basu BP, Kysela B et al (2003) Potential role for 53BP1 in DNA end-joining repair through direct interaction with DNA. J Biol Chem 278:36487–36495

Jeggo PA, Lobrich M (2005) Artemis links ATM to double-strand break rejoining. Cell Cycle 4:359–362

Kasten-Pisula U, Tastan H, Dikomey E (2005) Huge differences in cellular radiosensitivity due to only very small variations in double-strand break repair capacity. Int J Radiat Biol 81:409–419

Kasten-Pisula U, Menegakis A, Brammer I et al (2008) The extreme radiosensitivity of the squamous cell carcinoma SKX is due to a defect in double-strand break repair. Radiother Oncol DOI: 10.1016/j.radonc.2008.10.019

Kinner A, Wu W, Staudt C et al (2008) Gamma-H2AX in recognition and signaling of DNA double-strand breaks in the context of chromatin. Nucleic Acids Res 36:5678–5694

Komuro Y, Watanabe T, Hosoi Y et al (2002) The expression pattern of Ku correlates with tumor radiosensitivity and disease-free survival in patients with rectal carcinoma. Cancer 95:1199–1205

Lee SW, Cho KJ, Park JH et al (2005) Expressions of Ku70 and DNA-PKcs as prognostic indicators of local control in nasopharyngeal carcinoma. Int J Radiat Oncol Biol Phys 62:1451–1457

Lehmann AR (2005) The role of SMC proteins in the responses to DNA damage. DNA Repair (Amst) 4:309–314

Li CY, Nagasawa H, Dahlberg WK et al (1995) Diminished capacity for p53 in mediating a radiation-induced G1 arrest in established human tumor cell lines. Oncogene 11:1885–1892

Lieber MR, Ma Y, Pannicke U et al (2003) Mechanism and regulation of human non-homologous DNA end-joining. Nat Rev Mol Cell Biol 4:712–720

Little JB, Nagasawa H, Keng PC et al (1995) Absence of radiation-induced G1 arrest in two closely related human lymphoblast cell lines that differ in p53 status. J Biol Chem 270:11033–11036

Lobrich M, Jeggo PA (2007) The impact of a negligent G2/M checkpoint on genomic instability and cancer induction. Nat Rev Cancer 7:861–869

Lukas C, Melander F, Stucki M et al (2004) Mdc1 couples DNA double-strand break recognition by Nbs1 with its H2AX-dependent chromatin retention. EMBO J 23:2674–2683

Maacke H, Jost K, Opitz S et al (2000a) DNA repair and recombination factor Rad51 is over-expressed in human pancreatic adenocarcinoma. Oncogene 19:2791–2795

Maacke H, Opitz S, Jost K et al (2000b) Over-expression of wild-type Rad51 correlates with histological grading of invasive ductal breast cancer. Int J Cancer 88:907–913

Magne N, Chargari C, Castadot P et al (2008) The efficacy and toxicity of EGFR in the settings of radiotherapy: focus on published clinical trials. Eur J Cancer 44:2133–2143

Mailand N, Bekker-Jensen S, Faustrup H et al (2007) RNF8 ubiquitylates histones at DNA double-strand breaks and promotes assembly of repair proteins. Cell 131:887–900

Mansour WY, Schumacher S, Rosskopf R et al (2008) Hierarchy of nonhomologous end-joining, single-strand annealing and gene conversion at site-directed DNA double-strand breaks. Nucleic Acids Res 36:4088–4098

McMillan TJ, Cassoni AM, Edwards S et al (1990) The relationship of DNA double-strand break induction to radiosensitivity in human tumour cell lines. Int J Radiat Biol 58:427–438

Nagasawa H, Li CY, Maki CG et al (1995) Relationship between radiation-induced G1 phase arrest and p53 function in human tumor cells. Cancer Res 55:1842–1846

Narod SA, Foulkes WD (2004) BRCA1 and BRCA2: 1994 and beyond. Nat Rev Cancer 4:665–676

Nikjoo H, Uehara S, Wilson WE et al (1998) Track structure in radiation biology: theory and applications. Int J Radiat Biol 73:355–364

Nunez MI, Villalobos M, Olea N et al (1995) Radiation-induced DNA double-strand break rejoining in human tumour cells. Br J Cancer 71:311–316

Nussenzweig A, Nussenzweig MC (2007) A backup DNA repair pathway moves to the forefront. Cell 131:223–225

Nyati MK, Morgan MA, Feng FY et al (2006) Integration of EGFR inhibitors with radiochemotherapy. Nat Rev Cancer 6:876–885

Olive PL, Banath JP, MacPhail HS (1994) Lack of a correlation between radiosensitivity and DNA double-strand break induction or rejoining in six human tumor cell lines. Cancer Res 54:3939–3946

Paffett KS, Clikeman JA, Palmer S et al (2005) Overexpression of Rad51 inhibits double-strand break-induced homologous recombination but does not affect gene conversion tract lengths. DNA Repair (Amst) 4:687–698

Painter RB (1986) Inhibition of mammalian cell DNA synthesis by ionizing radiation. Int J Radiat Biol Relat Stud Phys Chem Med 49:771–781

Painter RB, Young BR (1980) Radiosensitivity in ataxia-telangiectasia: a new explanation. Proc Natl Acad Sci USA 77:7315–7317

Paull TT, Lee JH (2005) The Mre11/Rad50/Nbs1 complex and its role as a DNA double-strand break sensor for ATM. Cell Cycle 4:737–740

Powell SN, DeFrank JS, Connell P et al (1995) Differential sensitivity of p53$^-$ and p53$^+$ cells to caffeine-induced radiosensitization and override of G2 delay. Cancer Res 55:1643–1648

Prise KM, Davies S, Michael BD (1987) The relationship between radiation-induced DNA double-strand breaks and cell kill in hamster V79 fibroblasts irradiated with 250 kVp X-rays, 2.3 MeV neutrons or 238Pu alpha-particles. Int J Radiat Biol Relat Stud Phys Chem Med 52:893–902

Qiao GB, Wu YL, Yang XN et al (2005) High-level expression of Rad51 is an independent prognostic marker of survival in non-small-cell lung cancer patients. Br J Cancer 93:137–143

Riballo E, Kuhne M, Rief N et al (2004) A pathway of double-strand break rejoining dependent upon ATM, Artemis, and proteins locating to gamma-H2AX foci. Mol Cell 16:715–724

Richardson C, Stark JM, Ommundsen M et al (2004) Rad51 overexpression promotes alternative double-strand break repair pathways and genome instability. Oncogene 23:546–553

Ristic D, Modesti M, Kanaar R et al (2003) Rad52 and Ku bind to different DNA structures produced early in double-strand break repair. Nucleic Acids Res 31:5229–5237

Rodemann HP, Dittmann K, Toulany M (2007) Radiation-induced EGFR-signaling and control of DNA-damage repair. Int J Radiat Biol 83:781–791

Rothkamm K, Lobrich M (2003) Evidence for a lack of DNA double-strand break repair in human cells exposed to very low x-ray doses. Proc Natl Acad Sci USA 100:5057–5062

Rothkamm K, Kruger I, Thompson LH et al (2003) Pathways of DNA double-strand break repair during the mammalian cell cycle. Mol Cell Biol 23:5706–5715

Rübe C, Dong X, Kühne M et al (2008) DNA double-strand rejoining in complex normal tissues. Int J Radiat Biol Relat Stud Phys Chem Med 72:1180–1187

Ruiz de Almodovar JM, Nunez MI, McMillan TJ et al (1994) Initial radiation-induced DNA damage in human tumour cell lines: a correlation with intrinsic cellular radiosensitivity. Br J Cancer 69:457–462

Sartori AA, Lukas C, Coates J et al (2007) Human CtIP promotes DNA end resection. Nature 450:509–514

Schulte-Uentrop L, El-Awady RA, Schliecker L et al (2008) Distinct roles of XRCC4 and Ku80 in non-homologous end-joining of endonuclease- and ionizing radiation-induced DNA double-strand breaks. Nucleic Acids Res 36:2561–2569

Schultz LB, Chehab NH, Malikzay A et al (2000) p53 binding protein 1 (53BP1) is an early participant in the cellular response to DNA double-strand breaks. J Cell Biol 151:1381–1390

Shiloh Y (2006) The ATM-mediated DNA-damage response: taking shape. Trends Biochem Sci 31:402–410

Shrivastav M, De Haro LP, Nickoloff JA (2008) Regulation of DNA double-strand break repair pathway choice. Cell Res 18:134–147

Soderlund K, Stal O, Skoog L et al (2007) Intact Mre11/Rad50/Nbs1 complex predicts good response to radiotherapy in early breast cancer. Int J Radiat Oncol Biol Phys 68:50–58

Song G, Ouyang G, Bao S (2005) The activation of Akt/PKB signaling pathway and cell survival. J Cell Mol Med 9:59–71

Stark JM, Pierce AJ, Oh J et al (2004) Genetic steps of mammalian homologous repair with distinct mutagenic consequences. Mol Cell Biol 24:9305–9316

Stewart GS, Wang B, Bignell CR et al (2003) MDC1 is a mediator of the mammalian DNA damage checkpoint. Nature 421:961–966

Stiff T, O'Driscoll M, Rief N et al (2004) ATM and DNA-PK function redundantly to phosphorylate H2AX after exposure to ionizing radiation. Cancer Res 64:2390–2396

Stucki M, Clapperton JA, Mohammad D et al (2005) MDC1 directly binds phosphorylated histone H2AX to regulate cellular responses to DNA double-strand breaks. Cell 123:1213–1226

Taucher-Scholz G, Heilmann J, Kraft G (1996) Induction and rejoining of DNA double-strand breaks in CHO cells after heavy ion irradiation. Adv Space Res 18:83–92

Toulany M, Dittmann K, Kruger M et al (2005) Radioresistance of K-Ras mutated human tumor cells is mediated through EGFR-dependent activation of PI3K-AKT pathway. Radiother Oncol 76:143–150

Toulany M, Kasten-Pisula U, Brammer I et al (2006) Blockage of epidermal growth factor receptor-phosphatidylinositol 3-kinase-AKT signaling increases radiosensitivity of K-RAS mutated human tumor cells in vitro by affecting DNA repair. Clin Cancer Res 12:4119–4126

Valerie K, Yacoub A, Hagan MP et al (2007) Radiation-induced cell signaling: inside-out and outside-in. Mol Cancer Ther 6:789–801

Wang H, Zeng ZC, Bui TA et al (2001) Efficient rejoining of radiation-induced DNA double-strand breaks in vertebrate cells deficient in genes of the RAD52 epistasis group. Oncogene 20:2212–2224

Ward IM, Minn K, van Deursen J et al (2003) p53 Binding protein 53BP1 is required for DNA damage responses and tumor suppression in mice. Mol Cell Biol 23:2556–2563

Ward IM, Reina-San-Martin B, Olaru A et al (2004) 53BP1 is required for class switch recombination. J Cell Biol 165:459–464

Ward JD, Barber LJ, Petalcorin MI et al (2007) Replication blocking lesions present a unique substrate for homologous recombination. EMBO J 26:3384–3396

Weinstock DM, Richardson CA, Elliott B et al (2006) Modeling oncogenic translocations: distinct roles for double-strand break repair pathways in translocation formation in mammalian cells. DNA Repair (Amst) 5:1065–1074

West CM, Davidson SE, Elyan SA et al (2001) Lymphocyte radiosensitivity is a significant prognostic factor for morbidity in carcinoma of the cervix. Int J Radiat Oncol Biol Phys 51:10–15

Whitaker SJ, McMillan TJ (1992) Oxygen effect for DNA double-strand break induction determined by pulsed-field gel electrophoresis. Int J Radiat Biol 61:29–41

Wilson CR, Davidson SE, Margison GP et al (2000) Expression of Ku70 correlates with survival in carcinoma of the cervix. Br J Cancer 83:1702–1706

Windhofer F, Wu W, Wang M et al (2007) Marked dependence on growth state of backup pathways of NHEJ. Int J Radiat Oncol Biol Phys 68:1462–1470

Wurm R, Burnet NG, Duggal N et al (1994) Cellular radiosensitivity and DNA damage in primary human fibroblasts. Int J Radiat Oncol Biol Phys 30:625–633

Wyman C, Kanaar R (2006) DNA double-strand break repair: all's well that ends well. Annu Rev Genet 40:363–383

Xie A, Hartlerode A, Stucki M et al (2007) Distinct roles of chromatin-associated proteins MDC1 and 53BP1 in mammalian double-strand break repair. Mol Cell 28:1045–1057

Yacoub A, McKinstry R, Hinman D et al (2003) Epidermal growth factor and ionizing radiation up-regulate the DNA repair genes *XRCC1* and *ERCC1* in DU145 and LNCaP prostate carcinoma through MAPK signaling. Radiat Res 159:439–452

Yacoub A, Miller A, Caron RW et al (2006) Radiotherapy-induced signal transduction. Endocr Relat Cancer 13(Suppl):S99–S114

Yan CT, Boboila C, Souza EK et al (2007) IgH class switching and translocations use a robust non-classical end-joining pathway. Nature 449:478–482

You Z, Chahwan C, Bailis J et al (2005) ATM activation and its recruitment to damaged DNA require binding to the C terminus of Nbs1. Mol Cell Biol 25:5363–5379

Physiological Mechanisms of Treatment Resistance

PETER VAUPEL

CONTENTS

P. VAUPEL, Dr.med., M.A. / Univ. Harvard
Professor of Physiology and Pathophysiology, Institute of
Physiology and Pathophysiology, University Medical Center,
Duesbergweg 6, 55099 Mainz, Germany

KEY POINTS

- The unique, considerably dynamic and thus complex physiology of tumors can markedly influence the therapeutic response to standard irradiation, chemotherapy, photodynamic therapy, endocrine therapy and immunotherapy.
- Acquired treatment resistance due to the impact of the hostile microenvironment adds to the "classical" drug resistance based on the molecular biology of tumors.
- The chaotic microvasculature leads to a significant impediment of delivery, an uneven distribution and a compromised penetration of drugs from tumor capillaries to more distant tumor cells.
- Interstitial transport of larger molecules (monoclonal antibodies, cytokines) by convection is inhibited.
- Low cell proliferation rates and cell cycle arrest distant from tumor microvessels can protect tumor cells from the effects of cytotoxic therapies whose activity is selective for rapidly dividing cell populations.
- Hypoxia directly and/or indirectly confers resistance to therapy. Direct effects are mediated through reduced generation of free radicals (some chemotherapy, photodynamic therapy) or lacking fixation of DNA damage (X- and γ-rays).
- Indirect hypoxia-driven effects are mostly based on changes in the transcriptome, in differential regulations of gene expression and in alterations of the proteome and genome.
- Anemia can lead to therapeutic resistance through deepening hypoxia and reducing the transport capacity of red blood cells for various antineoplastic drugs.

- Tumor acidosis is involved in acquired treatment resistance through a series of mechanisms including, inter alia, inhibition of cell proliferation, reduced cellular uptake and activation or an increased efflux of drugs.

Abstract

It is generally accepted that tumor perfusion, microcirculation, characteristics of the interstitial space of tumors, oxygen (and nutrient) supply, tissue pH distribution and the bioenergetic status—factors that are usually closely linked and that define the so-called pathophysiological microenvironment—can markedly influence the therapeutic response of malignant tumors to sparsely ionizing radiation, chemotherapy, photodynamic therapy, hormonal therapy and immunotherapy. Besides more direct mechanisms involved in the development of acquired therapeutic resistance, there are in addition, obstacles in intratumor pharmacokinetics of antitumor agents due to delivery problems caused by an inadequate and heterogeneous perfusion and barriers within the interstitial compartment. Indirect effects causing therapeutic resistance include lower cell proliferation rates and cell cycle arrest. Changes in transcriptome, alterations in gene expression and in the genome, genomic instability and clonal selection can drive subsequent events that are known to further increase resistance to therapy, in addition to critically affecting long-term prognosis.

15.1
Introduction

The physiology of solid tumors is uniquely different to that of normal tissues. It is characterized, inter alia, by a chaotic microvascular structure and function, O_2 depletion (hypoxia and anoxia, respectively), extracellular acidosis, significant interstitial fluid flow, and interstitial hypertension, creating a hostile pathophysiological microenvironment (see Chap. 4). This microenvironment is not static, but instead is quite dynamic (and therefore more complex than previously assumed), describing a situation that is not compatible with earlier, conventional dogmas.

Hypoxia and the other microenvironmental parameters are known to directly or indirectly confer resistance to non-surgical treatment modalities through

limited access of therapeutics to the tumor, decreased radiosensitivity and drug action in the absence of O_2, critically reduced effects in tumor cells that are poorly proliferating and via changes in pH gradients, etc. Other mechanisms include the capacity of the hostile microenvironment to drive changes in gene expression, genomic instability and clonal selection.

15.2
Role of the Disorganized, Compromised Microcirculation as an Obstacle in Tumor Therapy

As already mentioned in Chap. 4, there is a disturbed balance of pro-angiogenic and anti-angiogenic molecules (yielding an unregulated angiogenesis), which leads to the development of a disorganized microvasculature and significant arterio-venous shunt perfusion and thus to an inefficient delivery of therapeutic molecules (e.g., drugs, cytokines and antibodies) and nutrients (e.g., oxygen and glucose) through the vascular system of the tumor (see Table 15.1). The situation is further aggravated by flow-dependent spatio-temporal heterogeneities in the distribution of plasma-borne drugs (and their metabolites).

The considerable impediment of fluctuating (intermittent) perfusion to successful cancer therapy has been comprehensively reviewed by DURAND (2001) and DURAND and AQUINO-PARSONS (2001 a,b).

The mean vascular density in most tumor areas is generally lower than that in normal tissues, and thus diffusion distances are enlarged. Penetration of drugs from tumor capillaries to tumor cells that are distant from them is therefore compromised. In these tumor regions distant to patent microvessels, some drugs (i.e., drugs with a short half-life within the circulation) cannot achieve sufficient concentrations to exert lethal toxicity for all of the viable cells further away from the tumor microvasculature system (MINCHINTON and TANNOCK 2006; DI PAOLO and BOCCI 2007). In addition, in these tumor regions, the concentrations of the key nutrients are also low, leading to marked gradients with higher cellular turnover rates close to blood vessels and lower cell proliferation rates (and cell cycle arrest) farther from the nearest microvessel before treatment and to repopulation of surviving tumor cells after/between treatments (TANNOCK 1968, 2001; HIRST and DENEKAMP 1979).

Cells dividing at a reduced rate would be protected from the effects of cytotoxic therapies whose activity is "selective" for rapidly dividing cell populations with a

Table 15.1. Role of chaotic tumor microcirculation in acquired treatment resistance (selection)

Pathophysiological condition	Leads via	To
Inadequate and heterogeneous perfusion	Inefficient and heterogeneous delivery of cytotoxic agents	Impaired pharmacokinetics of drugs, impaired delivery of therapeutic macromolecules and gene therapies
	Inefficient and heterogeneous nutrient supply yielding lower cell proliferation rates /cell cycle arrest	Protection from cytotoxic therapies whose activity is selective for rapidly dividing cells
Arterio-venous shunt vessels	Shunt perfusion (i.e., flow bypassing exchange vessels)	Impaired delivery of cytotoxic agents
Enlarged diffusion distances	Compromised penetration of cytotoxic agents	Insufficient concentrations of drugs and therapeutic macromolecules in tumor regions distant to patent blood vessels

short cell cycle, a large proportion of cells in S-phase and, therefore, a large growth fraction (Hall and Giaccia 2006; Trédan et al. 2007). There is a strong indication that the growth fraction decreases as tumor size increases, at least in experimental tumor systems.

Anti-angiogenic therapy for solid tumors using inhibition of VEGF-signaling can generate an early-phase of "normalization" of tumor vasculature (Jain 2001). This occurs via the recruitment of pericytes to the tumor microvasculature, an effect associated with a temporary, short-lived stabilization of the vessels and a (still hypothetic) improvement in blood flow. The latter may be accompanied by improved oxygen and drug delivery, creating a window of opportunity for higher sensitivity to ionizing radiation and the delivery of anti-cancer agents (Jain 2005). The postulated increase in pericyte recruitment is thought to be mediated by angiopoietin-1 and matrix metalloproteinases (Lin and Sessa 2004).

15.3

Interstitial Barriers to Delivery of Therapeutic Agents

As already outlined in Chap. 4, the interstitial compartment of tumors is significantly different from that of normal tissues. As a result of (a) vessel leakiness, (b) lack of functional lymphatics, (c) interstitial fibrosis and (d) contraction of the interstitial matrix mediated by stromal fibroblasts, most solid tumors have an increased interstitial (hydrostatic) fluid pressure (IFP; Jain 1987, 1990; Heldin et al. 2004; Milosevic et al. 2004; Cairns et al. 2006).

Increased interstitial fluid pressure (IFP) within solid tumors decreases extravasation and inhibits the extravascular transport of larger molecules (e.g., monoclonal antibodies, cytokines) by convection (see Table 15.2). Macromolecules rely more heavily on convection as opposed to simple diffusional transport. Interstitial transport of macromolecules is further impaired by a much denser network of collagen fibers in the extracellular matrix of tumors as compared to normal tissues. Collagen content in tumors is much higher and collagen fibers are much thicker than in normal tissues, leading to an increased mechanical stiffness of the tissue (Netti et al. 2000; Heldin et al. 2004).

IFP is almost uniform throughout a tumor and drops precipitously at the tumor/normal tissue interface. For this reason, the interstitial fluid oozes out of the tumor into the surrounding normal tissue and carries away anticancer agents with it (Fukumura and Jain 2007). As another consequence of this drop in IFP, blood may be diverted away from the tumor center toward the periphery where anticancer agents may be lost from larger vessels.

Transmural coupling between IFP and microvascular pressure can critically reduce perfusion pressure between up- and downstream tumor blood vessels (see Chap. 4, Sect. 4.6) leading to blood flow stasis and thus inadequate delivery of anticancer agents, in addition to the mechanisms impairing blood flow already mentioned.

Table 15.2. Interstitial barriers in acquired treatment resistance

Pathophysiological condition	Leads via	To
Interstitial hypertension	Decreased extravasation and compromised interstitial transport of macromolecules	Impaired delivery of therapeutic macro-molecules (e.g., passive immunotherapy) and gene therapies, disturbed immigration of immune effector cells
Dense network of collagen fibers	Compromised interstitial transport of macromolecules	Impaired delivery of therapeutic macro-molecules (e.g., passive immunotherapy)
IFP drop at the tumor/normal tissue interface	Centrifugal interstitial fluid flow Diversion of blood from tumor center to periphery	Loss of anticancer agents Loss of anticancer agents in the tumor periphery
Transmural coupling between IFP and microvascular pressure	Critical reduction in perfusion pressure	Flow stasis compromising intra-tumor pharmacokinetics
Expansion of the interstitial space	Increase in distribution space for anti-cancer (and diagnostic) agents	Time necessary for drug concentration equilibrium between vascular and interstitial space may be prolonged

IFP = interstitial fluid pressure

Interactions between cancer cells and the extracellular matrix can affect their response to chemotherapy. The basic mechanisms involved in the so-called adhesion-mediated drug resistance are rather complex and still under investigation. Agents that can modulate cell adhesion might enhance the effects of chemotherapy (TRÉDAN et al. 2007).

Several types of treatment have been shown to decrease tumor IFP in patients (LEE et al. 2000; WILLETT et al. 2004, 2005; BATCHELOR et al. 2007). This decrease in IFP has been attributed to a substantial reduction in vascular permeability (concomitant with a pruning of tumor vessels) after angiogenesis-inhibiting treatment with VEGF-receptor inhibitors (combined with radiation and/or chemotherapy).

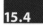

Hypoxia as an Obstacle in Tumor Therapy

Although resistance of human tumors to anticancer agents is mostly ascribed to gene mutations, gene amplification or epigenetic changes that influence the uptake, metabolism or export of drugs from single cells (TRÉDAN et al. 2007), tumor hypoxia plays a pivotal role in acquired treatment resistance, since O_2 depletion in solid tumors is classically associated with resistance to radiotherapy, but has also been shown to diminish the efficacy of certain forms of chemotherapy, of photodynamic therapy, immunotherapy and hormonal therapy (for reviews since 2000, see CHAPLIN et al. 2000; VAUPEL et al. 2001a,b, 2002, 2004; VAUPEL and MAYER 2005; SHANNON et al. 2003; VAUPEL 2004b; WEINMANN et al. 2004; BROWN 2002, 2007; TANNOCK et al. 2005; KUREBAYASHI 2005; HALL and GIACCIA 2006; LIAO et al. 2007; VAUPEL and HÖCKEL 2008; BRISTOW and HILL 2008).

15.4.1
General Aspects of Hypoxia-Driven Treatment Resistance

Hypoxia protects tumor cells from damage by nonsurgical anticancer therapies that are directly or indirectly O_2-dependent (or both; for reviews see MOULDER and ROCKWELL 1987; DURAND 1991, 1994; TANNOCK and HILL 1992; TEICHER 1993, 1994, 1995; HALL 1994; VAUPEL 1997b; CHAPLIN et al. 2000; HÖCKEL and VAUPEL 2001; see Table 15.3).

Table 15.3. Tumor hypoxia and acquired treatment resistance (selection of mechanisms)

Treatment affected	Mechanisms involved	Examples	References
A. Direct effects			
X- and γ-rays*	Reduced "fixation" of DNA damage		HALL and GIACCIA (2006)
Chemotherapy*	Reduced generation of free radicals	Antibiotics (bleomycin, doxorubin)	ERLICHMAN (1992)
Photodynamic therapy	Reduced generation of free radicals		SHANNON et al. (2003) HENDERSON and FINGAR (1987)
B. Indirect effects			
X- and γ-rays*	Cell cycle effects, modulation of proliferation kinetics Increased activity of repair enzymes Enhanced expression of anti-apoptotic proteins Selection of apoptosis-resistant cells Elevated intracellular levels of glutathione and associated nucleophilic thiols		HALL and GIACCIA (2006)
Chemotherapy**	Cell cycle effects, modulation of proliferation kinetics	Vinca alkaloids, methotrexate, platinum compounds, taxanes, doxorubicin	CHABNER et al. (1996)
	Increased activity of repair enzymes	Alkylating agents, platinum compounds, etoposide, anthracyclines	CHABNER et al. (1996) ZELLER (1995)
	Elevated intracellular levels of glutathione	Melphalan	
	Increased telomerase activity	Telomerase inhibitors	NISHI et al. (2004) ANDERSON et al. (2006)
	Development of an aggressive phenotype		LUNT et al. (2008)
	Amplification and increased synthesis of dihydrofolate reductase (DHFR)	Methotrexate	RICE et al. (1986)
	Increased synthesis of growth factors (e.g., TGF-β, bFGF)		WEI and AU (2005)
	Increased transcription of membrane transporters (e.g., GP-170, GLUT-1)	Vinca alkaloids, anthracyclines, etoposide, taxanes	VERA et al. (1991) COMERFORD et al. (2002)
	Increased expression of anti-apoptotic proteins, selection of apoptosis-resistant cells	Alkylating agents, cisplatin, anthracyclines, etoposide	COLE and TANNOCK (2005)
	Protection against drug-induced senescence	Anthracyclines	SULLIVAN et al. (2008)

*Anemia acts as a factor worsening tumor hypoxia

**Anemia acts as a factor that intensifies tumor hypoxia and that may impair transport of some cytotoxic drugs by red blood cells

Table 15.3. (*continued*) Tumor hypoxia and acquired treatment resistance (selection of mechanisms)

Treatment affected	Mechanisms involved	Examples	References
B. Indirect effects			
Endocrine therapy	Reduced expression of estrogen receptor	Hormonal therapy of breast cancer	Kurebayashi (2005)
	Enhanced androgen receptor function	Androgen-deprivation therapy	Park et al. (2006)
Immunotherapy	Reduced survival and proliferation of T-cells		Kim et al. (2008)
	Reduced production of cytokines by T-cells		Lukashev et al. (2007)
	Immunosuppression by adenosine		Sitkovsky and Lukashev (2005)
	Tumor-associated macrophages recruited to hypoxic sites can switch to a "protumor phenotype" leading to immune evasion of tumors		Lewis and Murdoch (2005)

15.4.1.1
Direct Effects

Direct effects (i.e., effects of hypoxia per se) are mediated via deprivation of molecular O_2 and thus reduced generation of free radicals that some chemotherapeutic agents (e.g., the antibiotics bleomycin and doxorubicin; Erlichman 1992) and photodynamic therapy require to be maximally cytotoxic. Sparsely ionizing radiation (X- and γ-rays) needs O_2 for "fixation" of DNA damage (Fig. 15.1).

15.4.1.2
Indirect Effects Based on Changes in the Transcriptome, in Differential Regulation of Gene Expression and in Alteration of the Proteome

Indirect effects, which to a great extent are reversible and which may occur upon exposure to oxygen levels <1% (pO_2 <7 mmHg), rely on the hypoxia-mediated modulation (stimulation or inhibition) of gene expression (see Fig. 15.1) and posttranscriptional or posttranslational effects resulting in changes in the proteome and leading, inter alia, to

(a) modulation of proliferation kinetics, perturbations of the cell cycle distribution, the number of tumor cells accumulating in G_1-phase (e.g., 5-FU; Yoshiba et al. 2008) and a reduction in the fraction of active S-phase cells (e.g., the vinca alkaloids and methotrexate exhibit cell-cycle-phase specificity; Chabner et al. 1996). As a rule, the portion of proliferating cells decreases with increasing hypoxia and increasing duration of hypoxia. Hereby, the fraction of hypoxic and not proliferating—but still viable—tumor cells is of special interest;

(b) quantitative changes in cellular metabolism (e.g., intensified glycolysis in hypoxic tumors with tissue acidosis, which in turn can have an impact on cellular activation, intracellular accumulation and membrane transport of drugs), increased enzyme activities, elevated intracellular concentrations of glutathione (GSH) and associated nucleophilic thiols that can compete with the target DNA for alkylation (see Table 15.3);

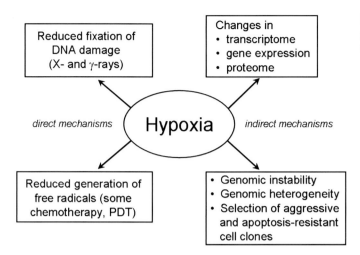

Fig. 15.1. Hypoxia-driven direct and indirect mechanisms leading to acquired treatment resistance

(c) increased transcription of membrane transporters (e.g., GLUT-1 facilitating the efflux of vinblastine, VERA et al. 1991), DNA repair enzymes, autocrine and paracrine growth factors (e.g., TGF-β), proteins involved in cell detachment and tumor invasiveness, and resistance-related proteins. Many hypoxia-inducible genes are controlled by the transcription factors HIF-1, nuclear factor κB (NFκB) and activator protein-1 (AP-1; KOONG et al. 1994; DACHS and TOZER 2000; LADEROUTE et al. 2002).

In addition to hypoxia, other epigenetic microenvironmental factors (e.g., acidosis, glucose depletion, lactate accumulation) may also be involved in the mechanisms described above. (For more details on hypoxia-mediated proteome changes, see RICE et al. 1986; LADEROUTE et al. 1992; AUSSERER et al. 1994; GRAEBER et al. 1994; SANNA and ROFSTAD 1994; GIACCIA 1996; MATTERN et al. 1996; RALEIGH 1996; BROWN and GIACCIA 1998; SUTHERLAND 1998; SEMENZA 2000a,b; HÖCKEL and VAUPEL 2001).

15.4.1.3
Indirect Effects
Based on Enhanced Mutagenesis, Genomic Instability and Clonal Selection

Therapeutic resistance can also result from (progressive) genome changes and clonal selection at tissue O_2 concentrations <0.1% (pO_2 <0.7 mmHg; VAUPEL 2004b, 2008).

Increasing resistance towards nonsurgical therapy concomitant with primary tumor growth can also be driven by transient or persistent genomic changes and clonal selection (often associated with subsequent clonal dominance) due to a hypoxia-related strong selection pressure (see Fig. 15.1). Hypoxia promotes genomic instability (through point mutations, gene amplification and chromosomal rearrangements), thus increasing the number of genetic variants and thereby promoting clonal and intrinsic tumor cell heterogeneity. Emancipative proliferation of resistant clonal variants in a "survival of the fittest" scenario and malignant progression are the final results (see Table 15.3).

Hypoxia-mediated clonal selection of tumor cells with persistent genomic changes can lead, inter alia, to a loss of differentiation and of apoptosis, which can stabilize or further aggravate tumor hypoxia and which in turn again promotes malignant progression (VAUPEL 2004a, 2008). Thus, hypoxia is involved in a vicious circle that is regarded as a fundamental biologic mechanism of malignant disease (for reviews, see HÖCKEL and VAUPEL 2001; VAUPEL et al. 2004; VAUPEL 2008). Other consequences of hypoxia-induced malignant progression are an increased locoregional spread and enhanced metastasis (HÖCKEL et al. 1996a, 1998). (For more details on hypoxia-mediated genome changes and expansion of aggressive tumor subclones, see YOUNG et al. 1988; STOLER et al. 1992; CHENG and LOEB 1993; STACKPOLE et al. 1994; RUSSO et al. 1995; GIACCIA 1996; GRAEBER et al. 1996; REYNOLDS et al. 1996; KIM et al. 1997; HÖCKEL et al. 1999; HÖCKEL and VAUPEL 2001).

15.4.2
Tumor Hypoxia
as an Obstacle in Radiotherapy

Tumor hypoxia may present a severe problem for radiation therapy (X- and γ-radiation), because radiosensitivity is progressively limited when the O_2 partial pressure in a tumor is less than 25–30 mmHg, the latter representing the median O_2 tensions in most normal tissues (VAUPEL et al. 2003; see Fig. 15.2). Hypoxia-associated resistance to photon radiotherapy is multifactorial. Molecular oxygen "fixes" (i.e., makes permanent) DNA damage produced by oxygen free radicals, which arise after the interaction of radiation with intracellular water (HALL and GIACCIA 2006). Thus, because of this so-called "oxygen-enhancement effect," the radiation dose required to achieve the same biologic effect is approximately three times higher in the absence of oxygen than in the presence of normal levels of oxygen (GRAY et al. 1953). Evidence suggests that hypoxia-induced proteome and genome changes (see Table 15.3) may also have a substantial impact on radioresistance by increasing the levels of heat shock proteins and repair enzymes or by increasing the number of cells in a tumor with diminished apoptotic potential or increased proliferation potential of selected clones, both of which have been linked to radioresistance (for a review, see HÖCKEL et al. 1996b; HÖCKEL and VAUPEL 2001).

Numerous clinical studies report an impaired radiocurability of anemic patients, most probably due to hypoxia-related radioresistance (EVANS and BERGSJØ1965; BUSH 1986; FROMMHOLD et al. 1998; HENKE et al. 1999; GRAU and OVERGAARD 2000; KUMAR 2000; HARRISON et al. 2002; DUNST 2004; DUNST and MOLLS 2008; HARRISON and BLACKWELL 2004; NOWROUSIAN et al. 2008; HAUGEN et al. 2004; HU and HARRISON 2005; LUDWIG

2004; PROSNITZ et al. 2005). A significant influence of hemoglobin level on the outcome of radiotherapy has been convincingly documented for carcinomas of the uterine cervix, head and neck, bladder and bronchus (for a review, see GRAU and OVERGAARD 2000). One major reason for these observations may be the fact that anemia can strongly aggravate tumor hypoxia (VAUPEL et al. 2006).

Carbon monoxide (CO) in tobacco smoke strongly binds to hemoglobin (formation of carboxyhemoglobin HbCO) and thus decreases the amount of "effective" hemoglobin. Furthermore, CO increases the hemoglobin affinity for O_2. The sum of these effects is a significant increase in tumor hypoxia and in radioresistance, resulting in a poorer treatment outcome after primary radiotherapy (for a review, see GRAU and OVERGAARD 2000).

15.4.3
Tumor Hypoxia
as an Adverse Parameter in Chemotherapy

Besides restricted delivery and uneven distribution (due to poor and heterogeneous blood flow) as well as reduced diffusional flux (due to enlarged diffusion distances), oxygen-dependency has been documented for a broad range of cytotoxic drugs (e.g., cyclophosphamide, carboplatin and doxorubicin) under in vitro and in vivo conditions (TEICHER et al. 1981, 1990; TEICHER 1994, 1995). However, these investigations have been qualitative, and clear hypoxic thresholds for O_2-dependent anticancer agents are still not available, although they presumably exist for each agent (WOUTERS et al. 2007). Thus, additional research is necessary to provide quantitative data on hypoxia-induced chemoresistance, although this information may be difficult to

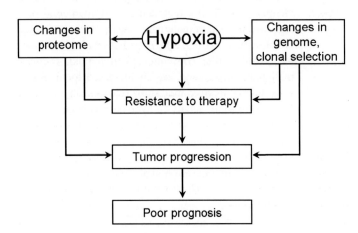

Fig. 15.2. Schematic representation of major hypoxia-induced mechanisms causing treatment resistance and malignant progression, finally leading to poor long-term prognosis

obtain under in vivo conditions. Multiple (direct and indirect) mechanisms are probably also involved in the hypoxia-induced resistance to chemotherapeutic agents, including a reduced generation of free radicals (e.g., bleomycin, anthracyclines), the increased production of nucleophilic substances such as glutathione, which can compete with the target DNA for alkylation (e.g., in the acquired resistance to alkylating agents), an increased activity of DNA repair enzymes (e.g., alkylating agents, platinum compounds; CHABNER et al. 1996), an inhibition of cell proliferation and tissue acidosis, which is often observed in hypoxic tumors with a high glycolytic rate (DURAND 1991, 1994). Furthermore, hypoxic stress proteins, the loss of apoptotic potential and multi-drug resistance proteins can impart resistance to certain chemotherapeutic drugs (SAKATA et al. 1991; HICKMAN et al. 1994; SHANNON et al. 2003). Clear hypoxic thresholds for chemotherapeutic agents are still not available, although resistance of hypoxic cells to conventional chemotherapy is well documented (WOUTERS et al. 2007).

Anemia is an independent risk factor for survival in most cancers treated with chemotherapy (e.g., HARRISON and BLACKWELL 2004; LUDWIG 2004; PROSNITZ et al. 2005; VAN BELLE and COCQUYT 2003). As with radiotherapy, the presence of anemia and its association with inferior results of chemotherapy may be—at least partially—linked to severe hypoxia and its profound effect on tumor biology (e.g., development of an aggressive phenotype). However, anemia as a result of a reduced red blood cell mass may also have a negative impact on the pharmacokinetics of chemotherapeutic agents (NOWROUSIAN 2008). RBCs have been reported to play an important role in storage, transport and metabolism of particular cytotoxic drugs. Anthracyclines, ifosfamide and its metabolites, and topoisomerase I/II inhibitors are incorporated in erythrocytes and may be transported by these cells to the tumor tissue and mobilized by active or passive mechanisms (HIGHLEY et al. 1997; RAMANATHAN-GIRISH and BOROUJERDI 2001; SCHRIJVERS 2003). 6-Mercaptopurine, methotrexate and aminotrexate are reported to accumulate in erythrocytes (COLE et al. 2006; HALONEN et al. 2006). As shown for oxaliplatin, platinum-derived cytotoxic agents are also bound to erythrocytes and transported by RBCs (LUO et al. 1999). In an animal model, a significant correlation was found between concentrations of melphalan in erythrocytes and the tumor availability of this drug (WILDIERS et al. 2002). Because of their potential ability to take up, transport and deliver various antineoplastic drugs, erythrocytes have increasingly become interesting objects to be evaluated as biological carriers in clinical oncology. Pretreatment elevation

and/or maintenance of Hb levels are therefore essential, irrespective of the way in which this goal is achieved (WILDIERS et al. 2002).

15.4.4
Tumor Hypoxia as an Obstacle in Chemoradiation

The combination of radiotherapy and chemotherapy is a promising approach because of its independent cell kill effect and the property of some cytotoxic agents to enhance the effect of radiotherapy. At the end of the 1970s, platinum complexes were described as being able to act as potent radiosensitizers of hypoxic tumor cells (DOUPLE and RICHMOND 1978, 1979). As an obstacle in this type of chemoradiation, KOUKOURAKIS et al. (2002) have suggested that (hypoxia-induced?) overexpression of HIF-1α in patients with head and neck cancer may be related to substantial resistance to carboplatin chemoradiotherapy. More in-depth research is needed to accurately characterize adverse effects of hypoxia in this type of combination therapy.

15.4.5
Tumor Hypoxia as a Barrier for Other Nonsurgical Anticancer Therapies

15.4.5.1
Photodynamic Therapy

Photodynamic therapy-mediated cell death requires the presence of oxygen, a photosensitizing drug, and light of the appropriate wavelength, both in vitro and in vivo (for a review see FREITAS and BARONZIO 1991). However, reports vary greatly on the extent to which photodynamic therapy with hematoporphyrin derivatives is dependent on oxygen (MOAN and SOMMER 1985; HENDERSON and FINGAR 1987). Cells were not killed under anoxic conditions. The critical threshold—below which progressively reduced cell death was observed—varied between 15 and 35 mmHg (MITCHELL et al. 1985; HENDERSON and FINGAR 1987; CHAPMAN et al. 1991), probably because of reduced production of singlet oxygen species ($^1O_2$) and different sensitivities from the treatment in different cell lines. Considering the reduced effectiveness of photodynamic agents at lower O_2 partial pressures, the rapid induction of tumor hypoxia by photodynamic therapy itself—either as a consequence of a photodynamic therapy-induced decrease in blood flow or as a result of oxygen consumption by the photodynamic therapy process itself—has to be considered under in vivo conditions, since it may mean that this therapy is self-limiting (CHAPMAN et al. 1991; CHEN et al. 2002). Photodynamic therapy involving prodrugs, such as aminolevulinic acid (ALA), may be further limited because conversion of the prodrug to the active photosensitizer appears to be less effective under hypoxic conditions.

15.4.5.2
Immunotherapy

As already described in Sects. 15.2 and 15.3, immunotherapy is heavily hampered by the morphologically aberrant tumor microvasculature and increased interstitial fluid pressure, which can impede the delivery of cytokines and monoclonal antibodies and can prevent immigration of immune effector cells into the established tumor parenchyma.

Tumor hypoxia can dramatically impede the effectiveness of certain (passive) immunotherapies using cytokines (interferon-γ and tumor necrosis factor-α). Hypoxia also reduces survival and proliferation of T-lymphocytes and the production of cytokines by these cells (KIM et al. 2008; LUKASHEV et al. 2007). Pharmacological studies have firmly established that high levels of adenosine, a pathophysiological feature of solid tumors (see Chap. 4, Sect. 4.11.12), have immunosuppressive effects (SITKOVSKY and LUKASHEV 2005; OHTA et al. 2006). In addition, hypoxia can alter IL-2-induced activation of lymphokine-activated killer (LAK) cells (reviewed by CHAPLIN et al. 2000; KIM et al. 2008; SITKOVSKY and LUKASHEV 2005). The potency of treatment started to decrease at oxygen partial pressures of less than approximately 35 mmHg ($\approx 5\%$ O_2).

15.4.5.3
Resistance to Hormonal Treatment

Endocrine therapy is the treatment of choice for patients with breast cancer expressing estrogen receptor (ER) and/or progesterone receptor (PR). A hypoxic microenvironment has been shown to posttranscriptionally reduce ER-α expression in breast cancer cells and thus decreases sensitivity to hormonal agents. ER-α-negative invasive breast cancer is more aggressive and in situ cancer is associated with increased risk of progression to invasive disease (KUREBAYASHI et al. 2001; KUREBAYASHI 2005; HELCZYNSKA et al. 2003; STONER et al. 2002). COOPER et al. (2004) have shown that the reduced ER-α expression in breast cancers is

caused by persistent changes in proteasome function as a response to intermittent hypoxia. As a consequence, the latter authors observed a diminished response to estradiol and development of resistance to endocrine therapy.

15.5
Tumor Acidosis and Treatment Resistance

As already outlined in Chap. 4, tumor cells have a lower extracellular pH (pH_e) than normal cells. This is an inherent characteristic of the tumor phenotype. Like normal cells, tumor cells have a neutral to slightly alkaline cytosolic ("internal") pH (pH_i), which is considered to be permissive for cell proliferation (GILLIES et al. 1992). The result is a reverse (or negative) pH gradient ($pH_i > pH_e$) across the tumor-cell plasma membrane in vivo compared with normal tissues where $pH_i < pH_e$ (≈ 7.2 vs. ≈ 7.4; reviewed in VAUPEL et al 1989; GRIFFITHS 1991).

The extracellular acidosis in tumors is not simply caused by excessive production of lactic acid and CO_2, but may also be the result of other mechanisms yielding H^+ ions that are exported into the extracellular space mainly via the H^+-monocarboxylate cotransporter (MCT1) and the Na^+/H^+ antiporter (NHE1), and—to a lesser extent—by a vacuolar type H^+-pump (H^+-ATPase; FAIS et al. 2007). Taking the various H^+ sources of the tumor metabolism into account, it is not surprising that hypoxia is not always correlated with a decrease in extracellular pH, i.e., acidic tumor regions and hypoxic tumor areas are not necessarily congruent.

pH effects on therapeutic modalities were summarized extensively prior to 2000 by WIKE-HOOLEY et al. (1984), TANNOCK and ROTIN (1989), DURAND (1991, 1994), SONG et al. (1993, 1999), VAUPEL (1997), GERWECK (1998) and STUBBS (1998). More recent reviews include STUBBS et al. (2000), EVELHOCH (2001) and ROEPE (2001).

15.5.1
Effects of Tumor Acidosis on Ionizing Radiation

Cell survival after ionizing radiation has been assessed at low extracellular pH for several mammalian cell lines. The results demonstrated increased radiation resistance at reduced pH_e, the effect, however, being much less than that due to hypoxia (HAVEMAN 1980; RÖTTINGER et al. 1980; FREEMAN et al. 1981; RÖTTINGER and MEN-DONCA 1982). The mechanisms involved may be due to either a greater capacity for DNA repair under low pH conditions or to an inhibition of the fixation of potentially lethal radiation damage (FREEMAN and SIERRA 1984; TANNOCK and ROTIN 1989). Furthermore, it has been reported that an acidic environment can suppress radiation-induced postmitotic apoptosis (LEE et al. 1987).

Low environmental pH has also been shown to inhibit cell proliferation, can exert substantial effects on cell cycle that also modify radiosensitivity and can select for a more aggressive phenotype (HILL et al. 2001; ROFSTAD et al. 2006; see Table 15.4).

Table 15.4. Tumor acidosis and acquired treatment resistance (selection of mechanisms)

Treatment affected	Mechanisms involved	Examples	References
X- and γ-rays	Reduced "fixation" of DNA damage		FREEMAN and SIERRA (1984)
	Increased capacity for DNA repair		HAVEMAN (1980) RÖTTINGER et al. (1980)
	Cell cycle effects, reduced cell proliferation rate		TAYLOR and HODSON (1984) EAGLE (1973)
	Development of an aggressive phenotype		HILL et al. (2001) ROFSTAD et al. (2006)
	Suppression of radiation-induced apoptosis		LEE et al. (1987)
Chemotherapy	Cell cycle effects, reduced cell proliferation rate		WIKE-HOOLEY et al. (1984) COLE and TANNOCK (2005) VALERIOTE and VAN PUTTEN (1975)
	Reduced active uptake due to ATP-depletion Reduced uptake by diffusion	Methotrexate Weakly basic drugs	GERWECK and SEETHARAMAN (1996)
	Increased DNA repair	Alkylating agents	SARKARIA et al. (2008)
	Over-expression of P-glycoprotein (P_{gp}), increased drug efflux	Anthracyclines vinca alkaloids	WEI and ROEPE (1994) LOTZ et al. (2007)
	Resistance to apoptosis	Overexpression of P_{gp}	ROBINSON et al. (1997)
Immunotherapy	Inhibition of cell-mediated anti-tumor immunity		LARDNER (2001)
	Decreased T-cell-mediated cytotoxicity through P_{gp}-overexpression		WEISBURG et al. (1996)
	Inhibition of LAK-cells		SEVERIN et al. (1994)
	Depression of NK-cells		LOEFFLER et al. (1991)

15.5.2
pH and Chemotherapy

The transport of drugs into tumor cells (either by diffusion or carrier-mediated mechanisms) and their intracellular metabolism are pH-dependent (TANNOCK and ROTIN 1989). Since the cellular uptake of drugs by diffusion is efficient only for the non-ionized form of compounds and since the extracellular pH in tumors is acidic with the cytosolic pH being maintained in the neutral/slightly alkaline range, the respective pH gradient acts to exclude weakly basic drugs and thus impairs their cellular uptake by diffusion. Since cell membranes are readily permeable only to uncharged drug molecules, weak bases tend to concentrate on the more acid side of the membrane, i.e., in the extracellular space, while weak acids accumulate on the more alkaline side of the membrane, i.e., in the cytosolic compartment. Weakly basic drugs include doxorubicin, idarubicin, epirubicin, daunorubicin, bleomycin, mitoxantrone and vinca alkaloids (RAGHUNAND and GILLIES 2000, 2001; GERWECK and SEETHARAMAN 1996; GERWECK 1998; GERWECK et al. 2006).

Multiple indirect mechanisms may additionally be involved in the acidosis-induced resistance to chemotherapeutic agents, including an increased efflux of drugs (WEI and ROEPE 1994) and resistance to apoptosis (ROBINSON et al. 1997), the latter mechanisms being mediated by overexpression of P-glycoprotein. Furthermore, an increased activity of DNA repair enzymes has been convincingly described (SARKARIA et al. 2008), and an inhibition of cell proliferation and cell cycle effects have extensively been discussed as mechanisms reducing the effectiveness of chemotherapeutic agents in acidic environments (e.g., VALERIOTE and VAN PUTTEN 1975; see Table 15.4).

15.5.3
pH and Immunotherapy

Although there are only relatively few studies on the effect of acidic extracellular pH on immune cells and their function, evidence of impaired lymphocyte cytotoxicity and proliferation at acidic pH is beginning to emerge (for a review see LARDNER 2001). There is a growing awareness among immunologists and oncologists of the potential modulatory role of the acidic tumor microenvironment on immune cell function (see Table 15.4). The majority of the work to date has focused primarily on cell-mediated immunity, with only a few studies on humoral immunity. Summarizing the few data available so far, the acidic microenvironment may be inhibitory

to the antitumor immunity (CAIRNS et al. 2006). Most of this evidence is experimental, and clinical demonstration of similar phenomena will be difficult. Furthermore, many data are still too preliminary for firm conclusions to be made and are thus speculative.

15.6
Conclusions

Besides "classical" drug resistance (mostly based on the molecular biology of tumors), which can only partly explain the lack of treatment efficacy, acquired therapeutic resistance due to the impact of hostile microenvironmental conditions is increasingly receiving attention in clinical practice. One of the goals of translational cancer research is to obtain a better understanding of the impact of these hostile microenvironmental parameters on tumor response to therapy, in order to improve patients' outcomes.

Based on the association between hostile microenvironmental parameters and treatment failure, further development and validation of noninvasive techniques for the repeated assessment of these factors are urgently needed to enable an application in the clinical routine and integration into general patient care. Pretreatment assessment of the hostile micromilieu and the pathophysiology of individual tumors should allow a selection of patients for more aggressive treatment and/or for individualization of therapy.

Acknowledgements

The valuable assistance of Dr. Debra K. Kelleher and Mrs. Anne Deutschmann-Fleck in preparing this manuscript is greatly appreciated.

This work has continuously been supported by grants from the Deutsche Krebshilfe (M 40/91Va1 and 106758).

References

Anderson CJ, Hoare SF, Ashcroft M, Bilsland AE, Keith WN (2006) Hypoxic regulation of telomerase gene expression by transcriptional and posttranscriptional mechanisms. Oncogene 25:61–69

Ausserer WA, Bourrat-Floeck B, Green CJ, Laderoute KR, Sutherland RM (1994) Regulation of c-jun expression during hypoxic and low-glucose stress. Mol Cell Biol 14:5032–5042

Batchelor TT, Sorensen AG, di Tomaso E, Zhang WT, Duda DG, Cohen KS, Kozak KR, Cahill DP, Chen PJ, Zhu M, Ancukiewicz M, Mrugala MM, Plotkin S, Drappatz J, Louis DN, Ivy P, Scadden DT, Benner T, Loeffler JS, Wen PY, Jain RK (2007) AZD2171, a pan-VEGF receptor tyrosine kinase inhibitor, normalizes tumor vasculature and alleviates edema in glioblastoma patients. Cancer Cell 11:83–95

Bristow RG, Hill RP (2008) Hypoxia, DNA repair and genetic instability. Nature 8:180–192

Brown JM (2002) Tumor microenvironment and the response to anticancer therapy. Cancer Biol Ther 1:453–458

Brown JM (2007) Tumor hypoxia in cancer therapy. Methods Enzymol 435:297–321

Brown JM, Giaccia AJ (1998) The unique physiology of solid tumors: Opportunities (and problems) for cancer therapy. Cancer Res 58:1408–1416

Bush RS (1986) The significance of anemia in clinical radiation therapy. Int J Radiat Oncol Biol Phys 12:2047–2050

Cairns R, Papandreou I, Denko N (2006) Overcoming physiologic barriers to cancer treatment by molecularly targeting the tumor microenvironment. Mol Cancer Res 4:61–70

Chabner B, Allegra CJ, Curt GA, Calabresi P (1996) Antineoplastic agents. In: Goodman and Gilman (eds) The pharmacological basis of therapeutics, 9th edn. McGraw-Hill, New York, pp 1233–1287

Chaplin DJ, Horsman MR, Trotter MJ, Siemann DW (2000) Therapeutic significance of microenvironmental factors. In: Molls M, Vaupel P (eds) Blood perfusion and microenvironment of human tumors. Implications for clinical radiooncology. Springer, Berlin, Heidelberg, New York, pp 133–143

Chapman JD, Stobbe CC, Arnfield MR, Santus R, Lee L, McPhee MS (1991) Oxygen dependency of tumor cell killing in vitro by light-activated Photofrin II. Radiat Res 126:73–79

Chen Q, Huang Z, Chen H, Shapiro H, Beckers J, Hetzel FW (2002) Improvement of tumor response by manipulation of tumor oxygenation during photodynamic therapy. Photochem Photobiol 76:197–203

Cheng KC, Loeb LA (1993) Genomic instability and tumor progression: Mechanistic considerations. Adv Cancer Res 60:121–156

Cole PD, Alcaraz MJ, Smith AK (2006) Pharmacodynamic properties of methotrexate and Aminotrexate™ during weekly therapy. Cancer Chemother Pharmacol 57:826–834

Cole SPC, Tannock IF (2005) Drug resistance. In: Tannock IF, Hill RP, Bristow RG, Harrington L (eds) The basic science of oncology, 4th edn. McGraw-Hill, New York, Chicago, San Francisco, pp 376–399

Comerford KM, Wallace TJ, Karhausen J, Louis NA, Montalto MC, Colgan SP (2002) Hypoxia-inducible factor-1-dependent regulation of the multidrug resistance (MDR1) gene. Cancer Res 62:3387–3394

Cooper C, Liu G-Y, Niu Y-L, Santos S, Murphy LC, Watson PH (2004) Intermittent hypoxia induces proteasome-dependent down-regulation of estrogen receptor α in human breast carcinoma. Clin Cancer Res 10:8720–8727

Dachs GU, Tozer GM (2000) Hypoxia modulated gene expression: Angiogenesis, metastasis and therapeutic exploitation. Eur J Cancer 36:1649–1660

Di Paolo A, Bocci G (2007) Drug distribution in tumors: mechanisms, role in drug resistance, and methods for modification. Curr Oncol Rep 9:109–114

Double EB, Richmond RC (1978) Platinum complexes as radiosensitizers of hypoxic mammalian cells. Br J Cancer Suppl 3:98–102

Double EB, Richmond RC (1979) Radiosensitization of hypoxic tumor cells cis- and trans-dichlorodiammineplatinum (II). Int J Radiat Oncol Biol Phys 5:1369–1372

Dunst J (2004) Management of anemia in patients undergoing curative radiotherapy. Erythropoietin, transfusions, or better nothing? Strahlenther Onkol 180:671–681

Dunst J, Molls M (2008) Incidence and impact of anemia in radiation oncology. In: Nowrousian MR (ed) Recombinant human erythropoietin (rhEPO) in clinical oncology—Scientific and clinical aspects of anemia in cancer, 2nd edn. Springer, Vienna, New York, pp 249–263

Durand RE (1991) Keynote address: The influence of microenvironmental factors on the activity of radiation and drugs. Int J Radiat Oncol Biol Phys 20:253–258

Durand RE (1994) The influence of microenvironmental factors during cancer therapy. In Vivo 8:691–702

Durand RE (2001) Intermittent blood flow in solid tumours—an under-appreciated source of drug resistance. Cancer Metastasis Rev 20:57–61

Durand RE, Aquino-Parsons C (2001a) Non-constant tumour blood flow: Implications for therapy. Acta Oncol 40:862–869

Durand RE, Aquino-Parsons C (2001b) Clinical relevance of intermittent tumour blood flow. Acta Oncol 40:929–936

Eagle H (1973) The effects of environmental pH on growth of normal and malignant cells. J Cell Physiol 82:1–8

Erlichman C (1992) Pharmacology of anticancer drugs. In: Tannock IF, Hill RP (eds) The basic science of oncology, 2nd edn. McGraw-Hill, New York, pp 317–337

Evans IC, Bergsjø P (1965) The influence of anemia on the results of radiotherapy in carcinoma of the cervix. Radiology 84:709–717

Evelhoch JL (2001) pH and therapy of human cancer. In: Goode JA, Chadwick DJ (eds) The tumour microenvironment: Causes and consequences of hypoxia and acidity. Novartis Foundation Symposium 240. John Wiley & Sons, Ltd, Chichester, New York, pp 68–84

Fais S, De Milito A, You H, Qin W (2007) Targeting vacuolar H+-ATPase as a new strategy against cancer. Cancer Res 67:10627–10630

Freeman ML, Holahan EV, Highfield DP, Raaphorst GP, Spiro IJ, Dewey WC (1981) The effect of pH on hyperthermic and X-ray induced cell killing. Int J Radiat Oncol Biol Phys 7:211–216

Freeman ML, Sierra E (1984) An acidic extracellular environment reduces the fixation of radiation damage. Radiat Res 97:154–161

Freitas I, Baronzio GF (1991) Tumor hypoxia, reoxygenation and oxygenation strategies: Possible role in photodynamic therapy. J Photochem Photobiol B 11: 3–30

Frommhold H, Guttenberger R, Henke M (1998) The impact of blood hemoglobin content on the outcome of radiotherapy. Strahlenther Onkol 174:31–34

Fukumura D, Jain RK (2007) Tumor microenvironment abnormalities: Causes, consequences, and strategies to normalize. J Cell Biochem 101:937–949

Gerweck LE (1998) Tumor pH: Implications for treatment and novel drug design. Semin Radiat Oncol 8:176–182

Gerweck LE, Seetharaman K (1996) Cellular pH gradient in tumor versus normal tissue: Potential exploitation for the treatment of cancer. Cancer Res 56:1194–1198

Gerweck LE, Vijayappa S, Kozin S (2006) Tumor pH controls the in-vivo efficacy of weak acid and base chemotherapies. Mol Cancer Ther 5:1275–1279

Giaccia AJ (1996) Hypoxic stress proteins: survival of the fittest. Semin Radiat Oncol 6:46–58

Gillies RJ, Martinez-Zaguilán R, Peterson EP, Perona R (1992) Role of intracellular pH in mammalian cell proliferation. Cell Physiol Biochem 2:159–179

Graeber TG, Osmanian C, Jacks T, Housman DE, Koch CJ, Lowe SW, Giaccia AJ (1996) Hypoxia-mediated selection of cells with diminished apoptotic potential in solid tumours. Nature 379:88–91

Graeber TG, Peterson JF, Tsai M, Monica K, Fornace AJ, Giaccia AJ (1994) Hypoxia induces accumulation of p53 protein, but activation of a G1-phase checkpoint by low-oxygen conditions is independent of p53 status. Molecular Cell Biol 14:6264–6277

Grau C, Overgaard J (2000) Significance of hemoglobin concentration for treatment outcome. In: Molls M, Vaupel P (eds) Blood perfusion and microenvironment of human tumors. Implications for clinical radiooncology. Springer, Berlin, Heidelberg, New York, pp 101–112

Gray LH, Conger AD, Ebert M, Hornsey S, Scott OCA (1953) The concentration of oxygen dissolved in tissues at the time of irradiation as a factor in radiotherapy. Br J Radiol 26: 638–648

Griffiths JR (1991) Are cancer cells acidic? Br J Cancer 64:425–427

Hall EJ (1994) Molecular biology in radiation therapy: The potential impact of recombinant technology on clinical practice. Int J Radiat Oncol Biol Phys 30:1019–1028

Hall EJ, Giaccia AJ (2006) Radiobiology for the radiologist, 6th edn. Lippincott Williams & Wilkins, Philadelphia, Baltimore, New York

Halonen P, Mattila J, Mäkipernaa A, Ruuska T, Schmiegelow K (2006) Erythrocyte concentrations of metabolites or cumulative doses of 6-mercaptopurine and methotrexate do not predict liver changes in children treated for acute lymphoblastic leukemia. Pediatr Blood Cancer 46:762–766

Harrison L, Blackwell K (2004) Hypoxia and anemia: Factors in decreased sensitivity to radiation therapy and chemotherapy? Oncologist 9:31–40

Harrison LB, Chadha M, Hill RJ, Hu K, Shasha D (2002) Impact of tumor hypoxia and anemia on radiation therapy outcomes. Oncologist 7:492–508

Haugen H, Magnusson B, Svensson M, Mercke C (2004) Pre-radiotherapy hemoglobin level but not microvessel density predicts locoregional control and survival in laryngeal cancer treated with primary radical radiotherapy. Clin Cancer Res 10:7941–7949

Haveman J (1980) The influence of pH on the survival after X-irradiation of cultured malignant cells. Effects of carbonyl-cyanide-3-chlorophenylhydrazone. Int J Radiat Biol Relat Stud Phys Chem Med 37:201–205

Helczynska K, Kronblad A, Jögi A, Nilsson E, Beckman S, Landberg G, Pahlman S (2003) Hypoxia promotes a dedifferentiated phenotype in ductal breast carcinoma in situ. Cancer Res 63:1441–1444

Heldin C-H, Rubin K, Pietras K, Östman A (2004) High interstitial fluid pressure - an obstacle in cancer therapy. Nature Rev Cancer 4:806–813

Henderson BW, Fingar VH (1987) Relationship of tumor hypoxia and response to photodynamic treatment in an experimental mouse tumor. Cancer Res 47:3110–3114

Henke M, Momm F, Guttenberger R (1999) Erythropoietin for patients undergoing radiotherapy: The Freiburg experience. In: Vaupel P, Kelleher DK (eds) Tumor hypoxia. Pathophysiology, clinical significance and therapeutical perspectives. Wissenschaftliche Verlagsgesellschaft, Stuttgart, pp 91–97

Hickman JA, Potten CS, Merritt AJ, Fisher TC (1994) Apoptosis and cancer chemotherapy. Philos Trans R Soc Lond B Biol Sci 345:319–325

Highley MS, Schrijvers D, van Oosterom AT, Harper PG, Momerency G, Van Cauwenberghe K, Maes RA, De Bruijn EA, Edelstein MB (1997) Activated oxazaphosphorines are transported predominantly by erythrocytes. Ann Oncol 8:1139–1144

Hill RP, De Jaeger K, Jang A, Cairns R (2001) pH, hypoxia and metastasis. In: Goode JA, Chadwick DJ (eds) The tumour microenvironment: Causes and consequences of hypoxia and acidity. Novartis Foundation Symposium 240. John Wiley & Sons, Ltd, Chichester, New York, pp 154–168

Hirst DG, Denekamp J (1979) Tumour cell proliferation in relation to the vasculature. Cell Tissue Kinet 12:31–42

Höckel M, Schlenger K, Aral B, Mitze M, Schäffer U, Vaupel P (1996a) Association between tumor hypoxia and malignant progression in advanced cancer of the uterine cervix. Cancer Res 56:4509–4515

Höckel M, Schlenger K, Höckel S, Aral B, Schäffer U, Vaupel P (1998) Tumor hypoxia in pelvic recurrences of cervical cancer. Int J Cancer 79:365–369

Höckel M, Schlenger K, Höckel S, Vaupel P (1999) Hypoxic cervical cancers with low apoptotic index are highly aggressive. Cancer Res 59:4525–4528

Höckel M, Schlenger K, Mitze M, Schäffer U, Vaupel P (1996b) Hypoxia and radiation response in human tumors. Semin Radiat Oncol 6:3–9

Höckel M, Vaupel P (2001) Tumor hypoxia: Definitions and current clinical, biological and molecular aspects. J Natl Cancer Inst 93:266–276

Hu K, Harrison LB (2005) Impact of anemia in patients with head and neck cancer treated with radiation therapy. Curr Treat Opt Oncol 6:31–45

Jain RK (1987) Transport of molecules across tumor vasculature. Cancer Metastasis Rev 6:559–593

Jain RK (1990) Physiological barriers to delivery of monoclonal antibodies and other macromolecules in tumors. Cancer Res 50:814s–819s

Jain RK (2001) Normalizing tumor vasculature with anti-angiogenic therapy: A new paradigm for combination therapy. Nat Med 7:987–989

Jain RK (2005) Normalization of tumor vasculature: An emerging concept in antiangiogenic therapy. Science 307:58–62

Kim CY, Tsai MH, Osmanian C, Graeber TG, Lee JE, Giffard RG, DiPaolo JA, Peehl DM, Giaccia AJ (1997) Selection of human cervical epithelial cells that possess reduced apoptotic potential to low-oxygen conditions. Cancer Res 57:4200–4204

Kim H, Peng G, Hicks JM, Weiss HL, von Meir EG, Brenner MK (2008) Engineering human tumor-specific cytotoxic T cells to function in a hypoxic environment. Mol Ther 16:599–606

Koong AC, Chen EY, Giaccia AJ (1994) Hypoxia causes the activation of nuclear factor κB through the phosphorylation of IκBα on tyrosine residues. Cancer Res 54:1425–1430

Koukourakis MI, Giatromanolaki A, Sivridis E, Simopoulos C, Turley H, Talks K, Gatter KC, Harris AL (2002) Hypoxia-inducible factor (HIF1A and HIF2A), angiogenesis, and chemoradiotherapy outcome of squamous cell head-and-neck cancer. Int J Radiat Oncol Biol Phys 53:1192–1202

Kumar P (2000) Tumor hypoxia and anemia: Impact on the efficacy of radiation therapy. Sem Hematol 37:4–8

Kurebayashi J (2005) Resistance to endocrine therapy in breast cancer. Cancer Chemother Pharmacol 56 (Suppl 1):s39–s46

Kurebayashi J, Otsuki T, Moriya T, Sonoo H (2001) Hypoxia reduces hormone responsiveness of human breast cancer cells. Jpn J Cancer Res 92:1093–1101

Laderoute KR, Calaoagan JM, Gustafson-Brown C, Knapp AM, Li G-C, Mendonca HL, Ryan HE, Wang Z, Johnson RS (2002) The response of c-Jun/AP-1 to chronic hypoxia is hypoxia-inducible factor 1α dependent. Mol Cell Biol 22:2515–2523

Laderoute KR, Grant TD, Murphy BJ, Sutherland RM (1992) Enhanced epidermal growth factor receptor synthesis in human squamous carcinoma cells exposed to low levels of oxygen. Int J Cancer 52:428–432

Lardner A (2001) The effects of extracellular pH on immune function. J Leukoc Biol 69:522–530

Lee CG, Heijn M, di Tomaso E, Griffon-Etienne G, Ancukiewicz M, Koike C, Park KR, Ferrara N, Jain RK, Suit HD, Boucher Y (2000) Anti-vascular endothelial growth factor treatment augments tumor radiation response under normoxic or hypoxic conditions. Cancer Res 60: 5565–5570

Lee HS, Park HJ, Lyons JC, Griffin RJ, Auger EA, Song CW (1987) Radiation-induced apoptosis in different pH environments in vitro. Int J Radiat Oncol Biol Phys 38:1079–1087

Lewis C, Murdoch C (2005) Macrophage responses to hypoxia: Implications for tumor progression and anti-cancer therapies. Am J Pathol 167:627–635

Liao YP, Schaue D, McBride WH (2007) Modification of the tumor microenvironment to enhance immunity. Front Biosci 12:3576–3600

Lin MI, Sessa WC (2004) Antiangiogenic therapy: Creating a unique "window" of opportunity. Cancer Cell 6:529–531

Loeffler DA, Juneau PL, Heppner GH (1991) Natural killer-cell activity under conditions reflective of tumor microenvironment. Int J Cancer 48:895–899

Lotz C, Kelleher DK, Gassner B, Gekle M, Vaupel P, Thews O (2007) Role of the tumor microenvironment in the activity and expression of the p-glycoprotein in human colon carcinoma cells. Oncol Rep 17:239–244

Ludwig H (2004) rHuEPO and treatment outcomes: The preclinical experience. Oncologist 9:48–54

Lukashev D, Ohta A, Sitkovsky M (2007) Hypoxia-dependent anti-inflammatory pathways in protection of cancerous tissues. Cancer Metastasis Rev 26:273–279

Lunt SJ, Chaudary N, Hill RP (2008) The tumor microenvironment and metastatic disease. Clin Exp Metastasis (DOI 10.1007/s10585-008-9182-2)

Luo FR, Wyrick SD, Chaney SG (1999) Pharmacokinetics and biotransformations of oxaliplatin in comparison with ormaplatin following a single bolus injection in rats. Cancer Chemother Pharmacol 44:19–28

Mattern J, Kallinowski F, Herfarth C, Volm M (1996) Association of resistance-related protein expression with poor vascularization and low levels of oxygen in human rectal cancer. Int J Cancer 67:20–23

Milosevic M, Fyles A, Haider M, Hedley D, Hill R (2004) The human tumor microenvironment: invasive (needle) measurement of oxygen and interstitial fluid pressure (IFP). Semin Radiat Oncol 14:249–258

Minchinton AL, Tannock IF (2006) Drug penetration in solid tumours. Nat Rev Cancer 6:583–592

Mitchell JB, McPherson S, De Graff W, Gamson J, Zabell A, Russo A (1985) Oxygen dependence of hematoporphyrin derivative-induced photo-inactivation of Chinese hamster cells. Cancer Res 45:2008–2011

Moan J, Sommer S (1985) Oxygen dependence of the photosensitizing effect of hematoporphyrin derivative in NHIK 3025 cells. Cancer Res 45:1608–1610

Moulder JE, Rockwell S (1987) Tumor hypoxia: Its impact on cancer therapy. Cancer Metastasis Rev 5:313–341

Netti PA, Berk DA, Swartz MA, Grodzinsky AJ, Jain RK (2000) Role of extracellular matrix assembly in interstitial transport in solid tumors. Cancer Res 60:2497–2503

Nishi H, Nakada T, Kyo S, Inoue M, Shay JW, Isaka K (2004) Hypoxia-inducible factor 1 mediates upregulation of telomerase (hTERT). Mol Cell Biol 24:6076–6083

Nowrousian MR (2008) Significance of anemia in cancer chemotherapy. In: Nowrousian MR (ed) Recombinant human erythropoietin (rhEPO) in clinical oncology, 2nd edn. Springer, Vienna, New York, pp 207–248

Nowrousian MR, Dunst J, Vaupel P (2008) Erythropoiesis-stimulating agents: Favorable safety profile when used as indicated. Strahlenther Onkol 184:121–136

Ohta A, Gorelik E, Prasad SJ, Ronchese F, Lukashev D, Wong MK, Huang X, Caldwell S, Liu K, Smith P, Chen JF, Jackson EK, Apasov S, Abrams S, Sitkovsky M (2006) A2A adenosine receptor protects tumors from antitumor T cells. Proc Natl Acad Sci USA 103:13132–13137

Park S-Y, Kim Y-J, Gao AC, Mohler JL, Onate SA, Hidalgo AA, Ip C, Park E-M, Yoon Sy, Park Y-M (2006) Hypoxia increases androgen receptor activity in prostate cancer cells. Cancer Res 66:5121–5129

Prosnitz RG, Yao B, Farrell CL, Clough R, Brizel DM (2005) Pretreatment anemia is correlated with the reduced effectiveness of radiation and concurrent chemotherapy in advanced head and neck cancer. Int J Radiat Oncol Biol Phys 61:1087–1095

Raghunand N, Gillies RJ (2000) pH and drug resistance in tumours. Drug Resist Updat 3:39–47

Raghunand N, Gillies RJ (2001) pH and chemotherapy. In: Goode JA, Chadwick DJ (eds) The tumour microenvironment: Causes and consequences of hypoxia and acidity. Novartis Foundation Symposium 240. John Wiley & Sons, Ltd, Chichester, New York, pp 199–211

Raleigh JA (ed) (1996) Hypoxia and its clinical significance. Semin Radiat Oncol 6:1–70

Ramanathan-Girish S, Boroujerdi M (2001) Contradistinction between doxorubicin and epirubicin: In vitro interaction with blood components. J Pharm Pharmacol 53:815–821

Reynolds TY, Rockwell S, Glazer PM (1996) Genetic instability induced by the tumor microenvironment. Cancer Res 56:5754–5757

Rice GC, Hoy C, Schimke RT (1986) Transient hypoxia enhances the frequency of dihydrofolate reductase gene amplification in Chinese hamster ovary cells. Proc Natl Acad Sci USA 83:5978–5982

Robinson LJ, Roberts WK, Ling TT, Lamming D, Sternberg SS, Roepe PD (1997) Human MDR1 protein overexpression delays the apoptotic cascade in Chinese hamster ovary fibroblasts. Biochemistry 36:11169–11178

Roepe PD (2001) pH and multidrug resistance. In: Goode JA, Chadwick DJ (eds) The tumour microenvironment: Causes and consequences of hypoxia and acidity. Novartis Foundation Symposium 240. John Wiley & Sons, Ltd, Chichester, New York, pp 232–250

Rofstad EK, Mathiesen B, Kindem K, Galappathi K (2006) Acidic extracellular pH promotes experimental metastasis of human melanoma cells in athymic nude mice. Cancer Res 66:6699–6707

Röttinger EM, Mendonca M (1982) Radioresistance secondary to low pH in human glial cells and Chinese hamster ovary cells. Int J Radiat Oncol Biol Phys 8:1309–1314

Röttinger EM, Mendonca M, Gerweck LE (1980) Modification of pH induced cellular inactivation by irradiation-glial cells. Int J Radiat Oncol Biol Phys 6:1659–1662

Russo CA, Weber TK, Volpe CM, Stoler DL, Petrelli NJ, Rodriguez-Bigas M, Burhans WC, Anderson GR (1995) An anoxia inducible endonuclease and enhanced DNA breakage as contributors to genomic instability in cancer. Cancer Res 55:1122–1128

Sakata K, Kwok TT, Murphy BJ, Laderoute KR, Gordon GR, Sutherland RM (1991) Hypoxia-induced drug resistance: Comparison to P-glycoprotein-associated drug resistance. Br J Cancer 64:809–814

Sanna K, Rofstad EK (1994) Hypoxia-induced resistance to doxorubicin and methotrexate in human melanoma cell lines in vitro. Int J Cancer 58:258–262

Sarkaria JN, Kitange GJ, James D, Plummer R, Calvert H, Weller M, Wick W (2008) Mechanisms of chemoresistance to alkylating agents in malignant glioma. Clin Cancer Res 14:2900–2908

Schrijvers D (2003) Role of red blood cells in pharmacokinetics of chemotherapeutic agents. Clin Pharmacokinet 42:779–791

Semenza GL (2000a) Hypoxia, clonal selection, and the role of HIF-1 in tumor progression. Crit Rev Biochem Mol Biol 35:71–103

Semenza GL (2000b) HIF-1: Mediator of physiological and pathophysiological response to hypoxia. J Appl Physiol 88:1474–1480

Severin T, Muller B, Giese G, Uhl B, Wolf B, Hauschildt S, Kreutz W (1994) pH-dependent LAK cell cytotoxicity. Tumour Biol 15:304–310

Shannon AM, Bouchier-Hayes DJ, Condron CM, Toomey D (2003) Tumour hypoxia, chemotherapeutic resistance and hypoxia-related therapies. Cancer Treat Rev 29: 297–307

Sitkovsky M, Lukashev D (2005) Regulation of immune cells by local-tissue oxygen tension: HIF-1α and adenosine receptors. Nat Rev Immunol 5:712–721

Song CW, Lyons JC, Luo Y (1993) Intra- and extracellular pH in solid tumors: Influence on therapeutic response. In: Teicher BA (ed) Drug resistance in oncology. Marcel Dekker, New York, Basel, Hong Kong, pp 25–51

Song CW, Park H, Ross BD (1999) Intra- and extracellular pH in solid tumors. In: Teicher BA (ed) Antiangiogenic agents in cancer therapy. Humana Press Inc., Totowa, NJ, pp 51–64

Stackpole CW, Groszek L, Kalbag SS (1994) Benign-to-malignant B16 melanoma progression induced in two stages in vitro by exposure to hypoxia. J Natl Cancer Inst 86: 361–367

Stoler DL, Anderson GR, Russo CA, Spina AM, Beerman TA (1992) Anoxia-inducible endonuclease activity as a potential basis of the genomic instability of cancer cells. Cancer Res 52:4372–4378

Stoner M, Saville B, Wormke M, Dean D, Burghardt R, Safe S (2002) Hypoxia induces proteasome-dependent degradation of estrogen receptor alpha in ZR-75 breast cancer cells. Mol Endocrinol 16:2231–2242

Stubbs M (1998) Tumour pH. In: Molls M, Vaupel P (eds) Blood perfusion and microenvironment of human tumors. Implications for clinical radiooncology. Springer, Berlin Heidelberg, New York, pp 113–120

Stubbs M, McSheehy PMJ, Griffiths JR, Bashford CL (2000) Causes and consequences of tumour acidity and implications for treatment. Mol Med Today 6:15–19

Sullivan R. Paré GC, Frederiksen LJ, Semenza GL, Graham CH (2008) Hypoxia-induced resistance to anticancer drugs is associated with decreased senescence and requires hypoxia-inducible factor-1 activity. Mol Cancer Ther 7: 1961–1973

Sutherland RM (1998) Tumor hypoxia and gene expression. Implications for malignant progression and therapy. Acta Oncol 37:567–574

Tannock IF (1968) The relation between cell proliferation and the vascular system in a transplanted mouse mammary tumour. Br J Cancer 22:258–273

Tannock IF (2001) Tumor physiology and drug resistance. Cancer Metastasis Rev 20:123–132

Tannock IF, Hill RP (eds) (1992) The basic science of oncology, 2nd edn. McGraw-Hill, New York

Tannock IF, Hill RP, Bristow RG, Harrington L (eds) (2005) The basic science of oncology, 4th edn. McGraw-Hill, New York

Tannock IF, Rotin D (1989) Acid pH in tumors and its potential for therapeutic exploitation. Cancer Res 49:4373–4384

Taylor IW, Hodson PJ (1984) Cell cycle regulation by environmental pH. J Cell Physiol 121:517–525

Teicher BA (1994) Hypoxia and drug resistance. Cancer Metast 13:139–168

Teicher BA (1995) Physiologic mechanisms of therapeutic resistance. Hematol Oncol Clin North Am 9:475–506

Teicher BA (ed) (1993) Drug resistance in oncology. Marcel Dekker, New York

Teicher BA, Holden SA, Al-Achi A, Herman TS (1990) Classification of antineoplastic treatments by their differential toxicity toward putative oxygenated and hypoxic tumor subpopulations in vivo in the FSaII murine fibrosarcoma. Cancer Res 50:3339–3344

Teicher BA, Lazo JS, Sartorelli AC (1981) Classification of antineoplastic agents by their selective toxicities toward oxygenated and hypoxic tumor cells. Cancer Res 41: 73–81

Trédan O, Galmarini CM, Patel K, Tannock IF (2007) Drug resistance and the solid tumor microenvironment. J Natl Cancer Inst 99:1441–1454

Valeriote F, van Putten L (1975) Proliferation-dependent cytotoxicity of anticancer agents: A review. Cancer Res 35:2619–2630

Van Belle SJP, Cocquyt V (2003) Impact of hemoglobin levels on the outcome of cancers treated with chemotherapy. Crit Rev Oncol Hematol 47:1–11

Vaupel P (1997) The influence of tumor blood flow and microenvironmental factors on the efficacy of radiation, drugs and localized hyperthermia. Klin Pädiatr 209:243–249

Vaupel P (2004a) The role of hypoxia-induced factors in tumor progression. Oncologist 9:10–17

Vaupel P (2004b) Tumor microenvironmental physiology and its implications for radiation oncology. Semin Radiat Oncol 14:198–206

Vaupel P (2008) Hypoxia and aggressive tumor phenotype: Implications for therapy and prognosis. Oncologist 13 (Suppl 3):21–36

Vaupel P, Briest S, Höckel M (2002) Hypoxia in breast cancer: Pathogenesis, characterization and biological/therapeutic implications. Wiener Med Wschr 152:334–342

Vaupel P, Höckel M (2008) Tumor hypoxia and therapeutic resistance. In: Nowrousian MR (ed) Recombinant human erythropoietin (rhEPO) in clinical oncology, 2nd edn. Springer, Vienna, New York, pp 283–306

Vaupel P, Kallinowski F, Okunieff P (1989) Blood flow, oxygen and nutrient supply, and metabolic microenvironment of human tumors: A review. Cancer Res 49:6449–6465

Vaupel P, Kelleher DK, Höckel M (2001a) Oxygenation status of malignant tumors: Pathogenesis of hypoxia and significance for tumor therapy. Sem Oncol 28 (Suppl 8): 29–35

Vaupel P, Mayer A (2005) Effect of anaemia and hypoxia in tumour biology. In: Bokemeyer C, Ludwig H (eds) Anaemia in cancer, 2nd edn. Elsevier, Edingburgh, London, pp 47–66

Vaupel P, Mayer A, Höckel M (2004) Tumor hypoxia and malignant progression. Methods Enzymol 381:335–354

Vaupel P, Mayer A, Höckel M (2006) Impact of hemoglobin levels on tumor oxygenation: the higher, the better? Strahlenther Onkol 182:63–71

Vaupel P, Thews O, Hoeckel M (2001b) Treatment resistance of solid tumors: Role of hypoxia and anemia. Med Oncol 18:243–259

Vaupel P, Thews O, Kelleher DK, Konerding MA (2003) O$_2$ extraction is a key parameter determining the oxygenation status of malignant tumors and normal tissues. Int J Oncol 22:795–798

Vera JC, Castillo GR, Rosen OM (1991) A possible role for a mammalian facilitative hexose transporter in the development of resistance to drugs. Mol Cell Biol 11:3407–3418

Wei LY, Roepe PD (1994) Low external pH and osmotic shock increase the expression of human MDR protein. Biochemistry 33:7229–7238

Wei Y, Au JL-S (2005) Role of tumour microenvironment in chemoresistance. In: Meadows GG (ed) Integration/interaction of oncologic growth. Springer, The Netherlands, pp 285–321

Weinmann M, Belka C, Plasswilm L (2004) Tumour hypoxia: Impact on biology, prognosis and treatment of solid malignant tumours. Onkologie 27:83–90

Weisburg JH, Curcio M, Caron PC , Raghu G, Mechetner EB, Roepe PD, Scheinberg DA (1996) The multidrug resistance phenotype confers immunological resistance. J Exp Med 183:2699–2704

Wike-Hooley JL, Haveman J, Reinhold HS (1984) The relevance of tumour pH to the treatment of malignant disease. Radiother Oncol 2:343–366

Wildiers H, Guetens G, de Boeck G, Landuyt W, Verbeken E, Highley M, de Bruijn EA, van Oosterom AT (2002) Melphalan availability in hypoxia-inducible factor-1$\alpha\alpha$+/+ and factor-1alpha-/- tumors is independent of tumor vessel density and correlates with melphalan erythrocyte transport. Int J Cancer 99:514–519

Willett CG, Boucher Y, di Tomaso E, Duda DG, Munn LL, Tong RT, Chung DC, Sahani DV, Kalva SP, Kozin SV, Mino M, Cohen KS, Scadden DT, Hartford AC, Fischman AJ, Clark JW, Clark JW, Ryan DP, Zhu AX, Blaszkowsky LS, Chen HX, Shellito PC, Lauwers GY, Jain RK (2004) Direct evidence that the VEGF-specific antibody bevacizumab has antivascular effects in human rectal cancer. Nat Med 10:145–147

Willett CG, Boucher Y, di Tomaso E, Duda DG, Munn LL, Tong RT, Kozin SV, Petit L, Jain RK, Chung DC, Sahani DV, Kalva SP, Cohen KS, Scadden DT, Fischman AJ, Clark JW, Ryan DP, Zhu AX, Blaszkowsky LS, Shellito PC, Mino-Kenudson M, Lauwers GY (2005) Surrogate markers for antiangiogenic therapy and dose-limiting toxicities for bevacizumab with radiation and chemotherapy: continued experience of a phase I trial in rectal cancer patients. J Clin Oncol 23:8136–8139

Wouters A, Pauwels B, Lardon F, Vermorken JB (2007) Implications of in vitro research on the effect of radiotherapy and chemotherapy under hypoxic conditions. Oncologist 12:690–712

Yoshiba S, Ito D, Nagumo T, Shirota T, Hatori M, Shintani S (2009) Hypoxia induces resistance to 5-fluorouracil in oral cancer cells via G_1 phase cell cycle arrest. Oral Oncol 45:109–115

Young SD, Marshall RS, Hill RP (1988) Hypoxia induces DNA overreplication and enhances metastatic potential of murine tumour cells. Proc Natl Acad Sci USA 85:9533–9537

Zeller WJ (1995) Bleomycin. In: Zeller WJ, zur Hausen H (Hrsg) Onkologie: Grundlagen, Diagnostik, Therapie, Entwicklungen. Ecomed, Landsberg, pp IV-3.12, 1–7

Influence of Time Factor and Repopulation on Treatment Resistance

Daniel Zips

CONTENTS

D. Zips, MD, PhD
Department of Radiation Oncology, OncoRay Centre for Radiation Research, Medical Faculty and University Hospital Carl Gustav Carus, Technische Universität Dresden, Fetscherstraße 74, 01307 Dresden, Germany

KEY POINTS

- Overall treatment time (OTT) is the time period between the first and the last day of treatment.
- Experimental and clinical evidence shows that OTT is an important parameter of curative radiotherapy and that many fractionated irradiated tumours exhibit a time factor.
- A meta-analysis of 12 randomized clinical trials including patients with squamous cell carcinomas of the head and neck revealed that accelerated radiotherapy resulted in significantly better local tumour control than conventional radiotherapy.
- Repopulation of tumour stem cells during fractionated irradiation is considered to be the major underlying mechanism of increased treatment resistance with longer OTT.
- The effective cell doubling time is determined by the rate of cell production and cell loss. Therefore, accelerated repopulation of tumour stem cells during radiotherapy could result from an increased production rate or reduced stem cell loss.
- While changes in microenvironment appear to passively affect repopulation, it has been postulated that an active regulatory element is involved in triggering accelerated repopulation in tumours. This view is supported by similar repopulation kinetics in squamous cell carcinomas and normal epithelium where reoxygenation is unlikely to contribute to accelerated repopulation. Several studies indicate a role of signalling via epidermal growth factor receptor (EGFR).
- In experimental studies, inhibition of EGFR by monoclonal antibodies has been shown to inhibit accelerated repopulation during fractionated irradiation.

- Clinical studies suggest that the concept of dose-dense chemotherapy, e.g. 2-week cycles instead of 3-week cycles, is more successful in patients with lymphoma and breast cancer than in those with small cell lung cancer.

Abstract

Delivering radiation treatment with identical total dose over a shorter as compared to a longer time period influences the clinical effects on both normal tissue and tumour cells. The concept of dose-dense chemotherapy is also based on reduction of overall treatment time by shortening the interval between cycles. This chapter reviews preclinical and clinical data on the influence of treatment time and cell kinetics on outcome.

16.1
Introduction

Conventional curative radiotherapy is given in 30–35 daily fractions of 1.8–2 Gy in an overall treatment time (OTT) of 6–7 weeks. OTT is the time period between the first and the last day of treatment. This standard regimen has been developed to treat the tumour with a high radiation dose and with acceptable side effects to normal tissues. It has been recognized that normal tissue tolerance to radiotherapy increases with the use of small doses per fraction and with a time interval between fractions long enough for regeneration. On the other hand, it was generally accepted among radiation oncologists that prolonged OTT did not reduce antitumour efficacy of curative radiotherapy. This view was based on the observation that tumours usually grow at a slow rate with volume doubling times of several months (reviewed in BEGG and STEEL 2002). Therefore it was assumed that prolongation of OTT by several days, e.g. because of acute side effects or machine breakdown, would not result in inferior tumour control probability. However, this view has changed dramatically during the last 20 years by experimental and clinical evidence showing that OTT is an important parameter of curative radiotherapy and that many fractionated irradiated tumours exhibit a time factor.

16.2
Time Factor of Fractionated Radiotherapy

In their seminal article published in 1988, Withers and colleagues reported that in patients with head and neck squamous cell carcinomas local tumour control after fractionated radiotherapy decreases with prolonged OTT (WITHERS et al. 1988). The loss in radiation dose was estimated to be as high as 0.6 Gy per day. Several experimental studies on tumours in mice supported the early clinical observation that OTT matters (BAUMANN et al. 1994; BECK-BORNHOLDT et al. 1991; SPEKE and HILL 1995a, b; SUIT et al. 1977). Consequently, the concept of shortening of the OTT (*accelerated radiotherapy*) as a therapeutic intervention counteracting the time factor of fractionated radiotherapy was tested in clinical trials. Today, data from numerous randomized clinical trials with several thousand patients, mainly with squamous cell carcinomas of the head and neck as well as with lung cancer, are available. A meta-analysis of 12 randomized clinical trials with 5,723 patients treated for squamous cell carcinomas of the head and neck revealed that accelerated radiotherapy resulted in significantly better local tumour control than conventional radiotherapy (BOURHIS et al. 2006). Although cancer-specific and overall survival were only slightly improved, the local tumour control data strongly support the existence of a time factor. Similar findings are reported from randomized trials in lung cancer (SAUNDERS et al. 1997, 1999; TURRISI et al. 1999). In other tumour types, such as bladder cancer, no benefit from accelerated radiotherapy was observed (HORWICH et al. 2005). Today radiation oncologists are obliged to prescribe OTT as well as dose and number of fractions. It has become the standard of care in curative radiotherapy of tumour types with proven time factor to compensate for unplanned treatment breaks, e.g. because of machine breakdown or holidays.

16.3
Mechanisms Underlying the Time Factor

Repopulation of tumour stem cells during fractionated irradiation is considered to be the major underlying mechanism of increased treatment resistance with longer OTT. Mechanisms other than repopulation could theoretically contribute to or modulate the time factor (Table 16.1). However, systematic experiments did not reveal supportive evidence for alternative mechanisms

Table 16.1. Biological mechanisms other than repopulation which may result in an increase of radiation resistance of tumour stem cells during fractionated radiotherapy and thereby contribute to the time factor

Resistance factor	Possible underlying radiobiological mechanisms
Increased tumour hypoxia	Progressive destruction of the tumour vasculature by radiotherapy results in impaired oxygen supply and thereby in an increased radiobiological hypoxia
Selection of radioresistant clones	Subpopulations of radioresistant and rapidly proliferating clonogenic cells are selected during radiotherapy
Increased capacity to recover from sublethal damage	Clonogenic tumour cells adapt to the repeated radiation-induced damage/stress by an increased capacity to recover from sublethal damage
Accumulation in radioresistant phases of the cell cycle	During fractionated radiotherapy clonogenic cells stop to proliferate and are blocked at radioresistant phases of the cell cycle

of accelerated repopulation (PETERSEN et al. 2001, 2005; ZIPS et al. 2003). Each fraction of radiation inactivates a proportion of tumour stem cells, i.e. the population of tumour stem cells in a tumour is reduced (depopulation). A complete depopulation of tumour stem cells is the aim of curative radiotherapy. The desired therapeutic effect of depopulation is abrogated by the proliferation of surviving tumour stem cells during treatment. This process has been named repopulation. Assuming a linear relationship between tumour volume and the number of tumour stem cells in untreated tumours, the doubling time of tumour stem cells would be in the range of several weeks to months which could not explain the time factor observed in experimental and clinical studies. Findings from early experimental studies suggest that in some but not all tumour types the tumour stem cell doubling time after single-dose irradiation is shortened (HERMENS and BARENDSEN 1969; JUNG et al. 1990; STEPHENS et al. 1978), i.e. repopulation apparently accelerates in some tumour types after radiotherapy. The concept of accelerated repopulation stimulated a number of experimental and clinical studies to explore the kinetics and underlying mechanisms of accelerated repopulation during fractionated radiotherapy (BAUMANN et al. 2003).

16.4
Mechanisms of Accelerated Repopulation

The effective cell doubling time (*net doubling time*) is determined by the rate of cell production and cell loss (BEGG and STEEL 2002). Therefore, accelerated repopulation of tumour stem cells during radiotherapy could result from an increased production rate or reduced stem cell loss (Table 16.2). Methods to determine cell loss or cell production such as immunohistochemistry or flow cytometry are plagued by the fact that tumour stem cells are morphologically not distinguishable from non-tumour stem cells and represent only a very small fraction (about 1%) of all tumour cells (implications of the tumour stem cell concept for radiotherapy were recently reviewed in BAUMANN et al. 2008). Even major changes in the tumour stem cell compartment during acceleration of repopulation might be easily overlooked. Radiobiological methods (tumour control assay, excision assay) allow determination of tumour stem cell survival after irradiation in vivo (BAUMANN et al. 2008; KRAUSE et al. 2006; ZIPS et al. 2005). Local tumour control data obtained from fractionated irradiated experimental tumours have been used to estimate repopulation rates of tumour stem cells (HESSEL et al. 2003, 2004a, b; PETERSEN et al. 2001; THAMES et al. 1996). However, using local tumour control assays, it still remains challenging to dissect mechanisms underlying accelerated repopulation of tumour stem cells. Therefore, data from local tumour control assays, studies into normal tissue response during fractionated irradiation and non-stem cell assays (histology, flow cytometry, etc.) were considered to hypothesize concepts of accelerated repopulation (FOWLER 1991; TROTT and KUMMERMEHR 1991).

Table 16.2. Determinants of production and loss of tumour stem cells

Cell production	Cell loss
Growth fraction	Probability of self-maintenance
Cell cycle time	Necrotic/apoptotic cell death

16.4.1
Increased Cell Production Rate of Tumour Stem Cells During Fractionated Radiotherapy

Experimental and clinical data on normal epithelia suggest that acceleration of stem cell divisions might contribute to repopulation during fractionated irradiation (Dorr 1997). Modelling of cell kinetic data implies a shorting of the cell doubling time of surviving stem cells during fractionated irradiation from 3.5 to 1.4 days (Dorr and Kummermehr 1991). It has been speculated that in some tumours, e.g. well-differentiated squamous cell carcinomas, repopulation is reminiscent of the normal epithelium (Kummermehr et al. 1992; Trott and Kummermehr 1991). This seems to be supported by clinical data showing a more pronounced time factor of fractionated radiotherapy in well-differentiated primary tumours with high expression of epidermal growth factor receptor (EGFR, see below) than in less well differentiated primaries or lymph node metastases (Eriksen et al. 2004; Overgaard et al. 2003). Taking the experimental and clinical data together, it is conceptually possible that an increased production of tumour stem cells contributes to accelerated repopulation during fractionated radiotherapy.

16.4.2
Reduced Cell Loss of Tumour Stem Cells During Fractionated Radiotherapy

Applying the hierarchal structure of epithelial or haemopoietic normal tissues to malignant tumours, after each tumour stem cell division, the progeny either remain in the stem cell compartment or differentiate into a non-stem cell (Kummermehr and Trott 1997). As malignant tumours grow and the number of tumour stem cells increases with tumour volume (Baumann et al. 1990; Kummermehr and Trott 1997; Suit et al. 1965) the average probability for a tumour stem cell daughter to remain a tumour stem cell after cell division (average probability of self-maintenance) is higher than 50%. Assuming a tumour stem cell fraction of 1%, model calculations suggest that the average probability of tumour stem cell self-maintenance is 51–65%, i.e. the average probability of cell loss would equal 35–49% (Kummermehr and Trott 1997). Based on data obtained from normal epithelia (Dorr 1997) and from studies on tumour cell kinetics (Begg and Steel 2002) it has been proposed that during fractionated radiotherapy the loss of tumour stem cells decreases and more cells remain in the stem cell compartment, which would result in accelerated repopulation (Fowler 1991; Kum-

mermehr et al. 1992; Trott and Kummermehr 1991). As an alternative mechanism of reduced cell loss, down-regulation of radiation-induced apoptotic cell death has been suggested as an underlying mechanism of accelerated repopulation (Thames et al. 1996).

16.4.3
Tumour Microenvironment and Accelerated Repopulation of Tumour Stem Cells

The microenvironment of malignant tumours is characterized by hypoxia, high interstitial fluid pressure, glucose and energy deprivation, high lactate levels and extracellular acidosis (Vaupel 2004). These hostile conditions contribute to the high cell loss occurring spontaneously in tumours. Cell loss factors between 89% and 97% have been estimated for carcinomas (Begg and Steel 2002). Experimental and clinical data indicate that tumours reoxygenate during fractionated irradiation (Horsman and Overgaard 2002). Based on these observations it has been hypothesized that reoxygenation during fractionated radiotherapy reduces cell loss and subsequently shortens the net doubling time of tumour stem cells (Fowler 1991). Experimental data support the hypothesis of a causative relationship between reoxygenation, cell loss and repopulation of tumour stem cells (Hessel et al. 2003, 2004a, b; Petersen et al. 2001, 2003; Speke and Hill 1995a, b). However, improved tumour microenvironment might also lead to a higher cell production rate.

16.4.4
Molecular Regulation of Accelerated Repopulation

While changes in microenvironment appear to passively affect repopulation, it has been postulated that an active regulatory element is involved in triggering accelerated repopulation in tumours (Trott and Kummermehr 1991). This view is supported by similar repopulation kinetics in squamous cell carcinomas and normal epithelium where reoxygenation is unlikely to contribute to accelerated repopulation. The molecular background of the hypothesized regulatory element has been explored in experimental and clinical studies. Several studies indicate that signalling via EGFR appears to be involved in accelerated repopulation of tumour stem cells during fractionated radiotherapy (Bentzen et al. 2005; Eriksen et al. 2004, 2005; Krause et al. 2005; Petersen et al. 2003; Schmidt-Ullrich et al. 1997; Zips et al. 2008). Activated EGFR signalling results in multiple biological responses potentially relevant for accelerated repopulation, e.g. increased cell proliferation and reduced cell death by antiapoptotic signalling or by improved DNA repair (BAUMANN et al. 2007). However, EGFR expression and signalling might also be associated with the tumour microenvironment and reoxygenation during radiotherapy (KRAUSE et al. 2005; ZIPS et al. 2008).

16.5
Time Factor of Fractionated Radiotherapy Combined with Other Treatment Modalities

Curative radiotherapy is often given combined with chemotherapy, surgery and biological modifiers. Radiotherapy after surgery is given to sterilize residual tumour stem cells. While it is clear that during the gap between surgery and start of radiotherapy the remaining tumour stem cells might repopulate, it remains controversial for example in patients with head and neck cancer whether accelerated postoperative radiotherapy improves locoregional control (ANG et al. 2001; AWWAD et al. 1992, 2002; SANGUINETI et al. 2005; SUWINSKI et al. 2008). Experimental data on repopulation rates of microscopic and macroscopic tumours suggest that in the postoperative situation the time factor of fractionated radiotherapy might be less pronounced (BECK-BORNHOLDT et al. 1991; RAABE et al. 2000).

In a large variety of advanced carcinomas curative radiotherapy is combined with chemotherapy. Experimental observations and some clinical studies indicate that chemotherapy as a single modality can induce accelerated repopulation in tumours (reviewed in DAVIS and TANNOCK 2000; KIM and TANNOCK 2005). Induced repopulation by induction chemotherapy may possibly explain the inferior results of induction chemotherapy before radiotherapy compared with concurrent chemoradiation in patients with non-small cell lung cancer (FOURNEL et al. 2005; FURUSE et al. 1999; ZATLOUKAL et al. 2004).

The evidence of a time factor of concurrent chemoradiation remains a controversial issue. A randomized clinical trial in patients with limited disease small cell lung cancer (SCLC) treated with chemoradiation demonstrated a significantly higher local tumour control when OTT was reduced from 33 to 19 days (TURRISI et al. 1999). A meta-analysis of four randomized clinical trials in patients with limited disease SCLC revealed that OTT is the most important predictive factor for outcome after chemoradiation (DE RUYSSCHER et al. 2006). In contrast to the results of this meta-analysis,

no impact of prolonged OTT on local tumour control rates after conventional fractionated chemoradiation for limited disease SCLC has been reported by others (BOGART et al. 2008). A time factor has been also hypothesized for postoperative chemoradiation in rectal cancer (FIETKAU et al. 2007). Comparison of results from randomized clinical trials in head and neck cancer given with and without prolonged OTT supports the evidence of a significant time factor of chemoradiation (BUDACH et al. 2006). Experimental data on human squamous cell carcinoma indicates that concurrent chemotherapy inhibits tumour cell repopulation (BUDACH et al. 2002). Based on this observation it could be speculated that concurrent chemotherapy reduces the time factor of fractionated radiotherapy and thereby diminishes the benefit from accelerated radiotherapy. Taken together, most observations support the evidence of a time factor during chemoradiation. In contrast to radiotherapy alone, the underlying mechanisms of the time factor during chemoradiation are poorly understood. The clinical benefit of accelerated radiotherapy compared with conventional radiotherapy in the context of chemoradiation has been demonstrated in SCLC but requires further studies in other cancer types such as head and neck cancer.

Epidermal growth factor receptor inhibition in combination with fractionated radiotherapy in patients with head and neck cancer significantly improved locoregional tumour control and survival (BONNER et al. 2006). In experimental studies, inhibition of EGFR by monoclonal antibodies has been shown to inhibit accelerated repopulation during fractionated irradiation (KRAUSE et al. 2005). Results from a subgroup analysis of a randomized clinical trial suggest that radiotherapy with and without EGFR inhibition is more effective when radiotherapy was given within shorter OTT, i.e. as accelerated and hyperfractionated-accelerated radiotherapy (BONNER et al. 2006). Although it is impossible to conclude on biological mechanisms of interaction from a subgroup analysis of a clinical trial, it appears that tumours treated with radiotherapy and EGFR inhibitor exhibit a time factor.

16.6
Dose-Dense Chemotherapy

Increased dose density is achieved by reducing the interval between each dose of chemotherapy. The cumulative drug dose remains constant, but the same amount of drug is administered over a shorter period. Mathematical models of tumour growth have provided the basis for the clinical application of dose-dense chemotherapy (NORTON 2005). The Norton-Simon model suggests that increasing the dose density of chemotherapy will increase efficacy by minimizing the opportunity for re-growth of tumour cells between cycles of chemotherapy. In patients with breast cancer, Intergroup trial 9741, coordinated by the Cancer and Leukemia Group B (CALGB), tested the two hypotheses that dose-dense and sequential administration of chemotherapy regimens incorporating doxorubicin, cyclophosphamide and paclitaxel would improve disease-free survival and overall survival. A statistically significant 4-year disease-free survival advantage was detected for the two dose-dense regimens compared with the regimens administered every 3 weeks (CITRON et al. 2003; MCARTHUR and HUDIS 2007; ORZANO and SWAIN 2005). In patients with non-Hodgkin's lymphoma, this concept has also been shown to improve the clinical outcome (reviewed in BROUSSAIS-GUILLAUMOT and COIFFIER 2007; HELD et al. 2006), while disappointing results were reported from a trial that included 318 patients with better-prognosis SCLC treated with ifosfamide, carboplatin and etoposide (LORIGAN et al. 2005).

16.7
Conclusion

Prolongation of overall treatment time has an adverse effect on outcome after fractionated radiotherapy. Accelerated repopulation of tumour stem cells during therapy, as the most likely explanation of this so-called time factor, is an established mechanism of treatment resistance. Understanding the underlying mechanisms and molecular regulation of accelerated repopulation resulted in successful therapeutic interventions. However, further investigations into accelerated repopulation in the context of combined treatments and into the clinical benefits of dose-dense chemotherapy without irradiation are necessary.

Acknowledgement

This work is supported by the German Research Council (DFG Ba1433-5).

References

Ang KK, Trotti A, Brown BW, et al (2001) Randomized trial addressing risk features and time factors of surgery plus radiotherapy in advanced head-and-neck cancer. Int J Radiat Oncol Biol Phys 51:571–578

Awwad HK, Khafagy Y, Barsoum M, et al (1992) Accelerated versus conventional fractionation in the postoperative irradiation of locally advanced head and neck cancer: influence of tumour proliferation. Radiother Oncol 25:261–266

Awwad HK, Lotayef M, Shouman T, et al (2002) Accelerated hyperfractionation (AHF) compared to conventional fractionation (CF) in the postoperative radiotherapy of locally advanced head and neck cancer: influence of proliferation. Br J Cancer 86:517–523

Baumann M, Dubois W, Suit HD (1990) Response of human squamous cell carcinoma xenografts of different sizes to irradiation: relationship of clonogenic cells, cellular radiation sensitivity in vivo, and tumor rescuing units. Radiat Res 123:325–330

Baumann M, Liertz C, Baisch H, et al (1994) Impact of overall treatment time of fractionated irradiation on local control of human FaDu squamous cell carcinoma in nude mice. Radiother Oncol 32:137–143

Baumann M, Dorr W, Petersen C, et al (2003) Repopulation during fractionated radiotherapy: much has been learned, even more is open. Int J Radiat Biol 79:465–467

Baumann M, Krause M, Dikomey E, et al (2007) EGFR-targeted anti-cancer drugs in radiotherapy: preclinical evaluation of mechanisms. Radiother Oncol 83:238–248

Baumann M, Krause M, Hill R (2008) Exploring the role of cancer stem cells in radioresistance. Nat Rev Cancer 8:545–554

Beck-Bornholdt HP, Omniczynski M, Theis E, et al (1991) Influence of treatment time on the response of rat rhabdomyosarcoma R1H to fractionated irradiation. Acta Oncol 30:57–63

Begg AC, Steel GG (2002) Cell proliferation and growth rate of tumors. In: Steel GG (ed) Basic clinical radiobiology, 3rd edn. Arnold, London, pp 8–21

Bentzen SM, Atasoy BM, Daley FM, et al (2005) Epidermal growth factor receptor expression in pretreatment biopsies from head and neck squamous cell carcinoma as a predictive factor for a benefit from accelerated radiation therapy in a randomized controlled trial. J Clin Oncol 23:5560–5567

Bogart JA, Watson D, McClay EF, et al (2008) Interruptions of once-daily thoracic radiotherapy do not correlate with outcomes in limited stage small cell lung cancer: Analysis of CALGB phase III trial 9235. Lung Cancer epub

Bonner JA, Harari PM, Giralt J, et al (2006) Radiotherapy plus cetuximab for squamous-cell carcinoma of the head and neck. N Engl J Med 354:567–578

Bourhis J, Overgaard J, Audry H, et al (2006) Hyperfractionated or accelerated radiotherapy in head and neck cancer: a meta-analysis. Lancet 368:843–854

Broussais-Guillaumot F, Coiffier B (2007) Strategies for improving outcomes with 14-day anthracycline-based regimens in patients with aggressive lymphomas. Clin Lymphoma Myeloma 8(suppl 2):S50–S56

Budach W, Paulsen F, Welz S, et al (2002) Mitomycin C in combination with radiotherapy as a potent inhibitor of tumour cell repopulation in a human squamous cell carcinoma. Br J Cancer 86:470–476

Budach W, Hehr T, Budach V, et al (2006) A meta-analysis of hyperfractionated and accelerated radiotherapy and combined chemotherapy and radiotherapy regimens in unresected locally advanced squamous cell carcinoma of the head and neck. BMC Cancer 6:28

Citron ML, Berry DA, Cirrincione C, et al (2003) Randomized trial of dose-dense versus conventionally scheduled and sequential versus concurrent combination chemotherapy as postoperative adjuvant treatment of node-positive primary breast cancer: first report of Intergroup Trial C9741/Cancer and Leukemia Group B Trial 9741. J Clin Oncol 21:1431–1439

Davis AJ, Tannock JF (2000) Repopulation of tumour cells between cycles of chemotherapy: a neglected factor. Lancet Oncol 1:86–93

De Ruysscher D, Pijls-Johannesma M, Bentzen SM, et al (2006) Time between the first day of chemotherapy and the last day of chest radiation is the most important predictor of survival in limited-disease small-cell lung cancer. J Clin Oncol 24:1057–1063

Dorr W (1997) Three A's of repopulation during fractionated irradiation of squamous epithelia: Asymmetry loss, Acceleration of stem-cell divisions and Abortive divisions. Int J Radiat Biol 72:635–643

Dorr W, Kummermehr J (1991) Proliferation kinetics of mouse tongue epithelium under normal conditions and following single dose irradiation. Virchows Arch B Cell Pathol Incl Mol Pathol 60:287–294

Eriksen JG, Steiniche T, Askaa J, et al (2004) The prognostic value of epidermal growth factor receptor is related to tumor differentiation and the overall treatment time of radiotherapy in squamous cell carcinomas of the head and neck. Int J Radiat Oncol Biol Phys 58:561–566

Eriksen JG, Steiniche T, Overgaard J (2005) The influence of epidermal growth factor receptor and tumor differentiation on the response to accelerated radiotherapy of squamous cell carcinomas of the head and neck in the randomized DAHANCA 6 and 7 study. Radiother Oncol 74:93–100

Fietkau R, Rodel C, Hohenberger W, et al (2007) Rectal cancer delivery of radiotherapy in adequate time and with adequate dose is influenced by treatment center, treatment schedule, and gender and is prognostic parameter for local control: results of study CAO/ARO/AIO-94. Int J Radiat Oncol Biol Phys 67:1008–1019

Fournel P, Robinet G, Thomas P, et al (2005) Randomized phase III trial of sequential chemoradiotherapy compared with concurrent chemoradiotherapy in locally advanced non-small-cell lung cancer: Groupe Lyon-Saint-Etienne d'Oncologie Thoracique-Groupe Francais de Pneumo-Cancerologie NPC 95-01 Study. J Clin Oncol 23:5910–5917

Fowler JF (1991) Rapid repopulation in radiotherapy: a debate on mechanism. The phantom of tumor treatment—continually rapid proliferation unmasked. Radiother Oncol 22:156–158

Furuse K, Fukuoka M, Kawahara M, et al (1999) Phase III study of concurrent versus sequential thoracic radiotherapy in combination with mitomycin, vindesine, and cisplatin in unresectable stage III non-small-cell lung cancer. J Clin Oncol 17:2692–2699

Held G, Schubert J, Reiser M, et al (2006) Dose-intensified treatment of advanced-stage diffuse large B-cell lymphomas. Semin Hematol 43:221–229

Hermens AF, Barendsen GW (1969) Changes of cell proliferation characteristics in a rat rhabdomyosarcoma before and after x-irradiation. Eur J Cancer 5:173–189

Hessel F, Petersen C, Zips D, et al (2003) Impact of increased cell loss on the repopulation rate during fractionated irradiation in human FaDu squamous cell carcinoma growing in nude mice. Int J Radiat Biol 79:479–486

Hessel F, Krause M, Helm A, et al (2004a) Differentiation status of human squamous cell carcinoma xenografts does not appear to correlate with the repopulation capacity of clonogenic tumour cells during fractionated irradiation. Int J Radiat Biol 80:719–727

Hessel F, Krause M, Petersen C, et al (2004b) Repopulation of moderately well-differentiated and keratinizing GL human squamous cell carcinomas growing in nude mice. Int J Radiat Oncol Biol Phys 58:510–518

Horsman M, Overgaard J (2002) The oxygen effect and tumour microenvironment. In: Steel GG (ed) Basic clinical radiobiology, 3rd edn. Arnold, London, pp 158–168

Horwich A, Dearnaley D, Huddart R, et al (2005) A randomised trial of accelerated radiotherapy for localised invasive bladder cancer. Radiother Oncol 75:34–43

Jung H, Kruger HJ, Brammer I, et al (1990) Cell population kinetics of the rhabdomyosarcoma R1H of the rat after single doses of X-rays. Int J Radiat Biol 57:567–589

Kim JJ, Tannock IF (2005) Repopulation of cancer cells during therapy: an important cause of treatment failure. Nat Rev Cancer 5:516–525

Krause M, Ostermann G, Petersen C, et al (2005) Decreased repopulation as well as increased reoxygenation contribute to the improvement in local control after targeting of the EGFR by C225 during fractionated irradiation. Radiother Oncol 76:162–167

Krause M, Zips D, Thames HD, et al (2006) Preclinical evaluation of molecular-targeted anticancer agents for radiotherapy. Radiother Oncol 80:112–122

Kummermehr J, Trott KR (1997) Tumour stem cells. In: Potten CS (ed) Stem cells. Academic, London, pp 363–399

Kummermehr J, Dorr W, Trott KR (1992) Kinetics of accelerated repopulation in normal and malignant squamous epithelia during fractionated radiotherapy. BJR Suppl 24:193–199

Lorigan P, Woll PJ, O'Brien ME, et al (2005) Randomized phase III trial of dose-dense chemotherapy supported by whole-blood hematopoietic progenitors in better-prognosis small-cell lung cancer. J Natl Cancer Inst 97:666–674

McArthur HL, Hudis CA (2007) Dose-dense therapy in the treatment of early-stage breast cancer: an overview of the data. Clin Breast Cancer 8(suppl 1):S6–S10

Norton L (2005) Conceptual and practical implications of breast tissue geometry: toward a more effective, less toxic therapy. Oncologist 10:370–381

Orzano JA, Swain SM (2005) Concepts and clinical trials of dose-dense chemotherapy for breast cancer. Clin Breast Cancer 6:402–411

Overgaard J, Hansen HS, Specht L, et al (2003) Five compared with six fractions per week of conventional radiotherapy of squamous-cell carcinoma of head and neck: DAHANCA 6 and 7 randomised controlled trial. Lancet 362:933–940

Petersen C, Zips D, Krause M, et al (2001) Repopulation of FaDu human squamous cell carcinoma during fractionated radiotherapy correlates with reoxygenation. Int J Radiat Oncol Biol Phys 51:483–493

Petersen C, Eicheler W, Frommel A, et al (2003) Proliferation and micromilieu during fractionated irradiation of human FaDu squamous cell carcinoma in nude mice. Int J Radiat Biol 79:469–477

Petersen C, Zips D, Krause M, et al (2005) Recovery from sublethal damage during fractionated irradiation of human FaDu SCC. Radiother Oncol 74:331–336

Raabe A, Eickholter S, Zieron J, et al (2000) Influence of dose per fraction and overall treatment time on the response of pulmonary micrometastases of the R1H-tumour to fractionated irradiation. Radiother Oncol 56:259–264

Sanguineti G, Richetti A, Bignardi M, et al (2005) Accelerated versus conventional fractionated postoperative radiotherapy for advanced head and neck cancer: results of a multicenter phase III study. Int J Radiat Oncol Biol Phys 61:762–771

Saunders M, Dische S, Barrett A, et al (1997) Continuous hyperfractionated accelerated radiotherapy (CHART) versus conventional radiotherapy in non-small-cell lung cancer: a randomised multicentre trial. CHART Steering Committee. Lancet 350:161–165

Saunders M, Dische S, Barrett A, et al (1999) Continuous, hyperfractionated, accelerated radiotherapy (CHART) versus conventional radiotherapy in non-small cell lung cancer: mature data from the randomised multicentre trial. CHART Steering committee. Radiother Oncol 52:137–148

Schmidt-Ullrich RK, Mikkelsen RB, Dent P, et al (1997) Radiation-induced proliferation of the human A431 squamous carcinoma cells is dependent on EGFR tyrosine phosphorylation. Oncogene 15:1191–1197

Speke AK, Hill RP (1995a) Repopulation kinetics during fractionated irradiation and the relationship to the potential doubling time, Tpot. Int J Radiat Oncol Biol Phys 31:847–856

Speke AK, Hill RP (1995b) The effects of clamping and reoxygenation on repopulation during fractionated irradiation. Int J Radiat Oncol Biol Phys 31:857–863

Stephens TC, Currie GA, Peacock JH (1978) Repopulation of gamma-irradiated Lewis lung carcinoma by malignant cells and host macrophage progenitors. Br J Cancer 38:573–582

Suit H, Shalek RJ, Wette R (1965) Radiation response of C3H mouse mammary carcinoma evaluated in terms of cellular radiation sensitivity. In: Shalek RJ (ed) Cellular radiation biology. Williams and Wilkins, Baltimore

Suit HD, Howes AE, Hunter N (1977) Dependence of response of a C3H mammary carcinoma to fractionated irradiation on fractionation number and intertreatment interval. Radiat Res 72:440–454

Suwinski R, Bankowska-Wozniak M, Majewski W, et al (2008) Randomized clinical trial on 7-days-a-week postoperative radiotherapy for high-risk squamous cell head and neck cancer. Radiother Oncol 87:155–163

Thames HD, Ruifrok AC, Milas L, et al (1996) Accelerated repopulation during fractionated irradiation of a murine ovarian carcinoma: downregulation of apoptosis as a possible mechanism. Int J Radiat Oncol Biol Phys 35:951–962

Trott KR, Kummermehr J (1991) Rapid repopulation in radiotherapy: a debate on mechanism. Accelerated repopulation in tumours and normal tissues. Radiother Oncol 22:159–160

Turrisi AT 3rd, Kim K, Blum R, et al (1999) Twice-daily compared with once-daily thoracic radiotherapy in limited small-cell lung cancer treated concurrently with cisplatin and etoposide. N Engl J Med 340:265–271

Vaupel P (2004) Tumor microenvironmental physiology and its implications for radiation oncology. Semin Radiat Oncol 14:198–206

Withers HR, Taylor JM, Maciejewski B (1988) The hazard of accelerated tumor clonogen repopulation during radiotherapy. Acta Oncol 27:131–146

Zatloukal P, Petruzelka L, Zemanova M, et al (2004) Concurrent versus sequential chemoradiotherapy with cisplatin and vinorelbine in locally advanced non-small cell lung cancer: a randomized study. Lung Cancer 46:87–98

Zips D, Petersen C, Junghanns S, et al (2003) Selection of genetically distinct, rapidly proliferating clones does not contribute to repopulation during fractionated irradiation in FaDu squamous cell carcinoma. Radiat Res 160:257–262

Zips D, Thames HD, Baumann M (2005) New anticancer agents: in vitro and in vivo evaluation. In Vivo 19:1–7

Zips D, Krause M, Yaromina A, et al (2008) Epidermal growth factor receptor inhibitors for radiotherapy: biological rationale and preclinical results. J Pharm Pharmacol 60:1019–1028

Molecular Tools, Expression Profiling

Angela M. Kaindl and Konrad Oexle

CONTENTS

A. M. Kaindl, MD
Klinik für Pädiatrie m. S. Neurologie, Charité – Universitäts-
medizin Berlin, Campus Virchow-Klinikum, Augustenburger
Platz 1, 13353 Berlin, Germany
and
Laboratoire de Neurologie du Développement, UMR 676
Inserm-Paris 7 & Service de Neuropédiatrie, Hôpital Robert
Debré, 48 Blvd. Serurier, 75019 Paris, France

K. Oexle, MD
Institut für Humangenetik, Klinikum Rechts der Isar,
Technische Universität München, Trogerstraße 32, 81675
München, Germany

KEY POINTS

- High-throughput technologies in genomics, epigenomics, transcriptomics, proteomics, and metabolomics may detect specific variation patterns and help to optimize individual medical decisions.
- Transcriptomics and proteomics quantify a large number of RNA and protein species, respectively, by using quantitative hybridization onto chips (microarrays) or signature sequencing of RNA and two-dimensional electrophoresis, mass spectrometry, or antibody array binding of proteins.
- High-throughput analyses are subject to problems of noise and multiple testing and involve the necessity to select reliable, informative, and biologically reasonable subsets.
- In the field of breast cancer, RNA expression profiles have been derived that achieve similar sensitivity but are more specific than are conventional algorithms in predicting distant metastasis, that is, less error-prone in recommending adjuvant systemic therapy.
- Meta-analysis of different prognostic RNA signatures revealed that genes associated with cell proliferation provide the driving force in all of them.
- While proteomics potentially oversees a larger space of expression variation than transcriptomics, proteomic profiling beyond the testing of individual markers has not yet been transferred successfully to the field of breast cancer.

Abstract

High-throughput technologies of modern biology provide "molecular portraits" of tissues and have entered the field of oncology. In the present chapter, we describe tools of high-throughput expression analysis in transcriptomics and proteomics, with an emphasis on microarrays, two-dimensional electrophoresis, and mass spectrometry. Options and limitations in data production, extraction, and interpretation are outlined. Problems of sensitivity, specificity, multiple testing, and noise are discussed. As a concrete example, we review the application of these tools to the field of breast cancer, where expression analyses already contribute to individual treatment decisions.

17.1
Introduction

Therapeutic algorithms in oncology depend on various clinical and pathologic parameters that provide information about the risk of disease recurrence and likelihood of response to specific treatment options. However, the predictive power of these parameters is still limited. Expression profiling offers a possibility to further classify tumor subtypes; to improve the prediction of survival, disease recurrence, and efficiency of therapeutic regimen; and to recognize more precisely the necessity of systemic and aggressive treatment in individual patients (Fig 17.1). Beyond refined disease subtyping and individualized treatment decision, it may provide molecular understanding of the disease and novel targets for therapy. Expression profiling may thus become relevant in all sections of oncology. This includes radiation oncology, e.g., the study of the radiation response of tumors and of normal tissues and the development of biomarkers that predict local disease control and toxicity after radiotherapy (NUYTEN et al. 2006).

From a methodological point of view, expression profiling belongs to a group of new high-throughput technologies that provide molecular portraits of cells and tissues (PEROU et al. 2000; SOTIRIOU and PICCART 2007). Such portraits can include data on genomic individuality, i.e., on DNA polymorphisms, mutations, copy number variations (*genomics*), and epigenetic modifications (*epigenomics*), as well as genome-wide quantitative data on gene expression at a specific point in time and under specific environmental circumstances (Fig. 17.2). Expression may be assessed in terms of *transcriptomics*, *proteomics*, or *metabolomics* by quantifying a large, if not exhaustive set of transcripts, proteins, or metabolites, respectively. RNA microarray expression studies look at responses on the transcript level. Thus, this methodical approach does not portrait alternative splicing or co- and posttranslational modifications. Proteomics, which encompasses an analysis of protein populations encoded by single genes, may offer further information at that level.

In this chapter, we review molecular tools of expression profiling that can be assigned to the field of *transcriptomics* and *proteomics*. We describe current techniques applied in these two research fields and, as an example, discuss advances that have been made or can be expected by their application to the field of breast cancer, the most frequently diagnosed cancer in women in Western countries (MILLER et al. 2006; SOTIRIOU and PICCART 2007).

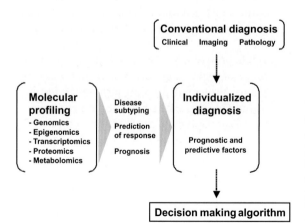

Fig 17.1. Prospect of an individualized therapy in oncology by the use of molecular profiles. Therapy of malignant tumors depends on clinical and pathological data such as tumor size, lymph node invasion, and distant metastasis. However, patients with similar clinicopathological features may have markedly different outcomes. Both the response of the tumor and that of normal tissue may vary substantially. Molecular profiling offers a possibility to further classify tumor subtypes, to improve the prediction of individual patient outcome, and to select the optimal therapeutic regimen

Genomics addresses the set of all genes (the "genome"). The field includes the elucidation of the entire DNA sequence of various organisms and the mapping of phenotypes (that may reveal pleiotropic effects and epistatic interactions of gene loci). In medicine, genomics serves to attribute disease features to common or rare variants with weak or strong effects, respectively. Variants may involve single genes only, submicroscopic copy number changes of chromosomal domains, or visible rearrangements. Microscopic analysis of chromosomes was the first form of genomics that achieved considerable relevance in all parts of genetics including tumor cytogenetics.

Epigenomics is the study of heritable modifications (marks) other than those in the DNA sequence that regulate gene expression, silence the activity of transposable elements, and stabilize adjustments of gene dosage as seen in X-chromosome inactivation and genomic imprinting. Epigenomics encompasses two major modifications of DNA and chromatin: DNA methylation and posttranslational histone modification.

Transcriptomics is the global study of gene expression at the RNA level. Generally, the transcriptome implies the set of all messenger RNA (mRNA) molecules, or "transcripts", produced in one or a population of cells. However, RNA-"omics" may also address the set of all microRNAs, transcripts that have regulative functions but are not translated into proteins.

Proteomics is the study of the entire spectrum of proteins (including co- and posttranslational modifications) of a cell, a tissue, or an organism.

Metabolomics is the study of the entire metabolic content of a cell, a tissue, or an organism addressing quantitatively the set of usually small molecules that are educts, intermediates, or products of metabolic pathways.

Interactomics is the study of interactions among proteins and other molecules within a cell by applying methods of biology, informatics, and engineering.

Fig. 17.2. Different forms of "-omics"

17.2
Transcriptomics

17.2.1
Data Production

Several methods are available to monitor transcription levels of tens of thousands of genes rapidly and simultaneously. The quantification of RNA species by sequence-specific annealing (hybridization) to complementary DNA probes arrayed on a substrate (microarray) was developed by SCHENA et al. (1995). Sample RNA was submitted to reverse transcription and fluorescent labeling. Thereby, a quantitative parameter was produced that could be measured as a localized signal after hybridization to the arrayed sensors. Comparison by competitive hybridization of two RNA samples labeled with two different dyes (Cy3 and Cy5) resulted in expression ratios of the two sources (e.g., of tumor and nontumor tissue). Whereas sensors were originally taken from libraries of DNA clones (cDNA), present-day microar-

ray technology prefers synthetic oligonucleotides, i.e., oligomers of single-stranded DNA. Oligonucleotides are designed *in silico* and can be synthesized *in situ* by a combinatorial sequence of photolithographic steps applied to the nascent microarray (Fig. 17.3; PEASE et al. 1994; HARDIMAN 2004).

Array technologies rely on representational labeling of the source RNA with reverse transcription and production of labeled or tagged molecules. This process may be coupled with a PCR amplification step. Arrays of oligonucleotides involve either the two-label scheme that results in ratios between two samples or a single-label method that attributes intensities to the RNA targets of a single source. In the two-label scheme, labels may be exchanged (dye swap) in order to neutralize artifacts associated with one of the dyes.

In most types of microarrays, the identity of a sensor is specified by its location and referenced *ex ante* by its Cartesian coordinates (Fig. 17.4). Alternatively, a sensor's identity may be referenced by an optical bar code or an address sequence. The array positions of the sensors may then be chosen randomly and identified

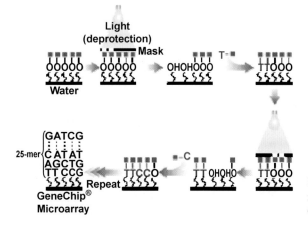

Fig. 17.3. Photolithographic in situ synthesis of an oligo-nucleotide microarray (courtesy of Affymetrix, Santa Clara, California)

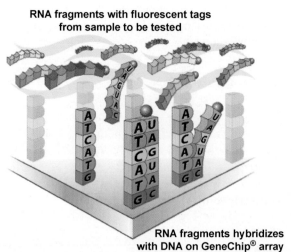

1.28 cm

1.28 cm

Actual size of GeneChip® array

Millons of DNA strands built up in each location

6.5 million locations on each GeneChip® array

Actual strand = 25 base pairs

RNA fragments with fluorescent tags from sample to be tested

RNA fragments hybridizes with DNA on GeneChip® array

Fig. 17.4. Design and function of a microarray expression chip. DNA oligonucleotides act as sensors. Sensors of the same sequence reside at one location. The hybridization intensity at this location depends on the concentration of complementary RNA in the sample. Quantification is achieved by laser-induced fluorescence of the label (courtesy of Affymetrix, Santa Clara, California)

ex post (STEEMERS et al. 2000). This method is used in bead technology, which allows for further miniaturization of the arrays.

Other methods of RNA monitoring exist that, in contrast to array techniques, are not based on quantitative hybridization. In serial analysis of gene expression ([SAGE] VELCULESCU et al. 1995), RNA fragments derived from a sample to be analyzed are ligated and cloned in a vector, which is then sequenced. The number of stretches in the vector sequence that belong to the same RNA species indicates the concentration of this RNA in the original sample. In massively parallel signature sequencing (MPSS), the relative amount of each RNA species in a sample is determined by mass sequencing of reversely transcribed DNA and subsequent counting of identical sequencing data.

17.2.2
Data Extraction

All methods of gene expression monitoring are subject to biological variability and experimental noise. Biological variability is due to endogenous, environmental, periodic, and stochastic causes. While factors such as daytime and feeding status may be controllable, others cannot be predicted. In the plant model *Arabidopsis*, for instance, touching has been shown to induce significant changes in gene expression (CHOTIKACHAROENSUK et al. 2006). In general, biological variability is reduced by randomization and replication. Replication of sampling may be more important than repeating the examination of a sample (BREITLING 2006). However, experimental noise has to be controlled as well. This can be achieved by a variance stabilization procedure such as log-transformation (Fig. 17.5).

RNA arrays need to be normalized since the distribution of the expression signal varies from array to array. Most simply, each signal y of an array a is replaced by a z-score with $z = (y - \mu_a)/\sigma_a$. Thereafter, all arrays have mean $\mu = 0$ and variance $\sigma^2 = 1$. Expression data of individual genes then can be compared across arrays. In many studies (e.g., STRANGER et al. 2005), section-wise normalization (quantile normalization) is performed, as the signal distribution of an array may be affected by skewness or other distortions. The method is motivated by the idea that two data vectors have the same distribution if the quantile–quantile plot is a straight diagonal line. The extension from two to n dimensions (i.e., arrays) is straightforward. BOLSTAD et al. (2003) provided a stepwise description of quantile normalization with standard spreadsheet software:

1. Given n arrays of p sensors (gene probes), form a spreadsheet X of dimension $p \times n$, where each array is a column.
2. Sort each column of X to give X_{sort}.
3. Take the means across rows of X_{sort} and assign this mean to each element in the row to get X^*_{sort}.
4. Get $X_{normalized}$ by rearranging each column of X^*_{sort} to have the same ordering as original X.

After normalization, individual replicates are averaged for each probe resulting in an expression data for each gene in each individual. However, the results have to be regarded cautiously. Thus, for instance, the normalized expression of the testis determining factor (SRY) in lymphoblastoid cells of the CEU and YRI parental HapMap samples (March 2007 release, www.sanger.ac.uk/humgen/genevar/) seems to be higher in women than in men (6.02 ± 0.05 versus 6.00 ± 0.07, $p = 0.03$, two-sided t-test). Of course, this is an artifact revealing that normalized expression levels of 6.02 do not indicate significant expression in this setting. For significance analysis of expression data, t-tests or rank products may be used (BREITLING et al. 2004). The seeming significance of the above example highlights the problem of multiple

---

Analysis of oligonucleotide-based microarray data revealed Poisson-like noise of gene expression data for a large range of expression levels (TU et al. 2002). This noise was mainly related to the hybridization process. Poisson noise occurs in signals that come about by a sequence of independent probabilistic events (Poisson process). The variance of such signals, i.e., the average squared distance from the mean, equals the mean signal intensity, $\sigma^2 = \mu$, and increases proportionally. Log-transformation of the data, $y(x) = \log(x)$, results in variance stabilization at higher expression levels. This is related to the property of the logarithm to compress distance with increasing number. Approximating y in the region surrounding μ_x by a Taylor expansion, $y(x) \approx \log(\mu_x) + \log'(\mu_x)(x - \mu_x) + ...$, with $\log'(\mu_x) = 1/\mu_x$, yields a rough estimate $\mu_y \approx \log(\mu_x)$ of the expectation (i.e., mean) of y if the zero-order approximation is used. The variance, i.e.,

the expectation of $(y - \mu_x)^2$ is then derived from the first-order approximation as $\sigma^2_y \approx \sigma^2_x/\mu^2_x$. In the case of a Poisson process where $\sigma^2_x = \mu_x$ logarithmic transformation thus results in a variance $\sigma^2_y \approx 1/\exp(\mu_y)$ that declines with increasing signal intensity. However, this "noise stabilization" is not effective at low expression levels. In the case of a Poisson process, for instance, the variance of the log-transformed signal becomes larger than the mean signal intensity μ_y if the latter is less than 0.57. Different methods of variance stabilization at low levels have been devised. As a most simple procedure started-log transformation has been recommended, i.e., $y = \log(x + b)$, which, in case of a Poisson process, implies an upper variance limit of about $1/(2b)$. Forgoing subtraction of the background from the raw signal may already have the desired effect of noise stabilization in the low expression range (BREITLING 2006).

Fig. 17.5. Variance stabilization

testing that occurs in all epidemiological investigations that run a large number of parameters on the same set of probands. In a microarray study that measures the expression of 30,000 genes, about 1,500 spurious results are to be expected purely due to chance if the "usual" significance level of $\alpha = 1/20 = 0.05$ is not corrected for multiple testing.

The classical *Bonferroni* correction divides the significance level acceptable for a single test ($p < \alpha$) by the number n of the tests in the multiplex assay ($p_i < \alpha/n$). This correction is too conservative, however, and implies an unnecessary decline of power. The *Simes* procedure is less conservative. It controls the false discovery rate (FDR), i.e., the expected fraction of false-positive results among all positive results (BENJAMINI and HOCHBERG 1995). After listing the n tests in an ascending order according to their p-values, the position with the largest k is identified which satisfies $p_k/k < \alpha/n$ and all tests up to this position are declared to be positive. Thus, the observed distribution of the p-values is taken into account. Multiple tests may be correlated; in case of

negative correlations, the limit of the *Simes* procedure can be relaxed even more. Permutation, e.g., random redistribution of proband labels, is another powerful method to control the probability of false-positive results as given by the actual data distributions and test correlations. For that purpose, each unadjusted p-value of the multiplex assay is replaced by the fraction (i.e., relative frequency) of random permutations that, by chance, produced smaller minimal p-values (WESTFALL and YOUNG 1993). The necessary number of permutations depends on the smallest p-value to be adjusted and may thus imply considerable computation time.

17.2.3
Data Interpretation

Results that are likely to be true positive still need to be interpreted (BREITLING 2006; SOTIRIOU and PICCART 2007). This is the expression-profiling step and involves dimensionality reduction of the large number of posi-

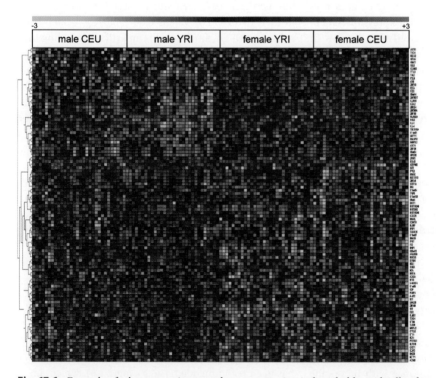

Fig. 17.6. Example of a heat map. Autosomal gene expression in lymphoblastoid cells of 2×60 men and women of African (*YRI*) and European (*CEU*) origin as listed in the Hap-Map gene variation project (log transformed and normalized across all samples; ftp.sanger. ac.uk/pub/genevar). 98 RefSeq-annotated genes (*right panel*) revealed a sex-dependent difference at a significance level of $p < 0.002$. Their average expression ranged from 5.7 to 12.0, with 8 genes not surpassing the average SRY expression in females, indicating substantial artifacts (see text). The heat map shows z-scores, i.e., deviations from the mean in standard deviation (SD) units. Hierarchical clustering of the 98 genes (complete linkage, Genesis®; *left panel*) recapitulates the sex difference

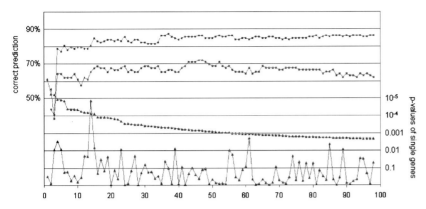

Fig. 17.7. Example of a predictive classifier. The autosomal genes shown in Fig. 17.6 were listed according to their significance level (*blue triangles*). Beginning with expression data (*z*-scores) of the two most significant genes a sex classifier (*blue squares*) was derived from the combined sample of 120 men and women (*CEU-YRI*) by a leave-one-out procedure: The gene expressions in each single individual were compared to the averages in the two groups of the remaining 59 or 60 men and women (Pearson coefficient of correlation between individual and average gene expressions). If the correlation with the group of the same sex was superior, then the prediction was counted as correct. The classifier reached a plateau after the top 40–50 genes had been included. Classification based on male and female averages in the CEU-YRI sample also worked in a sample of 90 Asian men and women (*CHN-JPN*) with a maximal predictive power of 70% (*brown squares*), that is, well above random prediction. However, only for a small number of genes the sex difference was replicated in the Asian sample (*brown triangles*). Technical artifacts, ethnical confounders, and random effects in multiple testing schemes have to be considered

tive results. Profiling may be *supervised*, that is, directed by a known grouping of the samples (e.g., probands versus control). In a "leave-one-out" procedure, an optimal set of genes may thus be selected that classifies correctly the largest number of left-out probands and controls (Figs. 17.6, 17.7). In *unsupervised* profiling, that is, grouping of similar expression patterns in a dataset without using any outside information, cluster analysis is the standard method. Clustering demands a measure of distance such as the correlation coefficient, for instance. Simple hierarchical clustering may proceed in an agglomerative way: Recursively, individuals and/or clusters with the smallest distance, i.e., highest correlation of gene expression, are united into a new cluster until a top cluster is formed that contains all individuals. Vice versa, genes may be clustered according to the correlation of their expression across probands. The following pitfall frequently occurs if clustering is applied in supervised analyses: if an outcome-related selection of genes is spurious, then a claim of correlation between clusters and clinical outcome is also spurious if the clustering is based on the expression of these genes (DUPUY and SIMON 2007).

Knowledge-driven dimensionality reduction according to the biological annotation of genes may be done before or after significance analysis, clustering, or classifier extraction. If it is done before, e.g., by focusing on a subset of genes only, it may help to uncover subtle effects that might remain insignificant otherwise. If it is done afterwards, e.g., by comparison with gene ontology databases (SMITH et al. 2007), it may help to recognize biological processes and to evaluate clusters or classifiers. Further conceptual integration may involve annealing with genome data and other "-omics" results, cross-species comparison, and network approach in terms of systems biology.

17.3
Proteomics

In the following, we review basic principles of proteomics as well as methods currently applied in this field and discuss the application of proteomic strategies in cancer research. The term *proteome*, a linguistic equivalent to the term *genome*, refers to the entire protein content encoded in the genome of a cell, a tissue, or an organism. In comparison to the genome that is believed to be similar in different cell types, the proteome of an or-

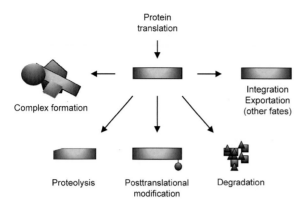

Fig. 17.8. Possible fates of proteins in the cell. The proteome is not stable, as there is constant turnover of proteins with a changing dynamic that depends on environmental and developmental conditions

ganism is a dynamic system that is constantly subject to changes. Protein composition changes from cell type to cell type, within subcellular compartments and between different stages of development and thus represents the functional status of a biological compartment (Fig. 17.8). Proteome research (proteomics) can be defined as the large-scale characterization of proteins expressed by the genome. Unlike the study of a single protein or pathway, proteomic methods enable a systematic overview of expressed protein profiles. An advantage of proteomics over transcriptomics is the ability to study posttranslational modifications. There is limited value, for example, in measuring signal transduction processes at the mRNA levels if they are characterized by protein phosphorylation or acetylation. Moreover, there are several genes with little correlation between RNA and protein expression levels.

Proteomics employs protein electrophoresis, mass spectrometry, and microarrays for the detection, identification, and characterization of proteins. These proteomic tools have their own individual advantages and limitations affecting their ability to assess the protein profile. Currently, the identification and characterization of all proteins in a given sample through high-resolution two-dimensional gel electrophoresis (2-DE) and subsequent analysis with mass spectrometry (MS) are expensive and time-consuming and, thus, not yet amenable to day-to-day use in the clinical setting. Routine approaches for obtaining protein data include enzyme-linked immunosorbent assay (ELISA) and immunohistochemistry. MS techniques have matured rapidly in recent years, due to the invention of two ionization techniques, electrospray ionization (ESI) and matrix-assisted laser desorption/ionization (MALDI). Protein arrays are being developed involving up to a few hundred antibodies or based on surface enhanced laser desorption/ionization (SELDI) for a wider coverage of the proteome.

Protein profiles could ultimately improve the diagnosis, prognosis, and management of patients by indicating protein markers of disease similar to the tumor markers already available (Healy et al. 2007), revealing the protein interactions affecting overall tumor progression, and identifying individual cancer profiles which are suitable for tailored chemotherapeutic strategies (Banks and Selby 2003; Alessandro et al. 2005).

In 2001, the Human Proteome Organization (HUPO) was launched. For information on international collaborations and training courses in proteomics, we refer to their webpage: http://www.hupo.org.

17.3.1
2-DE

2-DE, first introduced independently by Klose (1975) and O'Farrell (1975), still represents the most powerful tool for separating complex protein mixtures when combined with staining procedures and mass spectrometry (Fig. 17.8). The principle of 2-DE is to separate proteins according to the two parameters isoelectric point (pI; pH value at which the net charge on a protein is zero) and molecular weight. For this, it combines isoelectric focusing (IEF) in a polyacrylamide gel that has a pH gradient in the first dimension with a separation of proteins on a SDS polyacrylamide gel in the second dimension. After silver staining, protein spots in protein patterns of individual samples are compared among different 2-DE gels. The power of 2-DE lies in its high resolution of up to 10,000 proteins per sample and its ability to detect simultaneously vast amounts of proteins and to visualize co- and posttranslational modifications. Thereby, for instance, disease-associated proteins can be elucidated through subtractive analyses comparing disease with control protein patterns. At the stage of

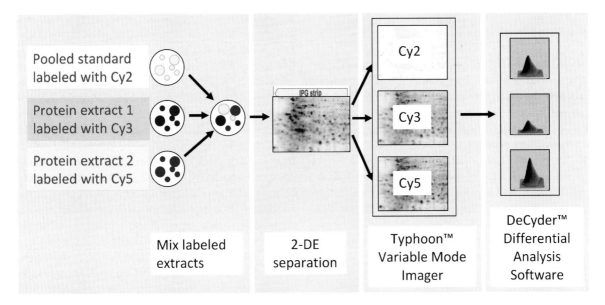

Fig. 17.9. Workflow for a standard two-dimensional difference gel electrophoresis (DIGE) experiment. After being labeling separately with different dyes, individual samples can be compared on a single gel. Thereby, experimental variation is reduced and spot matching is improved. Using an internal standard, i.e., a pool of all the samples within an experiment, each protein's abundances in different samples can be normalized and compared across different gels. Hence, the number of samples included in an experiment is not limited. Gels are imaged and analyzed quantitatively in order to identify protein differences among different samples (courtesy of GE Healthcare Life Sciences Little Chalfont, UK)

subtractive analysis, the approach has the potential to unravel complex networks of protein interactions. Individual stained protein spots can be digested into peptides, which can be analyzed by mass spectrometry and subsequent protein database searches. However, 2-DE in its current form has a number of serious disadvantages such as its lack of real high-throughput capability, for resolving hydrophobic and very low as well as very high molecular weight proteins.

Two-dimensional difference gel electrophoresis (DIGE) strengthened the 2-DE platform by allowing the detection and quantification of differences between three samples resolved on the same gel, or across multiple gels, when linked by an internal standard (Fig. 17.9; Issaq and Veenstra 2007). Samples (and standard) are labeled separately and then mixed to allow resolution on a single gel. This minimizes experimental variation and improves spot matching. Differentiation and comparison of samples is possible since they are labeled with different dyes (limited lysine labeling with DIGE Fluor Cy2, Cy3, and Cy5). The standard, a pool of all the samples within an experiment, enables normalizing the relative abundance of each protein and comparing abundances across different gels and sets of more than three samples. Protein detection levels span the linear

range of 0.125 ng to 10 μg. Image analysis with appropriate software allows for the identification of differences in protein abundance.

In classic 2-DE and DIGE approaches, highly alkaline and highly hydrophobic proteins are underrepresented since (1) in aqueous media, proteins have a minimum of solubility at their isoelectric point, may therefore precipitate there, and subsequently do not migrate into the SDS-PAGE gel; (2) hydrophobic proteins generally do not transfer easily from the first to the second dimension; and (3) non-ionic and zwitterionic detergents commonly used for isoelectric focusing have a lower power of solubilizing membrane proteins than ionic detergents. To bypass these limitations of 2-DE in resolving hydrophobic proteins such as membrane proteins, an alternative technique, the two-dimensional BAC/SDS-PAGE (2-DB), has been developed. Here, the first-dimension separation occurs according to molecular weight in an acidic discontinuous PAGE system (pH 4.0–1.5) using cationic benzyldimethyl-*n*-hexadecylammonium chloride (BAC) as detergent and the second-dimension separation is performed using the anionic detergent SDS (Zahedi et al. 2005, 2007; Braun et al. 2007).

17.3.2
MS-Based Proteomics

MS has become an indispensable analytical tool of proteomics (Sanz-Medel et al. 2008). Mass spectrometers measure the molecular mass of a sample through the following steps:

1. A protein sample is enzymatically digested into its constituent peptides.
2. The peptides of a sample are introduced to the ionization source of the instrument directly or are separated into a series of components, which then enter the mass spectrometer sequentially for individual analysis. Such en route separation can be performed, for example, through high-pressure liquid chromatography (HPLC).
3. Inside the ionization source, the sample molecules are ionized by ESI or MALDI.
4. The charged sample ions are accelerated into the vacuum-maintained mass analyzer region of the mass spectrometer where they are separated according to their mass (m) to charge (z) ratios (m/z). Mass analyzers currently available include quadrupoles and time-of-flight (TOF) analyzers; they differ in the covered m/z range, their mass accuracy, and their resolution.
5. Data on relative abundance and m/z ratios of detected ions are stored in the format of an m/z spectrum.
6. The m/z spectra are analyzed using protein databases and enable protein identification.

Since proteomics began with 2-DE methodology, the application of MS has been driven by the qualitative character of protein identification on a 2-DE gel. Indeed, MS techniques are very convenient for protein identification. However, their application to protein quantification is more complicated since there is no linear dependence between the concentrations of protein or peptides in a sample and the MS signals observed. While there are several promising gel-free MS-based approaches, presently available methods do not fulfill the increasing need for reliable methods of absolute quantification of proteins (Sanz-Medel et al. 2008).

17.3.3
Protein Arrays

Protein microarrays use either multiple capture antibodies dotted separately on a slide (forward microarrays) or multiple tissue/protein samples, again dotted and fixed together on single slides which then are stained with the different antibodies (reverse microarrays; Kopf and Zharhary 2007; Wingren and Borrebaeck 2007). Whereas these methods can detect the presence of numerous proteins or the level of expression in multiple tissue samples in a high-throughput manner, the technique is still limited by the availability of specific and sensitive antibodies. The latter proved to be an issue, for instance, in case of known lung cancer markers such as the cytokeratins (Conrad et al. 2008). Antibody specificity must be validated by immunoblotting, and internal controls may be required if the antibodies do not bind predictably. Detection of low-abundance proteins also remains a problem, as simple methods of multiple protein amplification, analogous to the polymerase chain reaction for DNA amplification, are not available. Moreover, the capacity of protein arrays to detect co- and posttranslational modifications is limited.

17.4
Expression Profiling in Breast Cancer

Expression analysis is applied in various medical fields. Here, we review some developments in the field of transcriptomics and proteomics concerning breast cancer. With a lifetime risk of 13%, breast cancer is the most frequently diagnosed cancer in women of Western countries (Miller et al. 2006). In a minor fraction of cases, the tumor develops due to the constitutional mutation of a breast cancer (*BRCA*) gene, whereas in general the genetic basis of breast cancer is complex and not sufficiently understood. Therapy is based on more or less radical surgery combined with radiation and adjuvant systemic treatment (chemotherapy, receptor-specific drugs). Adjuvant systemic therapy of patients with localized breast cancer reduces the risk of distant metastases by 30%, but 70–80% of these patients would survive without systemic therapy (van't Veer et al. 2002). Conventional clinical and pathological parameters such as age, menopausal status, tumor size, histological grade, lymph node involvement, and status of estrogen receptor (ER) and ERBB2 receptor (Her-2/neu) are used in algorithms such as Adjuvant!Online that prognosticate the course of the disease or provide recommendations for individual treatment decisions such as the St. Gallen criteria. However, the predictive power of these algorithms is limited. Expression profiling produces additional predictive information and, possibly, new treatment options (Rouzier et al. 2005; Sotiriou and Piccart 2007).

17.4.1
RNA Analyses

RNA microarray data of breast tumors have been analyzed in supervised or unsupervised manner. *Supervised* methods use outside information about the experimental condition (e.g., cases with metastases versus cases without) to shape the derivation of a model from the dataset. *Unsupervised* methods use information contained within the RNA data only and usually involve hierarchical clustering (see section on transcriptomics) to detect relationships among tumors, among genes, and connections between specific genes and specific tumors.

In *unsupervised* analyses, breast tumors have been found to cluster in at least four groups with specific composite expression profiles (PEROU et al. 2000; SOTIRIOU and PICCART 2007): Three major types related to a specific receptor status, ER⁻/ERBB2⁻, ERBB2⁺, or ER⁺, with the last type being subdivided in two groups that showed high or low proliferation resembling the luminal breast cancer subtypes A and B. Beyond this reproduction of the conventional histopathological classification, distinct expression patterns were found. In a subset of ER-negative tumors, for instance, a functional androgen receptor response was detected which eventually might serve as a novel therapeutic target (DOANE et al. 2006).

Supervised analyses produce expression classifiers on a set of tumors for which the outcome is known already. The endpoint, i.e., the definition of what is considered as outcome (e.g., metastasis-free survival or response to a specific treatment) may vary from study to study. For evaluation, classifiers are applied to an independent set of tumors and compared to conventional predictive algorithms such as Adjuvant!Online. VAN'T VEER et al. (2002) extracted a classifier from the expression data of 78 lymph-node negative breast cancer patients younger than 55 years of age, of whom 44 remained free of distant metastases for at least 5 years after diagnosis. By evidence of differential regulation and of correlation with disease outcome, 231 of 25,000 genes were selected. A leave-one-out procedure with the 78 samples then yielded an optimal classifier of 70 genes, which had maximal predictive power. Subsequent evaluation showed that the classifier is effective both in lymph node-negative and lymph node-positive patients (VAN DE VIJVER et al. 2002). Comparison with conventional predictive algorithms showed that the 70-genes signature (MammaPrint®) has similar sensitivity (>90%) but is more specific, that is, less patients are classified erroneously into the high-risk group where they would receive adjuvant systemic therapy.

Especially, patients in the ER-positive subgroup profit from this specification.

Recently, expression of SATB1 was found to have high prognostic value in both node-negative and node-positive breast cancer patients (HAN et al. 2008). SATB1 is a nuclear protein that acts as a cell-type-specific genome organizer and gene regulator essential for T-cell differentiation and activation. In breast cancer, SATB1 induces a metastatic gene expression pattern that correlates significantly with the 231 genes selected by VAN'T VEER et al. (2002) (see above) and with expression signatures for lung and for bone metastasis (HAN et al. 2008). However, the comparison of breast cancer classifiers among each other (including MammaPrint®, the Rotterdam signature, On*co*type DX®, and others) revealed little or no overlap although they have similar predictive values and carry similar prognostic information (WANG et al. 2005; FAN et al. 2006; SOTIRIOU and PICCART 2007). There are several reasons for this disparity. Methodical differences (microarray platforms, hybridization conditions, gene annotations, normalization methods, profiling strategies) have been identified which now are addressed in the US Food and Drug Administration (FDA)-launched microarray quality control (MAQC) project. Moreover, the different classifiers were not derived from the same patient sets. Most importantly, however, sets of selected genes may vary substantially among studies since on the one hand, the expression levels of different genes are correlated and, on the other hand, statistical power of small study groups is limited. Thus, genes from the same pathway that carry similar biological information are likely to rank differently in different expression studies based on relatively small numbers of tumors (DUPUY and SIMON 2007).

Supervised analyses may be developed bottom-up, that is, driven by a biological hypothesis and deriving an expression signature from a preselected subset of genes. Several subsets have been applied such as the wound-response signature, which was shown to be expressed in breast cancers of patients with markedly worse clinical outcome (CHANG et al. 2004) or the gene-expression grade index (GGI), a signature of 97 genes that consistently differed in expression between low- and high-grade breast cancers and which was used successfully to predict the clinical outcome in intermediate-grade tumors (SOTIRIOU et al. 2006).

A meta-analysis revealed that genes associated with cell proliferation provide the driving force in all previously reported prognostic signatures (SOTIRIOU and PICCART 2007). All of these classifiers provide useful information on the intrinsic properties of a tumor. However, tumor size and nodal status retain important prognostic information.

Besides prognostic signatures, predictive classifiers have been developed. Both top-down and bottom-up supervised analyses have been performed in order to find classifiers that—beyond the determination of the ER- and ERBB2-receptor status—predict the response to a specific treatment. Thereby, predictors of anti-estrogen treatment in patients with ER-positive tumors have been derived as well as classifiers that accurately predict the effect of chemotherapeutic agents that target specific pathways (Bild et al. 2006). Prediction of treatment response is complicated, however, by the heterogeneity and evolution of tumors, and by the individual biological properties of the host (Sotiriou and Piccart 2007).

17.4.2
Proteomics

Histological data, especially the receptor expression status, represents the protein level. Therefore, in a general sense, proteomics already has been taken successfully to the clinics of breast cancer. As yet, however, proteomics in the sense of multiprotein pattern analysis by 2-DE and MS has not (Harris et al. 2007). Proteomics is hampered by the heterogeneity of tissue biopsies, variability in time and space, and small volumes in focused sampling procedures such as microdissection or nipple aspiration. While some of these are shared with transcriptomics, proteomics lacks a PCR-like amplification method (Hondermarck et al. 2008). Of course, multiprotein analyses also encounter the multitesting problem, which might result in the generation of spurious results.

Thus, proteomics contributes to the understanding of factors in breast cancer biology such as the chaperone 14-3-3, which is involved in the control of proliferation and differentiation, the ubiquitinating activity of *BRCA1*, and the downstream effects of ERBB2 or tumor growth factor (TGF)β receptor activation, and may eventually reveal new therapeutic targets (Hondermarck et al. 2008). As of 2007, however, the clinical use of proteomic pattern analysis is not reliable enough and has not been recommended (Harris et al. 2007). Classifiers such as a 21-protein-signature of metastasis-free survival derived from unsupervised protein expression profiling (Jacquemier et al. 2005) still require confirmation in larger and well-designed prospective studies.

References

Alessandro R, Fontana S, Kohn E, De Leo G (2005) Proteomic strategies and their application in cancer research. Tumori 91:447–455

Banks R, Selby P (2003) Clinical proteomics—insights into pathologies and benefits for patients. Lancet 362:415–416

Benjamini Y, Hochberg Y (1995) Controlling the false discovery rate: a practical and powerful approach to multiple testing. J R Statist Soc B 57:289–300

Bild AH, Yao G, Chang JT et al (2006) Oncogenic pathway signatures in human cancers as a guide to targeted therapies. Nature 439:353–357

Bolstad BM, Irizarry RA, Astrand M, Speed TP (2003) A comparison of normalization methods for high density oligonucleotide array data based on variance and bias. Bioinformatics 19:185–193

Braun RJ, Kinkl N, Beer M, Ueffing M (2007) Two-dimensional electrophoresis of membrane proteins. Anal Bioanal Chem 389:1033–1045

Breitling R (2006) Biological microarray interpretation: the rules of engagement. Biochim Biophys Acta 1759:319–327

Breitling R, Armengaud P, Amtmann A, Herzyk P (2004) Rank products: a simple, yet powerful, new method to detect differentially regulated genes in replicated microarray experiments. FEBS Lett 573:83–92

Brenner S, Johnson M, Bridgham J et al (2000) Gene expression analysis by massively parallel signature sequencing (MPSS) on microbead arrays. Nat Biotechnol 18:630–634

Chang HY, Sneddon JB, Alizadeh AA et al (2004) Gene expression signature of fibroblast serum response predicts human cancer progression: similarities between tumors and wounds. PLoS Biol 2:E7

Chotikacharoensuk T, Arteca RN, Arteca JM (2006) Use of differential display for the identification of touch-induced genes from an ethylene-insensitive *Arabidopsis* mutant and partial characterization of these genes. J Plant Physiol 163:1305–1320

Conrad DH, Goyette J, Thomas PS (2008) Proteomics as a method for early detection of cancer: a review of proteomics, exhaled breath condensate, and lung cancer screening. J Gen Intern Med 23 Suppl 1:78–84

Doane AS, Danso M, Lal P et al (2006) An estrogen receptor-negative breast cancer subset characterized by a hormonally regulated transcriptional program and response to androgen. Oncogene 25:3994–4008

Dupuy A, Simon RM (2007) Critical review of published microarray studies for cancer outcome and guidelines on statistical analysis and reporting. J Natl Cancer Inst 99:147–157

Fan C, Oh DS, Wessels L et al (2006) Concordance among gene-expression-based predictors for breast cancer. N Engl J Med 355:560–569

Han HJ, Russo J, Kohwi Y, Kohwi-Shigematsu T (2008) SATB1 reprogrammes gene expression to promote breast tumour growth and metastasis. Nature 452:187–193

Hardiman G (2004) Microarray platforms—comparisons and contrasts. Pharmacogenomics 5:487–502

Harris L, Fritsche H, Mennel R et al (2007) American Society of Clinical Oncology 2007 update of recommendations for the use of tumor markers in breast cancer. J Clin Oncol 25:5287–5312

Healy DA, Hayes CJ, Leonard P et al (2007) Biosensor developments: application to prostate-specific antigen detection. Trends Biotechnol 25:125–131

Hondermarck H, Tastet C, El Yazidi-Belkoura I et al (2008) Proteomics of breast cancer: the quest for markers and therapeutic targets. J Proteome Res 7:1403–1411

Issaq HJ, Veenstra TD (2007) The role of electrophoresis in disease biomarker discovery. Electrophoresis 28:1980–1988

Jacquemier J, Ginestier C, Rougemont J et al (2005) Protein expression profiling identifies subclasses of breast cancer and predicts prognosis. Cancer Res 65:767–779

Kikuchi T, Carbone DP (2007) Proteomics analysis in lung cancer: challenges and opportunities. Respirology 12:22–28

Klose J (1975) Protein mapping by combined isoelectric focusing and electrophoresis of mouse tissues: a novel approach to testing for induced point mutations in mammals. Humangenetik 26:231–243

Kopf E, Zharhary D (2007) Antibody arrays—an emerging tool in cancer proteomics. Int J Biochem Cell Biol 39:1305–1317

Miller BA, Scoppa SM, Feuer EJ (2006) Racial/ethnic patterns in lifetime and age-conditional risk estimates for selected cancers. Cancer 106:670–682

Nuyten DS, Kreike B, Hart AA et al (2006) Predicting a local recurrence after breast-conserving therapy by gene expression profiling. Breast Cancer Res 8:R62

O'Farrell PH (1975) High resolution two-dimensional electrophoresis of proteins. J Biol Chem 250:4007–4021

Pease AC, Solas D, Sullivan EJ et al (1994) Light-generated oligonucleotide arrays for rapid DNA sequence analysis. Proc Natl Acad Sci USA: 5022–5026

Perou CM, Sorlie T, Eisen MB et al (2000) Molecular portraits of human breast tumours. Nature 406:747–752

Rouzier R, Rajan R, Wagner P et al (2005) Microtubule-associated protein tau: a marker of paclitaxel sensitivity in breast cancer. Proc Natl Acad Sci USA 102:8315–8320

Sanz-Medel A, Montes-Bayon M, del Rosario Fernandez de la Campa M et al (2008) Elemental mass spectrometry for quantitative proteomics. Anal Bioanal Chem 390:3–16

Schena M, Shalon D, Davis RW, Brown PO (1995). Quantitative monitoring of gene expression patterns with a complementary DNA microarray. Science 270:467–470

Smith JC, Lambert JP, Elisma F, Figeys D (2007) Proteomics in 2005/2006: developments, applications and challenges. Anal Chem 79:4325–4343

Sotiriou C, Piccart MJ (2007) Taking gene-expression profiling to the clinic: when will molecular signatures become relevant to patient care? Nat Rev Cancer 7:545–553

Sotiriou C, Wirapati P, Loi S et al (2006) Gene expression profiling in breast cancer: understanding the molecular basis of histologic grade to improve prognosis. J Natl Cancer Inst 98:262–272

Steemers FJ, Ferguson JA, Walt DR (2000) Screening unlabeled DNA targets with randomly ordered fiber-optic gene arrays. Nat Biotechnol 18:91–94

Stranger BE, Forrest MS, Clark AG et al (2005) Genome-wide associations of gene expression variation in humans. PLoS Genet 1:e78

Tu Y, Stolovitzky G, Klein U (2002) Quantitative noise analysis for gene expression microarray experiments. Proc Natl Acad Sci U S A 99:14031–14036

van de Vijver MJ, He YD, van't Veer LJ et al (2002) A gene-expression signature as a predictor of survival in breast cancer. N Engl J Med 347:1999–2009

van't Veer LJ, Dai H, van de Vijver MJ et al (2002) Gene expression profiling predicts clinical outcome of breast cancer. Nature 415:530–536

Velculescu VE, Zhang L, Vogelstein B, Kinzler KW (1995) Serial analysis of gene expression. Scienc. 270:484–487

Wang Y, Klijn JG, Zhang Y et al (2005) Gene-expression profiles to predict distant metastasis of lymph-node-negative primary breast cancer. Lancet 365:671–679

Westfall PH, Young SS (1993) Resampling-based multiple testing: examples and methods for *p*-value adjustment. Wiley, New York

Wingren C, Borrebaeck CA (2007) Progress in miniaturization of protein arrays—a step closer to high-density nano-arrays. Drug Discov Today 12:813–819

Zahedi RP, Meisinger C, Sickmann A (2005) Two-dimensional benzyldimethyl-n-hexadecylammonium chloride/SDS-PAGE for membrane proteomics. Proteomics 5:3581–3588

Zahedi RP, Moebius J, Sickmann A (2007) Two-dimensional BAC/SDS-PAGE for membrane proteomics. Subcell Biochem 43:13–20

Strategies of Gene Transfer and Silencing, and Technical Considerations

Kristoffer Valerie and Paul R. Graves

CONTENTS

K. Valerie, PhD
Department of Radiation Oncology, Virginia Commonwealth University, Richmond, Virginia 23112, USA

P. R. Graves, PhD
Department of Radiation Oncology, Virginia Commonwealth University, Richmond, VA 23112, USA

KEY POINTS

- Cancer gene therapy is based on the principle of altering a tumor cell genetically to improve cancer treatment. This strategy works because the tumor cells can be made to express a new gene, for example, from bacteria that other cells in the body do not express, that would render them susceptible to a drug or other treatment. In the years to come this technology is expected to make significant impact on how cancer patients are being treated.

Abstract

Cancer gene therapy is a relatively new modality that might ultimately revolutionize oncology. The basic principle is to alter the tumor genetically to enhance more traditional chemo- and radiation therapy schema. The last decade has seen tremendous progress and development of new technologies in the areas of vector delivery, tumor targeting, and numerous clever ways to increase tumor killing, including early attempts to modulate tumor gene expression by RNA interference. In recent years, attempts to image affected cells have also been part of these efforts. Many studies have proceeded to the preclinical stage and a fair number to early clinical testing with some showing encouraging results. However, real impact on patient survival remains to be seen. One major problem still to be overcome is the quantitative delivery of the vector into the tumor mass. The next decade is expected to resolve many of these technical issues and improve the treatment of patients. This chapter will discuss new technologies and provide a brief overview of the field.

18.1
Introduction

The last decade has seen tremendous growth of studies attempting to take gene therapy of cancer into the clinical arena. The major objective is to introduce genetic material into cancer cells with the intent of sensitizing them to chemo- and radiation therapy. A number of strategies have now reached phases I and II clinical trials, with some showing promise. In addition, using molecular tools and engineering, a major thrust in the field is to image affected cancer cells and their fate during therapy, for example by positron emission tomography (PET) or magnetic resonance imaging (MRI). Occasionally, this can be achieved by the conversion of an image probe by the therapeutic protein itself resulting in an imageable feature and sometimes a co-expressed protein can accomplish this. This chapter reviews the status of the cancer gene therapy field, with focus on new technology and directions, existing problems, and highlights and discusses areas with gene therapy applications in radiation therapy and imaging.

18.2
Vectors

The vector is the vehicle that carries the DNA into the cells (VALERIE 1999). One overriding technical diffi-

culty shared by all gene therapy vectors is the relative inefficient delivery of DNA into the tumor. *All* tumor cells need to be affected or the cancer would recur. Virus vectors including adenovirus (ADV), adeno-associated virus (AAV), and retrovirus (RV) have traditionally been the vectors of choice for introducing genetic material (e.g., suppressor genes, dominant-negative genes, and "suicide genes") into cancer cells to make them more sensitive to chemo- and radiation therapy. Viruses have evolved highly effective mechanisms for infecting cells, on which has been capitalized. However, each vector has its pros and cons (Table 18.1). By molecular engineering, these viruses have been altered to accommodate the therapeutic gene and at the same time allow for efficient growth and safe handling.

A significant problem using viral vectors for cancer gene therapy are production and quality control issues, safety, and cost associated with obtaining clinical grade preparations suitable for human use. In terms of the efficiency of delivery, ADV remains the most effective viral vector because of the ability to obtain high titers and higher multiplicities of infection ([MOI] i.e., virus per cell ratio) than other viral vectors, and the relative ease by which large quantities of virus can be isolated and purified (Table 18.1). Retrovirus, and more recently lentivirus (LV), remain promising vectors. However, whereas ADV is not typically integrated into the genome of infected cells, both RV and LV integrate and potentially could be a safety concern due to the possibility that a critical cellular gene is inactivated by insertion of the virus. Because of these advantageous properties,

Table 18.1. Vector properties

Vector(s)	Pros	Cons
ADV	Efficient gene transfer Infects nonreplicating cells High titers Transient expression Large gene capacity	Lack of cell type specificity
AAV	Single, site-specific integration Relatively small gene capacity	Difficult to purify
RV, LV	Efficient gene transfer Relatively small gene capacity Infects nonreplicating cells (LV)	Risk of insertional mutagenesis Relatively low titer and expression Cumbersome to purify for clinical use
Lipid–DNA	Unlimited gene capacity Excellent scale-up capability	Relatively poor in vivo gene transfer
Nanoparticles	Unlimited gene capacity Excellent scale-up capability Imageable Cell targeting	Relatively poor in vivo gene transfer Complicated preparation

ADV is considered a more suitable vector for cancer therapy than RV and LV. However, the efficient delivery of viruses into the tumor is still a major problem despite viruses' ability of infecting cells in culture at high levels. The effective delivery of virus or by any other means (physical or chemical) within the tumor bed remains a major technical hurdle (FREYTAG et al. 2004). Penetration of ADV within tissue rarely exceeds a volume larger than a cubic centimeter (BARTON et al. 2007), thus limiting potential success only to small tumors.

AAV has also been considered as a vector for cancer therapy (LI et al. 2005b). However, even though AAV supposedly is integrating at a specific chromosomal site, potentially avoiding mutagenesis, production issues and relatively low expression levels of therapeutic genes from AAV vectors are shared with RV and LV (Table 18.1).

Some studies have attempted direct injection of DNA into tumors, either alone or in complex with lipids. Introducing DNA or RNA directly into the tumor limits immune responses sometimes elicited when viral preparations are administered. However, the efficiency of lipid–DNA to enter cells in a tumor remains a problem, as does the relatively nonspecific cellular uptake of lipid–DNA complexes. Attempts to incorporate molecules in the lipid bilayer that bind to cell surface receptor to improve cell specificity have been investigated, but the differential effects seen in vitro are not generally duplicated in vivo. Along the same line and more recently, nanoparticles has also been considered as vector for delivering therapeutic genes. An added benefit with nanoparticles is that they can also be imaged (NIE et al. 2007).

18.2.1
ADV and AAV

Adenovirus is a relatively large DNA virus that infects a variety of epithelial and endothelial cells expressing the Coxsackie-adenovirus receptor and the integrin receptor (VALERIE 1999). Relatively large therapeutic genes can be transferred by ADV. First-generation viruses can harbor DNA inserts of more than 3-kb whereas "gutted" ADV is able to harbor up to 34-kb of DNA (NG and GRAHAM 2002; NG et al. 2002). This ability of ADV in addition to the relative ease by which the virus is propagated and purified in large quantities has made ADV an attractive vector choice for cancer gene therapy. In terms of targeting therapeutic ADVs to specific cells, a number of clever approaches have been devised including altering the viral penton protein necessary for infection to alter the propensity of infection to cancer cells

over normal cells (GLASGOW et al. 2006). Engineered ADV vectors remain the most biologically efficient and cost-effective viral cancer gene therapy vector.

AAV is a relatively small DNA virus that integrates at a specific chromosomal site on chromosome 19, infects both dividing and nondividing cells, transduces a broad range of tissues in vivo, and initiates long-term gene expression in these tissues (LI et al. 2005b). Furthermore, wild-type AAV does not cause any known disease and does not stimulate a cell-mediated immune response. In order for AAV to propagate, it requires a helper virus such as ADV. The relatively small genome size of 4.7-kb only allows smaller therapeutic genes to be transferred. Similar to ADV, attempts to change the cell tropism for AAV infection have been successful in vitro, but these approaches have not yet been fully tested in vivo. Thus, AAV is similar to RV and LV in its properties as gene therapy vector but may not be as significant mutagenesis threat as are these other two viruses (Table 18.1).

18.2.2
RV and LV

An engineered mouse leukemia retrovirus was the first viral vector developed for cancer gene therapy (CULVER et al. 1992). The retroviruses stably integrate randomly into the genome of infected cells, and thus would be a potential safety issue. Another major shortcoming of the RV as vector for cancer gene therapy is the relatively low expression levels compared with adenovirus. The typical LV used for gene therapy is a human retrovirus derived from human immunodeficiency virus (HIV-1) that is highly efficient in infecting cells. In contrast to the mouse retrovirus, human LV infects nondividing cells in addition to dividing cells, which makes this vector very attractive for somatic cell gene therapy and in vitro work. However, for *cancer* gene therapy, LV may not be advantageous since it infects indiscriminately, whereas RV only infects dividing cancer cells. RV and LV vectors have some very attractive features but are not ideal for human cancer gene therapy.

18.2.3
Lipids and Nanoparticles

The discovery that positively charged lipids could be used to introduce DNA into cells in vitro opened up the possibility of using lipid–DNA complexes for direct intratumoral injection. Lipid–DNA complexes efficiently transfect cells in vitro. However, the low yield of cellular uptake in vivo remains a problem. With the advent of using synthesized anti-sense oligonucleotides and RNA interference (see below) for manipulating gene expression, lipid vectors are probably the most promising vector in the long run, since viral vectors will most likely continue to have production and safety issues that have to be adequately addressed resulting in very high production costs. Entirely manmade DNA/RNA and lipids needed for human use would provide excellent scale-up capabilities, quality control, and increased safety, similar to the manufacturing of small molecule cancer drugs. However, the efficiency and specificity of lipids to deliver DNA into the tumor need improvement. Nanoparticles made of chemically synthesized, highly structured macromolecules able to entrap a drug, therapeutic DNA or RNA, and/or agents that can be imaged show enormous future potential (NIE et al. 2007). Completely synthetic nanoparticle vectors and DNA or RNA for gene therapy is likely the way of the future.

18.3
Strategies and Targets for Cancer Sensitization

Most cancer gene therapy studies have up until now used viral vectors, in particular ADV, to deliver the therapeutic DNA into the tumor cells. Many clever ways have been devised, and numerous cellular processes have been explored as targets for enhancing killing of cancer cells in vitro, for example by increasing apoptosis, and many times these strategies have also shown efficacy in animal tumor models. Herein, only the most significant studies and concepts will be discussed.

To improve the transmission and spread of ADV within the tumor and design a "magic bullet" for cancer cells, the oncolytic ONYX-015 ADV was developed (BISCHOFF et al. 1996). The basic idea is for this ADV to replicate only in cancer cells but not in normal cells, due to a mutation in a specific viral gene, *E1B*, that renders ADV replication dependent on mutant or abnormal *p53*, a condition found in about half of all cancers. When ONYX-015 infects a p53 mutant cancer cell, it subsequently lyses or breaks open the cell and releases new ADV available for infection of additional cancer cells, thus the name oncolytic. The tumor suppressor p53 was initially believed to make the decision whether replication occurred or not—mutant p53 allowed the oncolytic virus to replicate whereas wild type did not. Since normal somatic cells express wild-type p53 they would not allow the ADV to replicate and thus would be spared. However, it turns out that other p53-related processes and modulators of cell cycle checkpoints in-

cluding p14^{arf}/p16^{INK4a} may also play important roles in whether the oncolytic ADV replicates or not. Nevertheless, oncolytic ADV showed some positive initial clinical results, but it is not a magic bullet for cancer. However, the oncolytic virus concept remains a highly attractive strategy for cancer therapy in general since it would seek out cancer cells and destroy them, whereas normal cells would be left unharmed (ALEMANY 2007).

Additional permutations on the original oncolytic virus idea have been proposed and tested using a variety of different viruses. Some also include a therapeutic gene such as a tumor suppressor or suicide gene (see below) to produce a potential multi-prong therapeutic effect.

18.3.1
RNA Interference

RNA interference (RNAi) is a highly conserved mechanism by which small, nonprotein-coding RNA molecules interfere with, or modulate, gene expression. Although RNAi represents just one function of a variety of small noncoding RNA molecules, it has received the most attention largely because of its utility as a basic research tool to silence the expression of specific genes (ZAMORE and HALEY 2005). Moreover, because of its potency and high specificity, RNAi has now emerged as a promising new therapeutic strategy to reduce or eliminate gene expression in animals. Indeed, RNAi is already undergoing human clinical trials, including pioneering work for treating macular degeneration and respiratory syncytial viral infection (BUMCROT et al. 2006).

RNAi is catalyzed by RNA molecules approximately 22 nucleotides in length that can originate from both exogenous and endogenous sources (KIM 2005) (Fig. 18.1). The incredible specificity inherent in RNAi is derived from its basic mechanism of action, whereby the small interfering RNA (siRNA) molecule hybridizes specifically with its cognate messenger RNA, resulting in degradation of the mRNA. This endogenous silencing mechanism, found in all multicellular organisms, can be exploited to achieve silencing of specific genes by introduction of synthetic siRNA molecules predesigned to hybridize to target genes (Fig. 18.1). These siRNA molecules also hold significant promise for gene therapy approaches. (For a recent review of siRNA biogenesis and the mechanism of inhibition by RNAi, see LIU et al. 2008). In addition to extracellularly introduced siRNA, there exists another class of small RNA molecules, termed micro-RNA (miRNA), which is encoded by the genome of an organism. miRNA represent the most abundant class of naturally occurring small RNAs but differ from siRNA in their origins. Unlike siRNA, miRNA is initially transcribed as part of a much longer primary transcript and then processed to liberate a hairpin precursor of ~65 nucleotides in the nucleus (Liu et al. 2008). This precursor is then exported to the cytoplasm where it is processed by the enzyme Dicer to produce a ~22-bp RNA duplex. Thus, at this point, miRNA and siRNA is similar and both enter a common pathway in which one strand of the RNA duplex becomes incorporated into a protein complex known as RISC (for *RNA-induced silencing complex*). The function of RISC is to guide the interaction between the siRNA or miRNA and the mRNA and catalyze either the degradation of the mRNA or inhibit its translation (Fig. 18.1) (Hutvagner and Simard 2008).

Once the basic mechanism of RNAi was uncovered, it was clear that siRNA could be introduced into cells to silence the expression of specific genes. Indeed, synthetic siRNA is now commercially available to silence most human genes. Another strategy is the manipulation of miRNA to alter gene expression. It has been estimated that the human genome encodes hundreds of forms of miRNA, which regulate the expression of a large number of protein-coding genes (for review, see Ambros 2004). Indeed, miRNA has been found to control a wide range of biological processes, including development, metabolism, cell growth, cell death, and cell fate determination (Ambros 2004), and altered expression of miRNA has been associated with human diseases including cancer (Hammond 2006). One strategy to inhibit the function of miRNA is the use of antagomirs, which hybridize to miRNA and prevent its incorporation into RISC (Mattes et al. 2007) (Fig. 18.1). Using

this strategy, it is possible to increase the expression of specific genes (Mattes et al. 2007).

RNAi potentially has several major advantages compared with traditional therapeutics. First, siRNA can be designed to target genes with unparalleled specificity. Second, all proteins can be inhibited, including proteins that are not amenable for traditional drug inhibition such as structural proteins, etc. As a result, an increasing number of proof-of-principle studies have been conducted delivering siRNA to mice. Examples include systemic administration of siRNA in mouse models of hypercholesterolemia and rheumatoid arthritis (for a recent review, see Bumcrot et al. 2006). Along the same line, short hairpin RNA (shRNA) expressed from viral vectors such as RV or LV has been shown to inhibit specific gene expression, providing a more stable inhibition of gene expression than transiently transfected siRNA. siRNA delivered systemically to animals is degraded rapidly (Kim and Rossi 2007), making it more feasible to deliver siRNA with the help of a vector, e.g., lipids or nanoparticles.

The success of animal studies has now fueled the application of RNAi for use in primates and humans for the testing of treating various diseases (Dykxhoorn and Lieberman 2006). For example, it was shown that local delivery of siRNA to the lung was able to protect primates from the severe acute respiratory syndrome (SARS) coronavirus (Li et al. 2005a). Furthermore, human studies have shown that the delivery of uncomplexed, naked siRNA had success in the treatment of various human diseases (Dykxhoorn and Lieberman 2006). Survivin, telomerase, *MDR1*, and other genes critically involved in cancer growth and regulation, have been targeted by siRNA in vitro and in vivo with encouraging results (Martin and Caplen 2007; Putral et al. 2006).

Altogether, significant progress has been made in applying RNAi as a therapeutic strategy in a relatively short period since its initial discovery. Undoubtedly, the biggest challenge for successful application of RNAi-based therapy remains in its delivery like for all other approaches. However, a variety of strategies are being explored to address this problem (Kim and Rossi 2007), and it is clear that the potential of RNAi-based technology for the treatment of cancer and other human diseases has yet to be fully achieved.

18.3.2
Suppressor Genes

The introduction of a tumor suppressor gene into a cancer cell slows down growth and results in a more

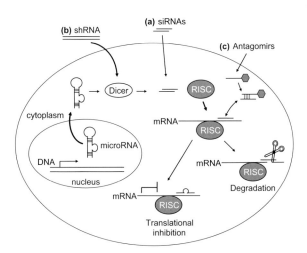

Fig. 18.1a–c. Mechanisms of RNAi. **a** synthetic siRNA, **b** shRNA-expressing viruses, and **c** antagomirs are externally introduced to inhibit the action of endogenous miRNA

manageable cancer or at least that is the underlying hypothesis. The suppressor gene is not likely affecting normal cells since most types of cells in the body are already growth suppressed. One of the first tumor suppressors that was considered for gene therapy was the *p53* gene (ROTH 2006). The introduction of the *p53* tumor suppressor gene into tumor cells results in a complete halt of proliferation and increases apoptosis. However, clinical trials have been disappointing, primarily because of insufficient administration of virus into the tumor (ROTH 2006). A number of different permutations of the p53 approach have been attempted but in general, these strategies have not been successful primarily because of the underlying problem of poor penetration of the vector into the tumor bed (TERNOVOI et al. 2006). Expression of other tumor suppressor genes such as retinoblastoma, and PTEN as therapeutic proteins, aimed at slowing tumor growth have not been pursued to clinical trials mainly because of similar reasons as why p53 has not moved forward. On the other hand, significant advances have been made with melanoma differentiation-associated gene-7 (*MDA-7/IL-24*) perhaps due to this molecule's multitude of attractive properties such as being a tumor suppressor and showing bystander effects that are specific for cancer cells (FISHER 2005; INOUE et al. 2006). In addition, cancer cells expressing MDA-7/IL-24 are also sensitized to chemo- and radiation therapy (FISHER 2005). A phase I trial in patients with solid tumors showed both clinical and biological effects (CUNNINGHAM et al. 2005; TONG et al. 2005), suggesting that MDA-7/IL-24 might be an excellent therapeutic molecule that might benefit patients with cancer.

18.3.3
Suicide Genes

The suicide gene concept is based on the expression of a heterologous gene coding for an enzyme that converts an inactive prodrug to an active drug that by itself or in combination with radiation results in increased cell kill (VALERIE 1999). Ideally and for maximum effect, the suicide gene should not exist in the target cells. The first suicide gene was the herpes simplex thymidine kinase (*HSV-TK*) gene used in combination with the antiherpes drug ganciclovir (CULVER et al. 1994). The improved utilization of acyclovir, a drug currently used for treating herpes-associated encephalitis in children, with mutant HSV-TK (ROSENBERG et al. 2002; VALERIE et al. 2001), and bacterial and yeast cytosine deaminase with 5-fluorocytosine (KIEVIT et al. 1999; TRINH et al. 1995), have also been shown in animal models to be effective

radiosensitizers. An added benefit of the suicide gene–prodrug concept is the fact that the active, toxic drug spreads to adjacent tumor cells by gap junctions or by cellular release that increases the toxicity to surrounding cells and improves the therapeutic effect about 10-fold. A number of phases I and II clinical studies have been conducted with suicide gene approaches. Focus here will be on those that combine the suicide gene concept with radiation therapy (see below).

18.3.4
Immunomodulatory Genes

To enhance tumor toxicity by using the cells own defense system, expression of various cytokines and other immunomodulatory proteins have been investigated as potential strategies for radiosensitization when expressed from various vectors. As with other combined modalities, the combinations of cytokine gene therapy with radiation or chemotherapy have shown some promise in clinical settings. The most advanced studies are those based on tumor necrosis factor-α (TNF-α) in combination with radiation (KUFE and WEICHSELBAUM 2003). TNF-α has potent antitumor and antiangiogenesis activities that synergize with radiation therapy. TNFerade™ was developed as an ADV that expressed TNF-α under control of a radiation-inducible promoter that limits toxicities to the irradiated area, which is not the case with the direct injection of TNF-α into the tumor.

Others studies have combined radiation therapy with IL-3 immunotherapy in preclinical models (CHIANG et al. 2000; TSAI et al. 2006). However, these studies and similar involving other immunotherapy-based approaches in combination with radiotherapy have not moved forward to clinical trials.

18.4
Clinical Applications Related to Radiotherapy and Imaging

The number of clinical trials aimed at determining the safety and/or efficacy of cancer gene therapy continue to grow. The discussion herein is limited to trials that focus on treatments combined with radiation therapy. TNFerade™ is an adenovirus expressing the cytokine TNF-α under control of a radiation-induced promoter (MUNDT et al. 2004). A phase I trial with TNFerade™ has been completed for metastatic solid tumors (SENZER et al. 2004). The treatment was well tolerated, with only minor toxicities with doses as high as 4×10^{11} particle units (PU) corresponding to approximately 1- to 2×10^{10} infectious units (IU). Controlled prospective clinical trials have been initiated with patients with locally advanced pancreatic cancer to better define the therapeutic contribution of TNFerade™ (CHANG et al. 2008).

Several phases I/II trials using a multiprong approach combining two suicide gene–prodrug approaches (CD+5-FC and HSV-TK+GCV) with the ONYX-015 conditionally replicating ADV and image-guided radiation therapy (IMRT) have been conducted, including one for patients with intermediate to high-risk prostate cancer that was recently completed (FREYTAG et al. 2007b). There were no dose-limiting toxicities or treatment-related serious adverse events in this trial. Relative to a previous trial using a first-generation ADV, there was no increase in hematologic, hepatic, gastrointestinal, or genitourinary toxicities. Posttreatment prostate biopsies yielded provocative preliminary results. When the results were categorized by prognostic risk, most of the treatment effect was observed in the intermediate-risk group, with 0 of 12 patients being positive for cancer at their last biopsy.

An improved ADV vector expressing yeast CD and mutant HSV-TK for better utilization of the prodrugs in an oncolytic ADV backbone were combined with co-expression of the ADV death protein (facilitates cell lysis and improves ADV spread) in a preclinical pancreatic cancer animal model. Because a substrate for HSV-TK labeled with [^{18}F], 9-(4-[^{18}F]-fluoro-3-hydroxy-methyl-butyl)guanine (^{18}F-FHBG), can be used as a probe for PET, infected tumor cells can be imaged (FREYTAG et al. 2007a). ADV was readily detected in the pancreas but not in other tissues, suggesting that this ADV can be combined with radiotherapy of the pancreas without resulting in excessive systemic toxicity. Currently, this novel ADV is undergoing a phase I trial in patients with pancreatic cancer. Other studies have tested the feasibility of using 8-[^{18}F]fluoroganciclovir (FGCV) as probe for imaging HSV-TK-expressing cells and tissues in preclinical animal models using microPET with similar positive results (LU et al. 2006).

Most times the therapeutic protein itself is not imageable. In this case, a second protein needs to be expressed that can be imaged, ideally with clinically suitable imaging technologies such as PET or MRI. The vector for such studies is usually limited to ADV or any other viral vector able to harbor larger DNA inserts. One example of this strategy is using the same double suicide gene prodrug with conditionally replicating ADV as mentioned above and co-expressing the human iodide symporter (*hNIS*) gene as a reporter for single-photon emission computed tomography (SPECT) (SID-DIQUI et al. 2007). hNIS will sequester the probe sodium pertechnetate (Na^{99m}TcO$_4$) to affected tissues, in this case the prostate (SIDDIQUI et al. 2007). Na^{99m}TcO$_4$ is an US Food and Drug Administration (FDA)-approved diagnostic imaging probe. It was found that SPECT images were readily detected up to 4 days after administering the ADV. Currently, such ADV is undergoing clinical testing. The ability to image the expression of the therapeutic gene increases the information gained from clinical trials tremendously. In the future, more, novel ways of imaging tumors by PET, MRI, or other clinically utilized imaging technologies of patients undergoing gene therapy, will likely continue to facilitate the assessment of vector penetration and treatment efficacy.

18.5
Conclusion

The idea of using cancer gene therapy to improve chemo- and radiotherapy was initially very exciting. Promising results were generated in various animal tumor models. However, clinical trials have so far shown little to no impact on patient survival, with a range of different types of cancers. Almost 20 years later, the field is still trying to deal with technical issues. Regardless of therapeutic strategy, the efficient delivery of therapeutic DNA or RNA into tumors needs to improve. RNAi-based strategies look very promising and so does the nanoparticles because of this vector's added benefit of being able to image the targeted cells and tissues. It is very likely that many of these technical hurdles will be overcome in the future, resulting in improved clinical outcome. In addition, more insights into the unique properties of cancer cells will continue to open up new targeting opportunities and move the field forward.

References

Alemany R (2007) Cancer selective adenoviruses. Mol Aspects Med 28:42–58

Ambros V (2004) The functions of animal microRNAs. Nature 431:350–355

Barton KN, Freytag SO, Nurushev T, Yoo S, Lu M, Yin FF, Li S, Movsas B, Kim JH, Brown SL (2007) A model for optimizing adenoviral delivery in human cancer gene therapy trials. Hum Gene Ther 18:562–572

Bischoff JR, Kirn DH, Williams A, Heise C, Horn S, Muna M, Ng L, Nye JA, Sampson-Johannes A, Fattaey A, McCormick, F (1996) An adenovirus mutant that replicates selectively in p53-deficient human tumor cells. Science 274:373–376

Bumcrot D, Manoharan M, Koteliansky V, Sah DW (2006) RNAi therapeutics: a potential new class of pharmaceutical drugs. Nat Chem Biol 2:711–719

Chang KJ, Lee JG, Holcombe RF, Kuo J, Muthusamy R, Wu ML (2008) Endoscopic ultrasound delivery of an antitumor agent to treat a case of pancreatic cancer. Nat Clin Pract Gastroenterol Hepatol 5:107–111

Chiang CS, Hong JH, Wu YC, McBride WH, Dougherty GJ (2000) Combining radiation therapy with interleukin-3 gene immunotherapy. Cancer Gene Ther 7:1172–1178

Culver KW, Ram Z, Wallbridge S, Ishii H, Oldfield EH, Blaese RM (1992) In vivo gene transfer with retroviral vector-producer cells for treatment of experimental brain tumors. [See comments.] Science 256:1550–1552

Culver KW, Van Gilder J, Link CJ, Carlstrom T, Buroker T, Yuh W, Koch K, Schabold K, Doornbas S, Wetjen B et al (1994) Gene therapy for the treatment of malignant brain tumors with in vivo tumor transduction with the herpes simplex thymidine kinase gene/ganciclovir system. Hum Gene Ther 5:343–379

Cunningham CC, Chada S, Merritt JA, Tong A, Senzer N, Zhang Y, Mhashilkar A, Parker K, Vukelja S, Richards D et al (2005) Clinical and local biological effects of an intratumoral injection of mda-7 (IL24; INGN 241) in patients with advanced carcinoma: a phase I study. Mol Ther 11:149–159

Dykxhoorn DM, Lieberman J (2006) Knocking down disease with siRNAs. Cell 126:231–235

Fisher PB (2005) Is mda-7/IL-24 a magic bullet for cancer? Cancer Res 65:0128–10138

Freytag SO, Kim JH, Brown SL, Barton K, Lu M, Chung M (2004) Gene therapy strategies to improve the effectiveness of cancer radiotherapy. Expert Opin Biol Ther 4:1757–1770

Freytag SO, Barton KN, Brown SL, Narra V, Zhang Y, Tyson D, Nall C, Lu M, Ajlouni M, Movsas B, Kim JH (2007a) Replication-competent adenovirus-mediated suicide gene therapy with radiation in a preclinical model of pancreatic cancer. Mol Ther 15:1600–1606

Freytag SO, Movsas B, Aref I, Stricker H, Peabody J, Pegg J, Zhang Y, Barton KN, Brown SL, Lu M et al (2007b) Phase I trial of replication-competent adenovirus-mediated suicide gene therapy combined with IMRT for prostate cancer. Mol Ther 15:1016–1023

Glasgow JN, Everts M, Curiel DT (2006) Transductional targeting of adenovirus vectors for gene therapy. Cancer Gene Ther 13:830–844

Hammond SM (2006) MicroRNAs as oncogenes. Curr Opin Genet Dev 16:4–9

Hutvagner G, Simard MJ (2008) Argonaute proteins: key players in RNA silencing. Nat Rev Mol Cell Biol 9:22–32

Inoue S, Shanker M, Miyahara R, Gopalan B, Patel S, Oida Y, Branch CD, Munshi A, Meyn RE, Andreeff M et al (2006) MDA-7/IL-24-based cancer gene therapy: translation from the laboratory to the clinic. Curr Gene Ther 6:73–91

Kievit E, Bershad E, Ng E, Sethna P, Dev I, Lawrence TS, Rehemtulla A (1999) Superiority of yeast over bacterial cytosine deaminase for enzyme/prodrug gene therapy in colon cancer xenografts. Cancer Res 59:1417–1421

Kim DH, Rossi JJ (2007) Strategies for silencing human disease using RNA interference. Nat Rev Genet 8:173–184

Kim VN (2005) MicroRNA biogenesis: coordinated cropping and dicing. Nat Rev Mol Cell Biol 6:376–385

Kufe D, Weichselbaum R (2003) Radiation therapy: activation for gene transcription and the development of genetic radiotherapy-therapeutic strategies in oncology. Cancer Biol Ther 2:326–329

Li BJ, Tang Q, Cheng D, Qin C, Xie FY, Wei Q, Xu J, Liu Y, Zheng BJ, Woodle MC et al (2005a) Using siRNA in prophylactic and therapeutic regimens against SARS coronavirus in Rhesus macaque. Nat Med 11:944–951

Li C, Bowles DE, van Dyke T, Samulski RJ (2005b) Adeno-associated virus vectors: potential applications for cancer gene therapy. Cancer Gene Ther 12:913–925

Liu X, Fortin K, Mourelatos Z (2008) MicroRNAs: biogenesis and molecular functions. Brain Pathol 18:113–121

Lu Y, Dang H, Middleton B, Zhang Z, Washburn L, Stout DB, Campbell-Thompson M, Atkinson MA, Phelps M, Gambhir SS et al (2006) Noninvasive imaging of islet grafts using positron-emission tomography. Proc Natl Acad Sci USA 103:11294–11299

Martin SE, Caplen NJ (2007) Applications of RNA interference in mammalian systems. Annu Rev Genomics Hum Genet 8:81–108

Mattes J, Yang M, Foster PS (2007) Regulation of microRNA by antagomirs: a new class of pharmacological antagonists for the specific regulation of gene function? Am J Respir Cell Mol Biol 36:8–12

Mundt AJ, Vijayakumar S, Nemunaitis J, Sandler A, Schwartz H, Hanna N, Peabody T, Senzer N, Chu K, Rasmussen CS et al (2004) A phase I trial of TNFerade biologic in patients with soft tissue sarcoma in the extremities. Clin Cancer Res 10:5747–5753

Ng P, Graham FL (2002) Construction of first-generation adenoviral vectors. Methods Mol Med 69:389–414

Ng P, Parks RJ, Graham FL (2002) Preparation of helper-dependent adenoviral vectors. Methods Mol Med 69:371–388

Nie S, Xing Y, Kim GJ, Simons JW (2007) Nanotechnology applications in cancer. Annu Rev Biomed Eng 9:257–288

Putral LN, Gu W, McMillan NA (2006) RNA interference for the treatment of cancer. Drug News Perspect 19:317–324

Rosenberg E, Hawkins W, Holmes M, Amir C, Schmidt-Ullrich RK, Lin PS, Valerie K (2002) Radiosensitization of human glioma cells in vitro and in vivo with acyclovir and mutant HSV-TK75 expressed from adenovirus. Int J Radiat Oncol Biol Phys 52:831–836

Roth JA (2006) Adenovirus *p53* gene therapy. Expert Opin Biol Ther 6:55–61

Senzer N, Mani S, Rosemurgy A, Nemunaitis J, Cunningham C, Guha C, Bayol N, Gillen M, Chu K, Rasmussen C et al (2004) TNFerade biologic, an adenovector with a radiation-inducible promoter, carrying the human tumor necrosis factor alpha gene: a phase I study in patients with solid tumors. J Clin Oncol 22:592–601

Siddiqui F, Barton KN, Stricker HJ, Steyn PF, Larue SM, Karvelis KC, Sparks RB, Kim JH, Brown SL, Freytag SO (2007) Design considerations for incorporating sodium iodide symporter reporter gene imaging into prostate cancer gene therapy trials. Hum Gene Ther 18:312–322

Ternovoi VV, Curiel DT, Smith BF, Siegal GP (2006) Adenovirus-mediated p53 tumor suppressor gene therapy of osteosarcoma. Lab Invest 86:748–766

Tong AW, Nemunaitis J, Su, D, Zhang Y, Cunningham C, Senzer N, Netto G, Rich D, Mhashilkar A, Parker K et al (2005) Intratumoral injection of INGN 241, a nonreplicating adenovector expressing the melanoma-differentiation associated gene-7 (*mda-7/IL24*): biologic outcome in advanced cancer patients. Mol Ther 11:160–172

Trinh QT, Austin EA, Murray DM, Knick VC, Huber BE (1995) Enzyme/prodrug gene therapy: comparison of cytosine deaminase/5-fluorocytosine versus thymidine kinase/ganciclovir enzyme/prodrug systems in a human colorectal carcinoma cell line. Cancer Res 55:4808–4812

Tsai CH, Hong JH, Hsieh KF, Hsiao HW, Chuang WL, Lee CC, McBride WH, Chiang CS (2006) Tetracycline-regulated intratumoral expression of interleukin-3 enhances the efficacy of radiation therapy for murine prostate cancer. Cancer Gene Ther 13:1082–1092

Valerie K (1999) Viral vectors for gene therapy. In: Wu-Pong S, Rojanasakul Y (eds) Biopharmaceutical drug design and development. Humana, Totowa, New Jersey, pp 69–105

Valerie K, Hawkins W, Farnsworth J, Schmidt-Ullrich R, Lin PS, Amir C, Feden J (2001) Substantially improved in vivo radiosensitization of rat glioma with mutant HSV-TK and acyclovir. Cancer Gene Ther 8:3–8

Zamore PD, Haley B (2005) Ribo-gnome: the big world of small RNAs. Science 309:1519–1524

Tumor Biology's Impact on Clinical Cure Rates

19

Michael Baumann and Mechthild Krause

CONTENTS

KEY POINTS

- While tumor grading might influence, for example, the need for postoperative radiotherapy, current data do not suggest a clear impact on local tumor control probability.
- Local tumor control probability decreases with increasing tumor volume, which is caused by the increase of the number of cancer stem cells with tumor volume.
- Other stem-cell-related parameters, such as cancer stem-cell density or intrinsic radiosensitivity, are currently not known for individual tumors; thus, predictive assays that could tailor the prescribed dose to the individual patient are not yet a clinical tool.
- Repair capacity substantially impacts radiosensitivity. As this parameter can also substantially vary within one tumor entity, research into predictive assays for repair capacity of individual tumors may contribute to further improvement of tumor control rates.
- Repopulation of cancer stem cells during fractionated radiotherapy is among the most important mechanisms of radioresistance of tumors.
- In addition to the intertumoral heterogeneity, strong evidence has accumulated that parameters of the tumor micromilieu that affect radiosensitivity may also be heterogeneously distributed within the individual tumor (intratumoral heterogeneity).

M. Baumann, MD, PhD,
Department of Radiation Oncology, OncoRay Centre for Radiation Research in Oncology, Medical Faculty and University Hospital Carl Gustav Carus, Technische Universität Dresden, Fetscherstraße 74, 01307 Dresden, Germany

M. Krause, MD, PhD
Department of Radiation Oncology, OncoRay Centre for Radiation Research in Oncology, Medical Faculty and University Hospital Carl Gustav Carus, Technische Universität Dresden, Fetscherstraße 74, 01307 Dresden, Germany

19.1
Introduction

Cure of cancer is defined as locoregional tumor control without distant metastases and without life-threatening treatment complications. Radiotherapy is one of the main cancer treatment modalities. As a local treatment, its aim is to achieve locoregional tumor control by inactivation of all cancer stem cells within the primary tumor and regional lymph nodes. Treatment effects on local tumor control are therefore the focus of this chapter; however, also potential indirect effects on the risk of distant metastases are briefly considered.

It is well recognized that the probability to permanently control tumors increases as a sigmoid function with increasing radiation dose. Below a threshold, the dose is not sufficient to inactivate all cancer stem cells in a tumor, i.e. all tumors recur. After this threshold, tumor control increases with increasing radiation dose, approaching 100% at high doses.

Even if some data suggest a higher metastatic potential of tumors during radiotherapy, successful radiotherapy is an effective way to stop metastasis at the source, thereby importantly contributing to overall survival of the patient.

Inclusion of biological parameters of the individual tumors is anticipated to further improve the results of radiotherapy by tailoring dose and treatment schedule, by combining radiotherapy with modern drugs, and by taking into account intratumoral heterogeneity based on biological imaging.

19.2
Inactivation of Cancer Stem Cells and Local Tumor Control

A cancer stem cell is defined as a cell within a tumor that possesses the capacity to self renew and to generate the heterogeneous lineages of cancer cells that comprise the tumor (Clarke et al. 2006). In the context of radiotherapy a cancer stem cell is defined as a cell that, if not killed by radiation, forms a tumor recurrence (Baumann et al. 2008, in press). Curative radiotherapy therefore aims at inactivation of all cancer stem cells in the primary tumor and locoregional lymph nodes. It is well recognized that the probability to permanently control tumors (tumor control probability, TCP) increases as a sigmoid function with increasing radiation dose. Below a threshold, the dose is never sufficient to inactivate all cancer stem cells in a tumor, i.e. all tumors recur. After

this threshold, tumor control increases relatively steeply with increasing radiation dose, approaching 100% at high doses. From the dose–response curves descriptors of their relative position, such as the radiation dose necessary to control 50% of the tumors (tumor control dose 50%, TCD50), can be easily derived. The sigmoid shape of the dose–response relationship for local control reflects the exponential inactivation of cancer stem cells by radiation and a Poisson distribution of surviving cancer stem cells (Munro and Gilbert 1961; Suit et al. 1987; Bentzen and Tucker 1997; Bentzen 2002; Baumann and Petersen 2005; Baumann et al. 2005).

For determination of the outcome of preclinical as well as clinical studies on radiation, it is important to discriminate local tumor control from volume-dependent endpoints such as tumor regression or tumor growth delay. Those cells which may form a recurrence after therapy, i.e. cancer stem cells, constitute only a small proportion of all cancer cells, whereas the bulk of tumor cells are non-tumorigenic (Baumann et al. 2008, in press); thus, changes in tumor volume after therapy are governed by the bulk of tumor cells, i.e. primarily by the non-stem cells. As outlined above, local tumor control is dependent on the complete inactivation of the subpopulation of cancer stem cells (Baumann et al. 2008). For a variety of reasons, including time and cost, volume-dependent endpoints are currently widely used for preclinical studies in cancer research. This carries a substantial risk that new treatments may be optimized for their effect on the bulk of non-stem cancer cells, with no improvement in the curative potential (Baumann et al. 2008). This has been demonstrated in several experiments which showed effects of novel combined radiation treatments on growth delay, but for the same treatment, not on the local tumor control (reviewed in Krause et al. 2006; Baumann et al. 2008). Overall, these experiments support the use of cancer-stem-cell-specific endpoints to test the effect of new treatment schedules or the predictive value of biological parameters in preclinical and clinical radiation oncology.

19.3
Heterogeneity Between Tumors and Steepness of Dose–Response Curves

A widely used method to quantify the steepness of dose–response relationships for local tumor control is the normalized dose–response gradient, or γ value (Brahme 1984; Bentzen and Tucker 1997). This value defines the percentage of increase in response for a 1% increase in dose at a specified response level in the steep part of the dose–response curve, e.g. 50% (γ50). It is important to note that dose–response curves for tumor control in experiments, and particularly in the clinical setting, are usually shallower than those calculated using biostatistical modelling. This is caused by heterogeneity in biological characteristics of the tumors. Figure 19.1 shows as an example the results of an experiment on nine different human head and neck squamous cell carcinomas (SCC) in nude mice. All tumors were irradiated at the same size with an identical fractionation schedule, i.e. 30 fractions within 6 weeks. Despite that all tumors are of the same entity, the dose relationships differ substantially in position and steepness. Four tumor lines are relatively sensitive with TCD50 values of 40–50 Gy. Two tumor lines exhibit intermediate resistance, whereas three lines, with TCD50 values of 90–130 Gy, are exquisitely radioresistant. The bold curve represents the composite dose–response relationship of all nine tumor lines. It is considerably less steep than most of the underlying dose–response relationships of the individual tumor models. The composite dose–response curve is close to the current clinical situation if strictly size-matched tumors of the same histology and origin (e.g. head and neck SCC) in different patients are evaluated. The reason for the relatively flat composite dose–response curve is that biological characteristics important for local tumor control, e.g. cancer-stem-cell, density or intrinsic radiosensitivity, are currently not known for the individual tumor. If we knew the biological parameters, which impact

the dose–response for individual tumors from predictive assays, with sufficient certainty, we could tailor the prescribed dose to the individual patient. For example, if we knew that a tumor in a given patient falls under the four sensitive tumor lines shown in Fig. 19.1, we could limit the radiation dose without jeopardizing local tumor control, thereby sparing normal tissues. If, in contrast, a given tumor falls under the three resistant lines, one would need to consider dose escalation, combination with radiosensitizing drugs, combination with surgery or LET beams if we want to achieve local control. The current status of determination of biological parameters to predict local tumor control is discussed in Sect. 19.5.

19.4
Heterogeneity Within Individual Tumors and Its Potential Importance for Optimizing Radiation Dose Distributions

In addition to differences of the overall radiosensitivity between different tumors (intertumoral heterogeneity), strong evidence has accumulated that biological parameters which affect radiosensitivity may also be heterogeneously distributed within the individual tumor (intratumoral heterogeneity). Figure 19.2 shows examples of heterogenous distribution of hypoxic tumor volumes detected by functional histology using the hypoxia marker pimonidazole (Fig. 19.2a) or by autoradiography using the hypoxia-specific tracer 18F-misonidazole (Fig. 19.2b) in an experimental SCC. Such intratumoral heterogeneity can also be detected by histology or functional imaging in patients. As an example, Fig. 19.2c shows a PET-CT after injection of 18-Fluordeoxyglucose or 18-F-misonidazole in a patient suffering from head and neck SCC. Knowledge of the spatial distribution of radioresistant vs radiosensitive tumor subvolumes, in principle, may be the basis for individualized, biologically adapted heterogeneous radiation dose distribution ("dose painting") to improve local tumor control (LING et al. 2000; BENTZEN 2005; BAUMANN 2006). Of interest in this context are recent reports that cancer stem cells may not be generally distributed evenly over the tumor but may accumulate preferentially in so-called microenvironmental niches (GILBERTSON and RICH 2007). These niches cannot yet be detected by imaging methods; however, it appears promising to explore the possibility of development of stem-cell-specific imaging modalities for development of irradiation techniques that allow inhomogeneous dose distributions adapted to both, inhomogeneous stem-cell density and inho-

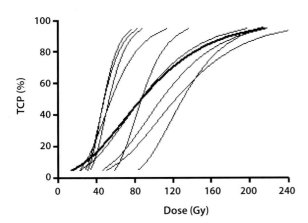

Fig. 19.1. Impact of heterogeneity in biological characteristics of tumors on dose–response for local tumor control probability (TCP). Nine different human head and neck squamous cell carcinomas in nude mice were irradiated at the same size with 30 fractions in 6 weeks. Despite that all tumors are of the same entity, the dose relationships differ substantially in position and steepness. The *bold curve* represents the composite dose–response relationship of all nine tumor lines

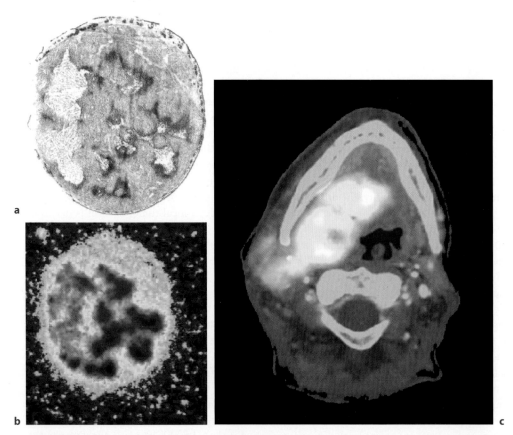

Fig. 19.2a–c. Heterogenous distribution of hypoxic tumor subvolumes detected by functional histology (pimonidazole; **a**) or by autoradiography (18F-misonidazole; **b**) in an experimental squamous cell carcinoma. Similar heterogeneity is regularly observed in patient tumors. **c** Heterogeneous distribution of the PET hypoxia marker 18F-misonidazole in comparison with the CT volume of the tumor

mogeneous distribution of microenvironment-driven radiosensitive and radioresistant tumor subvolumes.

19.5
Important Biological Parameters that Impact Local Tumor Control

19.5.1
Histology and Grading

It is well recognized that tumors of different histology, e.g. seminoma vs glioblastoma, are characterized by different radiosensitivity. Because of its strong predictive power, categorization of tumors by histology has been a major basis for dose prescription for already a century now (BECK-BORNHOLDT 1993). For a given histology, the importance of grading for local tumor control is more complex to judge. Poor differentiation has generally been associated with poor prognosis, but this ap-

pears more related to stage at diagnosis and to the rate of metastases than to the chance to locally control the tumor by radiation. Local subclinical extension of tumors is generally less in well-differentiated tumors than in poorly differentiated or undifferentiated tumors; therefore, grading is an important parameter to prescribe postoperative radiotherapy and to design margins in several tumor entities, e.g. soft tissue sarcoma, glioma, head and neck and endometrial carcinoma. The impact of grading on radiosensitivity of size-matched tumors of the same entity is less clear. It is often suspected that well-differentiated tumors are more radioresistant than undifferentiated tumors of the same histology (BERGONIE and TRIBONDEAU 1959). While such a correlation has been observed in some clinical series, it is overall not well supported by clinical outcome data (STUSCHKE et al. 1993). As others before (FLETCHER 1980, 1988), the authors of the present chapter suspect that the idea that well-differentiated tumors are radioresistant, historically originates from the experiments performed by BERGONIE and TRIBONDEAU on rat testis.

These experiments showed that irradiation destroyed germinal cells, whereas the interstitial tissue and sertoli syncytium remained unimpaired. They concluded that irradiation is more effective in cells that have a greater reproductive activity (Bergonie and Tribondeau 1959). Experimental investigations in vitro revealed that the dose necessary to eradicate tumor cell spheroids was higher in undifferentiated than in differentiated tumor lines, whereas the capacity to recover from sublethal radiation damage during fractionated irradiation was higher in better differentiated tumor lines (Stuschke et al. 1993). Another factor that may have contributed to the idea of radioresistance of well-differentiated tumors is that there is a correlation between speed of tumor growth and velocity of tumor regression (Fletcher 1980, 1988). This may lead to faster tumor regression in undifferentiated tumors and to the impression of higher radiosensitivity, which may vanish when permanent local tumor control is investigated; however, there is some suggestion that, as a reminder of their epithelial tissue of origin, well-differentiated head and neck SCCs may have a higher capacity for repopulation of cancer stem cells as a consequence of radiation injury (see Chap. 15). This would indeed lead to higher radioresistance of such tumors, but only after long fractionation schedules and not after accelerated treatments or single-dose stereotactic irradiation. In contrast, in prostate cancer, based on the results of randomized trials, higher doses are applied for intermediate-risk tumors than for low-risk tumors. Gleason score, as a measure of differentiation, is one of the parameters that determines the risk category (Jereczek-Fossa and Orecchia 2007). Overall, no general conclusion can currently be drawn regarding the impact of grading on local tumor control probability after radiotherapy. The often-heard statement that, based on examination of histological specimens, a tumor, because of good differentiation, would not be radiosensitive, should not be accepted by today's radiation oncologists. Better biological parameters for prediction are urgently needed.

19.5.2
Tumor Volume

It is the general experience of radiation oncologists that large tumors are more difficult to control by radiotherapy than small tumors. On the one hand, this is due to the often very large volumes of normal tissues irradiated to high doses, which can be dose- (and therefore success-) limiting in large tumors. On the other hand, the number of cancer stem cells increases with increasing tumor volume, leading to a higher radiation dose necessary for local tumor control (see sect. 19.2). A strong correlation between tumor control dose and the logarithm of tumor volume has been demonstrated in experimental tumor models as well as in clinical studies (Baumann et al. 1990a; Johnson et al. 1995; Bentzen and Thames 1996; Dubben et al. 1998). Exactly this correlation is predicted by an expected linear increase of the number of cancer stem cells with tumor volume and radiobiological models of stem-cell inactivation (Suit et al. 1965; Baumann et al. 1990a; Johnson et al. 1995; Bentzen and Thames 1996; Kummermehr and Trott 1997; Dubben et al. 1998).

19.5.3
Stem-Cell Density

It has been demonstrated in preclinical experiments that the number of cancer cells which need to be transplanted to achieve a tumor take in half of the recipient animals (tumor dose 50%, TD50) may vary by several logarithms between different tumor models (Hill and Milas 1989). The TD50 is a direct measure of stem-cell density in a given tumor (Hill and Milas 1989; Baumann et al. 1990a, in press). Experiments which show that the TCD50 after single doses correlates with the logarithm of TD50, implying that a higher stem-cell content per volume tumor leads to a higher radioresistance, are of great importance (Hill and Milas 1989). Recently published data on experimental SCC extend these studies and show a significant correlation of TCD50 after single doses with TCD50 after irradiation with 30 fractions over 6 weeks. These data suggest that pretreatment tumor stem-cell density and cellular radiosensitivity are major predictors of local control after clinically relevant radiation treatment.

19.5.4
Intrinsic Radiosensitivity

The above-mentioned experiments showing that TCD50 after fractionated irradiation correlates closely with TCD50 after single doses indicate that the number of cancer stem cells to be inactivated and their intrinsic radiosensitivity are major determinants of radioresistance of a given tumor. This is further supported by other experiments, which showed that only the combination of stem-cell density determined by TD50 and their intrinsic radiosensitivity significantly predict tumor radiocurability (Gerweck et al. 1994). Intrinsic radiosensitivity has widely been described by the SF2, i.e. the surviving fraction of tumor cells in vitro after irradiation with 2 Gy, a dose often used in the clinic. SF2 measures clonogenic survival, defined as colony formation under idealized growth conditions in vitro. It is noteworthy that the five to six cell divisions necessary for colony formation (usually defined as >50 cells) do not necessarily measure cancer stem cells, as these are defined as being able to form a complete tumor (see above). Re-evaluation of SF2 values for different tumor cell lines has shown that those histologies, which are expected to be radioresistant in the clinic, have, on average, higher SF2 values compared with more radio-sensitive tumors (MALAISE et al. 1986). Correlation of SF2 with survival or local tumor control in individual patients in some cases supported the importance of intrinsic radiosensitivity of clonogenic tumor cells for outcome of radiotherapy (RAMSAY et al. 1992; GIRINSKY et al. 1994; WEST et al. 1997); however, numerous other data sets did not confirm such a correlation (BROCK et al. 1990; ALLALUNIS-TURNER et al. 1992; TAGHIAN et al. 1993; ESCHWEGE et al. 1997; STAUSBOL-GRON and OVERGAARD 1999). Underlying reasons for these contradictory results include most likely that current clonogenic ex-vivo assays do not necessarily measure the radiosensitivity of cancer stem cells or yield different results because of differences between in-vivo and in-vitro microenvironmental conditions, including differences in cell–cell and cell–stroma interactions.

19.5.5
Apoptosis vs Other Cell-Death Mechanisms

Cells can die in several ways (OKADA and MAK 2004; BROWN and ATTARDI 2005), i.e. by apoptosis, mitotic catastrophe, senescence, necrosis and autophagy. Mitotic catastrophe caused by lethal chromosome damage is the most important cell-death mechanism for the effect of radiotherapy of solid tumors. After irradiation, cells can pass through few mitotic cycles before missegregation of chromosomes or cell fusion leads to the loss of the replicative potential of cells. While apoptosis has obtained much interest as a cell-death mechanism in neoplastic disease, it appears not to be the main mechanism of radiation-induced cell death, at least not in solid tumors. Apoptotic index or levels of proteins involved in apoptosis (e.g. p53, Bcl-2) are not predictive of the response of solid tumors to radiotherapy (BROWN and WOUTERS 1999; BROWN and WILSON 2003; BROWN and ATTARDI 2005). For example, the significantly decreased apoptotic fraction in Bcl-2 overexpressing cells after irradiation did not change clonogenic cell survival (WOUTERS et al. 1999). Thus far, no distinct radiation-dependent pathway for cellular necrosis has been de-

scribed; however, it is has been shown in a variety of studies that tumors after radiotherapy or radiochemotherapy often show massive necrosis, which sometimes correlates with improved prognosis (THOMAS et al. 1999; VECCHIO et al. 2005; DINCBAS et al. 2005). It can be speculated that this radiation-induced necrosis is the consequence of cell death by mitotic catastrophe in combination with effects of irradiation on the tumor microenvironment.

19.5.6
Repair Capacity and Fractionation Sensitivity

Both, tumors and normal tissues, repair the vast majority of radiation-induced DNA damage within hours after induction. Remaining, i.e. non- or falsely repaired, double-strand breaks are presently considered to be the most important mechanism for radiation-induced cell kill (FRANKENBERG-SCHWAGER 1989; ILIAKIS 1991; DIKOMEY et al. 2003; KASTEN-PISULA et al. 2005). Radiosensitivity of individual tumors might be predictable by evaluation of DNA repair-related proteins. Currently among the best investigated proteins is phosphorylated histone H2AX (γH2AX). Phosphorylation of H2AX occurs in response to DNA double-strand breaks, e.g. induced by irradiation. Foci formation of γH2AX around the double-strand breaks can be visualized microscopically after antibody labelling and correlates with the repair kinetics of DNA double-strand breaks. Recent preclinical data suggest a predictive value of residual γH2AX foci measured 24 h after irradiation with the individual radiosensitivity (KLOKOV et al. 2006) as well as a correlation with tumor hypoxia (BRISTOW et al. 2007). The capacity to repair sublethal damage between irradiation fractions can be expressed by the α/β value of different tumors. Generally, α/β values of many tumors are in the range of early-responding normal tissues or higher (WILLIAMS et al. 1985), whereas late-responding normal tissues usually have low α/β values, i.e. a better repair capacity (VAN DER KOGEL 2002). This differential has been the basis for successful clinical introduction of hyperfractionated irradiation schedules, particularly in head and neck SCC (BOURHIS et al. 2006); however, there are important exceptions, and some tumor entities appear to be characterized by significantly low α/β values in the range of late-responding normal tissues or even lower. Thus far, this has been clinically best investigated for breast cancer by several randomized clinical trials; however, also for prostate cancer, low-grade soft tissue sarcoma, melanoma and possibly other tumors low α/β values are suspected from clinical data (THAMES and SUIT 1986; BRENNER and HALL 1999; STUSCHKE and

Thames 1999; Williams et al. 2007; Bentzen et al. 2008a,b). For tumors with lower α/β values compared with the surrounding normal tissues, hypofractionation may be a viable option to improve the therapeutic ratio of radiotherapy, particularly as hypofractionation may also be a convenient way to accelerate the treatment, thereby counteracting repopulation (see below). Adaptation of the dose per fraction currently is limited to tumor entities and cannot be tailored to tumors in individual patients. As it is known that the repair capacity can also substantially vary within one tumor entity (Williams et al. 1985; Petersen et al. 1998), research into predictive assays for repair capacity of individual tumors may contribute to further improvement of tumor control rates.

19.5.7
Repopulation

Repopulation of cancer stem cells during fractionated radiotherapy is among the most important mechanisms of radioresistance of tumors. Repopulation has been best demonstrated for head and neck SCC where a host of preclinical and randomized clinical studies are available. Repopulation is extensively reviewed in Chap. 15. Because of its importance, and the recognized heterogeneity between different tumors (Petersen et al. 2001; Hessel et al. 2004a,b), intense efforts have been made to develop predictive assays for repopulation, which may be used to select patients for accelerated fractionation schedules. While initial studies on the potential doubling time of tumor cells, studied by flow cytometry after BrdU or IrdU labelling, showed promise, a large multicentre study did not reveal a predictive value for local tumor control or survival after radiotherapy (Begg et al. 1999). As outlined above, several studies in head and neck SCC suggest more pronounced repopulation in better-differentiated tumors. Also expression of the epidermal growth factor receptor (EGFR) might correlate with repopulation of cancer stem cells (Schmidt-Ullrich et al. 1997; Petersen et al. 2003; Eriksen et al. 2004a,b, 2005a,b; Bentzen et al. 2005; Krause et al. 2005; Baumann et al. 2007). In addition, TP53 mutations might predict local tumor control after accelerated radiotherapy in head and neck cancer (Alsner et al. 2001; Eriksen et al. 2005). As a large number of factors are involved in response of tumors to radiotherapy, it is likely that multiparametric approaches will better predict response to specific treatment schedules. While several studies were published on prognostic implications of molecular marker profiles (e.g. van't Veer et al. 2002; Seigneuric et al. 2007), studies on

the predictive value for radiotherapy are limited thus far; however, using the candidate-gene approach, which concentrates on genes or proteins that are known to be involved in tumor (or normal tissue) response, promising results for potential prediction of the response to accelerated radiotherapy schedules could be shown in two studies (Buffa et al. 2004; Eriksen et al. 2004).

19.5.8
Hypoxia and Other Factors of the Tumor Micromilieu

The chaotic vasculature of malignant tumors causes a heterogeneous oxygenation with well-oxygenated areas, hypoxic vital tumor regions and necrotic areas (Vaupel et al. 1989; Vaupel 2004). As hypoxic cancer stem cells are known to be more radioresistant, a number of studies tested the predictive value of tumor oxygenation on local tumor control after radiotherapy. Using polagraphic needle electrodes to measure pO2, the *prognostic* value of tumor hypoxia on local tumor control, and also on distant metastases, has been demonstrated for different tumor entities (Hockel and Vaupel 2001). In the largest study performed to date, a multicentric analysis of almost 400 patients with head and neck carcinoma, better oxygenation was prognostic for survival (Nordsmark et al. 2005). Preclinical data show that tumor hypoxia measured in histological sections of untreated tumors after injection of the hypoxia marker pimonidazole significantly correlates with local tumor control after fractionated irradiation (Yaromina et al. 2006). Also analysis of 43 tumors from head and neck cancer patients treated in a phase-II clinical trial indicates a correlation of pretherapeutic pimonidazole hypoxic fraction with local tumor control as well as with overall survival (Kaanders et al. 2002). In preclinical investigations plasminogen activator inhibitor-1 in tumor tissue correlated with hypoxia and tumor control after fractionated irradiation. Retrospective evaluation of plasma osteopontin levels, a protein which is activated by hypoxia, for head and neck cancer patients treated in the randomized DAHANCA 5 trial, showed a significant correlation with locoregional tumor control and disease-specific survival after radiotherapy (Overgaard et al. 2005). Furthermore, the outcome of patients with high, but not with low, osteopontin levels could be improved by the hypoxic cell sensitizer nimorazole, suggesting not only a prognostic but also a predictive value of osteopontin (Overgaard et al. 2005). It is still unclear which hypoxia marker has the highest relevance as a possible predictor for the outcome of radiotherapy (Nordsmark et al. 2007). Early experience is accumulating showing that hypoxia measured by PET imaging may yield predictive information useful for radiotherapy treatment planning and monitoring (THORWARTH and ALBER 2008). Independent of hypoxia, high tumor lactate levels have been shown to correlate with high TCD50 values after fractionated radiation in a preclinical study (QUENNET et al. 2006) and with prognosis in clinical investigations (WALENTA et al. 2000). As lactate levels can be mapped using specialized MRI, these results bear considerable promise for further studies assessing this technology for radiotherapy treatment planning.

19.6
Local Control and Distant Metastases

It has been speculated that cancer, at some very early stages, almost always reflects systemic disease. In addition, it has been hypothesized that those tumors which are radioresistant, and can currently not be locally controlled by radiation, are particularly malignant and therefore have a very high risk of subclinical distant metastases. Also, some experiments seem to suggest that radiation itself might increase the risk of tumors to metastasize (BAUMANN et al. 1990b; O'REILLY et al. 1994; CAMPHAUSEN et al. 2001). These three arguments seem to support the conclusion that improvement of local tumor control by more effective radiation treatments will have only negligible or no impact on survival. Nevertheless, there is ample experimental and clinical evidence that improved local tumor control improves survival. Several experiments demonstrate that the incidence of distant metastases in the same murine tumor lines is higher for local recurrences than in locally controlled tumors after radiotherapy or surgery (Table 19.1). The most likely explanation for this finding is that the overall integral tumor burden is higher in local recurrences. Even if the risk of a cancer cell to form a metastasis might be increased during radiation, e.g. because of altered gene expression or because of disturbance of tumor cell (stromal interactions), the overall number of tumor cells at risk decreases very rapidly during radiotherapy, which leads to a significant overall decrease in the risk to metastasize per tumor (RAMSAY et al. 1988; BAUMANN et al. 1990a,b). The observation of less-distant metastases in locally controlled tumors has been confirmed in extensive retrospective analysis of clinical results (SUIT et al. 1970; SUIT and WESTGATE 1986; SUIT 1992). Correlation analysis of radiosensitivity and metastasis has revealed that the cellular radiosensitivity measured ex vivo in head and neck, cervix or endometrial cancer was not different for patients with or without distant metastases. Furthermore, no correlation was found between TCD50 and incidence of distant metastases in a panel of 24 murine tumor models (SUIT et al. 1994). Last but not least, a number of randomized trials published in the past two decades clearly demonstrate that improved local control of, for example, breast can-

Table 19.1. Local tumor control and metastatic spread (murine tumors). *SCC* squamous cell carcinoma, *RT* radiotherapy, *OP* surgery

Reference	Tumor	Treatment	Lung metastases	
			Controlled (%)	Relapsed (%)
SHELDON et al. (1974)	Mammary carcinoma	RT	8	35
TODOROKI and SUIT (1985)	Sarcoma	OP	7	26
		RT	9	56
		OP + RT	7	45
RAMSAY et al. (1988)	SCC	RT	7	43
		RT	3	13
BAUMANN et al. (1990b)	SCC	RT	5	25
		RT	10	40

cer, rectal carcinoma, head and neck carcinoma, lung cancer, or cancer of the uterine cervix after intensified locoregional treatment approaches lead to better survival or decreased rates of distant metastases (Horiot et al. 1992; Gunderson and Martenson 1993; SRC Group 1997; Whelan et al. 2000; Bourhis et al. 2004); therefore, the overall conclusion of this chapter is that successful radiotherapy is an effective way to stop metastasis at their source, thereby significantly contributing to overall survival of the patient.

19.7
Conclusion

Several tumor biological parameters have been identified to impact local tumor control after radiotherapy in preclinical models as well as in clinical tumors. Some of these parameters are presently regularly considered for prescription of treatment in clinical practice, whereas for several other parameters predictive assays are still evolving. Inclusion of biological parameters of the individual tumors is anticipated to further improve the results of radiotherapy by tailoring dose and treatment schedule, by combining radiotherapy with modern drugs, and by consideration of intratumoral heterogeneity based on biological imaging. Improvement of local tumor control by these biology-driven approaches is expected to contribute significantly to improved survival.

Acknowledgements

This work is supported by the German Research Council (DFG Ba1433) and the German Federal Ministry of Education and Research (03ZIK041, 03ZIK042, 03NUK006B).

References

Allalunis-Turner MJ et al. (1992) Radiosensitivity testing of human primary brain tumor specimens. Int J Radiat Oncol Biol Phys 23(2):339–343

Alsner J, Sorensen SB, Overgaard J (2001) TP53 mutation is related to poor prognosis after radiotherapy, but not surgery, in squamous cell carcinoma of the head and neck. Radiother Oncol 59(2):179–185

Baumann M (2006) Keynote comment: radiotherapy in the age of molecular oncology. Lancet Oncol 7(10):786–787

Baumann M, Petersen C (2005) TCP and NTCP: a basic introduction. Rays 30(2):99–104

Baumann M, Dubois W, Suit HD (1990a) Response of human squamous cell carcinoma xenografts of different sizes to irradiation: relationship of clonogenic cells, cellular radiation sensitivity in vivo, and tumor rescuing units. Radiat Res 123(3):325–330

Baumann M, Suit HD, Sedlacek RS (1990b) Metastases after fractionated radiation therapy of three murine tumor models. Int J Radiat Oncol Biol Phys 19(2):367–370

Baumann M, Petersen C, Krause M (2005) TCP and NTCP in preclinical and clinical research in Europe. Rays 30(2):121–126

Baumann M et al. (2007) EGFR-targeted anti-cancer drugs in radiotherapy: preclinical evaluation of mechanisms. Radiother Oncol 83(3):238–248

Baumann M, Krause M, Hill R (2008) Exploring the role of cancer stem cells in radioresistance. Nat Rev Cancer 8(7):545–554

Baumann M et al. Cancer stem cells and radiotherapy. Int J Radiat Biol (in press)

Beck-Bornholdt HP (ed) (1993) Current topics in clinical radiobiology of tumors. 1st edn. Springer, Berlin, Heidelberg New York

Begg AC et al. (1999) The value of pretreatment cell kinetic parameters as predictors for radiotherapy outcome in head and neck cancer: a multicenter analysis. Radiother Oncol 50(1):13–23

Bentzen SM (2002) Dose–response relationships in radiotherapy. In: Steel GG (ed) Basic clinical radiobiology. Arnold, London, pp 94–104

Bentzen SM (2005) Theragnostic imaging for radiation oncology: dose-painting by numbers. Lancet Oncol 6(2):112–117

Bentzen SM, Thames HD (1996) Tumor volume and local control probability: clinical data and radiobiological interpretations. Int J Radiat Oncol Biol Phys 36(1):247–251

Bentzen SM, Tucker SL (1997) Quantifying the position and steepness of radiation dose–response curves. Int J Radiat Biol 71(5):531–542

Bentzen SM et al. (2005) Epidermal growth factor receptor expression in pretreatment biopsies from head and neck squamous cell carcinoma as a predictive factor for a benefit from accelerated radiation therapy in a randomized controlled trial. J Clin Oncol 23(24):5560–5567

Bentzen SM et al. (2008a) The UK Standardisation of Breast Radiotherapy (START) Trial A of radiotherapy hypofractionation for treatment of early breast cancer: a randomised trial. Lancet Oncol 9(4):331–341

Bentzen SM et al. (2008b) The UK Standardisation of Breast Radiotherapy (START) Trial B of radiotherapy hypofractionation for treatment of early breast cancer: a randomised trial. Lancet 371(9618):1098–1107

Bergonie J, Tribondeau L (1959) Interpretation of some results of radiotherapy and an attempt at determining a logical technique of treatment. Translation of original article in CR Acad Sci 143:983, 1906. Radiat Res 11:587–588

Bourhis J et al. (2004) Concomitant radiochemotherapy or accelerated radiotherapy: analysis of two randomized trials of the French Head and Neck Cancer Group (GORTEC). Semin Oncol 31(6):822–826

Bourhis J et al. (2006) Hyperfractionated or accelerated radiotherapy in head and neck cancer: a meta-analysis. Lancet 368(9538):843–854

Brahme A (1984) Dosimetric precision requirements in radiation therapy. Acta Radiol Oncol 23(5):379–391

Brenner DJ, Hall EJ (1999) Fractionation and protraction for radiotherapy of prostate carcinoma. Int J Radiat Oncol Biol Phys 43(5):1095–1101

Bristow RG et al. (2007) Homologous recombination and prostate cancer: a model for novel DNA repair targets and therapies. Radiother Oncol 83(3):220–230

Brock WA et al. (1990) Cellular radiosensitivity of primary head and neck squamous cell carcinomas and local tumor control. Int J Radiat Oncol Biol Phys 18(6):1283–1286

Brown JM, Attardi LD (2005) The role of apoptosis in cancer development and treatment response. Nat Rev Cancer 5(3):231–237

Brown JM, Wilson G (2003) Apoptosis genes and resistance to cancer therapy: What does the experimental and clinical data tell us? Cancer Biol Ther 2(5):477–490

Brown JM, Wouters BG (1999) Apoptosis, p53, and tumor cell sensitivity to anticancer agents. Cancer Res 59(7):1391–1399

Buffa FM et al. (2004) Molecular marker profiles predict locoregional control of head and neck squamous cell carcinoma in a randomized trial of continuous hyperfractionated accelerated radiotherapy. Clin Cancer Res 10(11):3745–3754

Camphausen K et al. (2001) Radiation therapy to a primary tumor accelerates metastatic growth in mice. Cancer Res 61(5):2207–2211

Clarke MF et al. (2006) Cancer stem cells: perspectives on current status and future directions: AACR Workshop on Cancer Stem Cells. Cancer Res 66(19):9339–9344

Dincbas FO et al. (2005) The role of preoperative radiotherapy in nonmetastatic high-grade osteosarcoma of the extremities for limb-sparing surgery. Int J Radiat Oncol Biol Phys 62(3):820–828

Dikomey E et al. (2003) Molecular mechanisms of individual radiosensitivity studied in normal diploid human fibroblasts. Toxicology 193(1–2):125–135

Dubben HH, Thames HD, Beck-Bornholdt HP (1998) Tumor volume: a basic and specific response predictor in radiotherapy. Radiother Oncol 47(2):167–174

Eriksen JG et al. (2004a) Molecular profiles as predictive marker for the effect of overall treatment time of radiotherapy in supraglottic larynx squamous cell carcinomas. Radiother Oncol 72(3):275–282

Eriksen JG et al. (2004b) The prognostic value of epidermal growth factor receptor is related to tumor differentiation and the overall treatment time of radiotherapy in squamous cell carcinomas of the head and neck. Int J Radiat Oncol Biol Phys 58(2):561–566

Eriksen JG et al. (2005a) The possible role of TP53 mutation status in the treatment of squamous cell carcinomas of the head and neck (HNSCC) with radiotherapy with different overall treatment times. Radiother Oncol 76(2):135–142

Eriksen JG, Steiniche T, Overgaard J (2005b) The influence of epidermal growth factor receptor and tumor differentiation on the response to accelerated radiotherapy of squamous cell carcinomas of the head and neck in the randomized DAHANCA 6 and 7 study. Radiother Oncol 74(2):93–100

Eschwege F et al. (1997) Predictive assays of radiation response in patients with head and neck squamous cell carcinoma: a review of the Institute Gustave Roussy experience. Int J Radiat Oncol Biol Phys 39(4):849–853

Fletcher GH (1980) Textbook of radiotherapy, 3rd edn. Lea and Febiger, Philadelphia

Fletcher GH (1988) Regaud lecture perspectives on the history of radiotherapy. Radiother Oncol 12(4):iii–v, 253–271

Frankenberg-Schwager M (1989) Review of repair kinetics for DNA damage induced in eukaryotic cells in vitro by ionizing radiation. Radiother Oncol 14(4):307–320

Gerweck LE, Zaidi ST, Zietman A (1994) Multivariate determinants of radiocurability. I: Prediction of single fraction tumor control doses. Int J Radiat Oncol Biol Phys 29(1):57–66

Gilbertson RJ, Rich JN (2007) Making a tumor's bed: glioblastoma stem cells and the vascular niche. Nat Rev Cancer 7(10):733–736

Girinsky T et al. (1994) In vitro parameters and treatment outcome in head and neck cancers treated with surgery and/or radiation: cell characterization and correlations with local control and overall survival. Int J Radiat Oncol Biol Phys 30(4):789–794

Gunderson LL, Martenson JA (1993) Postoperative adjuvant irradiation with or without chemotherapy for rectal carcinoma. Semin Radiat Oncol 3(1):55–63

Hessel F et al. (2004a) Differentiation status of human squamous cell carcinoma xenografts does not appear to correlate with the repopulation capacity of clonogenic tumor cells during fractionated irradiation. Int J Radiat Biol 80(10):719–727

Hessel F et al. (2004b) Repopulation of moderately well-differentiated and keratinizing GL human squamous cell carcinomas growing in nude mice. Int J Radiat Oncol Biol Phys 58(2):510–518

Hill RP, Milas L (1989) The proportion of stem cells in murine tumors. Int J Radiat Oncol Biol Phys 16(2):513–518

Hockel M, Vaupel P (2001) Tumor hypoxia: definitions and current clinical, biologic, and molecular aspects. J Natl Cancer Inst 93(4):266–276

Horiot JC et al. (1992) Hyperfractionation versus conventional fractionation in oropharyngeal carcinoma: final analysis of a randomized trial of the EORTC cooperative group of radiotherapy. Radiother Oncol 25(4):231–241

Iliakis G (1991) The role of DNA double strand breaks in ionizing radiation-induced killing of eukaryotic cells. Bioessays 13(12):641–648

Jereczek-Fossa BA, Orecchia R (2007) Evidence-based radiation oncology: definitive, adjuvant and salvage radiotherapy for non-metastatic prostate cancer. Radiother Oncol 84(2):197–215

Johnson CR et al. (1995) The tumor volume and clonogen number relationship: tumor control predictions based upon tumor volume estimates derived from computed tomography. Int J Radiat Oncol Biol Phys 33(2):281–287

Kaanders JH et al. (2002) Pimonidazole binding and tumor vascularity predict for treatment outcome in head and neck cancer. Cancer Res 62(23):7066–7074

Kasten-Pisula U, Tastan H, Dikomey E (2005) Huge differences in cellular radiosensitivity due to only very small variations in double-strand break repair capacity. Int J Radiat Biol 81(6):409–419

Klokov D et al. (2006) Phosphorylated histone H2AX in relation to cell survival in tumor cells and xenografts exposed to single and fractionated doses of X-rays. Radiother Oncol 80(2):223–229

Krause M et al. (2005) Decreased repopulation as well as increased reoxygenation contribute to the improvement in local control after targeting of the EGFR by C225 during fractionated irradiation. Radiother Oncol 76(2):162–167

Krause M et al. (2006) Preclinical evaluation of molecular-targeted anticancer agents for radiotherapy. Radiother Oncol 80(2):112–122

Kummermehr J, Trott KR (1997) Tumor stem cells. In: Potten CS (ed) Stem cells Academic Press, London, pp 363–400

Ling CC et al. (2000) Towards multidimensional radiotherapy (MD–CRT): biological imaging and biological conformality. Int J Radiat Oncol Biol Phys 47(3):551–560

Malaise EP et al. (1986) Distribution of radiation sensitivities for human tumor cells of specific histological types: comparison of in vitro to in vivo data. Int J Radiat Oncol Biol Phys 12(4):617–624

Munro TR, Gilbert CW (1961) The relation between tumor lethal doses and the radiosensitivity of tumor cells. Br J Radiol 34:246–251

Nordsmark M et al. (2005) Prognostic value of tumor oxygenation in 397 head and neck tumors after primary radiation therapy. An international multi-center study. Radiother Oncol 77(1):18–24

Nordsmark M et al. (2007) Differential risk assessments from five hypoxia specific assays: the basis for biologically adapted individualized radiotherapy in advanced head and neck cancer patients. Radiother Oncol 83(3):389–397

Okada H, Mak TW (2004) Pathways of apoptotic and non-apoptotic death in tumor cells. Nat Rev Cancer 4(8):592–603

O'Reilly MS et al. (1994) Angiostatin: a novel angiogenesis inhibitor that mediates the suppression of metastases by a Lewis lung carcinoma. Cell 79(2):315–328

Overgaard J et al. (2005) Plasma osteopontin, hypoxia, and response to the hypoxia sensitiser nimorazole in radiotherapy of head and neck cancer: results from the DAHANCA 5 randomised double-blind placebo-controlled trial. Lancet Oncol 6(10):757–764

Petersen C et al. (1998) Linear-quadratic analysis of tumor response to fractionated radiotherapy: a study on human squamous cell carcinoma xenografts. Int J Radiat Biol 73(2):197–205

Petersen C et al. (2001) Repopulation of FaDu human squamous cell carcinoma during fractionated radiotherapy correlates with reoxygenation. Int J Radiat Oncol Biol Phys 51(2):483–493

Petersen C et al. (2003) Proliferation and micromilieu during fractionated irradiation of human FaDu squamous cell carcinoma in nude mice. Int J Radiat Biol 79(7):469–477

Quennet V et al. (2006) Tumor lactate content predicts for response to fractionated irradiation of human squamous cell carcinomas in nude mice. Radiother Oncol 81(2):130–135

Ramsay J, Suit HD, Sedlacek R (1988) Experimental studies on the incidence of metastases after failure of radiation treatment and the effect of salvage surgery. Int J Radiat Oncol Biol Phys 14(6):1165–1168

Ramsay J, Ward R, Bleehen NM (1992) Radiosensitivity testing of human malignant gliomas. Int J Radiat Oncol Biol Phys 24(4):675–680

Schmidt-Ullrich RK et al. (1997) Radiation-induced proliferation of the human A431 squamous carcinoma cells is dependent on EGFR tyrosine phosphorylation. Oncogene 15(10):1191–1197

Seigneuric R et al. (2007) Impact of supervised gene signatures of early hypoxia on patient survival. Radiother Oncol 83(3):374–382

Sheldon PW et al. (1974) The incidence of lung metastases in C3H mice after treatment of implanted solid tumors with X-rays or surgery. Br J Cancer 30(4):342–348

SRC Trial Group (1997) Improved survival with preoperative radiotherapy in resectable rectal cancer. Swedish Rectal Cancer Trial. N Engl J Med 336(14):980–987

Stausbol-Gron B, Overgaard J (1999) Relationship between tumor cell in vitro radiosensitivity and clinical outcome after curative radiotherapy for squamous cell carcinoma of the head and neck. Radiother Oncol 50(1):47–55

Stuschke M, Thames HD (1999) Fractionation sensitivities and dose-control relations of head and neck carcinomas: analysis of the randomized hyperfractionation trials. Radiother Oncol 51(2):113–121

Stuschke M, Budach V, Sack H (1993) Radioresponsiveness of human glioma, sarcoma, and breast cancer spheroids depends on tumor differentiation. Int J Radiat Oncol Biol Phys 27(3):627–636

Suit HD (1992) Local control and patient survival. Int J Radiat Oncol Biol Phys 23(3):653–660

Suit HD, Westgate SJ (1986) Impact of improved local control on survival. Int J Radiat Oncol Biol Phys 12(4):453–458

Suit H, Shalek R, Wette R (1965) Radiation response of C3H mouse mammary carcinoma evaluated in terms of cellular radiation sensitivity. In: Cellular radiation biology. Williams and Wilkins, Baltimore, pp 514–530

Suit HD, Sedlacek RS, Gillette EL (1970) Examination for a correlation between probabilities of development of distant metastasis and of local recurrence. Radiology 95(1):189–194

Suit HD, Sedlacek R, Thames HD (1987) Radiation dose–response assays of tumor control, in rodent tumor models in experimental cancer therapy. In: Kallman RF (ed) Pergamon Press, New York, pp 138–148

Suit H et al. (1994) Is tumor cell radiation resistance correlated with metastatic ability? Cancer Res 54(7):1736–1741

Taghian A et al. (1993) Intrinsic radiation sensitivity may not be the major determinant of the poor clinical outcome of glioblastoma multiforme. Int J Radiat Oncol Biol Phys 25(2):243–249

Thames HD, Suit HD (1986) Tumor radioresponsiveness versus fractionation sensitivity. Int J Radiat Oncol Biol Phys 12(4):687–691

Thomas M et al. (1999) Impact of preoperative bimodality induction including twice-daily radiation on tumor regression and survival in stage III non-small-cell lung cancer. J Clin Oncol 17(4):1185

Thorwarth D, Alber M (2008) Individualised radiotherapy on the basis of functional imaging with FMISO PET. Z Med Phys 18(1):43–50

Todoroki T, Suit HD (1985) Therapeutic advantage in preoperative single-dose radiation combined with conservative and radical surgery in different-size murine fibrosarcomas. J Surg Oncol 29(4):207–215

Van der Kogel AJ (2002) Radiation response and tolerance of normal tissues. In: Steel GG (ed) Basic clinical radiobiology. Arnold, London, pp 30–41

Van't Veer LJ et al. (2002) Gene expression profiling predicts clinical outcome of breast cancer. Nature 415(6871):530–536

Vaupel P (2004) Tumor microenvironmental physiology and its implications for radiation oncology. Semin Radiat Oncol 14(3):198–206

Vaupel P, Kallinowski F, Okunieff P (1989) Blood flow, oxygen and nutrient supply, and metabolic microenvironment of human tumors: a review. Cancer Res 49(23):6449–6465

Vecchio FM et al. (2005) The relationship of pathologic tumor regression grade (TRG) and outcomes after preoperative therapy in rectal cancer. Int J Radiat Oncol Biol Phys 62(3):752–760

Walenta S et al. (2000) High lactate levels predict likelihood of metastases, tumor recurrence, and restricted patient survival in human cervical cancers. Cancer Res 60(4):916–921

West CM et al. (1997) The independence of intrinsic radiosensitivity as a prognostic factor for patient response to radiotherapy of carcinoma of the cervix. Br J Cancer 76(9):1184–1190

Whelan TJ et al. (2000) Does locoregional radiation therapy improve survival in breast cancer? A meta-analysis. J Clin Oncol 18(6):1220–1229

Williams MV, Denekamp J, Fowler JF (1985) A review of alpha/beta ratios for experimental tumors: implications for clinical studies of altered fractionation. Int J Radiat Oncol Biol Phys 11(1):87–96

Williams SG et al. (2007) Use of individual fraction size data from 3756 patients to directly determine the alpha/beta ratio of prostate cancer. Int J Radiat Oncol Biol Phys 68(1):24–33

Wouters BG et al. (1999) A p53 and apoptotic independent role for p21waf1 in tumor response to radiation therapy. Oncogene 18(47):6540–6545

Yaromina A et al. (2006) Pimonidazole labelling and response to fractionated irradiation of five human squamous cell carcinoma (hSCC) lines in nude mice: the need for a multivariate approach in biomarker studies. Radiother Oncol 81(2):122–129

20

Dose-Escalated High-Precision Radiotherapy: a Method to Overcome Variations in Biology and Radiosensitivity Limiting the Success of Conventional Approaches?

CARSTEN NIEDER and MINESH P. MEHTA

CONTENTS

C. NIEDER, MD
Medical Department, Nordlandssykehuset HF, Prinsensgate 164, 8092 Bodø, Norway

M. P. MEHTA, MD
Department of Human Oncology, University of Wisconsin Hospital Medical School, Madison, WI, 53792, USA

KEY POINTS

- The efficacy of clinically applied radiation treatment regimens might be limited by biologic parameters, such as tumor oxygenation, proliferation status, cell cycle distribution, DNA repair mechanisms, etc.
- Previous attempts to escalate the radiation dose or increase cell kill, e.g., by means of administration of more damaging types of radiation such as neutrons with high-linear-energy transfer, were often limited by the tolerance of normal tissues.
- Improved results appear to be seen, e.g., in early clinical trials with stereotactic radiotherapy for early stage non-small cell lung cancer. These improvements are likely to result from several different developments that influence our ability to stage tumors, to define the target volume, to predict target volume movement during treatment, and to administer highly conformal treatment in a precise manner.
- The technological basis of treatment is likely to broaden in the future. For example, the number of new facilities for proton and heavy-ion-beam treatment increases every year.
- As soon as the radiation oncology community has unequivocally demonstrated that current developments result in improved outcome, the challenge will be to enrich the patient population that is likely to respond, based, e.g., on gene signatures or specific pathologic or molecular features that might predict outcome.
- The ultimate goal would be to assign patients to individually tailored combinations of radiation and targeted drug treatment (if needed) in order to kill those tumor cells that are likely to survive monotherapy and give rise to recurrent and metastatic disease.

- Initial tumor volume or cell number profoundly influences local control and necessitates administration of higher radiation doses in large-volume disease. This poses a special challenge with regard to normal tissue exposure and dose limiting toxicities.

experience suggests that the local control rates, e.g., in limited stage non-small cell lung, nasopharyngeal, and uterine cervix cancers, are promising. It will be important to predict which patients can safely be treated with high-dose radiation alone and which patients should simultaneously receive radiosensitizers, hypoxia-modifying drugs or, in general, modifiers of the radiation response in order to optimize the cure rates.

Abstract

This chapter addresses the role of radiation dose escalation as a method to increase tumor cell eradication and to improve local control and thereby survival of cancer patients. While radiation treatment can be designed to cover the whole tumor with a homogeneously distributed full-radiation dose or a simultaneously integrated boost to defined subvolumes, the normal tissue exposure ultimately limits the dose that can safely be delivered. Exceeding certain dose thresholds to critical structures might result in unacceptable permanent dysfunction and sequelae, with profound consequences on quality of life. With improved methods of target volume definition, image-guided external beam radiotherapy, advanced brachytherapy applications, and the advent of proton and heavy-ion-beam facilities, the possibilities for safe radiation dose escalation have never been more promising than they are today. Whether such approaches ultimately will be able to overcome the substantial variability in radiation sensitivity and final treatment outcome remains to be demonstrated in sufficiently powered prospective studies. Preliminary

20.1
Introduction

If solid tumors are detected in nonmetastatic, localized stages, then effective local therapy can be curative. Depending on the risk of micrometastases, adjuvant or neoadjuvant treatment offers additional benefit. Besides surgery, radiotherapy has long been recognized as a curative modality. Potential advantages of radiotherapy over surgery include organ preservation, and the non-invasive nature of it is especially suitable for the treatment of elderly patients, or those with comorbidities, in whom the risks from surgery are greater. (We summarize representative results in Table 20.1.) While variable, but generally high rates of disease control are obtained, a certain number of failures continue to exist. Figure 20.1 illustrates potential sources of failure. Recurrence despite correctly administered treatment might result from survival of less radioresponsive cells, and factors such as oxygenation, DNA repair capacity, proliferation, etc., might impact radiosensitivity. This leads us to question whether radiation dose escalation will enable us to destroy less radioresponsive cells.

Table 20.1. Overview of treatment results with curative radiation therapy

Authors	Tumor	Treatment	Results
Garden et al. 2003	Glottic carcinoma T2N0	Various fractionation regimens	5-Year locoregional control without salvage surgery: 72% 5-Year disease-specific survival: 92%
Yamazaki et al. 2006	Glottic carcinoma T1N0	56–66 Gy, with different fraction sizes	5-Year locoregional control without salvage surgery: 86%, and cause-specific survival: 98%
Jones et al. 2004	Larynx carcinoma T1–2N0	60–66 Gy, conventional fractionation without CTx	5-Year tumor-specific survival: 87%
Fu et al. 2000	Stage II–IV head and neck tumors	Accelerated fractionation with concomitant boost, 72 Gy	5-Year locoregional control: 50%

Table 20.1. *(continued)* Overview of treatment results with curative radiation therapy

Authors	Tumor	Treatment	Results
Leung et al. 2008	Nasopharyngeal cancer T1–2b	Radiation with brachytherapy boost	5-Year progression-free survival: 95%
Wang et al. 1991	Nasopharyngeal cancer T1–2	Radiation with brachytherapy boost	5-Year local-control rate: 91%
Ortholan et al. 2005	Anal canal carcinoma T1	Various external beam or brachytherapy techniques	5-Year colostomy-free survival: 85% 5-Year disease-free survival: 89%
Deniaud-Alexandre et al. 2003	Anal canal carcinoma T1–4, stage I–IIIB	Various external beam or brachytherapy techniques, CTx in <10%	5-Year local-relapse-free survival: 86% 5-Year disease-free survival: 72%
Gerard et al. 1998	Anal canal carcinoma T1–4 N0–3	External beam radiotherapy plus implant and chemotherapy	5-Year colostomy-free survival: 72% 5-Year disease-specific survival: 90%
Papillon 1990	Rectal cancer T1–2	Intracavitary irradiation	Crude local failure rate 5%, pelvic lymph node metastases: 4%
	Rectal cancer T2–3	External beam plus intracavitary radiotherapy	5-Year cancer-specific survival: 84%
Groen et al. 2004	Non-small cell lung cancer stage IIIA/B	Conventional fractionation 60 Gy vs. 60 Gy plus carboplatin	2-Year local control rate: 38 vs. 72%
Onishi et al. 2004	Non-small cell lung cancer stage I	Hypofractionated stereotactic radiotherapy	Crude rate of local-disease recurrence: 13.5% 5-Year cause-specific survival: 78%
Zimmermann et al. 2005	Non-small cell lung cancer stage I	Hypofractionated stereotactic radiotherapy	2-Year-freedom-from-local-recurrence rate: 87% 2-Year disease-free survival: 72%
Xia et al. 2006	Non-small cell lung cancer stage I/II	Hypofractionated stereotactic radiotherapy	3-Year local control rate: 95% 3-Year overall survival: 78%
Sathya et al. 2005	T2–3 N0 prostate cancer	External beam radiotherapy plus implant	8-Year failure-free survival: 65% 8-Year overall survival: 82%
Wallner et al. 2003	T1c–2a low-risk prostate cancer	^{125}I or ^{103}Pd implant	3-Year biochemical-relapse-free survival: 89 vs. 91%
Pollack et al. 2002	T1–3 prostate cancer	External-beam radiotherapy, 78 Gy	6-Year failure-free survival: 70%
Lertsanguansinchai et al. 2004	Stage IB-IIIB cervical cancer	External-beam radiotherapy plus brachytherapy	3-Year pelvic control: 87% 3-Year relapse-free survival: 70%
Eifel et al. 2004	Stage IB/II cervical cancer and Stage III/IVA cervical cancer	Radiotherapy alone vs. chemoradiation	5-Year locoregional failure-free survival: 69 vs. 87% (IB/II), and 56 vs. 71% 5-Year disease-free survival: 46 vs. 74% (IB/II), and 37 vs. 54%
Milker-Zabel et al. 2005	Meningioma grade I vs. II	Stereotactic radiotherapy	5-Year recurrence-free survival: 90.5 vs. 89%
Selch et al. 2004	Meningioma grade I/II	Stereotactic radiotherapy	3-Year local control: 97%

CTx chemotherapy

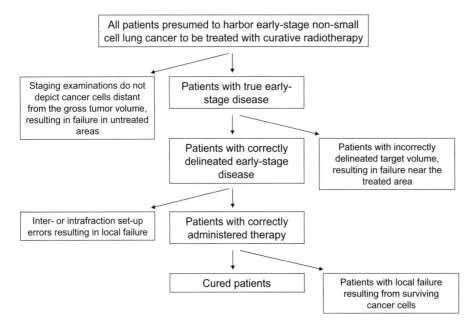

Fig 20.1. Factors associated with treatment success and failure

20.2

Staging and Target Volume Delineation

Noninvasive imaging techniques are a central component of treatment planning in radiation oncology. The information gained from different imaging modalities is usually of a complementary nature: MRI defines soft tissue with high resolution, computed tomography (CT) is important for the precise delineation of bony anatomy and for the accurate computation of radiation dose, PET and (SPECT) offer additional information about tumor biology, heterogeneity, and extent of spread. Thus, precise definition of the gross tumor volume (GTV) is dependent on proper integration of multimodal imaging information.

Delivery of sophisticated local treatment can only yield a survival advantage for patients with truly localized disease, or those with controlled or controllable systemic disease. The success of stereotactic radiotherapy, e.g., for early-stage non-small cell lung cancer (NSCLC) is critically dependent on the correct identification of node-negative patients. For this purpose, a hybrid PET–CT scanner and the tracer FDG might be used. Correct staging is also required for other diseases commonly treated with high-dose radiotherapy such as prostate cancer. In numerous clinical trials, PET and

PET–CT have been shown to improve the accuracy of staging and to result in treatment modification in approximately 20–30% of patients with diseases treated by curative radiotherapy (Mac Manus et al. 2001; Van Tinteren et al. 2002; Weber et al. 2003; Viney et al. 2004; Grosu et al. 2005a; Herder et al. 2006).

The principle of modern radiation therapy is to administer a curative dose to a precise and well-delineated target volume in a very accurate and reproducible fashion. The doses to critical organs must be kept at tolerable levels, because the normal tissue complication probability (NTCP) determines the ability to deliver a high dose (Belderbos et al. 2006). Beyond patient selection, the use of PET results in frequent and relevant modifications of the clinical target volume, mainly by exclusion of lymph nodes (Vanuytsel et al. 2000; Belderbos et al. 2006; Greco et al. 2007). Also with regard to the primary tumor, PET might improve the delineation, as shown, e.g., for intracranial tumors (Grosu et al. 2000, 2003, 2005a,b,c), head and neck tumors (Schinagl et al. 2007) and NSCLC (Mac Manus et al. 2001; Fox et al. 2005; Gondi et al. 2007). Furthermore, PET might reduce the interobserver variability if different radiation oncologists attempt to define the target volume in the same patient (Khoo et al. 2000; Weltens et al. 2001; Ashamalla et al. 2005; Cattaneo et al. 2005; Fox et al. 2005; Grosu et al. 2006a,b; Steenbakkers et al.

2006). The best-characterized tracers include FDG for extracranial tumors and L-(methyl-^{11}C) methionine for intracranial tumors. Currently, a number of questions around scanning protocols, image interpretation, image fusion, and choice of segmentation tool for treatment planning are not fully resolved (AERTS et al. 2008). In addition, the impact of PET-defined target volumes on local control and ultimately survival remains to be demonstrated in adequately designed prospective trials.

20.3
The Issue of Motion and Precise Targeting

It has long been recognized that the position of the target volume might change with, e.g., respiration, swallowing, bowel, and bladder activity, and that the patient's position on the treatment couch is also prone to variation (systematic and random errors, reviewed, e.g., by SONKE et al. 2008). This has led to the concept of an internal target volume to account for organ movement and an additional planning target volume, in other words, margins that expand the purely disease-defined target volumes in order to account for various types of uncertainties. It has been shown that patients who received suboptimal external-beam radiotherapy (geographical miss, protocol violation) had inferior outcome, e.g., in a prospective trial in Hodgkin's disease by the German Hodgkin Study Group, i.e., in a malignancy that is highly curable by moderate doses of radiation (DUHMKE et al. 2001). In stage I NSCLC,

the use of more sophisticated treatment, in this case of three-dimensional versus two-dimensional radiotherapy, contributed to improved outcome (FANG et al. 2006). Treatment toxicity is also dependent on the quality of radiotherapy, as demonstrated, e.g., in prostate cancer brachytherapy (KEYES et al. 2006). Some of the issues around organ motion and precise targeting apply to a lesser extent in brachytherapy, which makes this method attractive for dose escalation.

The exact margin expansion depends on several factors, such as the use of devices to track and/or minimize motion, to immobilize patients, etc. (BALTER and KESSLER 2007; NIJKAMP et al. 2008). The necessary margin expansion can now be determined for each individual patient, both prior to the first treatment and with serial controls during a course of fractionated radiotherapy. In addition, tumor shrinkage can be taken into account (WOODFORD et al. 2007; LIM et al. 2008), although questions regarding the safety of field reduction remain unanswered (SIKER et al. 2006). With improving technical capabilities, the step from CT-based three-dimensional conformal therapy to high-precision stereotactic or intensity-modulated techniques and inverse planning has recently been made (GALVIN and DE NEVE 2007; Fig. 20.2). A key feature of high-precision therapy is the determination of and correction for setup uncertainties that occur from fraction to fraction (interfraction movement), e.g., with megavoltage computed tomography (image-guided radiotherapy) (HONG et al. 2007). In addition, intrafraction tumor and organ movements, for example during the breathing cycle, can be quantified (often called four-dimensional radiother-

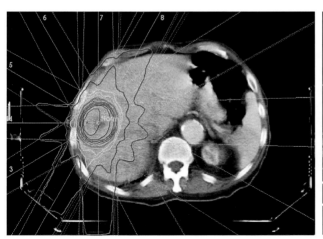
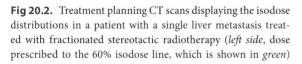
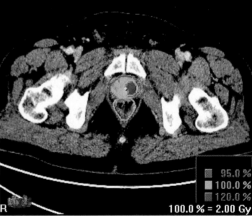

Fig 20.2. Treatment planning CT scans displaying the isodose distributions in a patient with a single liver metastasis treated with fractionated stereotactic radiotherapy (*left side*, dose prescribed to the 60% isodose line, which is shown in *green*)

and in a patient with prostate cancer (*right side*), in whom an intensity-modulated simultaneous integrated boost to a lesion in the left lobe is planned

apy). Reducing these uncertainties allows for tighter margins and better normal tissue sparing (DING et al. 2007; FENG and EISBRUCH 2007). It is also possible with intensity-modulated techniques to selectively reduce the dose to critical structures (conformal avoidance) (GUTIERREZ et al. 2007). It has been shown that control for respiratory motion and adaptive radiotherapy are feasible (RIETZEL et al. 2005; ZHANG et al. 2007). The same holds true for real-time assessment of rectum and bladder position for prostate cancer treatment. However, the patient population that will derive clinical benefit from such technology still needs to be defined. It is likely, that patients with otherwise high NTCP, for example, as a result of large target volumes, might benefit most from intrafraction movement adjustments.

The basis for clinical proton and heavy-ion-beam application was established years ago (WILSON 1946; LAWRENCE et al. 1963; SCHULZ-ERTNER and TSUJII 2007). While protons are characterized by superior physical properties, resulting in improved normal tissue sparing, their radiobiologic properties are not tremendously different from those of photons. In contrast, heavy-ion beams cause more severe biological effects (high-linear-energy transfer [LET]). Developments in the field of photon beam therapy such as intensity modulation are now also being translated to these applications; although, clinically robust devices and facilities able to deliver intensity modulated proton therapy are extremely scarce (LOMAX 2008). With increasing numbers of facilities, more and more patients are treated with this highly sophisticated and costly type of treatment. The controversy around the use of these technologies in the absence of clinical data from large prospective randomized trials (low level of evidence) has nicely been summarized in a recent review (BENTZEN 2008).

Although visualization and precise administration of treatment are key factors, the ultimate success of any cancer treatment is influenced by tumor cell number and biology, which has profound implications on radiosensitivity (LIND and BRAHME 2007). The key points are briefly discussed in the next paragraph.

20.4
The Influence of Cell Number and Biology

It is a well-known phenomenon that the success rate of radiation treatment is depended on tumor volume or cell number, as described, e.g., in studies of palliative radiotherapy for brain metastases and curative carbon ion therapy for stage I NSCLC (NIEDER et al. 1997; MIYAMOTO et al. 2007). For T1 NSCLC, the local control rate was 98% at a median follow-up of 39 months, while it was 80% for T2 tumors, which typically are larger. Both experimental and clinical observations have repeatedly confirmed the influence of initial tumor volume or cell number on local control (KHALIL et al. 1997; BELDERBOS et al. 2006; ZHAO et al. 2007; ONIMARU et al. 2008; WERNER-WASIK et al. 2008) and the need for administration of higher radiation doses in large-volume disease. The preclinical data of radiotherapy under hypoxic and ambient conditions also suggest that the dose–volume relationship is present under both conditions, i.e., not just related to increasing hypoxia in larger tumors.

Oxygen supply, number of clonogen cells, and proliferation rate are important determinants of outcome. Yet, typical treatment plans are developed with limited knowledge of tumor biology. The histology report provides information on some features, but is far from exhaustive. The tumor microenvironment influences expression of proteases, locally aggressive behavior, metastatic potential, and treatment resistance (MOLLS and VAUPEL 2000; ROFSTAD et al. 2000; STADLER et al. 2000; HEDLEY et al. 2003; NIEDER et al. 2003; ZIPS et al. 2004; NORDSMARK et al. 2005; WOUTERS et al. 2005). In vivo measurements suggest that hypoxia is still present in head and neck cancers at the end of radiation treatment. Killing of all remaining hypoxic tumor stem cells during the late treatment phase might therefore be very important. Tumor blood flow also is an interesting feature, e.g., in combined modality treatment because drug delivery depends on perfusion. Evaluation by dynamic MRI and other methods suggests that large differences exist between individual tumors (FELDMANN et al. 1993 and 1999; LONCASTER et al. 2002).

The induction of DNA damage is probably one of the most crucial events after irradiation of cells. In this regard, ionizing radiation triggers a wide array of lesions including base damage, single-strand breaks, and notably, double-strand breaks (DSB). After irradiation, different molecular systems are involved in recognition and repair of the damage. Whereas most of the induced damage is quickly repaired, DSB repair is slow, and unrepaired DSBs are considerably important for the final induction of cell death. Data from a subgroup of patients from the Stockholm breast cancer trials suggest that the magnitude of expression of certain DNA repair proteins (Mre11, Rad50, Nbs1) is associated with favorable response to radiotherapy (SÖDERLUND et al. 2007). In addition, striking differences in the radiation sensitivity occur as cells move through the different phases of the cell cycle. The use of radiation with greater LET circumvents some of the problems around damage that can be repaired and resistance of hypoxic and quiescent cells within a tumor (Masunaga et al. 2008).

Integration of biological information into treatment planning is desirable for treatment optimization. However, features such as oxygenation might be heterogeneously distributed within a tumor and vary during treatment (Lin et al. 2008). Certainly, repeat measurements with invasive approaches are inconvenient. Noninvasive methods, such as functional MRI, magnetic resonance spectroscopy (MRS), or PET with ^{18}F-fluoromisonidazole (FMISO) or ^{18}F-fluoroazomycin arabinoside (FAZA) might improve patient's acceptance and co-registration plus correlation with standard anatomical imaging (Grosu et al. 2007; Aerts et al. 2008). PET imaging was also shown to provide prognostic information (Vansteenkiste et al. 1999; Borst et al. 2005; Van Baardwijk et al. 2007). Ongoing studies will determine whether these approaches contribute to treatment individualization and ultimately improved cure rates.

20.5
What to Expect from Dose Escalation?

Under experimental conditions, researchers are able to kill all clonogenic cells and thereby control human tumors transplanted in mice with radiotherapy as long as the dose is high enough (Yaromina et al. 2007). Several randomized trials have demonstrated the benefits of dose escalation in prostate cancer (Pollack et al. 2002; Sathya et al. 2005; Zietman et al. 2005; Peeters et al. 2006; Dearnaley et al. 2007), but some tumor types, e.g., glioblastoma, were not successfully treated with higher doses of radiation (Lapperriere et al. 1998; Selker et al. 2002; Souhami et al. 2004). In NSCLC stage T1-3 N0 M0, dose escalation with 2.1-Gy fractions to a median dose of 84 Gy (maximum 102.9 Gy) resulted in 5-year local-progression-free survival of 42% in patients that received 92.4–102.9 Gy (Chen et al. 2006). Tumor volumes in this subgroup of patients were typically <60 cm³. These data suggest that dose escalation with fractionated radiotherapy is less successful than anticipated, although a 1-Gy increase in dose was associated with a 3% reduction of risk from death. Dose escalation with daily fractions of approximately 2 Gy leads to an increase in overall treatment time, which might reduce the anticipated additional cell kill because tumor cells start to repopulate faster

soon after initiation of treatment (Kim and Tannock 2005). To account for differences in dose per fraction and treatment time, the biologically equivalent dose of a certain radiotherapy regimen can be calculated. Increasing normal tissue complication probabilities pose huge challenges to treatment of patients with large volume disease, which, in addition, are at increased risk of metastatic spread.

In stereotactic radiotherapy of early-stage NSCLC, where high doses per fraction are administered to small volumes within a relatively short time interval, it was also demonstrated that dose escalation improves survival and local control (Onishi et al. 2004; Onimaru et al. 2008). Increasing the biologically equivalent dose to more than 100 Gy led to disappearance of significant differences in local tumor control between T1 and T2 NSCLC (Onishi et al. 2004). In early, stage Ib squamous cell carcinoma of the uterine cervix, radiation therapy alone resulted in 5-year survival of 93.5% and local control of 92% (Ota et al. 2007). Comparable findings were reported in nasopharyngeal carcinoma (Wang et al. 1991; Leung et al. 2008). Whether the remaining failures in such relatively small series of selected patients are the consequence of adverse biological features of the tumor or of the potential sources of errors discussed earlier cannot be decided. A comprehensive analysis of this question would require detailed data on both treatment accuracy and tumor biology. The latter would necessitate complete tumor removal, as biopsies might be prone to sampling errors, thereby eliminating the need for high-dose radiotherapy. If one tries to review data on tumor biology features such as oxygenation in early stage cancers, lung cancer is not a very attractive model, as data interpretation is hampered by the differences in histology and volume. The T2, -3, and -4 stages are composed of differently sized tumors. A recent study in prostate cancer patients suggests that increased staining for vascular endothelial growth factor and hypoxia inducible factor-1α is associated with a shorter time to biochemical failure, independent of tumor stage, Gleason score, serum prostate specific antigen, and radiation dose (Vergis et al. 2008). However, tumor volume differs within a given tumor stage. In tumors of the uterine cervix, dynamic contrast enhanced MRI appears to add information on oxygenation that complements the impact of tumor volume on outcome, but the stage distribution varied considerably in the relatively small study by Loncaster et al. (2002). A larger study on pimonidazole labeling and Eppendorf electrode measurements suggests that tumor size outperforms the other methods with regard to influence on local control (Nordsmark et al. 2006).

However, equally sized early-stage tumors might differ with regard to histologic grade, risk of nodal metastases, underlying causes, and genetic changes, etc., and are thus unlikely to represent a homogeneous biologic entity. Gene expression profile analysis can be used to divide early stage cancers into groups with different behavior (WATANABE et al. 2008), but it remains to be demonstrated that such strategies can be used to prescribe the radiation dose.

Dose escalation does not come without a price. Intensified treatment to conventional target volumes or certain anatomical areas might result in considerable, clinically unacceptable toxicity. These facts lead to the question whether selective intensification to certain, biologically relevant subvolumes might improve the therapeutic ratio and how such subvolumes should be defined. Currently, efforts are underway to validate suitable methods. Image fusion, for example of PET, MRI and CT scans, and hybrid PET–CT scans is being used for creation of individualized dose distributions, or so-called dose painting. The idea behind dose painting is to perform targeted dose escalation for less radiosensitive subvolumes (LING et al. 2000). It has been shown that this is technically feasible, although issues of temporal and spatial variations in target localization, the resolution of biological imaging, quality assurance, etc., remain evolutionary. The recent discovery of cancer stem cells and their role in radiation resistance (RICH 2007; KORKAYA and WICHA 2007) creates new questions around the issue of selective dose escalation. If such cells were the major source of treatment failure, would they not represent the logical target for dose escalation? If so, would we not need to know whether they are randomly distributed throughout the tumor or located in well-defined subvolumes that can be detected by some of the emerging biological imaging methods? How radioresistant are these cells in humans in vivo? We could not cure such a high number of small head and neck cancers, skin cancers, lung cancers, prostate cancers, etc., without killing all the cells that can give rise to a recurrence. What is the effect of high-LET radiation on these cells? Can we predict the need for treatment modification early during a course of radiotherapy, based on the response observed after a couple of fractions (SEIBERT et al. 2007)? In an ideal scenario, we would be able to apply a predictive test before the start of treatment (MINNA et al. 2007) that tells us whether our present patient can be cured and safely treated by relatively inexpensive photon beam therapy, whether, e.g., a hypoxia modifier should be added to this, or whether high-LET radiation is the only way to go. Yet another school of thought proposes that tumors may "mask" their potential to resist radiation until actually exposed to radiotherapy, and therefore, a reanalysis of tumor biology, either through repeat biopsies or imaging for molecular analysis, after a few fractions (one to five) might provide the most promising data to modify the delivery of radiotherapy; this concept is referred to as "theragnostic radiation therapy" (BENTZEN 2005).

References

Aerts HJ, Bosmans G, van Baardwijk AA et al (2008) Stability of ^{18}F-deoxyglucose uptake locations within tumor during radiotherapy for NSCLC: a prospective study. Int J Radiat Oncol Biol Phys (in press)

Ashamalla H, Rafla S, Parikh K et al (2005) The contribution of integrated PET/CT to the evolving definition of treatment volumes in radiation treatment planning in lung cancer. Int J Radiat Oncol Biol Phys 63:1016–1023

Balter JM, Kessler ML (2007) Imaging and alignment for image-guided radiation therapy. J Clin Oncol 25:931–937

Belderbos J, Heemsbergen WD, De Jaeger K et al (2006) Final results of a phase I/II dose escalation trial in non-small-cell lung cancer using three-dimensional conformal radiotherapy. Int J Radiat Oncol Biol Phys 66:126–134

Bentzen SM (2005) Theragnostic imaging for radiation oncology: Dose-painting by numbers. Lancet Oncol 6:112–117

Bentzen SM (2008) Randomized controlled trials in health technology assessment: overkill or overdue? Radiother Oncol 86:142–147

Borst GR, Belderbos JS, Boellaard R et al (2005) Standardised FDG uptake: a prognostic factor for inoperable non-small cell lung cancer. Eur J Cancer 41:1533–1541

Cattaneo GM, Reni M, Rizzo G et al (2005) Target delineation in post-operative radiotherapy of brain gliomas: interobserver variability and impact of image registration of MR(pre-operative) images on treatment planning CT scans. Radiother Oncol 75:217–223

Chen M, Hayman JA, Ten Haken RK et al (2006) Long-term results of high-dose conformal radiotherapy for patients with medically inoperable T1–3N0 non-small-cell lung cancer: is low incidence of regional failure due to incidental nodal irradiation? Int J Radiat Oncol Biol Phys 64:120–126

Dearnaley DP, Sydes MR, Graham JD et al (2007) Escalated-dose versus standard-dose conformal radiotherapy in prostate cancer: first results from the MRC RT01 randomised controlled trial. Lancet Oncol 8:475–487

Deniaud-Alexandre E, Touboul E, Tiret E et al (2003) Results of definitive irradiation in a series of 305 epidermoid carcinomas of the anal canal. Int J Radiat Oncol Biol Phys 56:1259–1273

Ding GX, Duggan DM, Coffey CW et al (2007) A study on adaptive IMRT treatment planning using kV cone-beam CT. Radiother Oncol 85:116–125

Duhmke E, Franklin J, Pfreundschuh M et al (2001) Low-dose radiation is sufficient for the noninvolved extended-field treatment in favorable early-stage Hodgkin's disease: long-term results of a randomized trial of radiotherapy alone. J Clin Oncol 19:2905–2914

Eifel PJ, Winter K, Morris M et al (2004) Pelvic irradiation with concurrent chemotherapy versus pelvic and para-aortic irradiation for high-risk cervical cancer: an update of Radiation Therapy Oncology Group Trial (RTOG) 90-01. J Clin Oncol 22:872–880

Fang LC, Komaki R, Allen P et al (2006) Comparison of outcomes for patients with medically inoperable stage I non-small-cell lung cancer treated with two-dimensional vs. three-dimensional radiotherapy. Int J Radiat Oncol Biol Phys 66:108–116

Feldmann HJ, Sievers K, Füller J et al (1993) Evaluation of tumor blood perfusion by dynamic MRI and CT in patients undergoing thermoradiotherapy. Eur J Radiol 16:224–229

Feldmann HJ, Molls M, Vaupel P (1999) Blood flow and oxygenation status of human tumors. Strahlenther Onkol 175:1–9

Feng M, Eisbruch A (2007) Future issues in highly conformal radiotherapy for head and neck cancer. J Clin Oncol 25:1009–1013

Fox JL, Rengan R, O'Meara W et al (2005) Does registration of PET and planning CT images decrease interobserver and intraobserver variation in delineating tumor volumes for non-small-cell lung cancer? Int J Radiat Oncol Biol Phys 62:70–75

Fu KK, Pajak TF, Trotti A et al (2000) A Radiation Therapy Oncology Group (RTOG) phase III randomized study to compare hyperfractionation and two variants of accelerated fractionation to standard fractionation radiotherapy for head and neck squamous cell carcinomas: first report of RTOG 9003. Int J Radiat Oncol Biol Phys 48:7–16

Galvin JM, De Neve W (2007) Intensity modulating and other radiation therapy devices for dose painting. J Clin Oncol 25:924–930

Garden AS, Forster K, Wong PF et al (2003) Results of radiotherapy for T2N0 glottic carcinoma: does the "2" stand for twice-daily treatment? Int J Radiat Oncol Biol Phys 55:322–328

Gerard JP, Ayzac L, Hun D et al (1998) Treatment of anal canal carcinoma with high dose radiation therapy and concomitant fluorouracil-cisplatinum. Long-term results in 95 patients. Radiother Oncol 46:249–256

Gondi V, Bradley K, Mehta M et al (2007) Impact of hybrid fluorodeoxyglucose positron-emission tomography/computed tomography on radiotherapy planning in esophageal and non-small-cell lung cancer. Int J Radiat Oncol Biol Phys 67:187–195

Greco C, Rosenzweig K, Cascini GL et al (2007) Current status of PET/CT for tumour volume definition in radiotherapy treatment planning for non-small cell lung cancer (NSCLC). Lung Cancer 57:125–134

Groen HJ, van der Leest AH, Fokkema E et al (2004) Continuously infused carboplatin used as radiosensitizer in locally unresectable non-small cell lung cancer: a multicenter phase III study. Ann Oncol 15:427–432

Grosu AL, Weber WA, Feldmann HJ et al (2000) First experience with I-123-alpha-methyl-tyrosine SPECT in 3-D radiation treatment planning of brain gliomas. Int Radiat Oncol Biol Phys 47:517–526

Grosu AL, Feldmann HJ, Dick S et al (2003) Implications of IMT-SPECT for postoperative radiotherapy planning in patients with gliomas. Int Radiat Oncol Biol Phys 54:842–854

Grosu AL, Weber WA, Franz M et al (2005a) Re-irradiation of recurrent high grade gliomas using amino-acids-PET(SPECT)/CT/MRI image fusion to determine gross tumor volume for stereotactic fractionated radiotherapy. Int J Radiat Oncol Biol Phys 63:511–519

Grosu AL, Weber AW, Riedel E et al (2005b) L-(Methyl-^{11}C) methionine positron emissions tomography for target delineation in resected high grade gliomas before radiation therapy. Int J Radiat Oncol Biol Phys 63:64–74

Grosu AL, Piert M, Weber WA et al (2005c) Positron emission tomography for radiation treatment planning. Strahlenther Onkol 181:483–499

Grosu AL, Molls M, Zimmermann FB et al (2006a) High-precision radiation therapy with integrated biological imaging and tumor monitoring—evolution of the Munich concept and future research options. Strahlenther Onkol 182:361–368

Grosu AL, Weber WA, Astner ST et al (2006b) ^{11}C-methionine PET improves the target volume delineation of meningiomas treated with stereotactic fractionated radiotherapy. Int J Radiat Oncol Biol Phys 66:339–344

Grosu AL, Souvatzoglou M, Roper B et al (2007) Hypoxia imaging with FAZA-PET and theoretical considerations with regard to dose painting for individualization of radiotherapy in patients with head and neck cancer. Int J Radiat Oncol Biol Phys 69:541–551

Gutierrez AN, Westerly DC, Tome WA et al (2007) Whole brain radiotherapy with hippocampal avoidance and simultaneously integrated brain metastases boost: a planning study. Int J Radiat Oncol Biol Phys 69:589–597

Hedley D, Pintilie M, Woo J et al (2003) Carbonic anhydrase IX expression, hypoxia, and prognosis in patients with uterine cervical carcinomas. Clin Cancer Res 9:5666–5674

Herder GJ, Kramer H, Hoekstra OS et al (2006) Traditional versus up-front ^{18}F- fluorodeoxyglucose-positron emission tomography staging of non-small-cell lung cancer: a Dutch cooperative randomized study. J Clin Oncol 24:1800–1806

Hof H, Muenter M, Oetzel D et al (2007) Stereotactic single-dose radiotherapy (radiosurgery) of early stage nonsmall-cell lung cancer. Cancer 110:148–155

Hong TS, Welsh JS, Ritter MA et al (2007) Megavoltage computed tomography: an emerging tool for image-guided radiotherapy. Am J Clin Oncol 30:617–623

Jones AS, Fish B, Fenton JE et al (2004) The treatment of early laryngeal cancers (T1–T2 N0): surgery or irradiation? Head Neck 26:127–135

Keyes M, Schellenberg D, Moravan V et al (2006) Decline in urinary retention incidence in 805 patients after prostate brachytherapy: the effect of learning curve? Int J Radiat Oncol Biol Phys 64:825–834

Khalil AA, Bentzen SM, Overgaard J (1997) Steepness of the dose-response curve as a function of volume in an experimental tumor irradiated under ambient or hypoxic conditions. Int J Radiat Oncol Biol Phys 39:797–802

Kim JJ, Tannock IF (2005) Repopulation of cancer cells during therapy: an important cause of treatment failure. Nat Rev Cancer 5:516–525

Khoo VS, Adams EJ, Saran F et al (2000) A comparison of clinical target volumes determined by CT and MRI for the radiotherapy planning of base of skull meningiomas. Int J Radiat Oncol Biol Phys 46:1309–1317

Korkaya H, Wicha MS (2007) Selective targeting of cancer stem cells: a new concept in cancer therapeutics. BioDrugs 21:299–310

Lawrence JH, Tobiascarborn JL, Gottschalk A et al (1963) Alpha particle and proton beams in therapy. JAMA 186:236–245

Lertsanguansinchai P, Lertbutsayanukul C, Shotelersuk K et al (2004) Phase III randomized trial comparing LDR and HDR brachytherapy in treatment of cervical carcinoma. Int J Radiat Oncol Biol Phys 59:1424–1431

Lind BK, Brahme A (2007) The radiation response of heterogeneous tumors. Phys Med 23:91–99

Ling CC, Humm J, Larson S et al (2000) Towards multidimensional radiotherapy (MD-CRT): biological imaging and biological conformality. Int J Radiat Oncol Biol Phys 47:551–560

Leung TW, Wong VY, Sze WK et al (2008) High-dose rate intracavitary brachytherapy boost for early T stage nasopharyngeal carcinoma. Int J Radiat Oncol Biol Phys 70:361–367

Lim K, Chan P, Dinniwell R et al (2008) Cervical cancer regression measured using weekly magnetic resonance imaging during fractionated radiotherapy: radiobiologic modeling and correlation with tumor hypoxia. Int J Radiat Oncol Biol Phys 70:126–133

Lin Z, Mechalakos J, Nehmeh S et al (2008) The influence of changes in tumor hypoxia on dose-painting treatment plans based on ^{18}F-FMISO positron emission tomography. Int J Radiat Oncol Biol Phys 70:1219–1228

Lomax AJ (2008) Intensity modulated proton therapy and its sensitivity to treatment uncertainties: parts I and II. Phys Med Biol 53:1027–1056

Loncaster JA, Carrington BM, Sykes JR et al (2002) Prediction of radiotherapy outcome using dynamic contrast enhanced MRI of carcinoma of the cervix. Int J Radiat Oncol Biol Phys 54:759–767

Mac Manus MP, Hicks RJ, Ball DL et al (2001) F-18 fluorodeoxyglucose positron emission tomography staging in radical radiotherapy candidates with nonsmall cell lung carcinoma: powerful correlation with survival and high impact on treatment. Cancer 92:886–895

Masunaga S, Ando K, Uzawa A et al (2008) Radiobiologic significance of response of intratumor quiescent cells in vivo to accelerated carbon ion beams compared with gamma-rays and reactor neutron beams. Int J Radiat Oncol Biol Phys 70:221–228

Milker-Zabel S, Zabel A, Schulz-Ertner D et al (2005) Fractionated stereotactic radiotherapy in patients with benign or atypical intracranial meningioma: long-term experience and prognostic factors. Int J Radiat Oncol Biol Phys 61:809–816

Minna JD, Girard L, Xie Y (2007) Tumor mRNA expression profiles predict responses to chemotherapy. J Clin Oncol 25:4329–4334

Miyamoto T, Baba M, Sugane T et al (2007) Carbon ion radiotherapy for stage I non-small cell lung cancer using a regimen of four fractions during 1 week. J Thorac Oncol 2:916–926

Molls M, Vaupel P (2000) Blood perfusion and microenvironment of human tumors. Springer, Berlin Heidelberg New York

Nieder C, Berberich W, Schnabel K (1997) Tumor-related prognostic factors for remission of brain metastases after radiotherapy. Int J Radiat Oncol Biol Phys 39:25–30

Nieder C, Milas L, Ang KK (2003) Modification of radiation response: cytokines, growth factors, and other biological targets. Springer, Berlin Heidelberg New York

Nijkamp J, Pos FJ, Nuver TT et al (2008) Adaptive radiotherapy for prostate cancer using kilovoltage cone-beam computed tomography: first clinical results. Int J Radiat Oncol Biol Phys 70:75–82

Nordsmark M, Bentzen SM, Rudat V et al (2005) Prognostic value of tumor oxygenation in 397 head and neck tumors after primary radiotherapy. An international multicenter study. Radiother Oncol 77:18–24

Nordsmark M, Loncaster J, Aquino-Parsons C et al (2006) The prognostic value of pimonidazole and tumour pO2 in human cervix carcinomas after radiation therapy: a prospective international multi-center study. Radiother Oncol 80:123–131

Onimaru R, Fujino M, Yamazaki K et al (2008) Steep dose-response relationship for stage I non-small-cell lung cancer using hypofractionated high-dose irradiation by real-time tumor-tracking radiotherapy. Int J Radiat Oncol Biol Phys 70:374–381

Onishi H, Araki T, Shirato H et al (2004) Stereotactic hypofractionated high-dose irradiation for stage I Nonsmall cell lung carcinoma. Cancer 101:1623–1631

Ortholan C, Ramaioli A, Pfeiffert D et al (2005) Anal canal carcinoma: early-stage tumors ≤10 mm (T1 or Tis): therapeutic options and original pattern of local failure after radiotherapy. Int J Radiat Oncol Biol Phys 62:479–485

Ota T, Takeshima N, Tabata T et al (2007) Treatment of squamous cell carcinoma of the uterine cervix with radiation therapy alone: long-term survival, late complications, and incidence of second cancers. Br J Cancer 97:1058–1062

Papillon J (1990) Present status of radiation therapy in the conservative management of rectal cancer. Radiother Oncol 17:275–283

Peeters ST, Heemsbergen WD, Koper PC et al (2006) Dose-response in radiotherapy for localized prostate cancer: results of the Dutch multicenter randomized phase III trial comparing 68 Gy of radiotherapy with 78 Gy. J Clin Oncol 24:1990–1996

Pollack A, Zagars GK, Starkschall G et al (2002) Prostate cancer radiation dose response: results of the M. D. Anderson phase III randomized trial. Int J Radiat Oncol Biol Phys 53:1097–1105

Rich JN (2007) Cancer stem cells in radiation resistance. Cancer Res 67:8980–8984

Rietzel E, Chen GT, Choi NC et al (2005) Four-dimensional image-based treatment planning: target volume segmentation and dose calculation in the presence of respiratory motion. Int J Radiat Oncol Biol Phys 61:1535–1550

Rofstad EK, Sundfor K, Lyng H, et al (2000) Hypoxia-induced treatment failure in advanced squamous cell carcinoma of the uterine cervix is primarily due to hypoxia-induced radiation resistance rather than hypoxia-induced metastasis. Br J Cancer 83:354–359.

Sathya JR, Davis IR, Julian JA et al (2005) Randomized trial comparing iridium implant plus external-beam radiation therapy with external beam radiation therapy alone in node-negative locally advanced cancer of the prostate. J Clin Oncol 23:1192–1199

Schinagl DA, Vogel WV, Hoffmann AL et al (2007) Comparison of five segmentation tools for ^{18}F-fluoro-deoxy-glucose-positron emission tomography-based target volume definition in head and neck cancer. Int J Radiat Oncol Biol Phys 69:1282–1289

Schulz-Ertner D, Tsujii H (2007) Particle radiation therapy using proton and heavier ion beams. J Clin Oncol 25:953–964

Schulz-Ertner D, Nikoghosyan A, Hof H et al (2007) Carbon ion radiotherapy of skull base chondrosarcomas. Int J Radiat Oncol Biol Phys 67:171–177

Seibert RM, Ramsey CR, Hines JW et al (2007) A model for predicting lung cancer response to therapy. Int J Radiat Oncol Biol Phys 67:601–609

Selch MT, Ahn E, Laskari A et al (2004) Stereotactic radiotherapy for treatment of cavernous sinus meningiomas. Int J Radiat Oncol Biol Phys 59:101–111

Selker RG, Shapiro WR, Burger P et al (2002) The Brain Tumor Cooperative Group NIH Trial 87–01: a randomised comparison of surgery, external radiotherapy, and carmustine versus surgery, interstitial radiotherapy boost, external radiation therapy, and carmustine. Neurosurgery 51: 343–353

Siker ML, Tome WA, Mehta MP (2006) Tumor volume changes on serial imaging with megavoltage CT for non-small-cell lung cancer during intensity-modulated radiotherapy: how reliable, consistent, and meaningful is the effect? Int J Radiat Oncol Biol Phys 66:135–141

Söderlund K, Stål O, Skoog L et al (2007) Intact Mre11/Rad50/Nbs1 complex predicts good response to radiotherapy in early breast cancer. Int J Radiat Oncol Biol Phys 68:50–58

Sonke JJ, Lebesque J, van Kerk M (2008) Variability of 4-dimensional computed tomography patient models. Int J Radiat Oncol Biol Phys 70:590–598

Souhami L, Seiferheld W, Brachman D et al (2004) Randomized comparison of stereotactic radiosurgery followed by conventional radiotherapy with carmustine to conventional radiotherapy with carmustine for patients with glioblastoma multiforme: report of Radiation Therapy Oncology Group 93–05 protocol. Int J Radiat Oncol Biol Phys 60:853–860

Stadler P, Becker A, Feldmann HJ et al (1999) Influence of the hypoxic subvolume on the survival of patients with head and neck cancer. Int J Radiat Oncol Biol Phys 44:749–754

Stadler P, Feldmann HJ, Creighton C et al (2000) Clinical evidence for correlation of insufficient tissue oxygen supply (hypoxia) and tumor-associated proteolysis in squamous cell carcinoma of the head and neck. Int J Biol Markers 15:235–236

Steenbakkers RJ, Duppen JC, Fitton I et al (2006) Reduction of observer variation using matched CT–PET for lung cancer delineation: a three-dimensional analysis. Int J Radiat Oncol Biol Phys 64:435–448

Tsuji H, Ishikawa H, Yanagi T et al (2007) Carbon-ion radiotherapy for locally advanced or unfavourably located choroidal melanoma: a phase I/II dose-escalation study. Int J Radiat Oncol Biol Phys 67:857–862

Van Baardwijk A, Dooms C, van Suylen RJ et al (2007) The maximum uptake of 18(F)-deoxyglucose on positron emission tomography scan correlates with survival, hypoxia inducible factor-1alpha and GLUT-1 in non-small cell lung cancer. Eur J Cancer 43:1392–1398

Vansteenkiste JF, Stroobants SG, Dupont PJ et al (1999) Prognostic importance of the standardized uptake value on 18(F)-fluoro-2-deoxy-glucose-positron emission tomography scan in non-small-cell lung cancer: an analysis of 125 cases. J Clin Oncol 17:3201–3206

Van Tinteren H, Hoekstra OS, Smit EF et al (2002) Effectiveness of positron emission tomography in the preoperative assessment of patients with suspected non-small-cell lung cancer: the PLUS multicentre randomised trial. Lancet 359:1388–1393

Vanuytsel LJ, Vansteenkiste JF, Stroobants SG et al (2000) The impact of ^{18}F-fluoro-2-deoxy-D-glucose positron emission tomography (FDG-PET) lymph node staging on the radiation treatment volumes in patients with non-small cell lung cancer. Radiother Oncol 55:317–324

Vergis R, Corbishley CM, Norman AR et al (2008) Intrinsic markers of tumour hypoxia and angiogenesis in localised prostate cancer and outcome of radical treatment: a retrospective analysis of two randomised radiotherapy trials and one surgical cohort study. Lancet Oncol in press

Viney RC, Boyer MJ, King MT et al (2004) Randomized controlled trial of the role of positron emission tomography in the management of stage I non-small-cell lung cancer. J Clin Oncol 22:2357–2362

Wallner K, Merrick G, True L et al (2003) [125]I versus [103]Pd for low-risk prostate cancer: preliminary PSA outcomes from a prospective randomized multicenter trial. Int J Radiat Oncol Biol Phys 57:1297–1303

Wang CC (1991) Improved local control of nasopharyngeal carcinoma after intracavitary brachytherapy boost. Am J Clin Oncol 14:5–8

Watanabe H, Mogushi K, Miura M et al (2008) Prediction of lymphatic metastasis based on gene expression profile analysis after brachytherapy for early-stage oral tongue carcinoma. Radiother Oncol in press

Weber WA, Dietlein M, Hellwig D et al (2003) PET with ^{18}F-fluorodeoxyglucose for staging of non-small cell lung cancer. Nuklearmedizin 42:135–144

Weber WA (2005) Use of PET for monitoring cancer therapy and for predicting outcome. J Nucl Med 46:983–995

Weltens C, Menten J, Feron M et al (2001) Interobserver variations in gross tumor volume delineation of brain tumors on computed tomography and impact of magnetic resonance imaging. Radiother Oncol 60:49–59

Werner-Wasik M, Swann RS, Bradley J et al (2008) Increasing tumor volume is predictive of poor overall and progression-free survival: secondary analysis of the Radiation Therapy Oncology Group 93-11 phase I-II radiation dose-escalation study in patients with inoperable non-small-cell lung cancer. Int J Radiat Oncol Biol Phys 70:385–390

Wilson RR (1946) Radiological use of fast protons. Radiology 47:491–498

Woodford C, Yartsev S, Dar AR et al (2007) Adaptive radiotherapy planning on decreasing gross tumor volumes as seen on megavoltage computed tomography images. Int J Radiat Oncol Biol Phys 69:1316–1322

Wouters BG, van den Beucken T, Magagnin MG et al (2005) Control of the hypoxic response through regulation of mRNA translation. Semin Cell Dev Biol 16:487–501

Xia T, Li H, Sun Q et al (2006) Promising clinical outcome of stereotactic body radiation therapy for patients with inoperable stage I/II non-small-cell lung cancer. Int J Radiat Oncol Biol Phys 66:117–125

Yamazaki H, Nishiyama K, Tanaka E et al (2006) Radiotherapy for early glottic carcinoma (T1N0M0): results of prospective randomized study of radiation fraction size and overall treatment time. Int J Radiat Oncol Biol Phys 64:77–82

Yaromina A, Krause M, Thames H et al (2007) Pre-treatment number of clonogenic cells and their radiosensitivity are major determinants of local tumour control after fractionated irradiation. Radiother Oncol 83:304–310

Zhang T, Lu W, Olivera GH et al (2007) Breathing-synchronized delivery: a potential four-dimensional tomotherapy treatment technique. Int J Radiat Oncol Biol Phys 68:1572–1578

Zhao L, West BT, Hayman JA et al (2007) High radiation dose may reduce the negative effect of large gross tumor volume in patients with medically inoperable early-stage non-small cell lung cancer. Int J Radiat Oncol Biol Phys 68:103–110

Zietman AL, DeSilvio ML, Slater JD et al (2005) Comparison of conventional-dose vs. high-dose conformal radiation therapy in clinically localized adenocarcinoma of the prostate: a randomized controlled trial. JAMA 294:1233–1239. Erratum in JAMA 299:899–900

Zimmermann FB, Geinitz H, Schill S et al (2005) Stereotactic hypofractionated radiation therapy for stage I non-small cell lung cancer. Lung Cancer 48:107–114

Zips D, Adam M, Flentje M et al (2004) Impact of hypoxia and the metabolic microenvironment on radiotherapy of solid tumors. Introduction of a multi-institutional research project. Strahlenther Onkol 180:609–615

21

Treatment of the Primary Tumor in Metastatic Cancer: Influence on Outcome

SATOSHI ITASAKA and MASAHIRO HIRAOKA

CONTENTS

KEY POINTS

- Tissue damage, blood loss, transfusions, anesthetics, hypothermia, pain, and/or anxiety that occurs perioperatively result in a mainly cell-mediated immunosuppressive state, which might influence the fate of cancer cells remaining after surgery.
- Changes in the expressed cytokine levels after treatment of a primary tumor can affect the tumor growth. Several cytokines are reported to correlate with distant effects outside of the area of treatment.
- The so-called abscopal effect as a positive influence of treatment outside of the target area is not often observed after radiotherapy.
- Suicide gene therapy has been reported to cause a distant bystander effect.

S. ITASAKA, MD

Assistant Professor, Department of Radiation Oncology and Image-applied Therapy, Kyoto University Graduate School of Medicine, 54 Shogoin Kawahara-cho, Sakyo-ku, Kyoto 606-8507, Japan

M. HIRAOKA, MD, PhD

Chairman and Professor, Department of Radiation Oncology and Image-applied Therapy, Kyoto University Graduate School of Medicine, 54 Shogoin Kawahara-cho, Sakyo-ku, Kyoto 606-8507, Japan

Abstract

Many cancer patients present with metastatic disease at the time of diagnosis. Usually, systemic therapy is the first choice of treatment; however, in some cases the primary tumor is treated first to relieve local symptoms, to reduce the tumor volume, or for other reasons. Surprisingly local therapy sometimes has a great impact on tumors outside of the treatment target: metastatic tumors grow more rapidly or shrink in conjunction with the local therapy directed at the primary lesion. These phenomena are reported for many types of cancer and treatments including radiation therapy, surgery, and other therapies. Although a few major theories have been proposed to explain these phenomena, they are not yet fully understood. Understanding of the mechanism would be useful to develop new treatment approaches for cancer patients with metastatic disease.

21.1
Introduction

It has been proposed by different authors that aggressive local treatment of an accessible, limited-stage primary tumor contributes to increased survival in patients diagnosed with synchronous distant metastases, e.g., selected patients with brain metastasis from non-small cell lung cancer (Hu et al. 2006; I et al. 2006; Yang et al. 2008). The question arises whether the occasional long-term success of such strategies results from actual removal of all malignant cells, or removal of all macroscopic manifestations followed by systemic chemotherapy, which might control micrometastases, or whether different mechanisms might be involved. Yet even negative consequences, e.g., of surgical procedures, cannot be ruled out. There have been a few major theories proposed to explain the possible consequences of radical treatment of the primary tumor in patients with metastatic cancer. For example, a systemic immune reaction generated against local tumor antigens has been described to affect distant tumor growth, and systemic release of specific cytokines generated against the primary tumor has also been reported to have a distant effect. Rapid growth of metastatic tumors is often observed and the development of new metastatic lesions might follow surgical resection of the primary tumor. The stress of surgery can reduce systemic immunity, and the immunosuppressive effects of surgery have been shown to increase the risk of metastasis. In the field of radiation therapy, the decrease of tumors outside of the radiation field is rarely observed after irradiation of the primary tumor and this phenomenon has been well known for a long time as the abscopal effect or bystander effect. Fifty years ago, Dr. R.H. Mole called this surprising phenomenon the "abscopal effect" (Mole 1953). The word "abscopal" is derived from the Latin prefix "ab" meaning "away from" and the Greek word "skopos" meaning "target." Multiple cases of the abscopal effect observed after radiotherapy have been reported for a variety of malignancies including lymphoma, leukemia, melanoma, papillary adenocarcinoma, and hepatocellular carcinoma. Radiation may have an advantage over surgery by providing local control and inducing a local inflammatory response with less systemic suppression of the immune system. The effects of radiation treatment on the immune system, cytokines, or other factors have been reported to be related to these distant effects.

21.2
Surgery

Rapid recurrence after surgical treatment can result from several possible mechanisms, including incomplete surgical excision, occult metastases, and potential seeding from surgical manipulation (Ben-Eliyahu 2002; Eschwege et al. 1995; Kassabian et al. 1993). Furthermore, suppression of immunity due to surgical stress, decreases in antiangiogenic factors released by the resected tumor, and the release of growth factors (e.g., epidermal growth factor or transforming growth factor-β) necessary for wound healing can enhance tumor proliferation (Ben-Eliyahu 2002). Tissue damage, blood loss, transfusions, anesthetics, hypothermia, pain, and/ or anxiety that occurs perioperatively result in a mainly cell-mediated immunosuppressive state (Shakhar and Ben-Eliyahu 2003; Vallejo et al. 2003). Carter et al. reported that open cecectomy was associated with significantly more lung metastases than anesthesia alone or laparoscopic-assisted cecectomy in a mouse model (Carter et al. 2003). Page and Ben-Eliyahu also demonstrated in a mouse model that surgery resulted in a 2- to 3.5-fold increase in lung tumor retention and that indomethacin significantly reduced the tumor retention (Page and Ben-Eliyahu 2002). The effect was associated with restoration of natural killer cell (NK cell) activity and/or reduction of interleukin (IL)-6. Decrease in NK cell activity through cytokines, such as IL-6 and immunosuppressive acidic protein (IAP), has been implicated in perioperative immunosuppression (Aso et al. 1992; Biffl et al. 1996; Carter and Whelan 2001; Oka et al. 1993; Schietroma et al. 2001). Other animal studies have also confirmed the correlation between high risk of metastasis and low NK cell activity induced by surgery (Ben-Eliyahu et al. 1999; Da Costa et al. 1998; Page and Ben-Eliyahu 1999; Wiltrout et al. 1985). Low NK cell activity during the perioperative period is associated with an increase in cancer recurrence and mortality in patients, e.g., for head and neck cancer (Schantz et al. 1987, 1989), lung cancer (Fujisawa and Yamaguchi 1997), colorectal cancer (Koda et al. 1997; Tartter et al. 1987), and breast cancer (Levy et al. 1985).

21.3
Radiation

Compared to surgery, radiation therapy appears to cause less immunosuppression (Tang et al. 1996).

Radiation-induced immune reaction or cytokines might affect tumors outside of the radiation field and under rare circumstances cause a significant outcome. Ohba et al. described a man who underwent radiation therapy for bone metastasis from hepatocellular carcinoma (OHBA et al. 1998). Surprisingly, regression of the non-irradiated primary tumor was observed. A rise in the serum tumor necrosis factor (TNF)-α after radiotherapy coincided with the response of the primary tumor and an immune response induced by TNF-α was suggested by the authors. Several cases of abscopal effects have been reported for leukemias and lymphomas after radiation therapy. One possible mechanism that is relevant mainly to leukemias and lymphomas is that the distant effect observed is due to the circulation of diseased lymphocytes through the field of local irradiation.

Radiation has the potential to enhance tumor immunogenicity by inducing an inflammatory response in tumor tissue and lead to the activation of the immune system. Radiation induces cell apoptosis and necrosis, and a dendritic cell mediated antitumor immunity can be induced by these necrotic and apoptotic cells in vitro and in vivo (ALBERT et al. 1998; BHARDWAJ 2001; KOTERA et al. 2001; SAUTER et al. 2000). It has been suggested that this cell death leads to the release of inflammatory cytokines, which may be responsible for the abscopal effect after radiation therapy (HONG et al. 1995; QUARMBY et al. 1999; WATTERS 1999). Radiation has direct effects on tumor blood vessels and can cause increased permeability. Increases in cytokines by radiation also cause increased permeability of tumor blood vessels, leading to greater access for dendritic and T cells to the tumor cells (GANSS et al. 2002; NIKITINA and GABRILOVICH 2001). Another mechanism is that radiation can induce antigen expression. Radiation has been shown to induce the expression of Death receptors (CD95), MHC class I expression, carcinoembryonic antigen, and a variety of adhesion molecules, such as ICAM-1 (HAREYAMA et al. 1991; SANTIN et al. 1998a, b).

To enhance the antitumor immunity, dendritic cell growth factor, Flt-3 ligand was combined with radiation therapy and there was greater induction of the abscopal effect compared with either treatment alone in certain tumor cell lines (CHAKRAVARTY et al. 1999; DEMARIA et al. 2004). Active variant of human macrophage inflammatory protein-1α also induced abscopal effects by radiation in several mouse tumor models and the accumulation of CD8+ and CD4+ lymphocyte and NK cells was observed in non-irradiated tumor sites (SHIRAISHI et al. 2008). There have also been a number of studies that have shown that radiation combined with cytokine

therapy reduces the risk of metastasis. IL-2 has been combined with lung irradiation and the rate of lung metastasis in renal cancer was studied. Although results in animal studies were promising, one phase II trial did not show a difference in metastatic rates between the patients treated with IL-2 alone or IL-2 with radiation (REDMAN et al. 1998; YOUNES et al. 1995a, b). These findings support the important role of the immune system in the abscopal effect.

The abscopal effect, however, is not often observed, possibly because of the weak immune reaction. The majority of cancer antigens are the same as those expressed on normal tissues or are slightly modified mutants (FRIEDMAN 2002) and tumors can escape from the immune system. Because of this, cancer cells are often unable to activate naive T cells independently because they lack co-stimulatory molecules (CHEN et al. 1992; TOWNSEND and ALLISON 1993). To induce abscopal effects efficiently, the development of new methods to induce cancer-specific antigens by radiation appears necessary.

21.4
Cytokines

Many types of cytokines are expressed by tumors. Changes in the expressed cytokine level by the treatment of a primary tumor can affect the tumor growth. Several cytokines are reported to correlate with distant effects outside of the area of treatment.

Overexpression of IL-6 and IL-6 receptor (IL-6R) is often observed in many types of cancer and is frequently correlated with the grade and stage of the tumor (TRIKHA et al. 2003). In most renal cell carcinomas, IL-6 is expressed and is necessary for proliferation (HORIGUCHI et al. 2002; MIKI et al. 1989; TAKENAWA et al. 1991). Large quantities of IL-6 are produced by the primary tumor and stimulate the growth of both primary and metastatic tumors (MIZUTANI et al. 1995). In addition, IL-6 increases the expression of glutathione S-transferase and makes renal cell carcinoma cells cisplatin resistant. The occasionally observed abscopal effects after nephrectomy may be attributed to the reduction of growth stimuli after removal of the primary tumor (SANCHEZ-ORTIZ et al. 2003).

IL-1α and IL-1β are inflammatory cytokines and are also expressed in a variety of cancer cell lines, including stomach, lung, ovary, breast, epithelium, and pancreas (BHAT-NAKSHATRI et al. 1998; CHEN et al. 2003; ITO et al. 1993; KAJI et al. 1995; KUMAR et al. 2003; KURTZMAN et al. 1999; LI et al. 1992; TSUYUOKA et al. 1994). IL-1α increases the expression of both adhesion molecules on vascular endothelial cells (LAFRENIE et al. 1994; LAURI et al. 1991) and proteases from tumor cell lines in vitro (MACKAY et al. 1992; TRAN-THANG et al. 1996) and thus enhances metastasis in some cancers (ANASAGASTI et al. 1997; TAKEDA et al. 1991). In addition, these interleukins induce cyclooxygenase-2 (COX-2) expression and lead to prostaglandin expression (DI MARI et al. 2003; FAN et al. 2001; LIU et al. 2003; MAIHOFNER et al. 2003; MIFFLIN et al. 2002). Overexpression of COX-2 in tumors can cause inflammation, immune response suppression, apoptosis inhibition, angiogenesis, carcinogenesis, tumor cell invasion, and metastasis (KOKI and MASFERRER 2002).

21.5
Angiogenesis Inhibition

Several kinds of intrinsic antiangiogenic molecules have been discovered, and the balance of angiogenic molecules and antiangiogenic molecules is one of the key factors behind tumor growth. Therefore, the decrease of these intrinsic angiogenesis inhibitors caused by the removal of a large primary tumor leads to angiogenesis and can enhance the growth of metastatic disease. For example rapid growth of liver metastases after resection of primary colon cancer is often observed in the clinic. Several experimental animal models indeed suggest that the growth of a primary tumor can inhibit the production of distant metastases (reviewed by GORELIK 1983 and by PREHN 1991). For example, a variant of Lewis lung carcinoma completely suppresses the growth of its metastases and angiostatin, a fragment of plasminogen, was purified from the urine of tumor-bearing mice (HOLMGREN et al. 1995; O'REILLY et al. 1994). Endostatin (BOEHM et al. 1997; O'REILLY et al. 1997), a carboxyl-terminal fragment of collagen XVIII, is also a specific inhibitor of endothelial cell proliferation and migration (YAMAGUCHI et al. 1999). Hartford et al. demonstrated in mice that irradiation of a primary tumor enhances inhibition of angiogenesis at a distal site, unlike surgery, which tended to increase distal angiogenesis. In addition, they also showed that endostatin levels were twice as high in irradiated mice as compared to surgically treated mice (HARTFORD et al. 2000). In another study, p53 appeared to mediate a radiation abscopal effect in mice that was dose dependent and the authors hypothesized that the systemic antiangiogenic effects were mediated through p53 (CAMPHAUSEN et al. 2003).

21.6
Other Therapies

Suicide gene therapy also has been reported to cause a distant bystander effect (AGARD et al. 2001; BI et al. 1997; CHIKARA et al. 2001, DONG et al. 2003; ENGELMANN et al. 2002; OKADA et al. 2001; PIERREFITE-CARLE et al. 2002). For example, Chikara et al. treated mouse prostate cancer xenografts with intratumoral injection of an adenoviral vector expressing herpes simplex-1 thymidine kinase (Ad-HSV-TK) and intraperitoneal injection of ganciclovir, followed by radiation (5 Gy), which resulted in decreased tumor growth and prolonged survival. The combination of gene therapy and radiation therapy also reduced the number of lung metastases compared to Ad-HSV-TK therapy alone, while radiation alone had no distant effect (CHIKARA et al. 2001). Suicide-gene-modified tumor cells can also induce a systemic antitumor effect that is mediated by NK cells (PIERREFITE-CARLE et al. 2002) or cytotoxic T lymphocytes (AGARD et al. 2001; OKADA et al. 2001). Overexpression of cytokines in tumor cells or cells like dendritic cells by transgenes expression also showed a distant bystander effect, including IL-2 (ASADA et al. 2002; FEARON et al. 1990; HILLMAN et al. 2004; HUANG et al. 1996), IL-4 (MORET-TATAY et al. 2003), TNF-α (KAWAKITA et al. 1997), IL-12 (TATSUMI et al. 2003), IL-15 (SUZUKI et al. 2001), IL-18 (TATSUMI et al. 2003), Flt-3 ligand (DONG et al. 2003), IFN-β (DONG et al. 1999), and GM-CSF (MORET-TATAY et al. 2003), or combinations of these (KAWAKITA et al. 1997). For example, Dong et al. demonstrated that murine squamous tumor cells (B4B8) expressing the soluble form of Flt-3 ligand were able to induce a distant bystander effect in naive cells in the contralateral flank (DONG et al. 2003). Vartak et al. showed in a mouse model that local hyperthermia of one leg prior to transplantation of a fibrosarcoma reduced the tumor growth not only in the heated but also in the unheated contralateral leg (VARTAK et al. 1993). Some studies showed that hyperthermia may enhance the immune response by increasing NK cell activity (YOSHIOKA et al. 1990) and cytokine production like interferon-gamma (DOWNING et al. 1988).

21.7
Conclusion

To understand the underlying mechanism of the distant effects on metastasis caused by local therapy, it is essential to understand such factors as the immune system and cytokine levels before, during, and after therapy. However, most clinical studies are more concentrated on treatment of the primary tumor and correlations between primary and metastatic tumors have not been of great interest. With cognizance of these correlations, we can minimize detrimental effects, while developing methods to stimulate the immune system and redirect inflammatory responses, or expression of cytokines to suppress primary tumor and metastasis. Although, radiation therapy causes less immunosuppression as compared to surgery and has the potential to induce tumor immunity, we do not know the method for making full use of abscopal effects. The development of a new approach to enhance abscopal effects is warranted for cancer patients with metastatic disease.

References

Agard C, Ligeza C, Dupas B, Izembart A, El Kouri C, Moullier P, et al. (2001) Immune-dependent distant bystander effect after adenovirus-mediated suicide gene transfer in a rat model of liver colorectal metastasis. Cancer Gene Ther 8:128–136

Albert ML, Darnell JC, Bender A, Francisco LM, Bhardwaj N, Darnell RB (1998) Tumor-specific killer cells in paraneoplastic cerebellar degeneration. Nat Med 4:1321–1324

Anasagasti MJ, Olaso E, Calvo F, Mendoza L, Martin JJ, Bidaurrazaga J, et al (1997) Interleukin 1-dependent and -independent mouse melanoma metastases. J Natl Cancer Inst 89:645–651

Asada H, Kishida T, Hirai H, Satoh E, Ohashi S, Takeuchi M, et al (2002) Significant antitumor effects obtained by autologous tumor cell vaccine engineered to secrete interleukin (IL)-12 and IL-18 by means of the EBV/lipoplex. Mol Ther 5:609–616

Aso H, Tamura K, Yoshie O, Nakamura T, Kikuchi S, Ishida N (1992) Impaired NK response of cancer patients to IFN-alpha but not to IL-2: correlation with serum immunosuppressive acidic protein (IAP) and role of suppressor macrophage. Microbiol Immunol 36:1087–1097

Ben-Eliyahu S (2002) The price of anticancer intervention. Does surgery promote metastasis? Lancet Oncol 3:578–579

Ben-Eliyahu S, Page GG, Yirmiya R, Shakhar G (1999) Evidence that stress and surgical interventions promote tumor development by suppressing natural killer cell activity. Int J Cancer 80:880–888

Bhardwaj N (2001) Processing and presentation of antigens by dendritic cells: implications for vaccines. Trends Mol Med 7:388–394

Bhat-Nakshatri P, Newton TR, Goulet Jr R, Nakshatri H (1998) NF-kappaB activation and interleukin 6 production in fibroblasts by estrogen receptor- negative breast cancer cell-derived interleukin 1alpha. Proc Natl Acad Sci U S A 95:6971–6976

Bi W, Kim YG, Feliciano ES, Pavelic L, Wilson KM, Pavelic ZP, et al (1997) An HSVtk-mediated local and distant antitumor bystander effect in tumors of head and neck origin in athymic mice. Cancer Gene Ther 4:246–252

Biffl WL, Moore EE, Moore FA, Peterson VM (1996) Interleukin-6 in the injured patient. Marker of injury or mediator of inflammation. Ann Surg 224:647–664

Boehm T, Folkman J, Browder T, O'Reilly MS (1997) Antiangiogenic therapy of experimental cancer does not induce acquired drug resistance. Nature 390:404–407

Camphausen K, Moses MA, Menard C, Sproull M, Beecken J, Folkman J, et al (2003) Radiation abscopal antitumor effect is mediated through p53. Cancer Res 63:1990–1993

Carter JJ, Whelan RL (2001) The immunologic consequences of laparoscopy in oncology. Surg Oncol Clin N Am 10:655–677

Carter JJ, Feingold DL, Kirman I, Oh A, Wildbrett P, Asi Z, et al (2003) Laparoscopic-assisted cecectomy is associated with decreased formation of postoperative pulmonary metastases compared with open cecectomy in a murine model. Surgery 134:432–436

Chakravarty PK, Alfieri A, Thomas EK, Beri V, Tanaka KE, Vikram B, et al (1999) Flt3-ligand administration after radiation therapy prolongs survival in a murine model of metastatic lung cancer. Cancer Res 59:6028–6032

Chen L, Ashe S, Brady WA, Hellstrom I, Hellstrom KE, Ledbetter JA, et al (1992) Costimulation of antitumor immunity by the B7 counterreceptor for the T lymphocyte molecules CD28 and CTLA-4. Cell 71:1093–1102

Chen WR, Jeong SW, Lucroy MD, Wolf RF, Howard EW, Liu H, et al (2003) Induced antitumor immunity against DMBA-4 metastatic mammary tumors in rats using laser immunotherapy. Int J Cancer 107:1053–1057

Chikara M, Huang H, Vlachaki MT, Zhu X, Teh B, Chiu KJ, et al (2001) Enhanced therapeutic effect of HSV-tk + GCV gene therapy and ionizing radiation for prostate cancer. Mol Ther 3:536–542

Da Costa ML, Redmond P, Bouchier-Hayes DJ (1998) The effect of laparotomy and laparoscopy on the establishment of spontaneous tumor metastases. Surgery 124:516–525

Demaria S, Ng B, Devitt ML, Babb JS, Kawashima N, Liebes L, et al (2004) Ionizing radiation inhibition of distant untreated tumors (abscopal effect) is immune mediated. Int J Radiat Oncol Biol Phys 58:862–870

Di Mari JF, Mifflin RC, Adegboyega PA, Saada JI, Powell DW (2003) IL-1alpha-induced COX-2 expression in human intestinal myofibroblasts is dependent on a PKCzeta-ROS pathway. Gastroenterology 124:1855–1865

Dong Z, Greene G, Pettaway C, Dinney CP, Eue I, Lu W, et al (1999) Suppression of angiogenesis, tumorigenicity, and metastasis by human prostate cancer cells engineered to produce interferon-beta. Cancer Res 59:872–879

Dong J, Bohinski RJ, Li YQ, Van Waes C, Hendler F, Gleich L, et al (2003) Antitumor effect of secreted Flt3-ligand can act at distant tumor sites in a murine model of head and neck cancer. Cancer Gene Ther 10:96–104

Downing JF, Martinez-Valdez H, Elizondo RS, Walker EB, Taylor MW (1988) Hyperthermia in humans enhances interferon-gamma synthesis and alters the peripheral lymphocyte population. J Interferon Res 8:143–150

Engelmann C, Heslan JM, Fabre M, Lagarde JP, Klatzmann Y, Panis Y (2002) Importance, mechanisms and limitations of the distant bystander effect in cancer gene therapy of experimental liver tumors. Cancer Lett 179:59–69

Eschwege P, Dumas F, Blanchet P, Le Maire V, Benoit G, Jardin A, et al (1995) Haematogenous dissemination of prostatic epithelial cells during radical prostatectomy. Lancet 346:1528–1530

Fan XM, Wong BC, Lin MC, Cho CH, Wang WP, Kung HF, et al (2001) Interleukin-1beta induces cyclo-oxygenase-2 expression in gastric cancer cells by the p38 and p44/42 mitogen-activated protein kinase signaling pathways. J Gastroenterol Hepatol 16:1098–1104

Fearon ER, Pardoll DM, Itaya T, Golumbek P, Levitsky HI, Simons JW, et al (1990) Interleukin-2 production by tumor cells bypasses T helper function in the generation of an antitumor response. Cell 60:397–403

Friedman EJ (2002) Immune modulation by ionizing radiation and its implications for cancer immunotherapy. Curr Pharm Des 8:1765–1780

Fujisawa T, Yamaguchi Y (1997) Autologous tumor killing activity as a prognostic factor in primary resected nonsmall cell carcinoma of the lung. Cancer 79:474–481

Ganss R, Ryschich E, Klar E, Arnold B, Hammerling GJ (2002) Combination of T-cell therapy and trigger of inflammation induces remodeling of the vasculature and tumor eradication. Cancer Res 62:1462–1470

Gorelik E (1983) Concomitant tumor immunity and the resistance to a second tumor challenge. Adv Cancer Res 39:71–120

Hareyama M, Imai K, Kubo K, Takahashi H, Koshiba H, Hinoda Y, et al (1991) Effect of radiation on the expression of carcinoembryonic antigen of human gastric adenocarcinoma cells. Cancer 67:2269–2274

Hartford AC, Gohongi T, Fukumura D, Jain RK (2000) Irradiation of a primary tumor, unlike surgical removal, enhances angiogenesis suppression at a distal site: potential role of host–tumor interaction. Cancer Res 60:2128–2131

Hillman GG, Slos P, Wang Y, Wright JL, Layer A, De Meyer M, et al (2004) Tumor irradiation followed by intratumoral cytokine gene therapy for murine renal adenocarcinoma. Cancer Gene Ther 11:61–72

Holmgren L, O'Reilly MS, Folkman J (1995) Dormancy of micrometastases: balanced proliferation and apoptosis in the presence of angiogenesis suppression. Nat Med 1:149–153

Hong JH, Chiang CS, Campbell IL, Sun JR, Withers HR, McBride WH (1995) Induction of acute phase gene expression by brain irradiation. Int J Radiat Oncol Biol Phys 33:619–626

Horiguchi A, Oya M, Marumo K, Murai M (2002) STAT3, but not ERKs, mediates the IL-6-induced proliferation of renal cancer cells, ACHN and 769P. Kidney Int 61:926–938

Hu C, Chang EL, Hassenbusch SJ 3rd, Allen PK, Woo SY, Mahajan A, et al (2006) Nonsmall cell lung cancer presenting with synchronous solitary brain metastasis. Cancer 106:1998–2004

Huang H, Chen SH, Kosai K, Finegold MJ, Woo SL (1996) Gene therapy for hepatocellular carcinoma: long-term remission of primary and metastatic tumors in mice by interleukin-2 gene therapy in vivo. Gene Ther 3:980–987

I H, Lee JI, Nam DH, Ahn YC, Shim YM, Kim K, et al (2006) Surgical treatment of non-small cell lung cancer with isolated synchronous brain metastases. J Korean Med Sci 21:236–241

Ito R, Kitadai Y, Kyo E, Yokozaki H, Yasui W, Yamashita U, et al (1993) Interleukin 1 alpha acts as an autocrine growth stimulator for human gastric carcinoma cells. Cancer Res 53:4102–4106

Kaji M, Ishikura H, Kishimoto T, Omi M, Ishizu A, Kimura C, et al (1995) E-selectin expression induced by pancreas-carcinoma-derived interleukin-1 alpha results in enhanced adhesion of pancreas carcinoma cells to endothelial cells. Int J Cancer 60:712–717

Kassabian VS, Bottles K, Weaver R, Williams RD, Paulson DF, Scardino PT (1993) Possible mechanism for seeding of tumor during radical prostatectomy. J Urol 150:1169–1171

Kawakita M, Rao GS, Ritchey JK, Ornstein DK, Hudson MA, Tartaglia J, et al (1997) Effect of canarypox virus (ALVAC)-mediated cytokine expression on murine prostate tumor growth. J Natl Cancer Inst 89:428–436

Koda K, Saito N, Takiguchi N, Oda K, Nunomura M, Nakajima N (1997) Preoperative natural killer cell activity: correlation with distant metastases in curatively research colorectal carcinomas. Int Surg 82:190–193

Koki AT, Masferrer JL (2002) Celecoxib: a specific COX-2 inhibitor with anticancer properties. Cancer Control 9(suppl 2):28–35

Kotera Y, Shimizu K, Mule JJ (2001) Comparative analysis of necrotic and apoptotic tumor cells as a source of antigen(s) in dendritic cell-based immunization. Cancer Res 61:8105–8109

Kumar S, Kishimoto H, Chua HL, Badve S, Miller KD, Bigsby RM, et al (2003) Interleukin-1 alpha promotes tumor growth and cachexia in MCF-7 xenograft model of breast cancer. Am J Pathol 163:2531–2541

Kurtzman SH, Anderson KH, Wang Y, Miller LJ, Renna M, Stankus M, et al (1999) Cytokines in human breast cancer: IL-1alpha and IL-1beta expression. Oncol Rep 6:65–70

Lafrenie RM, Gallo S, Podor TJ, Buchanan MR, Orr FW (1994) The relative roles of vitronectin receptor, E-selectin and alpha 4 beta 1 in cancer cell adhesion to interleukin-1-treated endothelial cells. Eur J Cancer A 30:2151–2158

Lauri D, Needham L, Martin-Padura I, Dejana E (1991) Tumor cell adhesion to endothelial cells: endothelial leukocyte adhesion molecule-1 as an inducible adhesive receptor specific for colon carcinoma cells. J Natl Cancer Inst 83:1321–1324

Levy SM, Herberman RB, Maluish AM, Schlien B, Lippman M (1985) Prognostic risk assessment in primary breast cancer by behavioral and immunological parameters. Health Psychol 4:99–113

Li BY, Mohanraj D, Olson MC, Moradi M, Twiggs L, Carson LF, et al (1992) Human ovarian epithelial cancer cell cultures in vitro express both interleukin 1 alpha and beta genes. Cancer Res 52:2248–2252

Liu W, Reinmuth N, Stoeltzing O, Parikh AA, Tellez C, Williams S, et al (2003) Cyclooxygenase-2 is up-regulated by interleukin-1 beta in human colorectal cancer cells via multiple signaling pathways. Cancer Res 63:3632–3636

Mackay AR, Ballin M, Pelina MD, Farina AR, Nason AM, Hartzler JL, et al (1992) Effect of phorbol ester and cytokines on matrix metalloproteinase and tissue inhibitor of metalloproteinase expression in tumor and normal cell lines. Invasion Metastasis 12:168–184

Maihofner C, Charalambous MP, Bhambra U, Lightfoot T, Geisslinger G, Gooderham NJ (2003) Expression of cyclooxygenase-2 parallels expression of interleukin-1beta, interleukin-6 and NF-kappaB in human colorectal cancer. Carcinogenesis 24:665–671

Mifflin RC, Saada JI, Di Mari JF, Adegboyega PA, Valentich DW, Powell DW (2002) Regulation of COX-2 expression in human intestinal myofibroblasts: mechanisms of IL-1-mediated induction. Am J Physiol Cell Physiol 282:C824–C834

Miki S, Iwano M, Miki Y, Yamamoto M, Tang B, Yokokawa K, et al (1989) Interleukin-6 (IL-6) functions as an in vitro autocrine growth factor in renal cell carcinomas. FEBS Lett 250:607–610

Mizutani Y, Bonavida B, Koishihara Y, Akamatsu K, Ohsugi O, Yoshida O (1995) Sensitization of human renal cell carcinoma cells to cis-diamminedichloroplatinum(II) by anti-interleukin 6 monoclonal antibody or anti-interleukin 6 receptor monoclonal antibody. Cancer Res 55:590–596

Mole RH (1953) Whole body irradiation: radiobiology or medicine. Br J Radiol 26:234–241

Moret-Tatay I, Diaz J, Marco FM, Crespo A, Alino SF (2003) Complete tumor prevention by engineered tumor cell vaccines employing nonviral vectors. Cancer Gene Ther 10:887–897

Nikitina EY, Gabrilovich DI (2001) Combination of gamma-irradiation and dendritic cell administration induces a potent antitumor response in tumor-bearing mice: approach to treatment of advanced stage cancer. Int J Cancer 94:825–833

Ohba K, Omagari K, Nakamura T, Ikuno N, Saeki S, Matsuo I, et al (1998) Abscopal regression of hepatocellular carcinoma after radiotherapy for bone metastasis. Gut 43:575–577

Oka M, Mitsunaga H, Hazama S, Yoshino S, Suzuki T (1993) Natural killer activity and serum immunosuppressive acidic protein levels in esophageal and gastric cancers. Surg Today 23:669–674

Okada T, Shah M, Higginbotham JN, Li Q, Wildner O, Walbridge S, et al (2001) AV.TK-mediated killing of subcutaneous tumors in situ results in effective immunization against established secondary intracranial tumor deposits. Gene Ther 8:1315–1322

O'Reilly MS, Holmgren L, Shing Y, et al (1994) Angiostatin: a novel angiogenesis inhibitor that mediates the suppression of metastases by a Lewis lung carcinoma. Cell 79:315–328

O'Reilly MS, Boehm T, Shing Y, et al (1997) Endostatin: an endogenous inhibitor of angiogenesis and tumor growth. Cell 88:277–285

Page GG, Ben-Eliyahu S (1999) A role for NK cells in greater susceptibility of young rats to metastatic formation. Dev Comp Immunol 23:87–96

Page GG, Ben-Eliyahu S (2002) Indomethacin attenuates the immunosuppressive and tumor promoting effects of surgery. J Pain 3:301–308

Pierrefite-Carle V, Baque P, Gavelli A, Brossette N, Benchimol D, Bourgeon A, et al (2002) Subcutaneous or intrahepatic injection of suicide gene modified tumour cells induces a systemic antitumour response in a metastatic model of colon carcinoma in rats. Gut 50:387–391

Prehn RT (1991) The inhibition of tumor growth by tumor mass. Cancer Res 51:2–4

Quarmby S, Kumar P, Kumar S (1999) Radiation-induced normal tissue injury: role of adhesion molecules in leukocyte-endothelial cell interactions. Int J Cancer 82:385–395

Redman BG, Hillman GG, Flaherty L, Forman J, Dezso B, Haas GP (1998) Phase II trial of sequential radiation and interleukin 2 in the treatment of patients with metastatic renal cell carcinoma. Clin Cancer Res 4:283–286

Sanchez-Ortiz RF, Tannir N, Ahrar K, Wood CG (2003) Spontaneous regression of pulmonary metastases from renal cell carcinoma after radio frequency ablation of primary tumor: an in situ tumor vaccine? J Urol 170:178–179

Santin AD, Hermonat PL, Ravaggi A, Chiriva-Internati M, Hiserodt JC, Pecorelli S, et al (1998a) Effects of retinoic acid combined with irradiation on the expression of major histocompatibility complex molecules and adhesion/costimulation molecules ICAM-1 in human cervical cancer. Gynecol Oncol 70:195–201

Santin AD, Hermonat PL, Ravaggi A, Chiriva-Internati M, Pecorelli S, Parham GP (1998b) Radiation enhanced expression of E6/E7 transforming oncogenes of human papillomavirus-16 in human cervical cancer. Cancer 83:2346–2352

Sauter B, Albert ML, Francisco L, Larsson M, Somersan S, Bhardwaj N (2000) Consequences of cell death: exposure to necrotic tumor cells, but not primary tissue cells or apoptotic cells, induces the maturation of immunostimulatory dendritic cells. J Exp Med 191:423–434

Schantz SP, Brown BW, Lira E, Taylor DL, Beddingfield N (1987) Evidence for the role of natural immunity in the control of metastatic spread of head and neck cancer. Cancer Immunol Immunother 25:141–148

Schantz SP, Savage HE, Racz T, Taylor DL, Sacks PG (1989) Natural killer cells and metastases from pharyngeal carcinoma. Am J Surg 158:361–366

Schietroma M, Carlei F, Lezoche E, Agnifili A, Enang GN, Mattucci S, et al (2001) Evaluation of immune response in patients after open or laparoscopic cholecystectomy. Hepatogastroenterology 48:642–646

Shakhar G, Ben-Eliyahu S (2003) Potential prophylactic measures against postoperative immunosuppression: could they reduce recurrence rates in oncological patients? Ann Surg Oncol 10:972–992

Shiraishi K, Ishiwata Y, Nakagawa K, Yokochi S, Taruki C, Akuta T, et al (2008) Enhancement of antitumor radiation efficacy and consistent induction of the abscopal effect in mice by ECI301, an active variant of macrophage inflammatory protein-1alpha. Clin Cancer Res 14:1159–1166

Suzuki K, Nakazato H, Matsui H, Hasumi M, Shibata Y, Ito K, et al (2001) NK cell-mediated antitumor immune response to human prostate cancer cell, PC-3: immunogene therapy using a highly secretable form of interleukin-15 gene transfer. J Leukoc Biol 69:531–537

Takeda K, Fujii N, Nitta Y, Sakihara H, Nakayama K, Rikiishi H, et al (1991) Murine tumor cells metastasizing selectively in the liver: ability to produce hepatocyte-activating cytokines interleukin-1 and/or -6. Jpn J Cancer Res 82:1299–1308

Takenawa J, Kaneko Y, Fukumoto M, Fukatsu A, Hirano T, Fukuyama H, et al (1991) Enhanced expression of interleukin-6 in primary human renal cell carcinomas. J Natl Cancer Inst 83:1668–1672

Tang JT, Yamazaki H, Nishimoto N, Inoue T, Nose T, Koizumi M, et al (1996) Effect of radiotherapy on serum level of interleukin 6 in patients with cervical carcinoma. Anticancer Res 16:2005–2008

Tartter PI, Steinberg B, Barron DM, Martinelli G (1987) The prognostic significance of natural killer cytotoxicity in patients with colorectal cancer. Arch Surg 122:1264–1268

Tatsumi T, Huang J, Gooding WE, Gambotto A, Robbins PD, Vujanovic NL, et al (2003) Intratumoral delivery of dendritic cells engineered to secrete both interleukin (IL)-12 and IL-18 effectively treats local and distant disease in association with broadly reactive Tc1-type immunity. Cancer Res 63:6378–6386

Townsend SE, Allison JP (1993) Tumor rejection after direct costimulation of CD8 + T cells by B7-transfected melanoma cells. Science 259:368–370

Tran-Thang C, Kruithof E, Lahm H, Schuster WA, Tada M, Sordat B (1996) Modulation of the plasminogen activation system by inflammatory cytokines in human colon carcinoma cells. Br J Cancer 74:846–852

Trikha M, Corringham R, Klein B, Rossi JF (2003) Targeted antiinterleukin-6 monoclonal antibody therapy for cancer: a review of the rationale and clinical evidence. Clin Cancer Res 9:4653–4665

Tsuyuoka R, Takahashi T, Sasaki Y, Taniguchi Y, Fukumoto A, Suzuki A, et al (1994) Colony-stimulating factor-producing tumours: production of granulocyte colony-stimulating factor and interleukin-6 is secondary to interleukin-1 production. Eur J Cancer A 30:2130–2136

Vallejo R, Hord ED, Barna SA, Santiago-Palma J, Ahmed S (2003) Perioperative immunosuppression in cancer patients. J Environ Pathol Toxicol Oncol 22:139–146

Vartak S, George KC, Singh BB (1993) Antitumor effects of local hyperthermia on a mouse fibrosarcoma. Anticancer Res 13:727–729

Watters D (1999) Molecular mechanisms of ionizing radiation induced apoptosis. Immunol Cell Biol 77:263–271

Wiltrout RH, Herberman RB, Zhang SR, Chirigos MA, Ortaldo KM, Green Jr KM, et al (1985) Role of organ-associated NK cells in decreased formation of experimental metastases in lung and liver. J Immunol 134:4267–4275

Yamaguchi N, Anand-Apte B, Lee M (1999) Endostatin inhibits VEGF-induced endothelial cell migration and tumor growth independently of zinc binding. EMBO J 18:4414–4423

Yang SY, Kim DG, Lee SH, Chung HT, Paek SH, Hyun Kim J, et al (2008) Pulmonary resection in patients with nonsmall-cell lung cancer treated with gamma-knife radiosurgery for synchronous brain metastases. Cancer 112:1780–1786

Yoshioka A, Miyachi Y, Toda K, Imamura S, Hiraoka M, Abe M (1990) Effects of local hyperthermia on natural killer activity in mice. Int J Hyperthermia 6:261–267

Younes E, Haas GP, Dezso B, Ali E, Maughan RL, Kukuruga MA, et al (1995a) Local tumor irradiation augments the response to IL-2 therapy in a murine renal adenocarcinoma. Cell Immunol 165:243–251

Younes E, Haas GP, Dezso B, Ali E, Maughan RL, Montecillo E, et al (1995b) Radiation-induced effects on murine kidney tumor cells: role in the interaction of local irradiation and immunotherapy. J Urol 153:2029–2033

Subject Index

List of Contributors

MITCHELL S. ANSCHER, MD, FACR, FACRO
Florence and Hyman Meyers Professor and Chair
Department of Radiation Oncology
Virginia Commonwealth University School of Medicine
401 College Street
P.O. Box 980058
Richmond, VA 23298-0058
USA

Email: manscher@mcvh-vcu.edu

SABRINA T. ASTNER, MD
Klinik und Poliklinik für Strahlentherapie
und Radiologische Onkologie
Klinikum rechts der Isar der
Technische Universität München
Ismaningerstraße 22
81675 München
Germany

Email: sabrina.astner@lrz.tu-muenchen.de

MICHAEL J. ATKINSON, PhD
Professor, Institute of Radiobiology
Helmholtz Centre Munich, German Research Centre
for Environmental Health
Ingolstädter Landstraße 1
85764 Neuherberg
Germany

Email: atkinson@gsf.de

MICHAEL BAUMANN, MD, PhD
Department of Radiation Oncology
OncoRay Centre for Radiation Research in Oncology
Medical Faculty and
University Hospital Carl Gustav Carus
Technische Universität Dresden
Fetscherstraße 74
01307 Dresden
Germany

Email: michael.baumann@uniklinikum-dresden.de

CLAUS BELKA, MD
Professor, Director
Clinic of Radiation Oncology
Ludwigs-Maximilians-Universität München
Marchioninistraße 15
81377 Munich
Germany

Email: claus.belka@med.uni-muenchen.de

NILS CORDES, MD, PhD
OncoRay-Center for Radiation Research in Oncology
Medical Faculty Carl Gustav Carus
Dresden University of Technology
Fetscherstraße 74
01307 Dresden
Germany

Email: nils.cordes@oncoray.de

JOCHEN DAHM-DAPHI, MD
Laboratory of Radiobiology and Experimental
Radio-Oncology
University Medical Center Hamburg-Eppendorf
Martinistraße 52
20246 Hamburg
Germany

Email: dahm@uke.uni-hamburg.de

PAUL DENT, PhD
Department of Biochemistry
Massey Cancer Center
Virginia Commonwealth University Health System
401 College Street
Richmond, VA 23298
USA

Email: pdent@vcu.edu

Ekkehard Dikomey, PhD
Laboratory of Radiobiology and Experimental
Radio-Oncology
University Medical Center Hamburg-Eppendorf
Martinistraße 52
20246 Hamburg
Germany

Email: dikomey@uke.uni-hamburg.de

Joachim Drevs, MD
Chefarzt und Ärztliche Direktion
Tumorklinik SanaFontis, Alpine GmbH
An den Heilquellen 2
79111 Freiburg
Germany

Email: drevs@sanafontis.com

Iris Eke, MD
OncoRay–Center for Radiation Research in Oncology
Medical Faculty Carl Gustav Carus
Dresden University of Technology
Fetscherstraße 74
01307 Dresden
Germany

Email: iris.eke@oncoray.de

Steven Grant, MD
Departments of Medicine and Biochemistry
Massey Cancer Center
Virginia Commonwealth University Health System
401 College Street
Richmond, VA 23298
USA

Email: stgrant@vcu.edu

Paul R. Graves, PhD
Department of Radiation Oncology
Virginia Commonwealth University
Richmond, VA 23112
USA

Email: prgraves@vcu.edu

Anca-Ligia Grosu, MD
Department of Radiation Oncology
Universitätsklinikum Freiburg
Robert-Koch-Straße 3
79106 Freiburg
Germany

Email: anca.grosu@uniklinik-freiburg.de

Miodrag Gužvić, MSc
Division of Oncogenomics
Department of Pathology
University of Regensburg
Franz-Josef-Strauss-Allee 11
93053 Regensburg
Germany

Email: miodrag.guzvic@klinik.uni-regensburg.de

Stephanie Hehlgans, PhD
OncoRay-Center for Radiation Research in Oncology
Medical Faculty Carl Gustav Carus
Dresden University of Technology
Fetscherstraße 74
01307 Dresden
Germany

Email: stephanie.hehlgans@oncoray.de

Masahiro Hiraoka, MD, PhD
Chairman and Professor
Department of Radiation Oncology and
Image-Applied Therapy
Kyoto University Graduate School of Medicine
54 Shogoin Kawahara-cho Sakyo-ku
Kyoto 606-8507
Japan

Email: hiraok@kuhp.kyoto-u.ac.jp

Georg Iliakis, PhD
Institute of Medical Radiation Biology
University of Duisburg–Essen Medical School
Hufelandstraße 55
45122 Essen
Germany

Email: georg.iliakis@uni-essen.de

SATOSHI ITASAKA, MD
Assistant Professor
Department of Radiation Oncology
and Image-Applied Therapy
Kyoto University Graduate School of Medicine
54 Shogoin Kawahara-cho Sakyo-ku
Kyoto 606-8507
Japan

Email: sitasaka@kuhp.kyoto-u.ac.jp

ISABEL L. JACKSON, B. S.
Department of Radiation Oncology
Box 3455 MSRB
Duke University Medical Center
Durham, NC 27705
USA

Email: lauren.jackson@duke.edu

ANGELA M. KAINDL, MD
Klinik für Pädiatrie m. S. Neurologie
Charité – Universitätsmedizin Berlin
Campus Virchow-Klinikum
Augustenburger Platz 1
13353 Berlin
Germany
and
Laboratoire de Neurologie du Développement
UMR 676 Inserm-Paris 7 & Service de Neuropédiatrie
Hôpital Robert Debré
48 Blvd. Serurier
75019 Paris
France

Email: angela.kaindl@inserm.fr

CHRISTOPH A. KLEIN, MD
Professor
Division of Oncogenomics
Department of Pathology
University of Regensburg
Franz-Josef-Strauss-Allee 11
93053 Regensburg
Germany

Email: christoph.klein@klinik.uni-regensburg.de

THOMAS KLONISCH, MD, PhD
Department of Human Anatomy and Cell Science
University of Manitoba
Winnipeg, MB
Canada

Email: klonisch@cc.umanitoba.ca

MECHTHILD KRAUSE, MD, PhD
Department of Radiation Oncology
OncoRay Centre for Radiation Research in Oncology
Medical Faculty and
University Hospital Carl Gustav Carus
Technische Universität Dresden
Fetscherstraße 74
01307 Dresden
Germany

Email: mechthild.krause@uniklinikum-dresden.de

MAREK LOS, MD, PhD
BioApplications Enterprises
34 Vanier Drive
Winnipeg, MB R2V2N6
Canada

Email: losmj@cc.umanitoba.ca; bioappl@gmail.com

MINESH P. MEHTA, MD
Department of Human Oncology
University of Wisconsin
Hospital Medical School
Madison, WI, 53792
USA

Email: mehta@humenc.wisc.edu

MICHAEL MOLLS, MD
Professor, Director
Klinik und Poliklinik für Strahlentherapie und
Radiologische Onkologie
Klinikum rechts der Isar der TU München
Ismaninger Straße 22
81675 Munich
Germany

Email: klinik-fuer-strahlentherapie@lrz.tu-muenchen.de

GABRIELE MULTHOFF, PhD
Klinik und Poliklinik für Strahlentherapie und
Radiologische Onkologie
Klinikum rechts der Isar der TU München
Ismaninger Straße 22
81675 Munich
Germany

Email: gabriele.multhoff@multimmune.de

Ursula Nestle, MD
Department of Radiation Oncology
Universitätsklinikum Freiburg
Robert-Koch-Straße 3
79106 Freiburg
Germany

Email: ursula.nestle@uniklinik-freiburg.de

Carsten Nieder, MD
Professor
Department of Medicine
Nordlandssykehuset HF
Prinsensgate 164
8092 Bodø
Norway

Email: carsten.nieder@nlsh.no

Jan Norum, MD
Professor
Department of Oncology
University Hospital Tromsø
Postboks, 9038 Tromsø
Norway

Email: jan.norum@unn.no

Konrad Oexle, MD
Institut für Humangenetik
Klinikum Rechts der Isar der
Technische Universität München
Trogerstraße 32
81675 München
Germany

Email: oexle@humangenetik.med.tum.de

Soumya Panigrahi, MD
Manitoba Institute of Cell Biology
CancerCare Manitoba and
Department of Physiology
University of Manitoba
ON6009-675 McDermot Avenue
Winnipeg, MB R3E0V9
Canada

Email: dspsts@gmail.com

Adam Pawinski, MD
Department of Medicine
Nordlandssykehuset HF
Prinsensgate 164
8092 Bodø
Norway

Email: adam.pawinski@nlsh.no

Iran Rashedi, MD
Manitoba Institute of Cell Biology
CancerCare Manitoba and
Department of Biochemistry and Medical Genetics
University Manitoba
ON 6009-675 McDermot Avenue
Winnipeg, MB, R3E0V9
Canada

Email: rashedi@cc.umanitoba.ca

Hans Christian Rischke, MD
Diagnostische Radiologie und PET/CT-Zentrum
Tumorklinik SanaFontis, Alpine GmbH
An den Heilquellen 2
79111 Freiburg
Germany

Email: rischke@sanafontis.com

Vesile Schneider, MD
Tumorklinik SanaFontis, Alpine GmbH
An den Heilquellen 2
79111 Freiburg
Germany

Email: VesileSchneider@web.de

Klaus Schulze-Osthoff, PhD
Institute of Molecular Medicine
University of Düsseldorf
Building 23.12, Universitätsstraße 1
40225 Düsseldorf
Germany

Email: kso@uni-duesseldorf.de

SHIYU SONG, MD
Department of Radiation Oncology
Massey Cancer Center
Virginia Commonwealth University Health System
401 College Street
Richmond, VA 23298
USA

Email: ssong@vcu.edu

SOILE TAPIO, PhD
Institute of Radiobiology
Helmholtz Centre Munich, German Research Centre
for Environmental Health
Ingolstädter Landstraße 1
85764 Neuherberg
Germany

Email: soile.tapio@gsf.de

KRISTOFFER VALERIE, PhD
Department of Radiation Oncology
Virginia Commonwealth University
Richmond, Virginia 23112
USA

Email: ckvaleri@vcu.edu

PETER VAUPEL, Dr. med., MA/Univ. Harvard
Professor of Physiology and Pathophysiology
Institute of Physiology and Pathophysiology
University of Mainz
Duesbergweg 6
55099 Mainz
Germany

Email: vaupel@uni-mainz.de

ZELJKO VUJASKOVIC, MD, PhD
Department of Radiation Oncology
Box 3455 MSRB
Duke University Medical Center
Durham, NC 27705
USA

Email: vujas@radonc.duke.edu

WOLFGANG A. WEBER, MD
Professor
Department of Nuclear Medicine
Universitätsklinikum Freiburg
Robert-Koch-Straße 3
79106 Freiburg
Germany

Email: wolfgang.weber@uniklinik-freiburg.de

DANIEL ZIPS, MD, PhD
Department of Radiation Oncology
OncoRay Centre for Radiation Research
Medical Faculty and
University Hospital Carl Gustav Carus
Technische Universität Dresden
Fetscherstraße 74
01307 Dresden
Germany

Email: daniel.zips@uniklinikum-dresden.de

MEDICAL RADIOLOGY Diagnostic Imaging and Radiation Oncology
Titles in the series already published

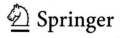

MEDICAL RADIOLOGY   Diagnostic Imaging and Radiation Oncology
Titles in the series already published

RADIATION ONCOLOGY

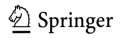

Springer

Printing and Binding: Stürtz GmbH, Würzburg